T0294390

VASCULAR AND ENDOVASCULAR SURGERY

Seventh Edition

A Companion to Specialist Surgical Practice

Series Editors
O. James Garden
Simon Paterson-Brown

Seventh Edition

VASCULAR AND ENDOVASCULAR SURGERY

Edited by

Ian Loftus, MBChB, MD, FRCS
Professor of Vascular Surgery, St George's NHS Trust, London, UK

Robert J. Hinchliffe, MD, FRCS
Professor of Vascular Surgery, University of Bristol, Bristol, UK

For additional online content visit eBooks+

ELSEVIER

© 2024, Elsevier Limited. All rights reserved.

First edition 1997
Second edition 2001
Third edition 2005
Fourth edition 2009
Fifth edition 2014
Sixth edition 2019
Seventh edition 2024

No part of this publication may be reproduced or transmitted in any form or by any means, electronic or mechanical, including photocopying, recording, or any information storage and retrieval system, without permission in writing from the publisher. Details on how to seek permission, further information about the Publisher's permissions policies and our arrangements with organizations such as the Copyright Clearance Center and the Copyright Licensing Agency, can be found at our website: www.elsevier.com/permissions.

This book and the individual contributions contained in it are protected under copyright by the Publisher (other than as may be noted herein).

Notices

Practitioners and researchers must always rely on their own experience and knowledge in evaluating and using any information, methods, compounds or experiments described herein. Because of rapid advances in the medical sciences, in particular, independent verification of diagnoses and drug dosages should be made. To the fullest extent of the law, no responsibility is assumed by Elsevier, authors, editors or contributors for any injury and/or damage to persons or property as a matter of products liability, negligence or otherwise, or from any use or operation of any methods, products, instructions, or ideas contained in the material herein.

ISBN: 978-0-7020-8462-1

Content Strategist: Alexandra Mortimer
Content Project Manager: Arindam Banerjee
Design: Ryan Cook
Art Buyer: Muthukumaran Thangaraj
Marketing Manager: Deborah Watkins

Printed in India

Last digit is the print number: 9 8 7 6 5 4 3 2 1

Working together
to grow libraries in
developing countries

www.elsevier.com • www.bookaid.org

Contents

Series Editors' preface

The *Companion to Specialist Surgical Practice* series has now reached its Seventh Edition and continues to remain popular for both surgeons in training as well as consultant surgeons in independent practice. The strength of this series has always been founded on contemporary, evidence-based information on the subspecialist areas relevant to their general surgical practice and this Seventh Edition has followed this plan.

This Edition continues to keep abreast of increasing sub-specialisation in general surgery. The ongoing developments in minimal access and increasingly robotic surgery are discussed, along with the desire of some subspecialities, such as breast and vascular surgery, to separate away from 'general surgery' in some countries. However, all volumes also underline the importance for all surgeons of being aware of current developments in their surgical field. The importance of evidence-based practice and in particular the management of emergency conditions remains throughout, and authors have provided recommendations and high-lighted key resources within each chapter. The ebook version of the textbook has also enabled improved access to the reference abstracts and links to video content relevant to many of the chapters.

As in all the previous editions, we are greatly indebted to the volume editors, and contributors, who have all put so much hard work into delivering such a high quality piece of work. We remain grateful for the support and encouragement of the team at Elsevier and we trust that our original vision of delivering an up-to-date, affordable text has been met and that readers, whether in training or independent practice, will find this Seventh Edition an invaluable resource.

We are grateful to Kathryn Rigby and Jonathan Michaels who wrote the guidelines on Evidence-based Practice in Surgery for previous editions of the series. These have been well received and have been retained again for this new edition in order to help guide readers in their assessment of the various levels of evidence discussed in each chapter.

O. James Garden, CBE, BSc, MBChB, MD, DSc(Hon), FRCS (Glas), FRCS(Ed), FRCP(Ed), FRACS(Hon), FRCSC (Hon), FACS(Hon), FCSHK(Hon), FRCSI(Hon), FRCS(Engl)(Hon), FRSE, MAMSE, FFST(RCSEd)
Professor Emeritus, Clinical Surgery, University of Edinburgh, UK.

Simon Paterson-Brown, MBBS, MPhil, MS, FRCS(Ed), FRCS (Engl), FCSHK, FFST(RCSEd)
Honorary Senior Lecturer, Clinical Surgery, University of Edinburgh, UK.

Editors' preface

The Seventh Edition of *Vascular and Endovascular Surgery* has been compiled by key opinion leaders in the field, using the most contemporary literature and experience. Our aim is to guide surgeons and allied health professionals with an interest in vascular disease in their everyday practice, as well as preparing for examinations.

Vascular surgery continues to evolve at pace, as some therapies emerge, and others become less relevant. The balance between open, endovascular and hybrid interventions throughout the vascular tree, causes debate and often controversy. We have aimed to give a balanced and evidence-based approach to these therapies. The epidemiology of vascular disease is also changing, with better medical therapies, screening programmes, reducing consumption of tobacco habits in many countries, and a globally increasing prevalence of diabetes, significantly changing the spectrum of patients we see in our practice. These changes challenge established vascular practitioners and those in training, to provide effective, safe and contemporary clinical practice.

In this edition, in response to previous feedback, we have added sample multiple choice questions, which we hope readers will find useful as an aide memoire. Each chapter also has a short list of key references as suggestions for further reading.

We are indebted to all the contributors to this edition of the *Companion to Specialist Surgical Practice* series. They have provided many hours of toil without compensation, other than the reward of continuing the tradition of teaching in vascular surgery, in which we are proud to play our part. It has been especially gratifying to work closely with new contributors who bring a fresh approach to many aspects of the text. We would also wish to acknowledge and thank the editorial team and all previous editions' contributors, without whom this new edition would not have been possible.

We hope you will continue to find this an invaluable resource, whether it be as part of surgical training, during preparation for an exam or complementing day-to-day clinical practice.

Ian Loftus
London
Robert J. Hinchliffe
Bristol

Evidence-based practice in surgery

Critical appraisal for developing evidence-based practice can be obtained from a number of sources, the most reliable being randomised controlled clinical trials, systematic literature reviews, meta-analyses and observational studies. For practical purposes three grades of evidence can be used, analogous to the levels of 'proof' required in a court of law:

1. **Beyond all reasonable doubt**. Such evidence is likely to have arisen from high-quality randomised controlled trials, systematic reviews or high-quality synthesised evidence such as decision analysis, cost-effectiveness analysis or large observational datasets. The studies need to be directly applicable to the population of concern and have clear results. The grade is analogous to burden of proof within a criminal court and may be thought of as corresponding to the usual standard of 'proof' within the medical literature (i.e. $P < 0.05$).

2. **On the balance of probabilities**. In many cases a high-quality review of literature may fail to reach firm conclusions due to conflicting or inconclusive results, trials of poor methodological quality or the lack of evidence in the population to which the guidelines apply. In such cases it may still be possible to make a statement as to the best treatment on the 'balance of probabilities'. This is analogous to the decision in a civil court where all the available evidence will be weighed up and the verdict will depend upon the balance of probabilities.

3. **Not proven**. Insufficient evidence upon which to base a decision, or contradictory evidence.

Depending on the information available, three grades of recommendation can be used:

Strong recommendation, which should be followed unless there are compelling reasons to act otherwise.

 a. A recommendation based on evidence of effectiveness, but where there may be other factors to take into account in decision-making, for example the user of the guidelines may be expected to take into account patient preferences, local facilities, local audit results or available resources.

 b. A recommendation made where there is no adequate evidence as to the most effective practice, although there may be reasons for making a recommendation in order to minimise cost or reduce the chance of error through a locally agreed protocol.

Evidence where a conclusion can be reached '**beyond all reasonable doubt**' and therefore where a **strong recommendation** can be given.

This will normally be based on evidence levels:

- Ia. Meta-analysis of randomised controlled trials
- Ib. Evidence from at least one randomised controlled trial
- IIa. Evidence from at least one controlled study without randomisation
- IIb. Evidence from at least one other type of quasi-experimental study.

Evidence where a conclusion might be reached '**on the balance of probabilities**' and where there may be other factors involved which influence the recommendation given. This will normally be based on less conclusive evidence than that represented by the double tick icons:

- III. Evidence from non-experimental descriptive studies, such as comparative studies and case–control studies
- IV. Evidence from expert committee reports or opinions or clinical experience of respected authorities, or both.

Evidence that is associated with either a **strong recommendation** or **expert opinion** is highlighted in the text in panels such as those shown above, and is distinguished by either a double or single tick icon, respectively. The references associated with double-tick evidence are listed as Key References at the end of each chapter, along with a short summary of the paper's conclusions where applicable. The full reference list for each chapter is available in the ebook.

The reader is referred to Chapter 1, 'Evaluation of surgical evidence' in the volume *Core Topics in General and Emergency Surgery* of this series, for a more detailed description of this topic.

Contributors

Julien Al Shakarchi, MBChB, MSc, MD
Consultant Vascular and Endovascular Surgeon
Worcestershire Acute Hospitals NHS Trust
Worcester, United Kingdom

Kirthi Bellamkonda, MD, MSc
Resident Physician
Vascular Surgery
Dartmouth Health
Lebanon, New Hampshire, United States

Romain Belmonte, MD
Vascular Surgeon
Department of Vascular Surgery
Clinique Esquirol Saint Hilaire
Agen, France

Martin Björck, MD, PhD
Professor Emeritus in Vascular Surgery
Department of Surgical Sciences
Uppsala University
Uppsala, Sweden;
Visiting Professor
Tartu University
Tartu, Estonia

Stephen Black, MD, FRCS
Department of Vascular Surgery
St Thomas' Hospital
London, United Kingdom

Patrick Coughlin, FRCS
Consultant
Vascular Surgery
Leeds Vascular Institute
Leeds, United Kingdom

Robert Fitridge, MBBS, MS, FRACS
Professor of Vascular Surgery
The University of Adelaide
Vascular and Endovascular Surgeon
Royal Adelaide Hospital
Adelaide, South Australia, Australia

Rachael O. Forsythe, MBChB, PhD, FRCS(Vasc)
Consultant Vascular Surgeon
Edinburgh Vascular Unit
Royal Infirmary of Edinburgh;
Honorary Senior Lecturer
University of Edinburgh
Edinburgh, United Kingdom

Fran Game, MBBCh, FRCP
Consultant Diabetologist and Director of R&D
University Hospitals of Derby and Burton NHS FT
Derby, United Kingdom

Andrew Garnham, MB BCh, FRCS(Ed), FRCS(Gen)
Consultant Vascular Surgeon
Royal Wolverhampton NHS Trust
Wolverhampton; United Kingdom;
Consultant Vascular Surgeon
Black Country Unit
Russells Hall Hospital
Dudley, United Kingdom

Michael Gawenda, PhD, MD
Professor of Surgery
University of Cologne;
Chief
Clinic of Vascular and Endovascular Surgery
St.-Antonius-Hospital
Academic Hospital of RWTH Aachen University
Eschweiler, Germany

Manjit S. Gohel, MB ChB, MD, FRCS, FEBVS
Consultant Vascular and Endovascular Surgeon
Cambridge Vascular Unit
Addenbrooke's Hospital
Cambridge, United Kingdom;
Honorary Senior Lecturer
Academic department of Vascular Surgery
Imperial College London
London, United Kingdom

Shigong Guo, LLM, MSc(Orth Eng), MRCS
Consultant in Rehabilitation Medicine
Major Trauma Centre
Major Arterial Centre
Hyperacute Rehabilitation Team
Southmead Hospital;
Clinical Specialty Lead
Bristol Centre for Enablement
Bristol, United Kingdom

Robert J. Hinchliffe, MD, FRCS
Professor of Vascular Surgery
University of Bristol
Bristol, United Kingdom

Peter Holt, PhD, FRCS
Professor of Vascular Surgery
St George's Vascular Institute
St George's Hospital
London, United Kingdom

Nedal Katib, MB, BCh, BAO, MS, FRACS
Vascular and Endovascular Surgeon
Prince of Wales Public and Private Hospitals;
Lecturer
School of Medicine
University of New South Wales
Sydney, NSW, Australia

Patrick D.W. Kiely, FRCP, PhD
Consultant Rheumatologist
St George's University Hospitals NHS Foundation Trust;
Professor of Practice
Clinical Rheumatology
Institute of Medical and Biomedical Education
St George's University of London
London, United Kingdom

Thanh-Phong Le, MD
Vascular Surgeon
Department of vascular surgery
Cho-Ray hospital
Hochiminh City, Vietnam

Dirk A. le Roux, MBChB(Pret), FCS(SA), CVS(SA)
Consultant and Lecturer of Vascular Surgery
University of the Witwatersrand
Johannesburg, Gauteng, South Africa

Iris Lebuhotel, MD
Vascular Surgeon
Department of vascular surgery
Clinique Esquirol Saint Hilaire
Agen, France

Mark E. Lloyd, MBChB, FRCP
Consultant Rheumatologist
Frimley Park Hospital
Frimley, United Kingdom

Ian Loftus, MBChB, MD, FRCS
Professor of Vascular Surgery
St George's NHS Trust
London, United Kingdom

Ian McCafferty, BSc, MBBS, MRCP, FRCR
Consultant Diagnostic and Interventional Radiologist
Imaging Department
Birmingham Women's & Children's Hospital
Birmingham, United Kingdom

Kurian J. Mylankal, MD, FRCS(Edin), FRACS
Vascular and Endovascular Surgeon
Royal Adelaide Hospital
Adelaide, South Australia, Australia

A. Ross Naylor, MBChB, MD, FRCSEd, FRCSEng
Professor
Leicester Vascular Institute
Glenfield Hospital
Leicestershire, United Kingdom

Jean-Baptiste Ricco, MD, PhD
Professor of Vascular Surgery
University of Poitiers
Poitiers, Vienne, France

Alexander Rolls, FRCS, PhD
Consultant Vascular and Trauma Surgeon
Department of Vascular Surgery
Imperial College Healthcare
London, United Kingdom

David Russell, MBChB, MD, FRCS(Gen Surg), FFST
Associate Professor
Clinical Trials Research Unit
University of Leeds;
Honorary Consultant Vascular Surgeon
Leeds Vascular Institute
Leeds Teaching Hospitals NHS Trust
Leeds, United Kingdom

Prakash Saha, PhD, FRCS
Academic Department of Vascular Surgery
St. Thomas' Hospital
King's College London
London, United Kingdom

Marc L. Schermerhorn, MD
Chief
Division of Vascular and Endovascular Surgery
Beth Israel Deaconess Medical Center;
George H.A. Clowes Jr. Professor of Surgery
Harvard Medical School
Boston, Massachusetts, United States

Peter A. Soden, MD, RPVI
Assistant Professor Brown University Medical School
Department of Vascular Surgery
Brown University Medical School;
Vascular Surgeon
Brown Surgical Associates
Providence, Rhode Island, United States

Rob H.W. Strijkers, MD, PhD
General Practitioner
Erasmus MC
Rotterdam, Zuid-Holland, The Netherlands

Jan David Süss, Dr. med.
Clinic of Vascular and Endovascular Surgery
St.-Antonius-Hospital
Academic Hospital of RWTH Aachen University
Eschweiler, Germany

Andrew L. Tambyraja, BMedSci, BM, BS, MD, FACS, FRCSEd
Consultant and Honorary Clinical Reader in Vascular
  Surgery
Royal Infirmary of Edinburgh
Edinburgh, United Kingdom

Ramesh Kaushal Tripathi, MD, FRCS, FRACS(Vasc.), DFSVS
Professor of Surgery
University of Queensland
Brisbane, QLD, Australia

Jos C. van den Berg, MD, PhD
Service of Interventional Radiology
Ospedale Regionale di Lugano
sede Civico, Lugano, Switzerland;
Ass. Professor of Radiology
Universitätsinstitut für Diagnostische, Interventionelle und
  Pädiatrische Radiologie Inselspital
Universitätsspital Bern
Bern, Switzerland

Jacobus van Marle, MBChB, MMed(Surg), FCS(SA)
Professor of Vascular Surgery
Department of Surgery
Sefako Makgatho Health Sciences University
Ga-Rankuwa, Gauteng, South Africa

Ramon L. Varcoe, MBBS, MS, FRACS, PhD, MMed(ClinEpi)
Associate Professor of Vascular Surgery
Faculty of Medicine
University of New South Wales;
Vascular Surgeon
Department of Vascular Surgery
Prince of Wales Hospital;
Director
The Vascular Institute
Prince of Wales
Sydney, NSW, Australia

Jacqueline E. Wade, MD
General Surgery Resident
Beth Israel Deaconess Medical Center
Boston, Massachusetts, United States

Cees H.A. Wittens, MD, PhD
Emeritus Professor and Head of Venous Surgery
Maastricht University Medical Centre
Maastricht, The Netherlands

Epidemiological risk factors and risk stratification for peripheral arterial disease

1

Patrick Coughlin

INTRODUCTION

Atherosclerotic peripheral artery disease (PAD) involving one or more major vessels of the lower limb is common.[1] The global spread of abdominal adiposity, its associated metabolic disorders and smoking has led to a significant increase in PAD, particularly in lower- and middle-income countries (LMIC). Current estimates suggest that over 200 million people globally are affected by PAD, with a marked increase in those affected over the last decade (LMIC 29% increase, high income countries (HIC) 13% increase). PAD tends to affect older patients and likely occurs because of both genetic and environmental interactions that result in the development of atherosclerotic disease. The natural history of the lower limb in patients with symptomatic PAD (intermittent claudication) is somewhat benign, with up to 75% of patients noticing stabilisation or some improvement of their symptoms.[2] Patients with PAD, however, are at significant risk of major adverse cardiovascular events (MACE), noticeably because of concomitant atherosclerotic disease within the coronary, carotid and cerebral circulation. Disability and mortality associated with PAD have increased over the last 20 years, and this increase in burden has been greater among women.[3]

There are a number of studies that highlight this link between PAD and MACE, predominantly using the ankle–brachial pressure index (ABPI) as a marker of disease severity. Data from the Ankle Brachial Index Collaboration group showed that a low ABPI (<0.9) was associated with an increased risk of subsequent all-cause mortality (pooled relative risk [RR] 1.60; 95% confidence interval [CI], 1.32–1.95), cardiovascular (CV) mortality (pooled RR 1.96; 95% CI, 1.46–2.64), coronary heart disease (pooled RR 1.45; 95% CI, 1.08–1.93) and stroke (pooled RR 1.35; 95% CI, 1.10–1.65) after adjustment for age, sex, conventional CV risk factors and prevalent CV disease.[4]

Medial artery calcification, associated with diabetes and renal disease leads to an inability to compress the arteries during ABPI measurement. An elevated ABPI (defined as >1.40) has also been identified with an increased risk of all-cause and CV disease mortality (adjusted risk estimates 1.77 all-cause mortality / 2.09 CV mortality).[5] This U-shaped relationship between ABPI and outcome is now well recognised (Fig. 1.1).

The aims of this chapter are to describe the epidemiology of lower limb PAD and analyse the role of reversible and irreversible risk factors on both disease progression and the incidence of MACE.

EPIDEMIOLOGY OF PERIPHERAL ARTERY DISEASE

Compared to coronary artery disease (CAD), there are few data available on the epidemiology of PAD. The incidence of PAD is defined as the rate of new (or newly diagnosed) cases of the disease (generally reported as the number of new cases occurring within a period of time). Prevalence is defined as the actual number of cases alive with the disease either during a period of time (period prevalence) or at a particular date in time (point prevalence). The true incidence and prevalence of PAD is difficult to determine accurately, in part because of methodological issues related to the diagnosis of PAD but also because of continuing changes in CV risk factor prevalence and management. Differences are also encountered depending on sampling criteria and whether the diagnosis of PAD is based purely on symptomatic patients (intermittent claudication/chronic limb threatening ischaemia [CLTI]) or whether one includes asymptomatic individuals.

The population may be screened using a questionnaire-based approach (Rose questionnaire/Edinburgh Artery Questionnaire). These questionnaires tend to underestimate the diagnosis of claudication and a more objective analysis of limb perfusion (ABPI/reactive hyperaemia) may be more appropriate. The ABPI has become an increasingly used diagnostic tool for PAD, with a value ≤0.9 signifying PAD. It is both a reproducible and reliable test although there are circumstances where a false-negative reading may be obtained, which includes patients with medial artery calcification where arterial compression is difficult, the presence of mild arterial lesions (often seen in the iliac artery) and where significant collateralisation has occurred. In such circumstances, pre- and post-exercise ABPI measurement can help, but these are impractical to perform in population-based studies. A number of the initial validation studies of ABPI were performed before the advent of arterial duplex. As such, intra-arterial lower limb angiography was used as the gold standard against which the ABPI was compared. As this is an invasive test, carrying some risk, ABPI was only determined in selected patients with significant symptoms who were more likely to have severe arterial disease, and this was compared against

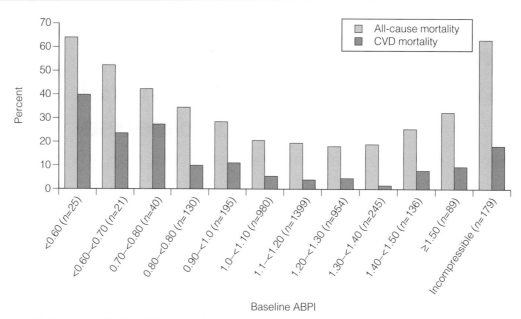

Figure 1.1 Relationship between ankle–brachial pressure index (ABPI) and survival in patients in the Strong Heart Study.[5] There is a U-shaped relationship such that both low (<0.9) and high (>1.4) ABPI is associated with increased risk of cardiovascular and all-cause mortality. *CVD*, Cerebrovascular disease.

younger 'normal' controls. As such, the observed sensitivity and specificity values obtained were between 97% and 100%.[6,7] In a more representative sample of patients seen in daily practice, the specificity of ABPI measurement is maintained at approximately 97%, the sensitivity falls to nearer 80%.[8] There can be confusion in such epidemiological studies when determining whether solely symptomatic PAD or PAD as a whole (symptomatic and asymptomatic) are included. This gains some importance when discussing the merits of screening for PAD.

In population studies using ABPI for the diagnosis of PAD, studies suggest a prevalence of PAD of approximately 3–10% in the population as a whole, with this increasing to between 15 and 20% when focusing on older patients (>70 years of age).[9–11] More recent studies include the PAD Awareness, Risk, and Treatment: New Resources for Survival (PARTNERS)study, the National Health and Nutritional Examination Survey (NHANES) and the REGICOR study[12–14] (Fig. 1.2). The PARTNERS study screened 6979 subjects for PAD using ABPI (included were people over 70 years OR age 50–69 years and at least one CV risk factor). PAD was detected in 29% of the population. The NHANES recruited an unselected cohort of subjects over 40 years of age and found a prevalence of PAD of 2.5% in those aged 50–59 years, rising to 14.5% in those aged >70 years. The REGICOR study, studying a purely Mediterranean population, found the prevalence of PAD to be 4.5% (5.2% in men and 3.9% in women). Other studies report prevalence of PAD from 3–20%, with variation depending upon methodology and the population examined. Interestingly, there appears to be little difference in prevalence between men and women, with ratios ranging from 0.8 to 1.2. The issue with regard to the method of assessment of PAD is borne out by the data from the British Regional Heart Study, where direct assessment of the femoral artery performed using ultrasound suggested that 64% of people aged 56–77 years have significant femoral atherosclerosis, of whom fewer than one-fifth were symptomatic.[15]

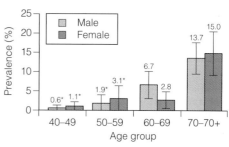

Figure 1.2 Recent information about the prevalence of peripheral artery disease (PAD) from the US National Health and Nutrition Survey, confirming a steep age-related prevalence.

Data on the incidence of PAD are more limited. The Limburg study, involving a cohort of 2327 patients selected from 18 primary care facilities in the Netherlands, found that after a follow-up period of 7.2 years the overall incidence rate for asymptomatic PAD was 9.9 (95% CI, 7.3–18.8) per 1000 person-years at risk. The rate was 7.8 (95% CI, 4.9–20.3) for men and 12.4 (95% CI, 7.7–24.8) for women and more marked in those patients over the age of 65 years.[16] The REGICOR study collected data on 5434 individuals aged between 35 and 79 years.[17] In total, 118 new cases of confirmed PAD were identified, resulting in a cumulative population incidence rate of 377 cases per 100 000 person years, lower than that seen in other areas.

Intermittent claudication is a symptom of muscular lower limb pain brought on by exertion and relieved by rest, with CLTI being at the more severe end of the symptom spectrum (night pain/rest pain/tissue loss). The prevalence of intermittent claudication varies, up to 3% at the age of 40 years and rising to 6% at 60 years. While some of the data are historic, the largest studies performed over 3 decades ago are probably still the most reliable. These include the

Edinburgh Artery Study, which screened large random samples of the general population using age/sex registers from general practices.[11] This study used both the World Health Organisation (WHO) questionnaire and the ABPI to determine the prevalence of both symptomatic and asymptomatic lower limb PAD in a sample of 1592 participants (men and women) aged between 55 and 74 years. They found that the prevalence of intermittent claudication was 4.5% (95% CI, 3.5–5.5) with major asymptomatic disease seen in 8.0% (95% CI, 6.6–9.4).

The incidence of claudication also varies, in part depending on geography, with values as low as 0.2% in Iceland, 1.0% in Israel and 1.6% from the Edinburgh Artery Study.[11,18,19] More detailed data come from the Framingham dataset that showed an overall incidence of 7.1 per 1000 years in men and 3.6 per 1000 years in women, although the gender differences were not seen between the ages of 65 and 75 years.[20] Data from the REGICOR dataset suggest an incidence for symptomatic PAD of 102 per 100 000 person years.[14] This suggests that the incidence of PAD is lower in the Mediterranean area than reported from other areas and warrants more in-depth analysis.

The incidence of CLTI has been estimated to be around 400 cases per million population per year, which equates to a prevalence of 1 in 2500 of the population annually.[21] For every 100 patients with intermittent claudication, approximately one new patient per year will develop critical ischaemia.[22]

What is clear is that the incidence of symptomatic PAD (intermittent claudication and CLTI) increases steeply with age.[11,16] When considering the effect of ethnicity, the most comprehensive data come from a study by Allison et al., who combined data from seven community-based studies within the USA.[23] The study showed that PAD was uncommon before the age of 50 years but was present in up to 20% of subjects over the age of 80 years. The rate of PAD in Black Americans was double that seen in non-Hispanic Whites (NHW), with the rates for Hispanics, Asian Americans and Native Americans similar to those in NHW.

NATURAL HISTORY OF PERIPHERAL ARTERY DISEASE: LIMB-SPECIFIC, CARDIOVASCULAR MORBIDITY AND MORTALITY

LIMB-SPECIFIC OUTCOMES

There are a number of important methodological issues in determining the natural history of lower limb PAD. This relates to a higher chance that significant disease progression may result in either revascularisation or limb loss, or if associated with more aggressive atherosclerotic progression in other arterial beds, then a higher mortality risk. When considering symptom progression, then this is in part related to the degree of collateralisation, muscle adaptation, allied physical function/ability and adaptability so that there may be marked differences seen between pathological disease progress and symptom progression. There is, however, a reasonable quantity of data on PAD progression using predominantly ABPI measurements as a marker of PAD.

The Cardiovascular Health Study, analysing a cohort of 5000 patients with normal ABPI, reported a 9.5% incidence of PAD over a 6-year follow-up period.[24] The Edinburgh Artery Study found between 7% and 15% of patients with initially asymptomatic PAD developed intermittent claudication over a 5-year follow-up period.[11] Nicoloff et al. reported a 37% deterioration in ABPI over a 5-year follow-up, which equated to clinical progression (defined as symptom change or need for revascularisation) in 22%.[25,26] A smaller study from Germany suggested lower limb PAD progression occurred in 18.6% over a 5-year follow-up period and 30% in a study from San Diego in a similar time period, using a six-category scale of disease severity.[27,28]

Large population studies from Edinburgh and Basle in people with claudication suggest that only a quarter of patients will have significant deterioration in symptoms, with this being most frequent within the first year after diagnosis (7–9%) and after this occurring in only 2–3%.[2] Specifically, the risk of amputation is rare, occurring in only 1–3% of patients with intermittent claudication at 5 years.[2]

ASSOCIATION OF PERIPHERAL ARTERY DISEASE WITH ATHEROSCLEROTIC DISEASE IN OTHER ARTERIAL BEDS

Atherosclerotic disease can be manifest in a number of arterial beds and as such PAD is associated with other vascular-related conditions, specifically within the coronary and cerebral circulations.

In a screening programme consisting of ultrasound screening of 3.6 million people in USA, the proportion of subjects with two or more affected arterial beds increased with age from 0.04% (40–50 yeas of age) to 3.6% (81–90 years of age).[29] In patients with a diagnosis of PAD (defined as an ABPI <0.9) between 25–70% of patients will have CAD, 14–19% of patients will have a carotid stenosis >70% and between 10–23% of patients will have a renal artery stenosis of >75%.[30]

These findings are supported by the Atherosclerosis Risk in Communities study, a study of 15000 middle-aged subjects.[31] A diagnosis of PAD (ABPI <0.9) was associated with a twofold increase in CAD. The association is starker in older patients. A study of 1800 older patients (mean age 80 years) from New York showed that a diagnosis of PAD was associated with coronary disease in 68% of patients and with a history of ischaemic stroke in 42%.[32]

Further corroboration comes from the Reduction of Atherothrombosis for Continued Health (REACH) registry, a large multinational registry collating observational data about the spectrum of disease progression, CV outcomes and patterns of treatment in patients with atherosclerotic disease. The registry encompasses a total of 67 888 patients, aged 45 years or more, from 44 countries with an inclusion criterion of either established CV disease or, if they were asymptomatic, with more than three risk CV risk factors (n = 12 389). Among the symptomatic group, patients were enrolled on the basis of CAD (n = 40 248), cerebrovascular disease (CVD; n = 18 843) or PAD (n = 8273), with 16% of this group having polyvascular disease.[33]

Between 7–16% of patient with a diagnosis of CAD will also have concomitant lower limb PAD. The PAD is commonly asymptomatic because of exercise limitations seen in patients with CAD, namely anginal and dyspnoea symptoms. Of note, patients with PAD in the coronary population exhibit more extensive, heavily calcified and progressive coronary atherosclerosis.[34]

ASSOCIATION OF PERIPHERAL ARTERY DISEASE WITH SUBSEQUENT CARDIOVASCULAR MORBIDITY AND MORTALITY

Given this association of PAD with atherosclerotic disease in the coronary and cerebral circulation, it is unsurprising therefore that such patients have a high CV event rate. To determine the true effect of PAD specifically on CV event rates, appropriate logistic or proportional hazards regression models, with multivariable adjustment for conventional CV risk factors, are required.[26]

PAD acts as a marker for underlying atherosclerotic processes affecting other vascular beds. This is prognostically important, to the extent that PAD has prognostic value independent of other known risk factors.

Data from 2 decades ago suggested that PAD was associated with a two- to threefold increased risk of stroke, a fourfold increase in the risk of fatal myocardial infarction (MI) or cardiac-related death and a sixfold risk of death from any CV cause.[35,36] CAD is the most common cause of death among patients with PAD (40–60%), with cerebral artery disease accounting for 10–20% of deaths. Other vascular events, including ruptured aortic aneurysm, cause approximately 10% of deaths.[2]

A more recent meta-analysis of 16 population-based cohort studies evaluated the association of ABPI with subsequent coronary events, CV mortality and total mortality.[37] An ABPI of ≤0.90 was associated with approximately twice the 10-year event rates in each of these three categories. In addition, these results held across the full range of Framingham Risk Score categories.

The Cardiovascular Health Study, a cohort-based study from the USA of 5000 Medicare patients, showed that the diagnosis of PAD was associated with a 2.5 increased risk of a history of MI, a twofold increased risk of angina and an approximately threefold increase in both congestive cardiac failure (× 3.3) and a previous stroke (× 3.1).[38]

When considering intermittent claudication specifically, there remains a link with high CV event rates. The Whitehall study analysed a cohort of 18 403 patients aged between 40 and 64 years who were followed up over a 17-year period.[39] Within this cohort, 322 were felt likely to have a diagnosis of intermittent claudication, with an associated 40% mortality rate in this group during the study period. The study concluded that intermittent claudication was independently related to increased mortality rates. Such correlations are also seen in more recent studies by Kollerits et al., and the SHIP study (n = 3995, median follow-up 8.5 years), where a diagnosis of intermittent claudication was associated with an increased risk of all-cause mortality (hazard ratio [HR] 1.79).[40,41] Data from the GetABI study showed that there was an increased risk of a composite endpoint of all-cause mortality and severe vascular event in patients with symptomatic PAD compared to those with asymptomatic disease.[42]

CLTI is associated with a higher burden of lower limb atherosclerotic disease. As such, mortality rates are notably higher in this specific cohort of patients. A recent meta-analysis of contemporary studies (n = 50 studies) showed that the estimated probability of all-cause mortality in patients with CLTI was 3.7% at 30 days, 17.5% at 1 year, 35.1% at 3 years and 46.2% at 5 years. Men had a statistically significant survival benefit at 30 days and 3 years. The presence of ischaemic heart disease, tissue loss and older age resulted in a higher probability of death at 3 years.[43]

What influence does the presence of lower limb PAD have in patients with coronary disease as their primary presenting condition, which is of significant relevance to cardiologists and cardiothoracic surgeons?

The coexistence of PAD in patient with CAD is associated with poor outcome. However, not all patients with coronary disease will also have PAD. The PEGASUS trial showed that in a coronary cohort, the presence of PAD was associated with a twofold increase in a mortality and major adverse CV outcomes at 3 years.[44] A similar finding has been identified in a number of acute coronary syndrome registries where patient with concomitant PAD had significantly higher rates of in-hospital mortality, acute heart failure and recurrent ischaemia.[45,46] It is also recognised that PAD is associated with poorer outcomes in patients undergoing percutaneous and open coronary revascularisation.[47,48]

SCREENING FOR LOWER PERIPHERAL ARTERY DISEASE

Screening refers to the use of simple tests across an apparently healthy population to identify individuals who have risk factors or early stages of disease, but do not yet have symptoms (WHO).

The criteria required for screening to be appropriate were defined by Wilson and Junger in 1968[49] (Table 1.1).

Lower limb PAD fits a number of these criteria with potential advantages of screening being an opportunity to slow

Table 1.1 Criteria required for screening to be appropriate

(i) the condition sought should be an important health problem,

(ii) there should be an accepted treatment for patients with recognised disease,

(iii) facilities for diagnosis and treatment should be available,

(iv) there should be a recognisable latent or early symptomatic stage,

(v) there should be a suitable test or examination,

(vi) the test should be acceptable to the population,

(vii) the natural history of the condition, including development from latent to declared disease, should be adequately understood,

(viii) there should be an agreed policy on whom to treat as patients,

(ix) the cost of case-finding (including diagnosis and treatment of patients diagnosed) should be economically balanced in relation to possible expenditure on medical care as a whole and

(x) case-finding should be a continuing process and not a 'once and for all' project.

any progression of PAD and earlier management of CV risk with a reduction in associated CV event rates.

The data relevant to screening to PAD has been analysed in two recent reviews. Firstly, a systematic review included studies that evaluated ABPI as the screening test for PAD in asymptomatic individuals.[50] The overall diagnosis of PAD averaged 17% (range, 1–42%) being lower in lower risk populations. Those patients diagnosed with PAD had higher adjusted risk of all-cause mortality (HR, 2.99; 95% CI, 2.16–4.12) and CV mortality (HR, 2.35; 95% CI, 1.91–2.89). Data quality overall was, however, poor with very limited evidence to support the cost-effectiveness of screening. This may well be that screened patients for PAD may already have other symptomatic CV disease and already be on appropriate CV risk modification therapy. This led the authors to conclude that the evidence did not support the benefit of routine ABPI screening. A similar conclusion was arrived from the updated evidence report for the US Preventive Services Task Force.[51] They also focused on the role of the ABPI as the screening method and found there to be no direct evidence and limited indirect evidence on the benefits of PAD screening in unselected or asymptomatic populations.

This has led to a number of vascular and CV authorities issuing the following guidance:

(i) Society for Vascular Surgery[52] recommend against routine screening for lower-extremity PAD in the absence of risk factors, history, or signs or symptoms of PAD. However, for asymptomatic individuals at elevated risk (i.e., those over age 70 years, smokers, diabetic patients, those with an abnormal pulse examination or other established CVD), screening for PAD may be reasonable if used to improve risk stratification, preventive care, and medical management.[56]

(ii) Joint recommendations from the American Heart Association/American College of Cardiology Foundation[53] recommended against PAD screening in adults who are not at increased risk and do not have a history or physical examination findings suggestive of PAD. Screening is reasonable in patients at increased risk of PAD (defined as those 65 years or older; those aged 50–64 years with risk factors for atherosclerosis, to include diabetes, history of smoking, hyperlipidaemia, hypertension, or family history of PAD; those younger than 50 years old with diabetes and one other risk factor for atherosclerosis; or those with known atherosclerotic disease in another vascular bed)[65,70]

More recent data that has not been considered as part of any guidelines or systematic review includes the Viborg Vascular screening trial.[54] They enrolled 50 156 men aged 65 to 74 years, randomized to screening versus no screening for a combination of conditions – namely hypertension, PAD and abdominal aortic aneurysm. Subsequent management then included counselling with regard physical activity, smoking cessation, lipid profile measurement and a low-fat diet, as well as prescription with aspirin and statin therapy where indicated. Analysis at a median follow-up of 4.4 years showed a small absolute risk reduction of 0.006 (95% CI, 0.001–0.011) in all-cause mortality in the screened group (HR, 0.93; 95% CI, 0.88–0.98) and a reduction in PAD-specific hospital days

(HR, 0.81; 95% CI, 0.76–0.87) within the study group suggesting that the majority of the benefits accrued were on the whole caused by preventive measures including statin and aspirin use. This type of screening programme also appeared to be cost-effective and compared favourably with other current screening programmes.[55] It is likely that data from other studies within other health systems are required before this becomes part of routine clinical practice.

EPIDEMIOLOGICAL RISK FACTORS FOR PERIPHERAL ARTERY DISEASE, RISK STRATIFICATION AND RISK FACTOR MANAGEMENT

Over the last 30 years, there have been significant advances in the understanding and management of a number of risk factors associated with the development and progression of atherosclerotic disease. This includes a high quality of evidence from a number of well-conducted randomised controlled trials. Data from such studies have had a major influence on day-to-day clinical practice, which has resulted in a decline in overall age-adjusted coronary mortality rates. Yet the onset of the 'diabetes epidemic' brings with it new challenges to maintain such reductions in CV morbidity and mortality.

Much of the data is from 'generic' CV studies, where patients with any form of atherosclerotic disease were recruited. Given both the significant association of PAD with coronary and CVD and the high MACE rate in PAD, extrapolation of such results into the PAD population is justified. As such, there is now overwhelming evidence that all patients with PAD should be receiving optimal secondary CV prevention strategies.

This is reflected in the most recent guidelines for the management of lower limb PAD issued by the National Institute for Health and Clinical Excellence (NICE) in the UK.[56] These guidelines delivered strategies for the management of recognised secondary CV risk factors. This guidance stated that all patients should be offered appropriate advice and treatment regarding these CV risk factors in line with the NICE guidance. This includes guidance regarding smoking cessation, diet, weight management and exercise, lipid modification/statin therapy, antiplatelet therapy and the prevention, diagnosis and management of diabetes and high-blood pressure.

AGE AND GENDER

A number of studies have highlighted the effect of increasing age with PAD risk irrespective of gender.[11,57] The effect of gender is, however, less clear, with some studies, notably the Framingham Study, suggesting that the risk of PAD is doubled in men compared to women. Such a relationship was not evident in the Edinburgh Artery Study and indeed the reverse was seen in the Limburg study.[11,16]

CIGARETTE SMOKING

Smoking is associated with increased mortality rates from cardiorespiratory disease and numerous cancers. It has a detrimental effect on the vascular and platelet function and promotes the inflammatory cascades that are associated with development of atherosclerotic disease.

True epidemiological assessment of its role can be somewhat problematic, specifically with regard to how one determines whether a subject is a smoker/ex-smoker (e.g., questionnaire-based/cotinine measurements) and an assessment of volume of smoking.

Smoking is, however, the strongest risk for PAD and all the largest epidemiological studies reported up to a fourfold increase in risk of PAD when compared to non-smokers.[26] There is also some evidence that suggests that even after having stopped smoking the risk of developing PAD is maintained for up to a further 20 years. However, the benefits of smoking cessation with regard to overall CV risk are evident within 5–7 years in men and 2–4 years in women.[58,59]

Once PAD has become evident, continued smoking is associated with up to a threefold increase in mortality risk and elevated risks of major amputation, need for revascularisation and progression to CLTI.[11] As such, smoking is the primary modifiable risk factor for the prevention of unfavourable CV outcomes, with mechanistic evidence of short- and longer-term benefits.

DIABETES MELLITUS

Increasing life expectancy allied to a global spread of obesity has resulted in a significant increase in the number of people with a diagnosis of diabetes mellitus (DM). The recent WHO data state that there are approximately 422 million adults with diabetes worldwide. Approximately 85–90% of such cases are classified as type 2 diabetes mellitus and it is estimated that this overall figure will double by the year 2030. Given the associated risks of DM, it is generally considered to be a coronary artery risk equivalent when it comes to determining those patients requiring intensive secondary risk factor management.

Apart from smoking, it is the most important risk factor for the development of PAD, with insulin resistance and hyperinsulinaemia also independent factors for PAD. Associated odds risk for developing PAD in patients with DM range from 1.89 to 4.05. In patients with DM, the distribution of atherosclerotic disease tends to be more distal, with a larger burden within the crural vessels, and this allied to the neuropathic complication seen results in a significantly increased lifetime risk of major amputation.[60]

There is strong evidence that glycaemic control is an independent predictor for macrovascular disease as well as microvascular disease. The UK Prospective Diabetes Study (UKPDS) showed a strong association of PAD with haemoglobin (Hb)A1c levels (a measure of glycaemic control), with a 1% increase equating to a 28% increase in the risk of developing PAD.[61]

Once PAD is established, there is less convincing evidence that strict glycaemic control reduces the risk of a subsequent CV event.[62] A meta-analysis of studies of glucose-lowering therapies suggested that intensive compared with standard glycaemic control reduces coronary events but did not affect cerebrovascular event rates or all-cause mortality. It is possible that both oral hypoglycaemics and insulin therapy may have differing effects on CV event rates. For example, the use of metformin in obese patients with diabetes has been shown to slow atherosclerotic progression and avert the development of DM in patients with insulin resistance.

What is evident is the benefit of modifying other CV risk factors in patients with DM. Specifically, statin therapy and blood pressure control have a greater effect in patients with diabetes than those without. Data from the UKPDS showed that for every 10-mmHg reduction in systolic blood pressure, there was a 12% reduction in overall CV risk as well as a 16% reduction in the risk of a major lower limb amputation or PAD-related mortality. This link between aggressive blood pressure control and reduction in CV events may be more relevant and effective clinically than tight glycaemic control.[63,64]

BLOOD PRESSURE MANAGEMENT

Hypertension is the most common CV risk factor worldwide.

There is overwhelming evidence of a direct relationship between levels of blood pressure control and associated CV event risk,[65] with more strict control of blood pressure associated with a greater reduction in risk. The aim is to achieve a target blood pressure of ≤140/90 mm Hg or down to 130/80 mmHg in patients with DM or chronic renal failure. Yet even a small reduction in blood pressure can make large clinical differences.

A number of epidemiological studies point to the direct effect that hypertension has on the incidence of PAD, patients with PAD tending to have more problems related to systolic hypertension because of the degree of arterial calcification and subsequent lack of arterial elasticity associated with PAD.

Data from the Framingham Study showed that a blood pressure of >160/95 mmHg was associated with a 2.5 increased risk in men and a fourfold increased risk of developing PAD in women over a follow-up period of 26 years. Furthermore, this is confirmed by a study, which showed that a 10-mmHg increase in systolic blood pressure was associated with an increase in risk of developing PAD (odds ratio, 1.3; 95% CI, 1.2–1.5). This link of hypertension and PAD is also evident in the fact that 5% of patients diagnosed with hypertension have clinical evidence of PAD at the time of diagnosis.

DYSLIPIDAEMIA

A link between cholesterol and the development of atherosclerotic disease has been evident for many years. There is now strong epidemiological evidence that a positive link exists between levels of total and low-density lipoprotein (LDL) cholesterol and the risk of major adverse CV events. Indeed, a reduction in LDL cholesterol levels of 1 mmol/L equates to a reduction in CV risk of 21%, irrespective of starting LDL cholesterol level.[66]

Recently, there has been recognition that the total cholesterol to high-density lipoprotein (HDL) cholesterol ratio is perhaps a better measure of CV risk and current NICE guidelines now focus on non-HDL cholesterol levels rather than more specific LDL cholesterol levels.

Cholesterol is derived from two sources: (i) endogenous synthesis within the liver, which is in part secreted into the gastrointestinal tract via the biliary system, and (ii) gastrointestinal absorption of dietary cholesterol as well as reabsorption of that excreted within the biliary salts (Fig. 1.3).

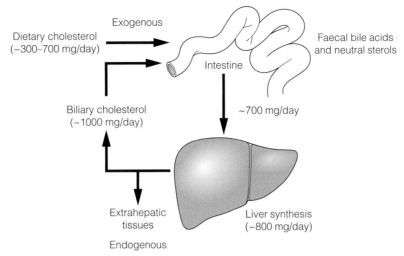

Figure 1.3 Circulating cholesterol is derived from endogenous synthesis in the liver and exogenous sources (dietary intake and bile acids) absorbed through the gut. Statins block synthesis, ezetimibe blocks gut absorption. The drugs have additive effects on serum cholesterol.

As such, pharmacological manipulation has been targeted at these processes. The most commonly used therapies are HMG-CoA reductase inhibitors (statins), with this being the rate-limiting enzyme in cholesterol biosynthesis. Other pharmacological agents include ezetimibe, which inhibits cholesterol absorption and is not systemically absorbed and proprotein convertase subtilisin kexin 9 inhibitors, which increase the concentration of LDL receptors (a plasma membrane glycoprotein that removes cholesterol-rich LDL particles from the plasma), which in turn leads to lower LDL cholesterol levels.

CONCLUSIONS

The prevalence of lower limb PAD is increasing and is a global problem. While the risk of limb loss is low, it does present major impairment of day-to-day activities. Of greatest concern is the significant additional CV risk that PAD confers and is considered to be a coronary heart disease risk equivalent. Epidemiological studies have identified numerous risk factors that, in longitudinal follow-up studies in large populations, are associated with a higher incidence and more rapid progression of PAD.

 References available at http://ebooks.health.elsevier.com/

KEY REFERENCES

[1] Fowkes FG, Rudan D, Rudan I, et al. Comparison of global estimates of prevalence and risk factors for peripheral artery disease in 2000 and 2010: a systematic review and analysis. Lancet 2013;382(9901):1329–40. 23915883.

[33] Bhatt DL, Steg PG, Ohman EM, et al. International prevalence, recognition and treatment of cardiovascular risk factors in outpatients with atherothrombosis. JAMA 2006;295:180–9. 16403930. The REACH registry is a large multinational observational study of >67 000 patients with cardiovascular disease, including patients with PAD.

[57] Alberts MJ, Bhatt DL, Mas J-L, et al. Three-year follow-up and event rates in the international REduction of atherothrombosis for continued health registry. Eur Heart J 2009;30:2318–26. 19720633. The first outcomes from the REACH registry, which suggested that PAD patients had a high risk for MI and stroke.

[59] Rosenberg L, Palmer JR, Shapiro S. Decline in the risk of myocardial infarction among women who stop smoking. N Engl J Med 1990;322:213–7. 2294448. Data identifying the benefits of smoking cessation.

[61] Adler A. Ukpds 59: hyperglycaemia and other potentially modifiable risk factors for peripheral arterial disease in type 2 diabetes. Diabetes Care 2002;25:894–9. 11978687. A large study conducted in the UK that showed a strong association between glycaemic control and PAD.

Key points

- There is a U-shaped relationship between ABPI and reduced life expectancy, with high ABPI measurements also associated with an increased risk of CV morbidity and mortality.
- The incidence of PAD increases steeply with advancing age and may be slightly more common in men.
- Although the risks of limb loss in most patients with PAD are low, the risk of premature death from other CV events is very high, as illustrated by the REACH registry.
- Risk factors for the development of PAD are similar to those for atherosclerotic disease in general but smoking and diabetes may have a more significant impact in the lower limbs.
- Glycaemic control for those with diabetes is important in the prevention of microvascular complications, but other factors in the diabetes syndrome, such as hypertension and dyslipidaemia, may be more important in the development of PAD.

2 Assessment of chronic lower limb ischaemia

Kurian J. Mylankal | Robert Fitridge

INTRODUCTION

Chronic lower limb ischaemia often referred to as peripheral arterial disease (PAD) is characterised by impaired circulation in the lower limb extremities. The worldwide prevalence of PAD is over 200 million and this disease burden is expected to increase with the aging global demographics and rise in diabetes.[1] The early assessment and recognition of PAD is crucial as these patients are at 2–4 times the risk for future cardiovascular and cerebrovascular events. Prompt treatment reduces longer-term risks of ischaemic events and major limb amputation.[2]

PAD is a consequence of systemic atherosclerosis, which involves the arterial tree throughout the body and commonly affects the coronary, carotid, iliac, femoral and infrainguinal arteries. For the purpose of this chapter, PAD will refer to its manifestations in the lower limb. PAD is a common disease and its prevalence can be as high as 20% over the age of 60 and two thirds of these patients remain asymptomatic and undiscovered without specific screening tests.[2–4] As the degree of arterial disease progresses, symptoms of PAD appear; the severity of which coincides with the extent of arterial bed involvement. These symptoms can range from exertional leg pain, which can subsequently progress to (or present as) severe limb threatening ischaemia.

Intermittent claudication (IC) is often the first symptom of PAD, most commonly located in calf muscles, and usually associated with atherosclerotic occlusion or stenosis involving the iliac or femoro-popliteal (FP) segments. More severe limb ischaemia is usually associated with PAD affecting the lower limb vasculature at two or three anatomical levels. This results in significantly impaired tissue perfusion with rest pain, ulceration or gangrene involving the toes or forefoot. This is referred to as *chronic limb-threatening ischaemia* (*CLTI*).[5] This chapter deals with the assessment of patients with chronic lower limb ischaemia, including the principles of vascular imaging.

Recent data from the Swedevasc Registry found that the risk of amputation in patients with claudication who had undergone revascularisation was 1.2% at 3 years, compared to a 12% risk of amputation in the first 6 months following revascularisation for those with CLTI and then 2% annually. After 3 years, the cumulative mortality rate for people with claudication was 12% and 41.4% in CLTI.[6]

Severity of PAD is commonly reported by two classification systems. The Fontaine classification is based on clinical symptoms alone (Table 2.1) and in contrast, the Rutherford classification is more detailed and takes into account clinical findings, including Doppler assessment and ankle pressure assessment (Table 2.2). These two classifications are inclusive of the asymptomatic and milder forms of PAD and useful for ensuring consistency in reporting standards.

INTERMITTENT CLAUDICATION

IC occurs because of inadequate augmentation of blood flow to the skeletal muscles, which fails to meet the increased metabolic requirements of the exercising muscle groups. IC is present in only 10–20% of patients with PAD with the majority of patients remaining asymptomatic. In addition to the reduced arterial perfusion from fixed atherosclerotic lesions, endothelial dysfunction with diminished vasodilator effect, inadequate angiogenesis combined with failure to develop collaterals, impaired skeletal muscle metabolism because of mitochondrial dysfunction and local inflammatory changes are also proposed as mechanisms for the pathogenesis of IC.[7] The classic feature of IC is of pain developing on walking in the muscle groups distal to the arterial obstruction, with relief of symptoms within 10 minutes of cessation of exercise (usually more quickly). This pain reappears after walking a similar distance and is not felt at rest or within the first few steps taken. The symptoms have a chronic history and are described as an ache, cramp or tightening in the muscle that usually forces the patient to stop. Exercise tolerance is dependent on the balance between tissue perfusion and energy expenditure. In mild PAD, claudication may be felt only while walking uphill or walking quickly. Conversely, in individuals with restricted mobility from other comorbidities, PAD may not manifest with claudication symptoms. Claudication pain most commonly affects the calf muscles, which are extensively used whilst walking. However, in the presence of aorto-iliac disease, pain may be felt more proximally in the buttocks or thigh, as well as in the calf.

DIFFERENTIAL DIAGNOSIS

Conditions such as osteoarthritis of the hip or knee, spinal canal stenosis and venous outflow obstruction may be mistaken for IC and should be considered in the differential diagnosis. Other relevant conditions to consider in the differential diagnosis of IC are described in Table 2.3.[8]

In osteoarthritis of the hip, pain may be referred down the leg to mimic claudication. However, these patients may also give a history of pain in the buttock or groin when turning their body and even in a sitting or supine position. Unlike the pain in IC, this is not relieved by standing still and requires easing the load off the arthritic joint. In addition, pain from

Table 2.1 Fontaine classification of the severity of PAD

Fontaine stage	Description
I Asymptomatic	PAD present but no symptoms
II Intermittent claudication	Cramping pain in leg muscles precipitated by walking and rapidly relieved by rest
III Rest pain	Constant pain in feet (often worse at night)
IV Tissue loss	Ischaemic ulceration or gangrene

PAD, Peripheral arterial disease

Table 2.2 Rutherford classification of the severity of PAD

Grade	Category	Description
0	0	Asymptomatic
I	1	Mild claudication
I	2	Moderate claudication
I	3	Severe claudication
II	4	Ischaemic rest pain (ankle pressure [AP] <40 mmHg of flat waveforms
II	5	Minor tissue loss (AP <40 mmHg, flat waveforms or toe pressure [TP] <40 mmHg)
III	6	Major tissue loss (AP <40 mmHg, flat waveforms or TP <40 mmHg)

PAD, Peripheral arterial disease

of iliofemoral deep vein thrombosis and inspection findings of lower limb oedema and other stigmata of chronic venous insufficiency will often help with the diagnosis.

The cornerstones in the assessment of chronic lower limb ischaemia are a careful history, palpation of pulses and ABI measurement. The important point is to verify that the clinical findings correlate well with the patient's symptoms. As the patients get older so does the arterial tree and the mere presence of PAD (i.e., reduced ABI, atherosclerosis visible on ultrasound examination) does not necessarily mean that it is the cause of the symptoms. The history should include the duration of symptoms and the mode of onset. Most patients gradually become aware of pain on walking, which is typical in progressive PAD.

The blood supply required by resting muscles is relatively small (130–150 mL/min) and may be increased five- to 10-fold during exercise.[10]

Arterial occlusions can be well tolerated when collaterals have developed, which may provide the same volume of blood flow at rest compared to normal individuals.[11] Examples include the thigh muscles, which are perfused by collaterals from the profunda femoris artery in superficial femoral artery occlusion and also occlusions of the iliac arteries, where collaterals develop through the pelvis and buttock and may even result in normal resting ABI and a palpable foot pulse. Significant PAD is usually associated with an ABI of <0.9 (see later), but in such cases, resting ankle pressures may be deceptively normal. However, an exercise challenge will result in a fall in ankle pressures and disappearance of the distal pulses. It is important to bear in mind that these patients may continue to remain asymptomatic if they undertake only limited physical activity below the threshold limit to induce claudication.

osteoarthritis typically begins when walking and gets better after some exercise. Although the diagnosis can usually be established by history and examination alone, non-invasive investigations including an exercise ankle–brachial index (ABI) test to exclude arterial disease will be reassuring.

Patients with spinal canal stenosis may also have symptoms that are very similar to IC although the history of pain may be inconsistent.[9] Postures such as sitting and leaning forward to straighten the lumbar lordosis relieves cord pressure although the pain symptoms may take 60 minutes or even longer to subside. A history of pain on standing as well as walking should raise the suspicion of neurogenic pain because of spinal stenosis.

Lumbar nerve route irritation may also cause aching in the calf or down the back of the leg from buttock to ankle. The sensation appears to be very similar to that of claudication, particularly when confined to the calf. Direct enquiry for these symptoms is helpful, but the key feature is again the need to sit or lie to obtain relief. Spinal flexion may release the involved nerve roots, whereas a straight leg raise will often precipitate the pain. When both sciatic nerve irritation or spinal canal stenosis and PAD coexist, it can be extremely difficult to identify which is contributing most to the patient's symptoms.

In venous outflow obstruction, exercise-induced arterial flow augmentation is not matched by the venous outflow, resulting in high venous pressures within the lower limbs. Tense dilatation of the veins can mimic claudication-like symptoms. However, this is often described as a severe bursting pain and is relieved slowly with rest or leg elevation. A previous history

CHRONIC LIMB-THREATENING ISCHAEMIA

CLTI represents the end stage of PAD.[5] Ischaemic rest pain, ischaemic ulceration or gangrene of the foot are the hallmarks of CLTI and this requires urgent investigation and revascularisation to avoid limb loss from progressive tissue necrosis and/or infection. Unlike IC, in CLTI the arterial perfusion is severely compromised to the degree that it is unable to meet the basal metabolic requirements of the ischaemic tissues or adequate perfusion to heal a foot wound. Severely compromised tissue perfusion causes pain even at rest and the inability for cellular repair and regeneration results in ulceration and gangrene commonly seen over areas of minor trauma. Untreated, the prognosis is poor with a higher risk of mortality, limb loss and associated pain and reduced quality of life. Recognition of CLTI is therefore very important in the assessment of chronic limb ischaemia.

The Global Vascular Guidelines for CLTI, which is a collaborative effort of the major vascular surgical societies worldwide, has proposed a revised model of care for CLTI.[5] These guidelines aim to redefine the nomenclature and propose a standardised disease staging and revascularisation approach (evidence-based revascularisation [EBR]). Adoption of the term *CLTI* addresses the shortcomings of the previous terms *"critical limb ischaemia"*, which was based on threshold values of ABI and toe pressures (TPs). CLTI aims to include a diverse group of patients with varying degrees of ischaemia, which can result in delayed wound healing or amputation. More importantly, this definition acknowledges the current global trend

Table 2.3   Differential diagnosis of intermittent claudication[8]

Condition	Location of pain or discomfort	Characteristic discomfort	Onset relative to exercise	Effect of rest	Effect of body position	Other characteristics
Intermittent claudication	Buttock, thigh or calf muscles and rarely the foot	Cramping, aching, fatigue, weakness or frank pain	After same degree of exercise	Rapid relief with rest	None	Reproducible
Nerve root compression (e.g., herniated disk)	Radiates down leg, usually posteriorly	Sharp lancinating pain	Soon, if not immediately, after onset	Not quickly relieved (also often present at rest)	Relief may be aided by adjusting back position	History of back problems
Spinal canal stenosis	Hip, thigh, buttocks (follows dermatome)	Motor weakness more prominent than pain	After walking or standing for variable lengths of time	Relieved by stopping only if position changed	Relief by lumbar spine flexion (sitting, using walking frame or stooping forward)	Frequent history of back problems, provoked by intra-abdominal pressure
Arthritic, inflammatory processes	Foot, arch	Aching pain	After variable degree of exercise	Not quickly relieved (and may be present at rest)	May be relieved by not bearing weight	Variable, may relate to activity level
Hip arthritis	Hip, thigh, buttocks	Aching discomfort, usually localised to hip and gluteal region	After variable degree of exercise	Not quickly relieved (and may be present at rest)	More comfortable sitting, weight taken off legs	Variable, may relate to activity level, weather changes
Symptomatic Baker's cyst	Behind knee, down calf	Swelling, soreness, tenderness	With exercise	Present at rest	None	Not intermittent
Venous claudication	Entire leg, but usually worse in thigh and groin	Tight, bursting pain	After walking	Subsides slowly	Relief speeded by elevation	Often history of iliofemoral deep vein thrombosis, signs of venous congestion, oedema
Chronic compartment syndrome	Calf muscles	Tight, bursting pain	After much exercise (e.g., jogging)	Subsides very slowly	Relief speeded by elevation	Typically occurs in heavy muscled athletes

Norgren L, Hiatt WR, Dormandy JA, Nehler MR, Harris KA, Fowkes FG, et al. Inter-Society Consensus for the Management of Peripheral Arterial Disease (TASC II). Eur J Vasc Endovasc Surg. 2007;33 Suppl 1:S1-75.

of PAD and its close association with diabetes and recognises this as an important risk factor that can result in limb loss.

CLTI is defined as objectively documented PAD **and** any of the following clinical symptoms or signs:

- Ischaemic rest pain present for longer that 2 weeks and associated with ABI <0.4, ankle pressure (AP) <50 mmHg, TP, <30 mmHg, transcutaneous partial pressure of oxygen ($TcPO_2$) <30 mmHg or flat waveforms on pulse volume recordings.
- Diabetic foot ulcer (DFU) or any lower limb ulceration present for at least 2 weeks
- Gangrene involving any portion of the lower limb or foot.

Pure venous ulcers, pure traumatic wounds, acute limb ischaemia (symptoms less than 2 weeks) embolic disease and non-atherosclerotic chronic vascular conditions of the lower limb extremity (e.g., vasculitis, Buerger's disease, radiation arteritis) are excluded in this definition.

STAGING OF CHRONIC LIMB-THREATENING ISCHAEMIA – WOUND, ISCHAEMIA AND FOOT INFECTION

CLTI encompasses a wide range of clinical disease burden and anatomical complexity. Staging of CLTI therefore becomes paramount not only to estimate risk of amputation and effectiveness of treatment strategies but also in making objective comparisons in research trials and for a uniform and reliable reporting mechanism of disease severity. The Society for Vascular Surgery Lower Extremity Guideline

Table 2.4 Wound grading (W) in wound, ischaemia and foot infection (WIfI) classification[12]

Grade (W)	Ulcer	Gangrene
0	No ulcer *Clinical description: ischaemic rest pain (requires typical symptoms + ischaemia grade 3); no wound.*	No gangrene
1	Small, shallow ulcer on distal leg or foot; no exposed bone, unless limited to distal phalanx *Clinical description: minor tissue loss. Salvageable with simple digital amputation (1 or 2 digits) or skin coverage.*	No gangrene
2	Deeper ulcer with exposed bone, joint or tendon; generally not involving the heel; shallow heel ulcer, without calcaneal involvement *Clinical description: major tissue loss salvageable with multiple (>3) digital amputations or standard TMA ± skin coverage.*	Gangrenous changes limited to digits
3	Extensive, deep ulcer involving forefoot and/or midfoot; deep, full-thickness heel ulcer ± calcaneal involvement *Clinical description: extensive tissue loss salvageable only with a complex foot reconstruction or non-traditional TMA (Chopart, or Lisfranc amputation); flap coverage or complex wound management needed for large soft tissue defect.*	Extensive gangrene involving forefoot and/or midfoot; full-thickness heel necrosis ± calcaneal involvement

TMA, Transmetatarsal amputation
Mills JL, Sr., Conte MS, Armstrong DG, Pomposelli FB, Schanzer A, Sidawy AN, et al. The Society for Vascular Surgery Lower Extremity Threatened Limb Classification System: risk stratification based on wound, ischemia, and foot infection (WIfI). J Vasc Surg. 2014;59(1):220-34 e1-2.

Table 2.5 Ischaemia grading (I) in wound, ischemia, and foot infection (WIfI) classification[12] haemodynamics/perfusion: Measure TP or TcPO$_2$ if ABI incompressible (>1.3) SVS grades 0 (none), 1 (mild), 2 (moderate), and 3 (severe)

Grade (I)	ABI	Ankle systolic pressure	TP, TcPO$_2$
0	≥0.80	>100 mmHg	≥60 mmHg
1	0.6–0.79	70–100 mmHg	40–59 mmHg
2	0.4–0.59	50–70 mmHg	30–39 mmHg
3	≤0.39	<50 mmHg	<30 mmHg

ABI, Ankle-brachial index; *TcPO$_2$*, transcutaneous oximetry; *TP*, toe pressure.
Flat or minimally pulsatile forefoot pulse volume recording is grade 3. Measure TP or TcPO$_2$ if ABI incompressible (>1.3). Patients with diabetes should have TP measurements. If arterial calcification precludes reliable ABI or TP measurements, ischaemia should be documented by TcPO$_2$, skin perfusion pressure, or pulse volume recording. If TP and ABI measurements result in different grades, TP will be the primary determinant of ischaemia grade.
Mills JL, Sr., Conte MS, Armstrong DG, Pomposelli FB, Schanzer A, Sidawy AN, et al. The Society for Vascular Surgery Lower Extremity Threatened Limb Classification System: risk stratification based on wound, ischemia, and foot infection (WIfI). J Vasc Surg. 2014;59(1):220-34 e1-2.

Committee published the Threatened Limb Ischaemia Classification System in 2014 and this staging system takes into account the three major risk factors that determine the probability of lower limb amputation –**w**ound, **i**schaemia and **f**oot **i**nfection (**WIfI**).[12] Each of the three risk factors are graded from 0–3 based on severity, where 0 represents none, 1 mild, 2 moderate and 3 severe (Tables 2.4–2.6).[12] The scores derived from each component are combined and analysed using two tables: one which estimates the risk of amputation at 1 year and the second table, which estimates the benefit from revascularisation (Table 2.7 A&B).[12] Accordingly, the limb is stratified into clinical stages 1, 2 , 3 or 4 as very low, low,

medium and high risk of amputation and also the likely benefit from revascularisation. Stage 5 is clinically assessed as a non-salvageable limb. Several studies have now validated WIfI as a reliable staging system in predicting lower limb outcome in CLTI. It is recommended that all patients with CLTI are staged with WIfI initially and this should be repeated after vascular intervention or foot surgery, treatment of infection or when there is a clinical deterioration.

Rest pain often presents with pain in the forefoot at night sufficient to disturb the patient's sleep when the patient is supine.[13] When the patient hangs the leg out of bed, sits in a chair or if they stand up and walk (thereby increasing the blood flow to the foot), the pain is often relieved. If the patient constantly hangs their feet out of bed at night, or even sleeps sitting in a chair, the limb tends to swell because of dependent oedema. This oedema in turn increases the hydrostatic pressure of the peripheral tissue and compresses the already compromised capillaries and further interferes with tissue perfusion and nutrition. These patients may often require inpatient treatment with analgesia (usually including opiates) so that the limb can be kept in the supine position overnight to relieve the oedema before arterial reconstruction.

To the experienced eye, the diagnosis of CLTI seems obvious, but it is often easy to miss a small ischaemic lesion on the heel or between the toes. When established necrosis or gangrene is present with absent limb pulses, there is no doubt about the diagnosis. The stage of CLTI without necrosis or gangrene is characterised by pallor when the leg is elevated above the heart and changing to a deep red colour when hanging down (Buerger's test-positive). The red colour is caused by the dilated capillaries of the foot. In CLTI, the natural compensatory mechanisms for ischaemia including angiogenesis (new capillary formation) and arteriogenesis (enlargement of pre-existing capillaries) are exhausted and the capillaries are maximally vasodilated and hence unresponsive to pro-vasodilatory stimuli.[13,14] Therefore it may take a while for pallor on elevation to occur but capillary refill will be abolished immediately.

Table 2.6 Foot infection grading (fI) in wound, ischaemia, and foot infection (WIfI) classification[12] SVS grades 0 (none), 1 (mild), 2 (moderate), and 3 (severe: limb and/or life-threatening) SVS adaptation of Infectious Diseases Society of America (IDSA) and International Working Group on the Diabetic Foot (IWGDF)

Clinical manifestation of infection	SVS	IDSA/PEDIS infection severity
No symptoms or signs of infection	0	Uninfected
Local infection involving only the skin and the subcutaneous tissue (without involvement of deeper tissues and without systemic signs as described later).	1	Mild
Infection present, as defined by the presence of at least 2 of the following items:		
• Local swelling or induration		
• Erythema >0.5 to ≤2 cm around the ulcer		
• Local tenderness or pain		
• Local warmth		
• Purulent discharge (thick, opaque to white or sanguineous secretion)		
Exclude other causes of an inflammatory response of the skin (e.g., trauma, gout, acute Charcot neuro-osteoarthropathy, fracture, thrombosis, venous stasis)		
Local infection (as described earlier) with erythema >2 cm, or involving 2 structures deeper than skin and subcutaneous tissues (e.g., abscess, osteomyelitis, septic arthritis, fasciitis), and no systemic inflammatory response signs (as described later)	2	Moderate
Local infection (as described earlier) with the signs of SIRS, as manifested by two or more of the following:	3	Severe
• Temperature >38°C or <36°C		
• Heart rate >90 beats/min		
• Respiratory rate >20 breaths/min or $PaCO_2$ <32 mmHg		
• White blood cell count >12 000 or <4000 cu/mm or 10% immature (band) forms		

$PaCO_2$, Partial pressure of arterial carbon dioxide; *SIRS*, systemic inflammatory response syndrome.
Ischaemia may complicate and increase the severity of any infection. Systemic infection may sometimes manifest with other clinical findings, such as hypotension, confusion, vomiting, or evidence of metabolic disturbances, such as acidosis, severe hyperglycemia, new-onset azotemia.
Mills JL, Sr., Conte MS, Armstrong DG, Pomposelli FB, Schanzer A, Sidawy AN, et al. The Society for Vascular Surgery Lower Extremity Threatened Limb Classification System: risk stratification based on wound, ischemia, and foot infection (WIfI). J Vasc Surg. 2014;59(1):220-34 e1-2.

Table 2.7 A. Estimate risk of amputation for each combination at 1 year[12]

	Ischaemia - 0				Ischaemia - 1				Ischaemia -2				Ischaemia - 3			
W-0	VL	VL	L	M	VL	L	M	H	L	L	M	H	L	M	M	H
W-1	VL	VL	L	M	VL	L	M	H	L	M	H	H	M	M	H	H
W-2	L	L	M	H	M	M	H	H	M	H	H	H	H	H	H	H
W-3	M	M	H	H	H	H	H	H	H	H	H	H	H	H	H	H
	fl-0	fl-1	fl-2	fl-3	fl-0	fl-1	fl-2	fl-3	fl-0	fl-1	fl-2	fl-3	fl-0	fl-1	fl-2	fl-3

B. Estimate benefit of/requirement for revascularisation (after control of infection first)[12]

	Ischaemia - 0				Ischaemia - 1				Ischaemia -2				Ischaemia - 3			
W-0	VL	VL	VL	VL	VL	L	L	M	L	L	M	M	M	H	H	H
W-1	VL	VL	VL	VL	L	M	M	M	M	H	H	H	H	H	H	H
W-2	VL	VL	VL	VL	M	M	H	H	H	H	H	H	H	H	H	H
W-3	VL	VL	VL	VL	M	M	H	H	H	H	H	H	H	H	H	H
	fl-0	fl-1	fl-2	fl-3	fl-0	fl-1	fl-2	fl-3	fl-0	fl-1	fl-2	fl-3	fl-0	fl-1	fl-2	fl-3

W, Wound; *I*, ischaemia; *fl*, foot infection.
VL = Very Low = Stage 1
L = Low = Stage 2
M = Medium = Stage 3
H = High = Stage 4
Stage 5 represents an unsalvageable foot
Mills JL, Sr., Conte MS, Armstrong DG, Pomposelli FB, Schanzer A, Sidawy AN, et al. The Society for Vascular Surgery Lower Extremity Threatened Limb Classification System: risk stratification based on wound, ischemia, and foot infection (WIfI). J Vasc Surg. 2014;59(1):220-34 e1-2.

RARE CAUSES OF ISCHAEMIA

Although the vast majority of cases of chronic lower limb isch-aemia are caused by atherosclerotic PAD, other rare conditions exist and these are more frequently seen in the younger age group of patients. History of IC in a patient who is young and also in older patients without risk factors for atherosclerosis should alert one to the possibility of these rare diagnoses. Thorough history and meticulous examination including peripheral pulses and resting ABIs should be recorded. In patients giving a convincing history of IC with palpable foot pulses or normal ABI, onset of symptoms with exercise testing and post-exercise ABI's may help clinch the diagnosis.

POPLITEAL ARTERY ENTRAPMENT SYNDROME

This condition should be suspected particularly when a young patient, especially an athletic individual complains of claudication symptoms or CLTI. There is a male preponderance for popliteal artery entrapment syndrome (PAES) with 85% being male and over 60% of cases occur in athletes.[15,16] The presentation is bilateral in 30% of cases.[17] During embryonic development, the medial head of the gastrocnemius muscle (MHG) migrates medially from the posterior aspect of the fibula and lateral tibia across the popliteal fossa to its attachment to the posterior aspect of the medial femoral condyle. The popliteal artery simultaneously develops superficial to the popliteus muscle during this stage. These complex and dynamic changes associated with the foetal limb bud rotation and knee extension raises the chance for various anatomical variations to develop in the relationship between the popliteal artery and the MHG. There are six variants of popliteal entrapment described (Table 2.8). Fig. 2.1 demonstrates the anatomical variants of PAES.

Continuous compression of the artery can result in fibrotic change, which progresses from the outer adventitial layer of the artery to the intima. As a consequence, aneurysmal

---

Table 2.8   Anatomical classification of popliteal artery entrapment (based on[52])

Type 1	The popliteal artery takes an aberrant medial course around the normally placed medial head of the gastrocnemius muscle (MHG)
Type II	The MHG has a more lateral insertion on the femoral condyle and hence the popliteal artery runs medially and inferiorly
Type III	Abnormal muscle slips or fibrous bands tether the artery to the medial or lateral femoral condyles
Type IV	Popliteal artery is entrapped by the popliteus muscle and here a persisting axial artery replaces the popliteal artery
Type V	The popliteal artery and vein are involved in any of the aforementioned subtypes
Type VI	(Functional variant): Muscle hypertrophy causes functional compression of the popliteal artery and vein. No anatomical abnormality is noted

Pillai J. A current interpretation of popliteal vascular entrapment. J Vasc Surg. 2008;48(6 Suppl):61S-5S; discussion 5S.

---

degeneration and/or thrombosis may develop. Examination may reveal reduction or obliteration of pedal pulses during active plantar flexion. Duplex scanning or arteriography using this manoeuvre may also demonstrate kinking or compression of the popliteal artery. Computed tomography (CT) or magnetic resonance (MR) scanning can also demonstrate the anatomical abnormality. Symptomatic patients should be treated by the division of the medial head of gastrocnemius and/or reconstruction of the popliteal artery. Surgery may be indicated for an asymptomatic contralateral limb whenever anatomical entrapment is detected.[18] The functional variant of the condition, unlike the anatomical variant, should only be treated when symptomatic.[19]

CYSTIC ADVENTITIAL DISEASE

Cystic adventitial disease (CAD) is caused by cyst formation in the adventitia of the artery because of implantation of mucin-secreting mesenchymal cells on the adventitial wall during development. CAD commonly affects the popliteal artery and less often the external iliac and femoral vessels. It predominantly affects males in the mid-30s, is unilateral in presentation and patients commonly present with IC. The contents of the cyst resemble that of a ganglion and the cysts may be connected to the synovium of the knee joint. IC may be severe and of rapid onset. The condition should be particularly suspected in young patients without significant risk factors for PAD. Pedal pulses sometimes disappear on knee flexion (Ishikawa's sign). Arteriography may show an unusually smooth 'hourglass' stenosis referred to as the 'scimitar' sign (Fig. 2.2). Ultrasound scanning will demonstrate the cystic abnormality with absence of flow within it and CT may help delineate CAD from popliteal entrapment syndrome and aneurysm. The appearance of CAD on MR imaging (MRI) is distinctive. CAD demonstrates homogenous low intensity signal on T1-weighted images and high signal intensity on T2-weighted images. On post-contrast T1-weighted images, the cyst does not enhance and can be seen compressing the arterial lumen.[20] The distinctive findings on MRI make this modality the imaging technique of choice when the condition is suspected or diagnosed on ultrasound. Resection of the affected segment of artery and repair with an interposition vein graft via a posterior approach is the most widely practised technique and is mandatory in popliteal artery thrombosis or in extensive arterial involvement.[21] Non-resectional techniques such as cyst excision or evacuation have been described with some success although a high incidence of recurrence has been observed with these techniques.

PERSISTENT SCIATIC ARTERY

This is a rare congenital anomaly with only a couple of hundred cases reported in the literature. In early embryonic development, the sciatic artery, which is the embryonic limb artery, disappears when the superficial femoral artery has developed. However, in persistent sciatic artery (PSA), the sciatic artery does not obliterate and remains continuous with the popliteal artery, providing the major blood supply to the lower limb. The anomaly is bilateral in approximately 30% of cases and is commonly associated with failure of the iliofemoral vessels to develop normally. The presenting symptoms

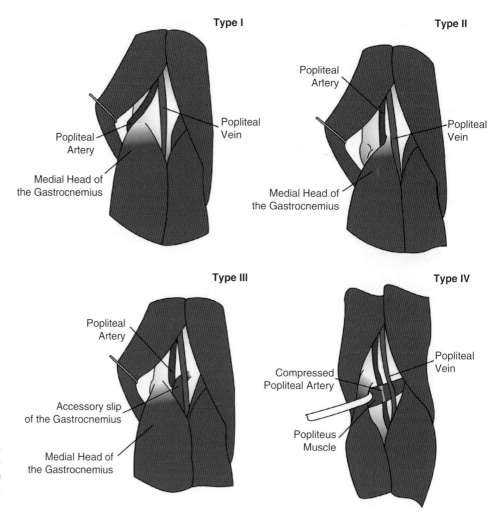

Figure 2.1 Types of popliteal entrapment syndrome showing anatomical variation in the course of the popliteal artery in relation to the medial head of gastrocnemius.[52]

are variable and include IC, limb ischaemia, a pulsatile mass in the buttock or neurological symptoms from sciatic nerve compression. Aneurysmal degeneration of the artery as it emerges from the sciatic foramen is a common presentation and thrombosis or distal embolism may lead to acute ischaemia. In a review of 159 patients with PSA, the mean patient age at the time of diagnosis was 59 years and 80% were symptomatic.[22] Although pedal pulses may be present, the femoral pulse will be reduced or absent if the iliofemoral vessels are hypoplastic (Cowie's sign) and IC will result if neither system has developed properly (Fig. 2.3). Symptomatic patients can be treated by combined bypass grafting and endovascular exclusion of the aneurysm.[23] Asymptomatic patients should be monitored for aneurysm development.

FIBROMUSCULAR DYSPLASIA

Fibromuscular dysplasia (FMD) is a non-atherosclerotic and non-inflammatory arterial disease, which is more commonly seen in middle-aged women and usually affects the renal, carotid and vertebral arteries. It can also affect the iliac, femoral or popliteal arteries although this is less common. In younger patients, FMD can cause IC or microembolisation and rarely severe limb ischaemia from arterial dissection. Depending on the layer of the arterial wall that is predominantly affected, three varieties of FMD

are recognised – medial fibroplasia (most common type), intimal fibroplasia and adventitial fibroplasia. It is characterised by luminal fibrotic webs that give rise to stenoses and post-stenotic dilatations giving the classic beaded appearance. The external iliac artery is the commonest site of involvement in the lower limb vasculature (Fig. 2.4). Patients with iliac FMD should be screened for renal and carotid/vertebral involvement. Symptomatic stenoses usually respond well to angioplasty. Stenting should be reserved for cases with suboptimal angioplasty results or procedural complications following angioplasty.[24]

ENDOFIBROSIS OF THE ILIAC ARTERY

This is a rare cause of arterial stenosis seen particularly in the external iliac artery among competitive cyclists. It is thought to develop as a result of repetitive trauma to the external iliac artery and the commonest presentation is IC with maximal exertion. Clinical examination may be normal and occasionally, a femoral bruit may be heard. Exercise testing with immediate post-exercise ABIs and duplex ultrasound (DUS) help confirm the lesion. DUS and contrast angiography may demonstrate concentric stenosis but the lesions may be very subtle at rest. Techniques widely reported for repair are endarterectomy and patch angioplasty and interposition graft.[25,26]

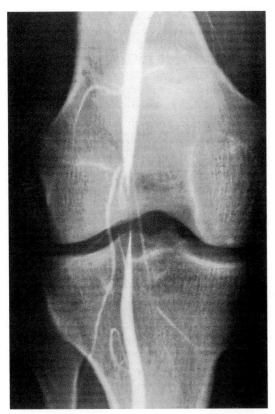

Figure 2.2 Smooth 'hourglass' stenosis of popliteal artery caused by cystic adventitial disease. A similar appearance may be seen in popliteal entrapment, especially during active plantar flexion.

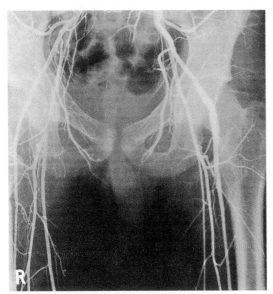

Figure 2.3 Persistent bilateral sciatic arteries arising from the common iliac arteries with dilatation and intimal irregularity of the left sciatic artery at the level of the acetabulum.

BUERGER'S DISEASE

Buerger's disease (thromboangiitis obliterans) is a systemic vasculopathy associated with tobacco use that affects medium-sized arteries and veins in both the upper and lower limbs. It

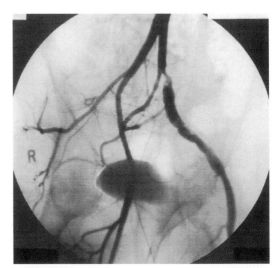

Figure 2.4 Fibromuscular dysplasia affecting the left external iliac artery of a 12-year-old boy.

should be considered in any heavy-smoking young male patient with claudication, especially if they are of Middle or Far Eastern origin.[27] Vasospastic symptoms and superficial thrombophlebitis commonly occur and patients may progress rapidly to, or present with, CLTI. The pathophysiology and management of this condition and other causes of vasculitis such as Takayasu's are covered in Chapter 12. Patients who smoke large quantities of cannabis may present with symptoms and imaging indistinguishable from those of Buerger's disease.

The crural vessels are usually severely affected, with patent arteries to the knee joint and typical 'corkscrew' collaterals in the calf.[28]

DIAGNOSIS OF PERIPHERAL ARTERIAL DISEASE

A meticulous approach to the patient presenting with suspected arterial disease is paramount in the diagnosis of PAD. This includes a detailed history to delineate symptoms from other conditions, clinical examination and non-invasive hemodynamic tests to stage severity followed by dedicated vascular imaging for those presenting with CLTI or disabling claudication.

HISTORY

Duration of symptoms and factors that relieve or aggravate these symptoms usually help in diagnosing PAD and a meticulous history will often delineate other causes discussed in differential diagnosis. Localising pain to the forefoot, calf, thigh or buttocks will help ascertain the anatomical level of atherosclerotic disease and subsequent clinical examination can further confirm this. Quantifying walking distance can help ascertain the limitations imposed on the quality of life and document progression of symptoms over a period of time. Pain interrupting sleep, pain alleviated by dependency and sleeping in a chair are all features suggestive of CLTI. It is also important to establish the impact of these symptoms on the patient's daily activities, ability to work and ability to remain independent.

As all patients with PAD are at risk of myocardial infarction or stroke, a full history for other cardiovascular diseases and risk factors is essential (see Chapter 1).

All cardiovascular risk factors including smoking, diabetes mellitus, hypertension, dyslipidaemia, chronic kidney disease and a detailed drug and family history should be documented. The patient must be asked about a history of ischaemic heart disease, coronary stenting or bypass grafting and cerebrovascular disease, including transient ischaemic attacks and stroke. Although approximately 30% of patients with symptoms of limb ischaemia will have a history of myocardial infarction, it is not uncommon that angina or transient ischaemic attacks are diagnosed for the first time at initial vascular assessment. The investigation and treatment algorithm for these symptoms are usually based on a rational approach of prioritisation dependent on the severity of other comorbidities (see Chapter 3). Upper extremity exertional pain, postprandial abdominal pain and erectile dysfunction in men are important clues to the presence of significant occlusive atherosclerotic disease in other vascular territories.

A systematic approach to history taking helps establish the correct diagnosis and institute optimal strategies/therapy to counter concomitant cardiac and cerebrovascular risks. In addition, it also helps develop a safe management strategy for PAD taking into account patient's functional status, health related quality of life and fitness to undergo interventions.

EXAMINATION

A thorough and systematic approach to examination aims to establish the site and severity of PAD and elicit signs of atherosclerosis in the cardiovascular system. General inspection should focus on peripheral stigmata of cardiovascular disease such as cigarette staining of fingernails, scars from previous surgery, amputated limbs and toes, and xanthelasma. Measurement of blood pressure in both arms and the inter-arm difference, palpation of radial and brachial pulses (rhythm, rate and volume) and cardiac and pulmonary auscultation are mandatory to assess the extent of atherosclerotic involvement. Careful inspection of the feet for skin integrity including the interdigital web spaces and heel pressure points, skin colour and changes with elevation and dependency and skin surface temperature are noted. Abnormal femoral and foot pulses, lower extremity bruits, unilateral cool extremities, prolonged venous refill time and Buerger's test are findings highly suggestive of underlying PAD. Capillary refill test, foot discolouration, atrophic skin and hairless extremities are generally unhelpful in the diagnosis of PAD.[29]

The body mass index should be calculated by measuring height and weight. This is a good estimate of obesity, which may affect the patient's walking capacity, risk from anaesthesia and also the likelihood of surgical complications. In some cases, weight loss will reduce the patient's symptoms substantially.

Palpation of pulses is subjective and influenced by the sensitivity of the fingers, the experience of the examiner, the obesity of the patient and the warmth of the room. This should commence with a preliminary examination of the abdomen, assessing the aorta for the presence of an aneurysm and palpation for other abdominal masses. The femoral artery should be palpable in all subjects. If it is occluded, it can often be palpated as a hard cord because of calcific

atherosclerosis. A weak femoral pulse is indicative of a proximal stenosis or obstruction causing reduced femoral artery pressure. The popliteal pulse is more difficult to palpate, particularly in a well-built or obese subject, but should always be examined to exclude an aneurysm. Palpation of the foot pulses should be performed and recorded although it may be difficult when the foot is swollen, or the room is cold. Presence or absence of foot pulses on physical examination is a 'weak' and subjective sign of PAD and should always be supplemented by objective measurements (ABI). The absence of a single foot pulse may have little clinical significance and, although it should be recorded, it is not an indication for more detailed investigation. Auscultation of the neck, abdomen and groin should be performed to assess for bruits that may suggest stenoses of the carotid, renal/mesenteric and femoral arteries.

In patients with CLTI and diabetes, assessment of neuropathy – sensory, motor and autonomic should be documented. Glove and stocking distribution of neuropathy may manifest as tingling, numbness, burning pain or weakness. Neuropathy is tested with a monofilament and tuning fork test. Other characteristic features of abnormal foot biomechanics and weight loading associated with neuropathy are discussed in Chapter 5. Presence of a foot ulcer should trigger a probe-to-bone test to assess depth of the ulcer, likelihood of osteomyelitis and for accurate assessment of WIfI status.

RISK FACTORS

Identifying the risk factors for PAD is critical for implementing strategies to modify this risk and reduce both fatal and non-fatal cardiovascular events and the need for arterial reconstruction. The risk factors associated with PAD are essentially the same as those for ischaemic heart disease, and include smoking, dyslipidaemia, diabetes mellitus, hypertension, age, lack of exercise, unhealthy dietary habits and male sex (see Chapter 1).

All patients with PAD require a full blood count, electrolytes, renal function, a random blood glucose and lipid levels. Anaemia as well as polycythaemia can present with symptoms of leg ischaemia. Renal impairment is often associated with PAD and requires detection before contemplating both imaging and intervention. Arterial thromboembolism is relatively infrequent in patients under the age of 50 years and young patients presenting with PAD should raise suspicion of the presence of a thrombophilia. This cohort of patients merit screening for antiphospholipid antibodies or antithrombin III deficiency, which may lead to rethrombosis following either angioplasty or reconstruction. Hyperhomocysteinaemia can cause accelerated atherosclerosis and should be excluded in young patients with PAD.

EXERCISE CHALLENGE

Occasionally, patients present with a classic history of IC, but with palpable foot pulses. These patients may have been extensively investigated for joint disease or lumbar nerve root irritation even though their history is 'typical' of claudication. Most often, there is proximal aorto-iliac disease with collaterals through the pelvis, sufficient to produce adequate or even normal pulses at rest. In patients who complain of symptoms only on exercise, it is useful to examine the leg following an exercise challenge. The Strandness protocol of treadmill testing at a speed of 3 km/h and 10% slope gives an objective assessment of maximal walking distance and is helpful in differentiating claudication from pain because of non-ischaemic causes. This can also be done quite simply by asking the patient to walk up and down the corridors of the outpatient clinic or on a treadmill if available. The patient returns to the couch so that the pulses can be examined immediately after exercising for 1 minute. More importantly, the post-exercise ABI is measured and a drop in ABI of >20% from baseline and/or drop in ankle pressure >30 mmHg is considered significant.[30] In moderate to severe PAD, a sustained drop in post-exercise ABI is noted, which persists for the observation period of 10–15 minutes.

NON-INVASIVE HAEMODYNAMIC TESTS

ANKLE–BRACHIAL INDEX AND ANKLE PRESSURE MEASUREMENT

The perfusion pressure at the ankle can be measured using a tourniquet and insonating the pedal arteries with a Doppler ultrasound. The patient should be rested for more than 5 minutes, lying supine, and a standard blood pressure tourniquet applied just above the ankle, with the tourniquet being 50% wider than the limb diameter. The tourniquet cuff is inflated above the systolic pressure when the pedal Doppler signal should disappear. On gradually lowering the cuff pressure, the Doppler signal reappears at the ankle systolic pressure (Fig. 2.5). The probe should be held at a 30–60-degree angle to the vessel to achieve the optimal signal. The systolic blood pressure is then taken from the brachial artery in the same way and the ABI calculated as the ratio of the ankle to the brachial systolic pressures. Blood pressures should be assessed on both arms at the patient's first visit as 3–5% of PAD patients may also have supra-aortic occlusive disease. The higher of the two brachial blood pressures should be used as the reference for calculating ABI.

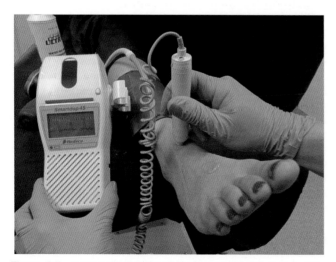

Figure 2.5 Hand-held Doppler detecting an arterial signal at the ankle. Assessment of the waveform and measurement of the ankle-brachial index (ABI).

An ABI of <0.9 confirms the presence of arterial disease. An ABI of <0.4 is often associated with CLTI.[5]

An ankle pressure of 50 mmHg is required for ulcer healing in patients without diabetes and a higher pressure of 80 mmHg is generally required in patients with diabetes. Falsely elevated ankle pressures may be present if the calf arteries are rigid because of calcification in diabetes and chronic kidney disease. Ankle pressures on their own failed to identify 42% of CLTI in one study.[31] Very high or incompressible ankle pressures (systolic >200 mmHg or ABI >1.4) should always raise suspicion of a false result. In such cases, measurement of TPs (see later) will reveal a pressure more reflective of foot perfusion as the small digital arteries are less frequently affected by medial calcification. Alternatively, if TP measurement is not possible, the pedal Doppler signal should be assessed for normal triphasic or biphasic waveforms (see later, Waveform assessment). A combination of monophasic doppler signals caused by proximal disease and APs above brachial pressures is highly suggestive of a falsely high reading because of vascular calcification.

ABI is recommended as the first-line non-invasive haemodynamic test in all patients suspected to have CLTI. It is particularly important in diabetic 'neuropathic' ulcers or infection involving the toes or feet, where missed proximal arterial disease may lead to avoidable amputation. The ABI is also useful in elderly patients referred with foot symptoms that do not appear to be vascular in aetiology and in these instances, a normal measurement is reassuring.

TOE PRESSURES

TP measurements may be useful when the calf arteries are incompressible or when severe distal arterial disease is suspected in the foot, that is, in cases with high ABI but absent or equivocal foot pulses, or non-healing toe or forefoot ulcers.

A small toe cuff should be used and placed around the proximal phalanx of the great or second toe with a photoelectric cell on the toe distally[32] (Fig. 2.6).

TP is most commonly measured using photoplethysmography or continuous-wave Doppler techniques to detect the disappearance and reappearance of the pulse as the cuff is inflated and deflated. Laser Doppler, which utilises the Doppler shift phenomenon of reflected light from moving blood cells to measure microcirculatory blood perfusion, is an alternative technique for TP assessment. A warm room is essential to avoid vasospasm and most often the feet need a 15- to 20-minute warm-up period. TP are expressed as an absolute value in mmHg and also as a ratio to brachial artery pressure referred to as toe–brachial index (TBI).

TP is normally 20–40 mmHg less than the ankle pressures, which may be caused by the sensitivity of the measurement technique. The International Working Group for the Diabetic Foot recommendations state that, in a patient with PAD and a DFU that a TP <30 mmHg (or an AP <50 mmHg), there is unlikely to be adequate foot perfusion for ulcer healing to occur and thus there is an increased risk of amputation without revascularisation. This is also consistent with Grade 3 (severe) ischaemia in WIfI.[31] In general, superficial foot ulcers are more likely to heal with TP greater than 40 mmHg; the higher the TP, the more confident one can be that healing will occur. A normal TBI ranges from 0.75 to 0.9.

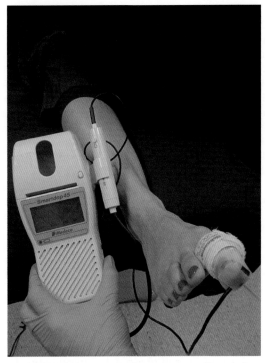

Figure 2.6   Measurement of toe pressure with waveform.

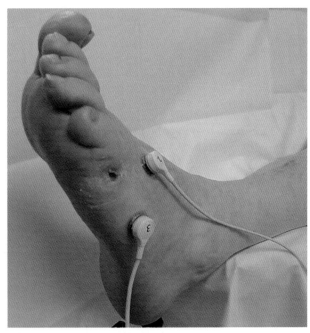

Figure 2.7   Measurement of transcutaneous oxygen pressure.

WAVEFORM ASSESSMENT

The use of Doppler waveforms with hand-held continuous-wave Doppler devices, still has an important role in the investigation of PAD. The elasticity in normal arteries gives a characteristic triphasic waveform (see Figs. 2.5 and 2.6). The blood pressure may be reduced distal to a stenosis and consequently, the resistance in the peripheral vascular bed is reduced, changing the shape of this waveform. Distal to a moderate stenosis (50% diameter reduction), the waveform is usually biphasic, and with a >70% stenosis, the distal waveform generally becomes monophasic.[33] Waveform shape can be affected by distal disease, dilatation of arteries, multisegment disease, complete occlusion of an artery and also ambient temperature.

TRANSCUTANEOUS OXIMETRY

This technique measures the partial pressure of oxygen diffusing through the surface of the skin as an indirect measure for oxygen tension in the underlying tissue (Fig. 2.7). It was hoped that $TcPO_2$ measurements of calf skin would help determine the likelihood of healing a below knee amputation wound. Unfortunately, $TcPO_2$ is unreliable for this purpose as the changes in the proximal skin perfusion after amputation of the limb cannot be predicted. A $TcPO_2$ value of <25–30 mmHg is defined as the threshold for CLTI and <10 mmHg significantly increases the risk of major amputation. A recent systematic review suggested that $TcPO_2$ ≥25 mmHg is a favourable indicator for ulcer healing and combined with a TP ≥45 mmHg, a predictor of a positive outcome.[34]

Two algorithms for investigating patients with (a) suspected claudication and (b) suspected CLTI are given in Fig. 2.8a, b.

ANATOMICAL IMAGING FOR CHRONIC LOWER LIMB ISCHAEMIA

A methodical approach to vascular anatomical imaging is important in all patients presenting with CLTI and also in patients with claudication where intervention is contemplated. This allows the clinician to assess the extent and severity of arterial disease and carefully plan a revascularisation strategy taking into account the endovascular and/or open surgical options available. The Global Limb Anatomic Staging System (GLASS) is a novel concept developed by the Global Vascular Guidelines for CLTI in an attempt to introduce a unified and standardised strategy to classify the anatomical pattern of arterial disease, which in turn serves as a robust foundation for EBR.[5]

History and clinical examination often help the clinician make decisions regarding the choice of imaging modality. A weak or absent femoral pulse may suggest proximal iliac disease, which is often better visualised with a CT angiogram (CTA) than DUS. However, a CTA may not be the ideal imaging modality in patients with diabetes or renal failure where information of the tibial vasculature is sought. Extensive vessel wall calcification in these scenarios may justify a diagnostic angiogram for a detailed mapping of the tibial/foot vasculature for pre-operative planning and this can be performed with a smaller volume of contrast than a CTA in patients with renal impairment. Table 2.9 compares the advantages and limitations of the various imaging modalities available to the vascular surgeon. In accordance with the GLASS principles in PAD staging, the flow chart details the recommended anatomical imaging algorithm in patients with chronic lower limb ischaemia who are being considered for intervention (Fig. 2.9).

DUPLEX ULTRASOUND

DUS has emerged as the most important first-line non-invasive anatomical imaging modality to assess severity of

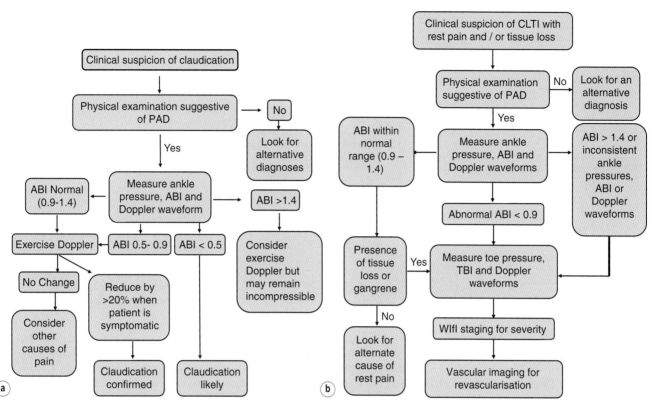

Figure 2.8 **(a)** Algorithm for investigating patients with suspected claudication. **(b)** Algorithm for investigating patients with suspected chronic limb-threatening ischaemia (based on [5]). *ABI*, Ankle–brachial index; *CLTI*, chronic limb-threatening ischaemia; *PAD*, peripheral arterial disease; *TBI*, toe–brachial index; *WIfI*, Wound, ischaemia, and foot infection.

Table 2.9 Comparison of the different imaging modalities for chronic lower limb ischaemia[5]

Modality	Advantages	Limitations
Duplex Ultrasound	Non-invasive Inexpensive Widely available Useful to monitor success of intervention	Operator dependent Poor visualisation of iliac arteries because of body habitus, bowel gas Poor visualisation in calcified vessels Validity in CLTI patients is uncertain as most DUS studies performed on mixed populations
CT Angiography	Non-invasive Patient compliance Imaging of stented arteries Can be used in most patients where MRA is contraindicated Rapidly images aorta to foot	Poor visualisation in calcified arteries Post-contrast acute kidney injury Radiation exposure Uncertain value for assessing below knee disease in CLTI
MR Angiography	Non-invasive Eliminates radiation exposure Not limited by arterial calcification Entire arterial tree can be presented as a maximum intensity projection (MIP)	Contra-indicated in patients with pacemakers, defibrillators, cerebral clips Overestimates arterial stenosis Artefact effect by metal can mimic vessel occlusion (e.g., stents) Venous contamination of arterial phase imaging
Digital Subtraction Angiography	Complete map of the lower limb arteries Images are easily displayed and interpreted Selective catheterisation allows enhanced images with reduced contrast volume Intervention can be performed at time of imaging	Ionising radiation Post-contrast acute kidney injury Catheterisation-related complications

CLTI, Chronic limb-threatening ischaemia; *DUS*, duplex ultrasound; *MRA*, magnetic resonance angiography
Conte MS, Bradbury AW, Kolh P, White JV, Dick F, Fitridge R, et al. Global Vascular Guidelines on the Management of Chronic Limb-Threatening Ischemia. Eur J Vasc Endovasc Surg. 2019;58(1S):S1-S109 e33.

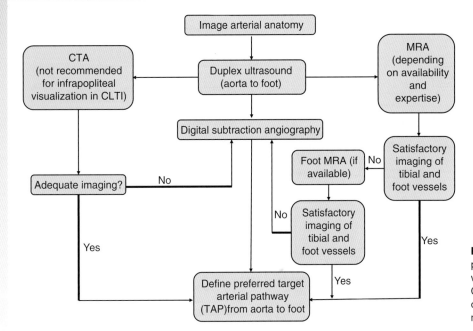

Figure 2.9 Anatomical imaging algorithm in patients with chronic lower limb ischaemia in whom revascularisation is considered.[5] *CLTI*, Chronic limb-threatening ischaemia; *CTA*, computed tomographic angiography; *MRA*, magnetic resonance angiography.

PAD. DUS allows the visualisation of arteries in real time using grey-scale (B-mode) imaging and detailed haemodynamic evaluation of blood flow by colour-flow Doppler mapping, power Doppler and spectral Doppler. DUS is a non-invasive and cost-effective imaging modality, which has also resulted in its widespread use in serial imaging to assess disease progression and surveillance following intervention. It is an operator-dependent examination and reliability of DUS is dependent on the experience and knowledge of the operator and interpreting clinician.

Current recommendations are to consider DUS imaging as the first-line vascular imaging modality in patient with suspected CLTI.[5,35]

Lower extremity scanning requires a variety of transducers. Lower frequency transducers (2 MHz or 3 MHz) are suitable for deeper structures, such as the abdominal aorta and iliac arteries and a higher frequency (5 MHz or 7 MHz) is required for the infra-inguinal segments. In general, the higher the probe frequency, the greater will be the resolution and hence the highest frequency transducer that provides satisfactory depth of view should be used for the examination.

DUS of lower limb arterial disease is dependent on high quality B-mode, which visualises echogenic plaques and the anatomy of the artery/disease. Colour-flow Doppler and spectral Doppler are two types of ultrasound displays, which are often used simultaneously during arterial imaging. Colour flow Doppler depicts both direction of blood flow and mean velocity and is used to visualise blood flow by colour encoding Doppler information and displaying the colour through the colour box positioned within the grey-scale image. The colour box is subdivided into small sample regions or colour pixels and represents the mean velocity within that region. By convention, flow towards the transducer is depicted in red and flow away from the transducer in blue. The display of blood flow includes different shades of blue and red to represent the flow velocity and this colour allocation is dependent on the colour map provided by the manufacturer. Colour filling will only occur where

blood is moving and can therefore be used to enhance the grey-scale image by identifying 'soft' echolucent atheroma or thrombus as an area of absent colour filling. Colour flow allows identification of increased blood velocity by a change in colour within the lumen of the artery. Severe stenosis can be seen as grey echoes reducing the diameter of the colour filling and a 'mosaic' of colours indicates increased velocity and turbulence. However, colour flow Doppler does not provide a quantitative means of determining the severity of a stenosis other than by direct luminal diameter or area loss measurement (Fig. 2.10a, b).

Accurate quantification of the severity of the stenosis requires the use of spectral Doppler. In this form of ultrasound image display, flow velocities are graphically represented on the Y axis against time on the X axis. Continuous wave Doppler and pulse wave Doppler are two types of spectral Doppler with some differences. As the name implies, in continuous wave Doppler, the transducer is emitting and receiving ultrasound waves continuously and hence can measure velocities along an entire line of interrogation. For the same reason, it can detect very high velocity flow although it cannot pinpoint where along the line this arises from. In contrast, in pulse wave Doppler, the transducer emits a pulsed ultrasound signal, which is pinpointed to a specific depth by the sampling box. The change of frequency (Doppler shift) in the reflected signal is determined by the transmitted frequency, angle of insonation and the velocity of blood flow. Modern DUS machines allow automated calculation of blood velocity but the accuracy of this relies heavily on the correct positioning of the pulsed-wave Doppler box and angling of the central cursor to the axis of blood flow. The peak systolic velocity is measured in the normal artery proximal to a stenosis and then in the stenosis identified by colour flow. The shape of the Doppler waveform (triphasic, biphasic or monophasic), degree of spectral broadening (range of velocity profiles within the wave spectra secondary to turbulence) and change in peak systolic velocity relative to the upstream normal artery all help to determine the severity

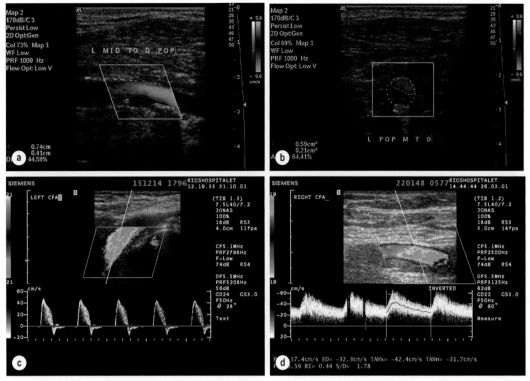

Figure 2.10 **(a)** A longitudinal colour Doppler image of a mid to distal left popliteal artery stenosis with a diameter reduction of approximately 50%. **(b)** The area reduction of the same lesion on axial imaging is 60–70%. **(c, d)** Doppler waveforms from common femoral artery, just proximal to stenosis **(c)** and distal to stenosis **(d)**. Notice how the waveform **(c)**, is triphasic with steep acceleration phase signalling high resistance and monophasic **(d)** and dampened distal to the stenosis, where the stenosis has caused a pressure drop with reduction in resistance.

Table 2.10 Diagnostic criteria for peripheral artery diameter reduction

Degree of stenosis	Velocity ratio (Vr)	Spectral waveform of artery
Normal	<1.5	Triphasic
30–49%	1.5–2	Triphasic or multiphasic waveform
50–74%	2–4	Biphasic, spectral broadening
≥75%	>4	Damped, monophasic
Occlusion		No flow in occluded segment, proximal and distal collaterals help estimate occlusion length. Damped, monophasic waveform distally

PSV=peak systolic velocity; Vr=PSV ratio across a stenosis
Adapted from: Cossman DV, Ellison JE, Wagner WH, Carroll RM, Treiman RL, Foran RF, et al. Comparison of contrast arteriography to arterial mapping with color-flow duplex imaging in the lower extremities. J Vasc Surg. 1989;10(5):522-8; discussion 8-9; and Kim ES, Sharma AM, Scissons R, Dawson D, Eberhardt RT, Gerhard-Herman M, et al. Interpretation of peripheral arterial and venous Doppler waveforms: A consensus statement from the Society for Vascular Medicine and Society for Vascular Ultrasound. Vasc Med. 2020;25(5):484-506.

of a given stenosis (Table 2.10).[36,37] In the peripheral arteries, a twofold increase in the peak systolic velocity generally indicates a 50% narrowing of the artery, while a fourfold increase in velocity ratio with monophasic waveform indicates a high-grade stenosis. Distal to a stenosis, the Doppler waveform changes shape because of dampening with reduction in peak systolic velocity and a slower acceleration time (time from end diastole to peak systole; Fig. 2.10c, d).

Differentiating complete occlusion from high-grade stenosis with trickle flow within an artery may be difficult and depends heavily on the experience of the sonographer. The shape of the Doppler waveform proximally and distally, colour-flow images and the presence of collaterals all contribute to separating these two lesions. Difficulties can arise with deep or tortuous arteries, where signal return is reduced and optimum angles of insonation are difficult to obtain. Multiple stenoses along the length of an artery reduce the accuracy of flow velocity measurements in the assessment of more distal stenoses. Power Doppler imaging, which is dependent on the amplitude of Doppler signals and independent of flow velocity and direction, is a sensitive imaging technique that can help in such situations to differentiate arterial occlusion from high-grade stenosis. The sonographer must use valuable experience and knowledge of more subtle changes in blood velocity to determine the severity of a given stenosis when there are tandem or multiple stenoses.

ASSESSMENT OF SUPRA-INGUINAL ARTERIES

This can be achieved by direct assessment of the iliac arteries although this poses challenges because of respiratory movements, the depth of arteries, arterial tortuosity, overlying bowel gas and arterial wall calcification obscuring the vessel lumen. Changing the plane of insonation may often help find an acoustic window through obscuring and distracting anatomy and pathology. It is critical that sonographers communicate difficulties encountered during scanning to the referring physician.

Changes in the Doppler waveform proximal and distal to an inadequately viewed segment often give an indication of the extent of disease and the need for further investigation. Evaluation of the Doppler waveform in the common femoral artery is an indirect method for assessing the iliac arteries. If it is triphasic, the likelihood of a severe obstructive lesion in the aorto-iliac segment is very low.[38]

In comparison to catheter angiography, aorto-iliac DUS has a sensitivity of 82% and specificity of 92% in detecting a >50% stenosis using the criteria of peak systolic velocity ratio >2.[39]

ASSESSMENT OF FEMORO-POPLITEAL AND TIBIAL ARTERIES

DUS assessment of the superficial femoral artery can give accurate information regarding flow and stenoses although insonation at the level of the adductor canal may pose technical challenges. The crural arteries can be more difficult, especially when there is severe proximal disease. In large calves, the depth of insonation attenuates the signal return, making it difficult to visualise the proximal crural arteries. Accuracy can be improved by using a low-frequency transducer such as a curved-array abdominal probe, which allows for deeper penetration albeit at the cost of reduced image quality. Alternatively, power Doppler, which is more sensitive to slow flow, can help detect the optimum tibial artery for revascularisation.

In experienced hands, DUS is accurate at identifying >50% stenosis of the FP segment with a sensitivity of 80% and specificity of 96%. However, in the infra-genicular arteries, this reduces to 83% sensitivity and 84% specificity.[40]

Most vascular centres use DUS as the first-line imaging modality to investigate PAD because of availability, lower cost and lack of risks associated with the study. However, relying solely on DUS before lower limb revascularisation risks underestimation of the severity and number of sites of vascular disease, particularly difficult-to-reach anatomical areas such as the iliac and proximal infra-genicular crural arteries. Alternative imaging modalities such as CTA or MR angiogram and digital subtraction angiography (DSA) may address these limitations.

COMPUTED TOMOGRAPHIC ANGIOGRAPHY

Multislice (multidetector) CT enables scanning a large tissue volume with multiple separate slices simultaneously. The slices can be reconstructed in any plane (multiplanar and curved planar reconstructions). It allows acquisition of high-resolution images of less than 0.6 mm^3 voxel (volume element) size. Multidetector CT scanners with 256 slice capabilities are currently in routine use. CTA enables visualisation of vessels by administration of intravenous contrast and the acquisition speed of spiral CT helps chase the bolus of contrast as it passes through the tissue imaged.

Complex reconstructions can be performed, with the subtraction of bone or other detail that may obscure the arteries. As the Hounsfield unit of arterial wall calcification is close to that of arterial blood opacified by contrast, care must be taken to ensure that part of the normal vessel has not been erroneously subtracted when using automated subtraction algorithms. This also applies to vessels that lie in close proximity to bone, for example the tibial arteries, which may be subtracted if the bones are automatically

removed. The radiologist must therefore review the source data in the plane of greatest spatial resolution as well as the reconstructions. Calcification within the lower limb arterial tree has limited the use of CTA for the assessment of chronic lower limb ischaemia, particularly in the calf arteries in patients with diabetes and renal failure.

Maximum intensity projection (MIP) images can be constructed by selecting the highest-density voxel along a given plane or planes (Fig. 2.11a). This produces a two-dimensional (2D) angiography-like image that can be rotated to allow multiple viewing angles. A variety of three-dimensional (3D) volume-rendered reconstructions can also be displayed in colour, with preset colour maps to display the anatomy (Fig. 2.11b, c). These images are useful for surgical and endovascular planning – reproducing accurate vessel diameters, preselection of optimal catheter configurations ahead of interventions or planning the angulation of tube positions for fluoroscopy and DSA. Metanalysis comparing the accuracy of CTA with DSA to assess extent of arterial disease in patients with claudication showed a sensitivity and specificity of 95% and 96% in the aorto-iliac segment, 97% and 94% in the FP segment and 95% and 91% in tibial vessels, respectively.[41]

CONTRAST MEDIA AND NEPHROTOXICITY

Iodinated intravascular contrast media, whether for use in catheter angiographic procedures or CT examinations poses risks of nephrotoxicity. Post-contrast acute kidney injury (PC-AKI) or contrast-associated AKI (CA-AKI) can be defined as an increase in serum creatinine of ≥0.3 mg/dL (26.5 μmol/L) or of ≥1.5–1.9 times baseline in the 48–72 hours following contrast media administration.[42] A substantial proportion of AKI that occurs after contrast utilisation is not attributable to the contrast or the aetiology of the AKI is likely multifactorial. Contrast-induced AKI (CI-AKI) refers to the cases of AKI that can be causally linked to the contrast utilisation. Impaired renal function is the primary patient-related risk factor for PC-AKI.[43]

Methods to reduce the incidence of PC-AKI include the use of alternative imaging techniques, minimising contrast volume, pharmacological manipulation by stopping nephrotoxic drugs and intravenous volume expansion.[44] Prehydration remains the cornerstone in the management strategy to prevent PC-AKI although evidence to support a particular hydration strategy, fluid composition (sodium bicarbonate vs. sodium chloride) is lacking.[45–47] Current guidelines recommend pre- and post-contrast hydration for patients with estimated glomerular filtration rate (eGFR) <30 mL/min who are not undergoing dialysis. Pre- and post-hydration should also be considered in individual high-risk patients (e.g., in intensive care unit, recent AKI) with an eGFR of <45 mL/min. There appears to be no difference in the risk of AKI associated with low- or iso-osmolar contrast.

To reduce the risk of PC-AKI in at-risk patients, the European Society of Urogenital Radiology Contrast Media Safety Committee guidelines[48] recommend:

1) Measuring eGFR in at-risk patients or all patients
2) Consider alternative imaging to avoid contrast exposure
3) Preventative hydration for patients with eGFR <30 mL/min/1.73 m^2– intravenous normal saline (0.9%), 1 mL/kg/h for 3–4 hours before and 4–6 hours after contrast

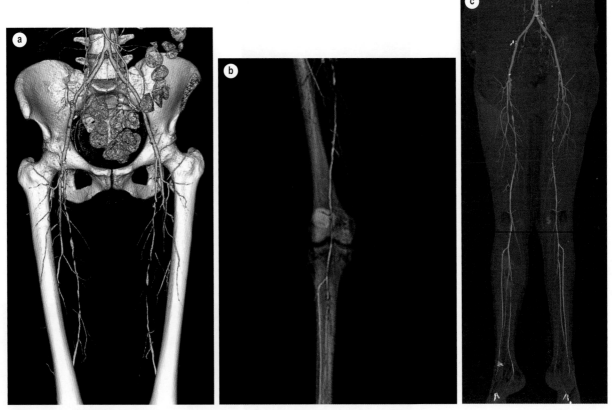

Figure 2.11   Volume-rendered three-dimensional computed tomographic angiography (CTA) of the **(a)** aorta to femoral and **(b)** femoro-popliteal segment in a young patient with diabetes and renal failure presenting with chronic bilateral lower limb ischaemia. Bilateral multifocal high-grade stenosis of both the superficial femoral arteries is noted. **(c)** Composite stitched coronal maximum intensity projection (MIP) of bilateral lower limb CTA from aorta to ankle.

medium or sodium bicarbonate (1.4%): 3 mL/kg/h for 1 hour before and 1 mL/kg/h for 4–6 hours after contrast medium

4) Use low or iso-osmolar contrast media and the lowest dose possible

5) Discontinue metformin from the time of contrast administration if eGFR <30 or receiving first pass renal exposure of contrast (contrast medium reaches the renal arteries in an undiluted form as in contrast injection into the left heart, descending or suprarenal aorta) or in AKI. Check eGFR at 48 hours and restart metformin if eGFR is stable.

6) For direct intra-arterial injection, it is advisable to keep the ratio of contrast dose (in grams of iodine) / absolute eGFR<1.

MAGNETIC RESONANCE ANGIOGRAPHY

The basic principles of MRI rely on a large external magnetic field, which magnetises the tissue protons to align parallel to the field, a magnetic field gradient, which helps alter the direction of the external magnetic field and a radiofrequency field provided by resonant coils placed in close proximity to the area of interest. The resonant frequency of the protons is tapped into by the receivers to process the final image by a complex mathematical algorithm. The contrast seen in MRI depends on the characteristics of the imaging object. They are referred to as *T1-weighted* and *T2-weighted images*. MR angiography (MRA) and MR venography (MRV) are dependent on T1-weighted images and fat, methaemoglobin, flow and contrast agents will appear bright. T2-weighted images display fluids as bright and are not used for MRA. There are several MR techniques for the assessment of vessels and vessel patency, all of which continue to evolve at a rapid pace. Modern MR scanners are capable of high-quality angiographic images without exposing the patient to radiation. In addition, MRA avoids the need for image manipulation to remove overlying bone and calcification from the arterial wall. MRA can be performed by contrast-enhanced techniques (CE-MRA) and also non-contrast techniques such as time of flight (TOF) MRA and phase contrast MRI. The non-contrast techniques utilise the ability to differentiate signal characteristics of flowing blood from static tissues for image acquisition. TOF MRA poses significant challenges with inadequate signals from deeper vessels with poor image resolution, flow-related artefacts especially in areas of stenosis, and prolonged scan time. Phase contrast MRI, although has >90% sensitivity and specificity for detection of stenosis compared to DSA, once again is limited by prolonged image acquisition time.[49]

In recent years, these two techniques have been supplanted by 3D CE-MRA. CE-MRA provides a non-invasive, 3D luminal assessment of vessels without the risk of iodine-based contrast agents and ionising radiation and it has now become the preferred first-line imaging technique in some centres for the investigation of PAD (Fig. 2.12). However, the widespread adoption of MRA for arterial imaging has

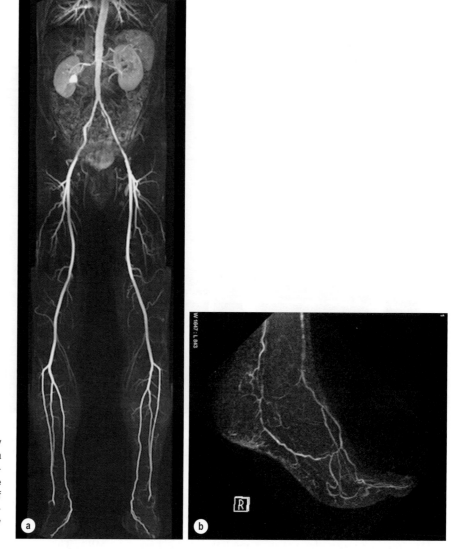

Figure 2.12 **(a)** Coronal maximum intensity projection (MIP) of contrast-enhanced aorta and lower limb magnetic resonance angiography (MRA) at 3 T using a stepping, bolus chase technique and image fusion. **(b)** Sagittal MIP of optimal arterial filling during dynamic contrast-enhanced MRA of the foot. (Images provided by Dr A. Holden, Auckland City Hospital.)

been hampered by the limitations in local expertise to generate high resolution images. In addition, safety concerns related to gadolinium-based CE-MRA and nephrogenic systemic fibrosis (see later) over the last decade has further undermined interest in CE-MRA.

In a meta-analysis of 32 studies including 1022 patients, CE-MRA was noted to have high accuracy for identifying or excluding clinically relevant arterial stenoses or occlusions in adults with PAD symptoms.[50]

CONTRAINDICATIONS TO MAGNETIC RESONANCE ANGIOGRAPHY

Contraindications include the presence of a pacemaker or certain types of metallic prosthetic cardiac valve implants, intracranial aneurysm clips, cochlear implants or metallic intraocular foreign bodies. Up to 5% of patients may be claustrophobic in the MR bore, which may be overcome using open bore systems or by using psychotherapy relaxation techniques. Occasionally, sedation or rarely, a general anaesthetic may be required.

Nephrogenic systemic fibrosis (NSF) is a phenomenon of skin, muscle and organ fibrosis that occurs in a setting of severe chronic or acute renal failure following exposure to gadolinium-based contrast agents (GBCA), which are widely used in MRI. Clinical features include skin manifestations such as skin plaques, joint contractures, cobblestone skin appearance, marked induration or peau d'orange, skin puckering and dermal papules to multi-organ involvement, which is associated with an increased mortality.

Impaired gadolinium clearance by the kidney leads to tissue accumulation of gadolinium and the toxicity is primarily caused by competitive binding of gadolinium ion (Gd^{3+}) with components of the extracellular matrix and these deposit in tissues such as skin, kidney, liver and brain.

The worldwide incidence of NSF has significantly reduced since the United States Food and Drug Administration and European Medicine Agency alert in 2007. Only restoration of renal function by renal transplantation and recovery of acute renal failure has been shown to slow or arrest the progression of NSF.[51] Hence there is a greater emphasis on preventative measures. General recommendations for avoidance of NSF in patients with AKI, those with GFR <30 mL/min, and those on dialysis, are to avoid gadolinium administration.

DIGITAL SUBTRACTION ANGIOGRAPHY

DSA is often referred to as the gold standard in the investigation of PAD because of superior image resolution and also the ability to perform both diagnostic and interventional procedures at the same sitting. However, as an invasive procedure placing patients at some risk of harm, this has now given way to non-invasive imaging modalities and is no longer recommended for routine diagnostic imaging of PAD. Diagnostic angiography is also expensive, requires a day-case bed, ties up numerous members of angiography suite staff and negatively impacts on time available for planned therapeutic interventions. Modern practice has thus changed and the use of DSA is reserved for situations where there is an intention to proceed to endovascular intervention or before open reconstructive surgery, or where non-invasive imaging has not provided adequate diagnostic accuracy.

TECHNIQUE OF DIGITAL SUBTRACTION ANGIOGRAPHY

An initial standard X-ray exposure is captured and digitised, and this is referred to as the *mask image*. This mask image is subsequently subtracted from subsequent images known as the *live images*. This allows for the display of contrast opacifying the arterial lumen without the visual distraction of adjoining anatomy.

There are various applications of DSA that facilitate optimal visualisation and improve procedural success. Road mapping is one such technique where an unsubtracted fluoroscopic image is superimposed over a live fluoroscopic image. This enables the observation and manipulation of guide wires and catheters in real time through a virtual image of the vessel. Image overlay or fade is superimposition of a live fluoroscopic image on a reference image and this again provides a virtual image of the vessel during intervention.

Single injection multi-linear arteriography or bolus chase angiography permits visualisation of entire lower limb arteries in sequence from a single injection of contrast agent. Image acquisition occurs during a continuous longitudinal movement of the image intensifier. As this technique takes a considerably longer time, patient movement can affect the image quality. In addition, asymmetrical disease severity in the lower limbs can limit its use.

Cone-beam CT is an advanced application where a 3D image data set is created by rotating the C-arm around the patient and this allows for CT images during interventions, 3D angiography and 3D road mapping.

Pre-procedural planning is critical to the outcome of any intervention. The access vessel and puncture site are chosen based on a likely low risk of complications and reasonable proximity to the site of intervention (frequently the common femoral artery). Standard angiographic access is by the modified Seldinger technique. Arterial puncture under ultrasound guidance is widely accepted as safe practice and an 18-gauge puncture needle is used. Once pulsatile backbleeding is confirmed through the needle, a floppy tip guidewire, usually a J-tip, is advanced via the central lumen of the needle into the artery lumen under fluoroscopic guidance. A sheath is advanced over this wire or alternatively a catheter may be used 'bareback'. Intraluminal position of sheath/catheter is checked by assessing back bleeding and a small trial injection of contrast. A flush catheter with multiple side holes allows for even distribution of contrast in diagnostic studies. Injection of contrast can be performed by power injector or by manual injection and both have distinct advantages. Large high-flow arteries such as the aorto-iliac segments may require a higher pressure to dispense the contrast for satisfactory images. A micropuncture set with a 21-gauge needle may be used in scarred groins, pulseless arteries, calcified arteries or for antegrade access to the femoral artery. With care, diagnostic angiography is safe with 4-Fr catheters in most patients. Adequate analgesia is essential to ensure a pain-free and cooperative patient who will comply with the instructions to avoid movement artefacts, especially during imaging of the crural (tibial) arteries and plantar arch.

CARBON DIOXIDE ANGIOGRAPHY

Carbon dioxide (CO_2) creates a negative radiographic contrast image because of its reduced radiodensity. With modern advances in digital subtraction technology, it is now possible to achieve good quality angiographic images. The use of CO_2 is not associated with nephrotoxicity and allergic reactions and hence valuable in patients with renal impairment requiring endovascular intervention and patients with contrast allergy. Complications related to CO_2 angiography are extremely rare during investigations of the lower limb arteries. However, caution needs to be exercised in the use of CO_2 in situations where there is a risk of gas trapping and ischaemia as in mesenteric imaging. CO_2 should not be used for cerebral and coronary imaging.

RISKS AND LIMITATIONS

The risks of conventional DSA are related to contrast media or technique.

Contrast-related risks and limitations

- Allergic: Allergic reactions are not dose related and probably result from mast cell degranulation. The incidence of severe anaphylactic reactions caused by ionic contrast media is 0.01–0.02%, but non-ionic low-osmolar iodinated contrast agents are 5–10 times safer than their predecessors. Patients with severe asthma or hay fever are at increased risk of an allergic reaction, which may be severe. Steroid prophylaxis should be considered. Patients with known contrast allergy should be imaged using alternative techniques.
- Toxic: These are dose related and manifest themselves as a metallic taste in the mouth, feelings of warmth, nausea or vomiting, cardiac arrhythmias and pulmonary oedema. They are more likely to occur in patients with severe vascular disease.
- Renal (PC-AKI – see earlier).

Technique related

- Pseudoaneurysm/haematoma: Haematoma around the puncture site is common. This can be reduced by using smaller catheters and a good manual haemostatic arterial compression technique for at least 10 minutes. Arterial closure devices are rarely indicated for diagnostic angiography although this may allow faster ambulation of patients and be useful in patients with uncorrected clotting profiles.

- Dissection: A dissection flap is usually caused by poor technique using undue force or hydrophilic guidewires or from closure devices, which may disrupt the integrity of plaques. Although small flaps are rarely a problem, larger or antegrade flaps may significantly slow blood flow or occlude the artery.
- Infection is rare with good aseptic technique.
- Arteriovenous fistula: As the femoral artery and vein are contained within the femoral sheath, they may both be punctured during arterial access when a blind puncture is performed. Where ultrasound is available, this should be used to avoid anterior wall plaques and accurately identify the common femoral artery.
- Embolisation: If atheroma lining the artery is inadvertently dislodged, it will embolise distally. This may be retrieved using suction aspiration but may need surgical embolectomy or bypass surgery.

RADIATION SAFETY

Clinicians should have a clear understanding of the risks involved with radiation exposure to the patient and staff, as well as measures to reduce radiation dose. The main source of radiation to the operator is scatter and this decreases by the inverse square of the distance from the source. In addition, fluoroscopic field size significantly affects scatter radiation. Image intensifier positioning close to the patient, beam collimation, minimising fluoroscopic screening time and number of angiographic runs, and protective personal equipment including lead shields, lead aprons, thyroid shields and eye protection, are all important strategies to limit radiation exposure.

PERFUSION ANGIOGRAPHY

This is a novel imaging technology, which allows quantification of tissue perfusion and aims to help determine if a revascularisation procedure is likely to achieve wound healing in CLTI. This requires dedicated software for post-processing on a 2D perfusion enabled angiography workstation. A time-density curve produced by the first pass of the contrast agent during DSA generates indices for inflow time, maximal contrast density and blood volume for a pre-selected area of tissue under investigation. The perfusion status is represented in a colour coded display with different colours denoting a corresponding perfusion level (Fig. 2.13). This imaging technique is early in its development and holds promise in determining the adequacy of interventions real time and allows for a targeted approach for improved outcomes in CLTI.

CLASSIFICATION OF AORTO-ILIAC, FEMORAL, POPLITEAL AND INFRA-POPLITEAL DISEASE

Atherosclerotic arterial lesions in PAD may be focal or extensive and involve multiple segments of the lower limb arteries. Hence it is important to have a universally acceptable classification system that clearly defines the extent and complexity of these lesions for the purpose of standardised reporting and also planning intervention.

The **Trans-Atlantic Inter-Society Consensus** for the management of peripheral artery disease (TASC II) document described a simplified nomenclature to classify lesions in the aorto-iliac, FP and the infra-popliteal (IP) arterial regions.[8] The TASC classification reflects the location and extent of arterial lesions and also gives recommendations for the revascularisation options most suited, taking into consideration the risks of a specific intervention and its durability. The TASC classification of aorto-iliac lesions in used in clinical practice (Fig. 2.14). Progressively more complex aorto-iliac lesions are being treated by endovascular approaches in contemporary practice.

Global Anatomic Staging System (GLASS) is a novel approach to anatomical staging of lower limb arterial disease.[5] This was designed as a refinement to the existing staging systems, which are focused on the severity of an individual lesion or arterial segment. However, the pattern of disease in CLTI is usually multi-segmental with distal vessel involvement; and GLASS offers a holistic approach to revascularisation taking into consideration the anatomic complexity of the entire lower limb vasculature. The current TASC aorto-iliac staging system (see Fig. 2.14), is deemed appropriate and hence the focus of GLASS is on the infra-inguinal disease. The common femoral artery and deep femoral artery

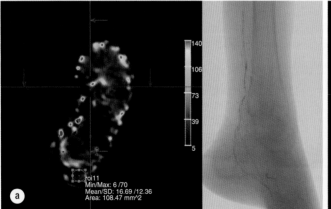
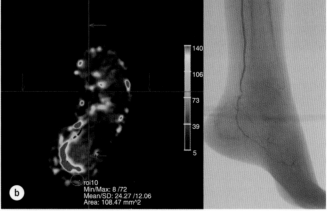

Figure 2.13   Revascularisation of the posterior tibial artery in a patient with heel ulceration. The posterior tibial artery is the only artery with direct outflow to the foot. Three-dimensional (3D) perfusion angiography pre-intervention and post-intervention show strong improvement of flow to the hindfoot after revascularisation. The scale on the right side of the images shows increasing perfusion. **(a)** 3D perfusion angiography pre-posterior tibial artery angioplasty. **(b)** 3D perfusion angiography post-posterior tibial artery angioplasty.

Type A lesions

• Unilateral or bilateral stenoses of CIA
• Unilateral or bilateral single short (≤3 cm) stenosis of EIA

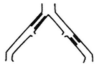

Type B lesions:

• Short (≤3cm) stenosis of infrarenal aorta
• Unilateral CIA occlusion
• Single or multiple stenosis totaling 3–10 cm involving the
  EIA not extending into the CFA
• Unilateral EIA occlusion not involving the origins of
  internal iliac or CFA

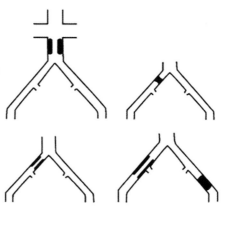

Type C lesions

• Bilateral CIA occlusions
• Bilateral EIA stenoses 3–10 cm long not extending into
  the CFA
• Unilateral EIA stenosis extending into the CFA
• Unilateral EIA occlusion that involves the origins of
  internal iliac and/or CFA
• Heavily calcified unilateral EIA occlusion with or without
  involvement of origins of internal iliac and/or CFA

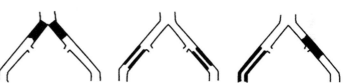

Type D lesions

• Infra-renal aortoiliac occlusion
• Diffuse disease involving the aorta and both iliac arteries
  requiring treatment
• Diffuse multiple stenoses involving the unilateral CIA,
  EIA, and CFA
• Unilateral occlusions of both CIA and EIA
• Bilateral occlusions of EIA
• Iliac stenoses in patients with AAA requiring treatment
  and not amenable to endograft placement or other
  lesions requiring open aortic or iliac surgery

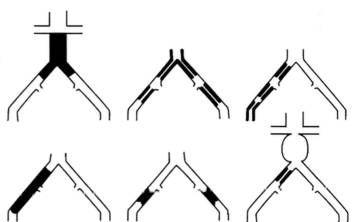

Figure 2.14 The Trans-Atlantic Inter-Society Consensus for the management of peripheral artery disease (TASC II) classification of aortoiliac lesions.[8] *AAA,* Abdominal aortic aneurysm; *CFA,* common femoral artery; *CIA,* common iliac artery; *EIA,* external iliac artery.

(Profunda femoris) are defined as inflow vessels. The Target Arterial Path (TAP) is a new concept that has been introduced, which is the anatomical route from the groin to the foot to ensure in-line flow. High-quality imaging is a prerequisite for ensuring that the appropriate crural artery is selected for TAP. However, the preferred TAP for endovascular revascularisation may not always align with the selected artery for open surgical reconstruction. The best approach

to revascularisation should be based on comparative risks and benefits in the context of patient fitness, availability of suitable venous conduit and likely long-term durability.

The GLASS stages are determined by taking into account the complexity of the multiple lesions in the FP and IP segment along the TAP traversed during intervention. The FP segment grades 0–4 (Fig. 2.15) are combined with the IP segment grades 0–4 (Fig. 2.16) to generate

FP Grade 0	Mild or no significant (<50%) disease	
FP Grade 1	• Total length SFA disease < 1/3 (< 10 cm) • May include single focal CTO (< 5 cm) as long as not flush occlusion • Popliteal artery with mild or no significant disease	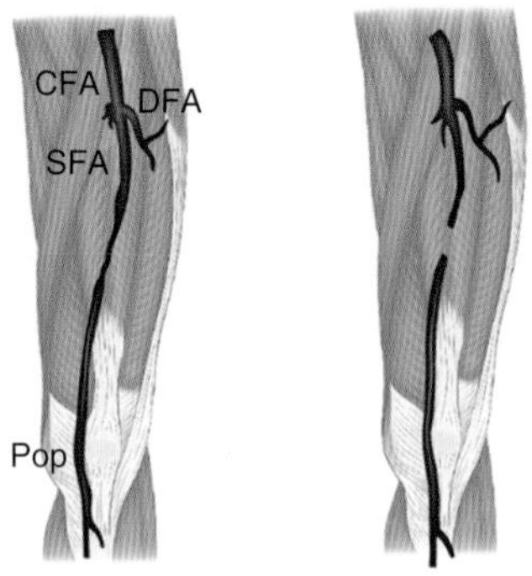
FP Grade 2	• Total length SFA disease 1/3-2/3 (10-20 cm) • May include CTO totaling < 1/3 (10 cm) but not flush occlusion • Focal popliteal artery stenosis < 2 cm, not involving trifurcation	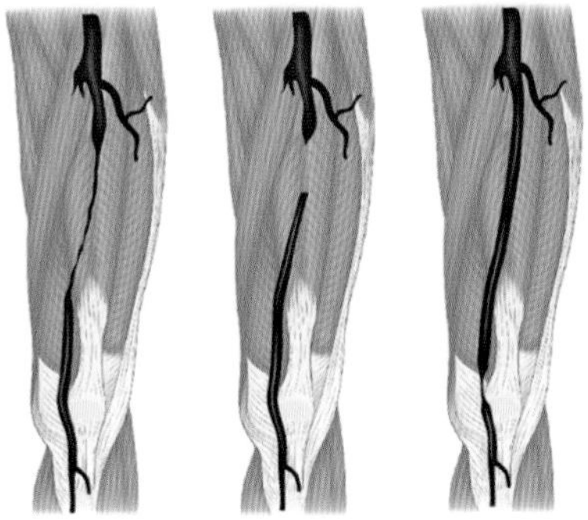
FP Grade 3	• Total length SFA disease > 2/3 (> 20 cm) length • May include any flush occlusion < 20 cm or non-flush CTO 10-20 cm long • Short popliteal stenosis 2-5 cm, not involving trifurcation	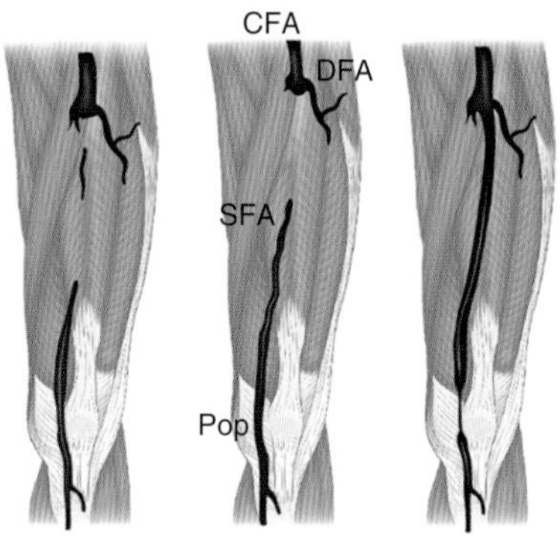
FP Grade 4	• Total length SFA occlusion > 20 cm • Popliteal disease > 5 cm or extending into trifurcation • Any popliteal CTO	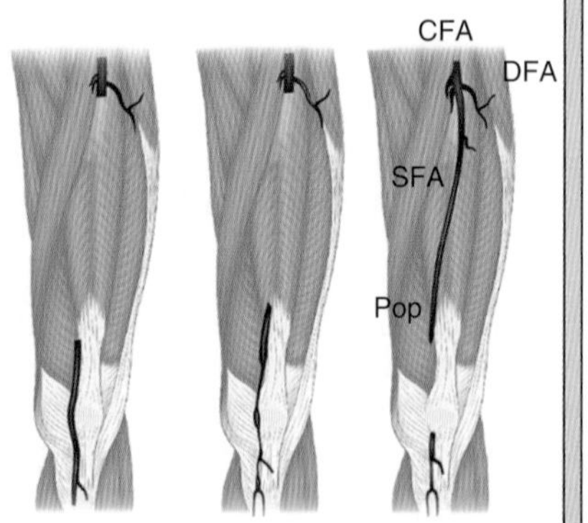

Figure 2.15 The Global Limb Anatomic Staging System (GLASS) grading of femoropopliteal lesions.[5] *CFA,* Common femoral artery; *CTO,* chronic total occlusion; *DFA,* deep femoral artery; *Pop,* popliteal artery; *SFA,* superficial femoral artery.

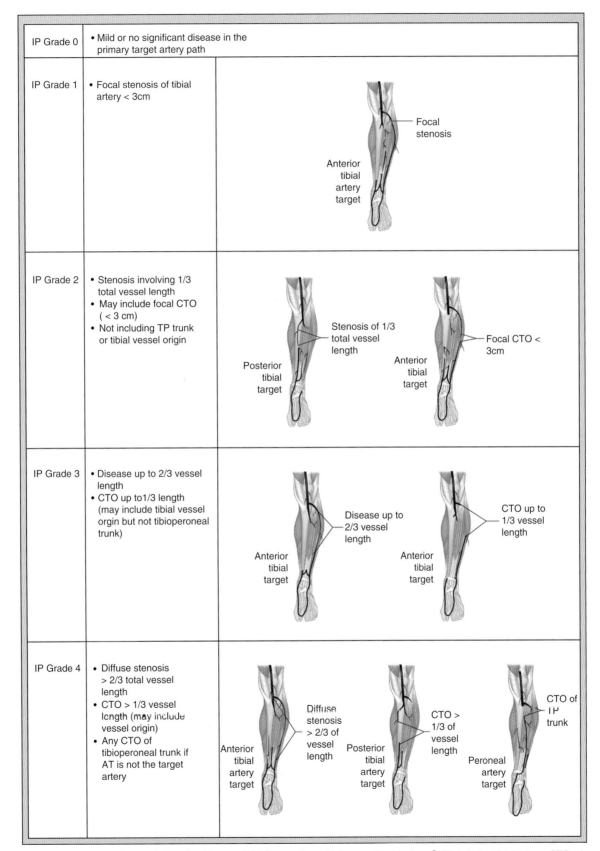

IP Grade 0	• Mild or no significant disease in the primary target artery path
IP Grade 1	• Focal stenosis of tibial artery < 3cm
IP Grade 2	• Stenosis involving 1/3 total vessel length • May include focal CTO (< 3 cm) • Not including TP trunk or tibial vessel origin
IP Grade 3	• Disease up to 2/3 vessel length • CTO up to 1/3 length (may include tibial vessel orgin but not tibioperoneal trunk)
IP Grade 4	• Diffuse stenosis > 2/3 total vessel length • CTO > 1/3 vessel length (may include vessel origin) • Any CTO of tibioperoneal trunk if AT is not the target artery

Figure 2.16   The Global Limb Anatomic Staging System (GLASS) grading of infra-popliteal lesions.[5] *AT,* Anterior tibial artery, *CTO,* chronic total occlusion, *TP,* tibio peroneal.

Table 2.11 Assignment of stage in the Global Limb Anatomic Staging System (GLASS)[5]

Femoro-popliteal grade	Infra-popliteal grade				
	0	1	2	3	4
4	III	III	III	III	III
3	II	II	II	III	III
2	I	II	II	II	III
1	I	I	II	II	III
0	NA	I	I	II	III

The femoro-popliteal (FP) grade and infra-popliteal (IP) grade are determined once the target arterial pathway (TAP) is selected. The combination of the IP grade and FP grade gives the GLASS stage, which can be used to estimate procedural outcomes.
GLASS stage I; predicted technical failure <10%, 1 year limb-based patency >70%
GLASS stage II; predicted technical failure 10–20%, 1 year limb-based patency 50–70%
GLASS stage III; predicted technical failure >20%, 1 year limb-based patency <50%
Conte MS, Bradbury AW, Kolh P, White JV, Dick F, Fitridge R, et al. Global Vascular Guidelines on the Management of Chronic Limb-Threatening Ischemia. Eur J Vasc Endovasc Surg. 2019;58(1S):S1-S109 e33.

Table 2.12 Infra-malleolar (IM)/pedal disease descriptor in Global Limb Anatomic Staging System (GLASS)[5]

P0	Target artery crosses the ankle into foot and pedal arch is intact
P1	Target artery crosses the ankle into foot and the pedal arch is severely diseased
P2	No target artery crossing ankle into the foot

Conte MS, Bradbury AW, Kolh P, White JV, Dick F, Fitridge R, et al. Global Vascular Guidelines on the Management of Chronic Limb-Threatening Ischemia. Eur J Vasc Endovasc Surg. 2019;58(1S):S1-S109 e33.

the GLASS stages I, II and III and they reflect the technical complexity of intervention from low, intermediate to high risk (Table 2.11). The interventionist can assign a higher difficulty score (by one numeric level) for the FP or IP segment for the presence of severe calcification with >50% reduction in circumference, diffuse or bulky plaques. There is also provision to assign a modifier to correlate with the presence of infra-malleolar (pedal) disease (Table 2.12). In addition, GLASS stages are also predicted to correlate with likelihood of procedural technical success and likely limb-based patency with stage 1 >70%, stage II – 50–70% and stage III <50% patency at the end of 1 year.

GLASS aims to standardise the anatomical staging for infra-inguinal endovascular intervention and will be useful for future research and trials, which can contribute to the evidence regarding revascularisation strategies in clinical practice.

Key points

- The Fontaine classification for the severity of PAD has the benefit of simplicity and is clinically useful.
- Atherosclerotic risk factors must be identified and treated in all patients with PAD.
- A careful history of exertional leg pain is essential, especially in patients with coexisting spinal problems.
- Patients with a good history of claudication and palpable pulses should be examined after exercise and an exercise ABI test should be performed.
- Rare causes of ischaemia should be considered, especially in younger patients.
- Documentation of the severity of ischaemia by Doppler pressures/waveforms is mandatory in all patients with absent or weak pulses who are complaining of leg pain, weakness or numbness.
- Further anatomical investigation of PAD is not warranted unless revascularisation is being considered.
- Chronic limb-threatening ischaemia requires urgent investigation and revascularisation to avoid limb loss because of progressive tissue necrosis and/or infection.
- Offer DUS as the first-line imaging to all people with peripheral artery disease for whom revascularisation is being considered. Consider performing CTA or MRA for patients with peripheral artery disease who need further imaging before considering revascularisation.
- Post-contrast–induced AKI remains a serious concern for all procedures requiring iodinated contrast medium. Serum creatinine or eGFR must be known and provided on all patients at risk for developing this complication and must also be checked at 48 hours post-contrast injection.
- Nephrogenic systemic fibrosis is a rare but serious condition occurring in chronic kidney disease patients receiving GBCA. Serum creatinine levels or eGFR must be known and provided on all patients referred for CE-MRA who are at risk of developing this condition (stage 3, 4 and 5 chronic kidney disease).
- CTA provides detailed angiographic imaging in peripheral artery disease but is limited in severely calcified arteries. It is particularly useful in the acute assessment of limb ischaemia where potentially embolising sources may be identified.
- DSA is invasive and is no longer recommended as a first-line imaging modality in the diagnosis of PAD. It should be limited to patients in whom therapeutic intervention is planned at the same time and when inadequate information is obtained from non-invasive investigations.
- TASC II classification of aorto-iliac segment reflects the location and extent of the arterial lesions.
- Global Limb Anatomical Staging System (GLASS) can be used to stage FP and IP arterial occlusive disease when defining the Target Arterial Pathway from groin to foot and for staging the complexity of revascularisation and likelihood of success in restoring in-line flow to the foot.

References available at http://ebooks.health.elsevier.com/

KEY REFERENCES

[5] Conte MS, Bradbury AW, Kolh P, White JV, Dick F, Fitridge R, et al. Global vascular guidelines on the management of chronic limb-threatening ischemia. Eur J Vasc Endovasc Surg 2019;58(1S):S1–109 e33.
A collaboration of major vascular societies from around the globe have produced this Global Vascular Guideline to standardise the management of PAD and improve the overall outcome of patients with chronic limb-threatening ischaemia.

[8] Norgren L, Hiatt WR, Dormandy JA, Nehler MR, Harris KA, Fowkes FG, et al. Inter-society consensus for the management of peripheral arterial disease (TASC II). Eur J Vasc Endovasc Surg 2007;33(Suppl. 1):S1–75.

A working group comprised of members from sixteen societies from around the world collaborated in producing this abbreviated document which focuses on diagnosis and management of PAD based on available evidence at the time.

[12] Mills Sr JL, Conte MS, Armstrong DG, Pomposelli FB, Schanzer A, Sidawy AN, et al. The society for vascular surgery lower extremity threatened limb classification system: risk stratification based on wound, ischemia, and foot infection (WIfI). J Vasc Surg 2014;59(1). 220-234 e1-2.

WIfI risk stratification for CLTI and the diabetic foot published by The Society for Vascular Surgery.

[31] Salaun P, Desormais I, Lapebie FX, Riviere AB, Aboyans V, Lacroix P, et al. Comparison of ankle pressure, systolic toe pressure, and transcutaneous oxygen pressure to predict major amputation after 1 year in the COPART Cohort. Angiology 2019;70(3):229–36.

A study involving 556 patients where three non-invasive haemodynamic tests were compared for their accuracy in predicting major limb amputation.

[34] Brownrigg JR, Hinchliffe RJ, Apelqvist J, Boyko EJ, Fitridge R, Mills JL, et al. Performance of prognostic markers in the prediction of wound healing or amputation among patients with foot ulcers in diabetes: a systematic review. Diabetes Metab Res Rev 2016;32(Suppl. 1):128–35.

A systematic review of the prognostic markers for wound healing and amputation in diabetes.

3 Medical treatment of chronic lower limb ischaemia

Jacqueline E. Wade | Peter A. Soden | Marc L. Schermerhorn

INTRODUCTION

The number of patients with peripheral artery disease (PAD) is continuously increasing in the setting of an aging population and increasing global disease burden of diabetes.[1] A recent meta-analysis of 34 studies estimated that over 202 million people worldwide suffer from PAD.[2] In the Edinburgh Artery Study of men and women aged 55–74 years, 4.5% had symptomatic PAD.[3] However, a further 8% had evidence of major asymptomatic disease and 17% had abnormal hemodynamic parameters suggesting minor PAD. Five years later, all new cases of intermittent claudication in the study group were in patients who were previously found to have asymptomatic disease.[4] It is believed that the current ratio of asymptomatic to symptomatic PAD is approximately 3:1.[5,6]

As discussed in Chapter 1, the risk factors associated with PAD are similar to those in coronary artery disease (CAD) and cerebrovascular disease. These include both demographic and comorbid conditions (Fig. 3.1).[5,7–10] Patients older than 64 years appear to be at highest risk for having PAD.[5] PAD is also a strong risk factor for cardiovascular disease, which has been estimated to be at least as great as for patients with a history of previous myocardial infarction (MI).[11] In a survey of 1886 patients with PAD, 58% had CAD and 34% had suffered a cerebrovascular event.[12]

The key aims for treatment of PAD should include reduction of cardiovascular risk factors, improvement of symptoms, and disruption of disease progression. This chapter will address the concepts and guidelines for medical management of all stages of PAD, including asymptomatic PAD, symptomatic PAD, and chronic limb-threatening ischaemia (CLTI).

UNDERTREATMENT OF PERIPHERAL ARTERY DISEASE

Studies have consistently reported the undertreatment of patients with PAD, especially when compared to patients with cardiovascular disease.[13] The suboptimal management of vascular risk in patients with PAD is well-documented to result in an unacceptably high incidence of MI, stroke, and cardiovascular death.[14] Recent data suggests that there are both sex- and race-specific patterns of medical undertreatment of cardiovascular risk factors[15,16] that lead to differences in clinical disease burden at the time of presentation,[17] and the interventions performed.[18–20]

The US PARTNERS program demonstrated medical under-diagnosis and under-treatment of patients with PAD among primary care practices.[6] The GetABI study showed that patients with PAD were under-treated in comparison to those with cerebrovascular disease including

CAD and stroke.[21] Two out of three patients with CAD were given antiplatelet drugs, but only around a half of patients with PAD. The situation was similar in regard to lipid lowering statins. Some 46% of patients with CAD received statins compared with only 23% of those with symptomatic PAD. The differences were even more pronounced in the prescription of beta-blockers.[22] The international REACH registry of patients at increased cardiovascular risk, most being treated in the primary care setting, also showed that patients with PAD received suboptimal medical treatment and few were controlled within target ranges for blood pressure, cholesterol and glucose control, regardless of geographic region.[23,24] Furthermore, in patients referred to specialists, only 70% were on antiplatelet therapy and 44% were taking a statin.[25] Multiple other studies continue to show disproportionate levels of fatal and non-fatal cardiovascular events in patients with PAD, while others document failures in diagnosis and risk management.[26,27] Overall, the mortality of PAD patients at 5 years is high and exceeds that of some common cancers (Fig. 3.2). As awareness around the importance of cardiovascular risk reduction increases, the proportion of at-risk patients on appropriate medical therapy has increased but opportunities remain for improvement.[28]

PERIPHERAL ARTERY DISEASE DIAGNOSIS AND SCREENING

Given the associated cardiovascular risk with PAD, it is not surprising that ankle–brachial pressure index (ABPI) alone can be used as a marker for future cardiovascular risk.[31] The Atherosclerotic Risk in Communities Study found that the lower the ABPI the greater the risk of cardiac and cerebrovascular disease.[32] Despite this, however, general screening of the adult population for PAD is not currently recommended but there may be specific at-risk groups where screening may be helpful (see Chapter 1).[33]

MODIFYING CARDIOVASCULAR RISK

A key aim of medical therapy in the management of patients with any stage of PAD is to reduce the risk of future cardiovascular events. There is strong evidence that patients with any stage of PAD have increased cardiovascular risk and are

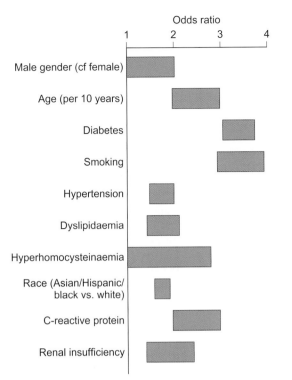

Figure 3.1 Approximate range of odds ratios for risk factors for symptomatic peripheral artery disease.[5]

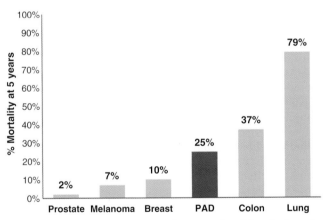

Figure 3.2 Five-year relative mortality rates of peripheral artery disease (PAD)[29] and common cancers in the United States 2010–2016.[30] (Adapted from Heiss, 2019.[13])

therefore likely to benefit from risk reduction strategies, which include exercise, smoking cessation, curbing obesity, antiplatelet agents, and treatment of diabetes, hypertension, and dyslipidaemia.

Many of the current recommendations for risk-factor modification in PAD have been extrapolated from studies on secondary prevention in patients primarily with CAD. There is a significant gap in the evidence regarding treatment of PAD patients specifically. However, the strength of the association between PAD and coronary disease makes such extrapolations clinically highly credible.

SMOKING CESSATION

Smoking is associated with worsening atherosclerosis, increases the risk of cardiovascular death, and accelerates

bypass graft failure.[34,35] For patients with PAD, smoking cessation has been shown to reduce death from coronary disease, and decrease lower extremity interventions and amputations.[36] Advising and assisting patients to quit smoking is a beneficial intervention that healthcare professionals can deliver in the population with PAD. Supplementing counselling on smoking cessation with nicotine replacement and the antidepressant bupropion has been shown to be most effective in 12-month abstinence from smoking rates compared to each alone.[37] This has led some clinical guidelines to recommend prescribing pharmacological interventions such as varenicline, bupropion and nicotine replacement to assist in smoking cessation.[38]

MANAGEMENT OF DYSLIPIDAEMIA

Elevated total cholesterol concentrations, increased levels of low-density lipoprotein cholesterol (LDL-c), triglycerides and decreased high-density lipoprotein (HDL) levels are independent risk factors for the development of PAD.[39] The term *dyslipidaemia* refers to abnormal concentrations in LDL, HDL and triglycerides, however, there are currently no data to suggest treating elevated triglyceride levels and low HDL cholesterol values leads to a reduction in morbidity and mortality in people with PAD. Therefore the treatment of dyslipidaemia remains focused on lowering LDL levels, primarily through the use of HMG-CoA reductase inhibitors (statins).

The ideal target values for LDL cholesterol levels in at-risk patients remains unknown. An inverse correlation has been shown between the level of LDL cholesterol and the ABPI in patients with newly diagnosed PAD.[40] In one large randomised control trial (RCT), lowering LDL reduced the risk of a cardiovascular event in patients with atherosclerosis, even in patients with 'normal' starting cholesterol values.[41]

Indeed, the international guidelines for treatment of dyslipidaemias diverge on this point. In the United States, a fixed-dose strategy utilising moderate- to high-dose statins for all adults with a 10-year cardiovascular disease event risk of 7.5% or greater has been recommended instead of a goal-targeted therapy to a particular lipid target level.[42,43] The UK National Institute for Health and Care Excellence (NICE) has adopted a similar recommendation for statin therapy in at-risk populations without the goal of a particular lipid level target.[44] The European Society of Cardiology guidelines recommend lowering LDL cholesterol levels to <100 mg/dL (<2.58 mmol/L) in high-risk patients and to <70 mg/dL (<1.81 mmol/L), or reduced by ≥50% in those at a very high risk including PAD patients.

Recently, high-intensity statin therapy versus low-intensity statin therapy has been shown to improve graft patency[45] and reduce adverse limb outcomes including amputation.[46] In addition to providing cardiovascular protection, there is some evidence that statins may alter vasomotor tone, stimulate angiogenesis and they have been shown to improve pain-free walking distance in patients with claudication.[47,48] It appears that the benefits of statins go beyond their lipid-lowering properties and are linked with their ability to decrease oxidative stress and vascular inflammation, as well as their protection against thrombosis through platelet influence.[49]

High-dose statin therapy (e.g., atorvastatin 40–80 mg daily or rosuvastatin 20–40 mg daily) should be considered for all patients with symptomatic vascular disease who are <75 years old and not on haemodialysis. Moderate statin doses should be considered for all other patients with symptomatic PAD or with >7.4% 10-year risk of atherosclerotic vascular disease.

NON-STATIN AGENTS FOR LOWERING LOW-DENSITY LIPOPROTEIN CHOLESTEROL LEVELS

The most common adverse effect limiting the use of statin therapy is associated with muscle aching. This may be difficult to interpret in people with claudication. If muscle aches occur, the statin dose can be lowered to the maximum tolerated dose, and a second non-statin cholesterol-lowering agent can be added. Similarly, for very high-risk patients who do not achieve adequate reduction in LDL levels while on high-dose statin therapy, the addition of a second agent is reasonable. In either scenario, the addition of the selective cholesterol-absorption inhibitor ezetimibe is recommended.[43,50]

In addition, monoclonal antibodies against pro-protein convertase subtilisine Kesine 9 (PCSK9), which direct the degradation of LDL receptors in the liver, have recently gained traction in clinical practice. Reduction in PCSK9 activity by two monoclonal antibodies approved for use in the United States, alirocumab and evolocumab, available as injections once every 2 or 4 weeks, have demonstrated substantial reductions in LDL cholesterol levels, when administered as either monotherapy or in addition to statin therapy. The Further Cardiovascular Outcomes Research with PCSK9 Inhibition in Subjects with Elevated Risk (FOURIER) trial demonstrated evolocumab also reduced major adverse cardiovascular events (MACE) including MI and stroke, as well as a reduction in the risk of acute limb ischemia and major amputation.[51] The cost of these two agents currently limits their generalizability, however, recent cost-benefit analyses suggest they can be cost-effective in select high-risk patients with symptomatic PAD on maximum tolerated statin therapy, plus ezetimibe, who do not reach a target LDL.[52]

TREATMENT OF DIABETES

Type 2 diabetes mellitus is an important risk factor for the development of asymptomatic and symptomatic PAD.[53] The severity and duration of diabetes is related to the extent of PAD. Every 1% increase in haemoglobin A1c (HbA1C) level has been associated with a 28% increased relative risk for the development of PAD[54] and has been shown to increase the risk of adverse outcomes among patients with PAD, including progression to CLTI, amputation and death.[55,56] Diabetes mellitus is thought to worsen atherosclerosis as a consequence of arterial wall degeneration and inflammation, in addition to increases in platelet aggregation, blood viscosity and fibrinogen levels.[57]

Good glucose control, with a HbA1C level between 6.5–7.5% is recommended.[18,58] In elderly vascular patients, a range of 7–8%, may be used generally to avoid hypoglycaemic events. In addition, intensive glycaemic control has been shown to reduce the development of microvascular complications such as neuropathy.[59]

Biguanides, specifically metformin monotherapy is generally recognised as the best initial oral hypoglycaemic agent for patients with an estimated glomerular filtration rate (eGFR) >30 mL/min.[60] Furthermore, an observational study has shown that the use of metformin was associated with a lower prevalence of below-the-knee arterial calcification.[61] While metformin is associated with improved survival and decreased incidence of major adverse cardiac and limb events in patients with PAD compared with insulin or other hypoglycaemics, it does not appear to improve limb salvage or patency rates after open or endovascular interventions.[62] People with diabetes and abnormal renal function treated with metformin may be at higher risk for contrast-induced nephropathy and lactic acidosis and may benefit from withholding metformin for 24 to 48 hours following delivery of iodinated contrast.[63]

When additional therapy is needed, other classes of oral hypoglycaemic agents can be added without significant differences in all-cause mortality,[64] however, each comes with important considerations:

Glucagon-like peptide 1 (GLP-1) receptor agonists such as dulaglutide, liraglutide and semaglutide have recently been shown to decrease MACE, reduce hospitalisations for heart failure and slow the progression of chronic kidney disease (CKD) in high-risk patients with type 2 diabetes, whether or not they have a prior history of established cardiovascular disease. Furthermore, in the LEADER study, liraglutide was associated with reduced amputation rates. The American Diabetes Association now recommends GLP-1 receptor agonists can also be considered in patients with type 2 diabetes with or without established cardiovascular disease if they have other indicators of high risk, specifically, patients aged 55 years or older with coronary, carotid or lower extremity artery stenosis >50%, left ventricular hypertrophy, an eGFR <60 mL min−1[1.73 m]−2 or albuminuria to reduce risk of MACE, regardless of baseline or target HbA1c level.[65] It should be noted, however, semaglutide should be avoided in patients with diabetic retinopathy, as rates of retinopathy complications were significantly higher even though rates of new or worsening nephropathy were decreased overall.[66]

Sodium-glucose co-transporter 2 (SGLT-2) inhibitors are a newer class of agents that have been associated with beneficial effects in patients with heart failure and CKD on cardiovascular complications, renal disease and mortality in type 2 diabetics. However, one large trial (>10 000 subjects) demonstrated an almost twofold increased risk of lower limb amputations associated with the use of the SGLT-2 inhibitor, canaglifozin,[67] prompting a warning from the US Food and Drug Administration.[68] We advise against the use of canaglifozin in diabetic patients with foot ulcers, advanced PAD and/or CLTI.

Sulphonylureas including glyburide may elevate the risk of cardiovascular disease among patients with diabetes. Caution is advised in the use of these agents as they have a high risk of hypoglycaemia, weight gain, and may have negative effects in patients with coronary heart disease.[69]

Thiazolidinediones (PPAR γ agonists) such as pioglitazone, cardiovascular survival was improved in patients with diabetes and pre-diabetes in the PROactive[70] and IRIS trials.[71] These studies have also suggested pioglitazone therapy is associated with higher risks of weight gain and fracture. Early analyses within the PROactive trial suggested pioglitazone decreased amputation rates, however, after 10 years, no differences remained in amputation rates compared with the control group.[72]

Dipeptidyl peptidase 4 (DPP4) inhibitors such as saxagliptin and alogliptin may reduce the risks of MI and stroke, however, significantly more hospitalisations for heart failure was observed in patients receiving saxagliptin, so this substance should be used with caution in patients with known heart failure. The impact of DPP4 inhibitors on patients with PAD and CLTI is not yet well defined.[73,74]

Insulin-providing therapies such as basal insulin, sulfonylureas, repaglinide or nateglinide, are recommended for use in patients with type 2 diabetes only after the initiation of an optimised oral or GLP-1 based therapy. Post-hoc analyses of the BARI-2D trial displayed lower incidence of lower extremity arterial disease among patients assigned to insulin-sensitising therapy (metformin or thiazolidinedione) compared with those assigned to insulin-providing therapy.[75] For basal insulin therapy, no endpoint studies are available for patients with type 2 diabetes and PAD.

MANAGEMENT OF HYPERTENSION

Antihypertensive therapy reduces cardiovascular events and mortality. Current guidelines recommend a target blood pressure of 120–129/70–80 mmHg in patients below 65 years, and 130–139/70–80 mmHg for older patients and in patients with concomitant cardiovascular disease, PAD and diabetes.[76]

Angiotensin converting enzyme (ACE) inhibitors, angiotensin receptor blockers (ARB), calcium antagonists, and diuretics are all first-line options for blood pressure lowering treatment in patients with PAD.[77] ACE inhibitors and ARB have been shown to reduce cardiovascular events in patients with arterial peripheral vascular diseases.[78,79] Initially, ACE inhibitors were thought to improve symptoms in patients with intermittent claudication but this view has since been revised.[80,81] If blood pressure remains uncontrolled, the addition of spironolactone may be considered.

Studies of the use of beta-blockade for treatment of hypertension show a smaller reduction in blood pressure overall and somewhat less risk reduction for cardiovascular events than when compared with other antihypertensive drug classes. Of note, beta-blockers are well tolerated in patients with PAD or CLTI and there is no evidence that this medication reduces walking distance or worsens claudication pain, as was previously suspected.[82–84] Thus, beta-blockers are useful in PAD patients with concomitant cardiovascular disorders, as in the case of atrial fibrillation.

ANTIPLATELET THERAPY

Antiplatelet therapy is recommended in all patients with symptomatic PAD if not otherwise contraindicated. The Antiplatelet Trialists' Collaboration, which included 135 000 patients with cardiovascular disease, reported a nearly 25% reduction in cardiovascular events for those treated with an antiplatelet agent.[85] This result has been replicated for both aspirin and clopidogrel in lowering the risk of MI and stroke in patients with symptomatic PAD.[86,87] In the CAPRIE study, at 3 years, clopidogrel was shown to be superior to aspirin with lower rates of MI, stroke and cardiovascular mortality. The overall benefit in the PAD subgroup compared with acetyl salicylic acid (ASA) was a 24% relative risk reduction.[87] In the current European Society of Cardiology PAD guidelines, clopidogrel was therefore recommended over aspirin in PAD patients.[88]

In the randomised Effects of Ticagrelor and Clopidogrel in Patients with Peripheral Artery Disease (EUCLID) trial, ticagrelor was compared to clopidogrel in 13 885 patients ≥50 years of age with symptomatic LEAD. Ticagrelor and clopidogrel were equivalent in effect, though there were more drug discontinuations with ticagrelor in the setting of side effects.[89]

More recently, there has been a suggestion that certain high-risk patients with symptomatic PAD may benefit from dual antiplatelet therapy.[90,91] However, evidence for prolonged dual-therapy is lacking. The combination of ASA and clopidogrel in high-risk patients with multiple risk factors including PAD and cardiovascular disorders resulted in an increased bleeding risk and no benefit over aspirin alone.[92]

It should be noted to date, no specific trial has addressed the role of antiplatelet agents in the full spectrum of LEAD (asymptomatic, intermittent claudication and CLTI). For patients with asymptomatic PAD, the benefits of antiplatelet agents are unknown at this point. The Aspirin for Asymptomatic Atherosclerosis Trial randomised 3350 patients to aspirin versus placebo and found no difference in vascular events through 8 years, although there were criticisms regarding the measurement of ABPI used to stratify patients.[93]

ANTICOAGULANTS

Investigations into the use of direct oral anticoagulants in patients with PAD and CLTI are ongoing. Recently, the Cardiovascular Outcomes for People Using Anticoagulation Strategies (COMPASS) trial, a multicenter randomised trial, which compared the oral factor Xa inhibitor rivaroxaban monotherapy (5 mg twice a day) with dual therapy (aspirin plus rivaroxaban 2.5 mg twice a day) and with aspirin monotherapy in 27 395 patients with CAD or PAD, demonstrated rivaroxaban plus aspirin resulted in a 24% relative risk reduction in major cardiac and limb events compared with aspirin alone.[94] This drug combination was associated with a small but statistically significant increase in clinically relevant bleeding, suggesting careful consideration of individualised patient factors and remains the topic of future studies.

The Vascular Outcomes studY of ASA alonG with rivaroxaban in Endovascular or surgical limb Revascularisation for Peripheral Artery Disease (VOYAGER-PAD) evaluated the efficacy and safety of low-dose rivaroxaban used together with aspirin in patients undergoing lower extremity revascularisation. They found rivaroxaban significantly reduces the risk of acute limb ischemia, major amputation, MI, ischemic stroke or cardiovascular death, compared with aspirin alone in high-risk CLTI patients.[95]

Currently, there is no evidence to suggest that oral anticoagulation with the vitamin K antagonist warfarin decreases the rate of adverse cardiovascular events in patients with PAD and it has been associated with increased bleeding complications in other patient populations. Therefore unless indicated for other reasons, warfarin should not be prescribed for the treatment of PAD to reduce cardiovascular risk.

ADDITIONAL LIFESTYLE MODIFICATIONS

Other potentially modifiable behaviours include dietary indiscretion and inactivity as they relate to cardiovascular health. Diet can have a profound effect on lipid metabolism and atherogenesis, as well as on weight and diabetes mellitus. Exercise also plays an important role in cardiovascular health and will be discussed further subsequently.

EXERCISE

Exercise therapy is thought to be the best initial therapy for claudication.[96] It has been clearly demonstrated to improve pain-free ambulation and walking performance.[5,97] There is good evidence that exercise leads to improvement in muscle and vascular endothelial cell function and increases collateral vessel growth.[97] Beyond improving the symptoms of claudication, exercise also reduces cardiovascular risk.[98] This benefit is lost when a sedentary lifestyle is resumed and therefore sustained exercise regimens are key to achieving long-term results. There is also a correlation between ABPI and a patient's exercise routine, suggesting that a sustained active lifestyle could help prevent PAD.[99] This has led multiple professional societies to recommend formal exercise therapy in patients with claudication.[5,38,100]

Walking, compared to other forms of lower extremity exercise (e.g., cycling, stair climbing, static and dynamic leg exercises), has been shown to be superior.[101] In fact, independent predictors of increased walking distance with an exercise programme from a meta-analysis of 21 rehabilitation studies included the type of claudication pain endpoint used (meaning walking distance until maximum pain instead of onset of pain), mode of exercise (walking vs. other), and duration of the exercise programme.[96] Current recommendations are for supervised walking exercise programmes 3 ×/week for >30 minutes, each session for more than 6 months. Neither lower extremity strength training nor upper extremity aerobic exercise appear to augment the benefits of walking exercise programmes.[102]

Intervention (angioplasty and stenting) has been studied as both a supplement and an alternative to exercise therapy for claudication. Multiple studies have shown that after both endovascular lower extremity intervention and bypass, supplementing with a structured exercise regimen improves long-term maximal claudication and walking distance.[103,104] The CLEVER trial randomised 111 patients with claudication to optimal medical care, optimal medical care with supervised exercise or optimal medical care with stent revascularisation and found that at 6 months peak walking time was greatest in the supervised exercise group, whereas improvements in quality of life were greatest in the stent revascularisation group.[105] However, at 18 months, there was no difference in quality of life metrics between the supervised exercise and stent revascularisation groups.[106] Markov models on a 5-year time horizon have found structured exercise therapy to be more cost-effective than endovascular revascularisation.[107]

The data supporting benefits of exercise are mostly from structured and supervised programmes; however, reimbursement for such therapy ranges widely across the United States and Europe and is rarely fully covered. Given this, for those patients placed on home-based walking regimens, frequent assessment of progress by patient and provider is needed to ensure adherence.

Patients with CLTI may have more physical restrictions on their ability to walk but low-intensity exercise should be encouraged in those patients who are able. This would likely involve close attention to footwear and foot care as well as involvement of physical therapy services to assist in establishing a suitable regimen tailored to the individual patient with CLTI.

ADDITIONAL PHARMACOLOGICAL INTERVENTIONS

Pharmacological management of PAD is aimed at symptom control and slowing the progression of atherosclerotic disease. In addition to cardiovascular risk reduction, primary pharmacological intervention is utilised most often in patients with claudication whereas it is often used as a supplement to revascularisation or after failed intervention in those with CLTI.

CILOSTAZOL

This vasoactive drug is more commonly used in the United States. It is a phosphodiesterase inhibitor that suppresses platelet aggregation and promotes vasodilatation. RCTs have shown its benefit in 6-month maximum and pain-free walking distance compared to pentoxifylline (mean change from baseline: cilostazol 107 m vs. pentoxifylline 64 m, $P < 0.001$ and cilostazol 94 m vs. pentoxifylline 74 m, $P < 0.001$, respectively) and placebo (cilostazol 107 m vs. placebo 65 m, $P < 0.001$ and cilostazol 94 m vs. placebo 57 m, $P < 0.001$, respectively).[108,109] Treatment should be discontinued if symptoms fail to improve after 3 months.

NAFTIDROFURYL

This vasoactive drug works by enhancing aerobic glycolysis and oxygen consumption in ischaemic tissues. A meta-analysis based on individual patient data reported that individuals with PAD receiving naftidrofuryl walked 37% further than those getting placebo at 6 months.[110] This benefit in claudication was further verified in a subsequent Cochrane review.[111] NICE evaluated the evidence of four vasoactive drugs used in the treatment of intermittent claudication – cilostazol (Pletal), naftidrofuryl oxalate (Praxilene), pentoxifylline (Trental) and inositol nicotinate (Hexopal) – and found that there was no conclusive evidence of an advantage of one agent over the other; however, naftidrofuryl oxalate was more cost-effective.[112] As a result, naftidrofuryl was recommended by this group as the only vasoactive agent to be used out of this group of medications for treatment of symptoms related to claudication. Treatment should be discontinued if symptoms fail to improve after 3 months.

PENTOXIFYLLINE

This was one of the first medications used to treat symptoms related to PAD and works through reducing blood viscosity and interrupting platelet aggregation, which results in improved oxygenation to compromised areas in PAD. Port et al. in 1982 demonstrated that it improved both pain-free and maximal walking distance versus placebo.[113] However, later placebo controlled and comparative studies have not shown improvement in PAD symptoms from pentoxifylline and therefore it is currently not commonly used in either Europe or the United States.[109,114]

HOMOCYSTEINE-LOWERING MEDICATIONS

Roughly 30% of patients with PAD have elevated homocysteine levels compared with only 1% of the general population.[5] Elevated homocysteine levels are thought to be associated with endothelial dysfunction and injury. In addition, people with PAD also exhibit increased production of hydrogen peroxide, increases in Factor XII and V and decreases in Protein C, thrombomodulin and heparin sulphate activity.[115] This led some to believe that folic acid and cobalamin (Vitamin B12) may help reduce the risk of cardiovascular events in those with hyperhomocysteinemia. However, no data to date have proved this and currently, there are no level 1 recommendations to prescribe these medications in the setting of PAD.[5,116,117]

LEVOCARNITINE

This is a carrier molecule involved in the transport of long-chain fatty acids. Supplementation with levocarnitine results in an increase in the availability of energy substrate for skeletal muscle metabolism. It has been shown to improve pain-free and maximum walking distance compared to placebo but not to exercise alone.[118,119] Currently, there are no strong recommendations for its use.

PROSTANOIDS

Prostanoids or prostaglandins, are thought to work in PAD through vasodilatation and inhibition of platelet aggregation. In recent trials, this group of medications showed mixed results, especially in patients with claudication.[120,121] A recent RCT has failed to show any significant benefit from alprostadil in CLTI.[122] Buflomedil, an alpha-1 and -2 antagonist resulting in vasodilatation, has shown positive effects on treadmill performance in PAD patients; however, these findings were from small studies and need further confirmation before conclusions about its use in PAD can be made.[123,124] L-Arginine, an amino acid precursor of endothelial-derived nitric oxide, which acts through vasodilatation of vascular smooth muscle cells has also been studied, with inconsistent results, and is also currently not recommended for PAD.[125]

INTERMITTENT PNEUMATIC COMPRESSION

Intermittent pneumatic compression of the calf and foot has been shown to increase popliteal artery blood flow. It is thought to accomplish this through increases in the arteriovenous pressure gradient, reversal of vasomotor paralysis and enhanced release of nitric oxide. The role of this therapy is not clearly defined yet but studies have shown its benefit in patients with both claudication and CLTI who do not have good revascularisation options.[126,127] An additional benefit is that this therapy can be used by patients in the comfort of their own homes. Further research is needed to establish where this therapy is most effectively utilised.

ANGIOGENESIS AND STEM CELL THERAPY

There is much hope for pro-angiogenic factors to help in symptomatic PAD, but this research is still in its infancy. In early human trials, the use of growth factors, including vascular endothelial growth factor, fibroblast growth factor and platelet-derived growth factor, has been associated with increased vascularity and limb blood flow. However, these trials were small and without controls.[128] There are also potential risks with such a therapy, such as new vessel growth at other sites including the eye and malignant lesions.

In addition to injecting growth factors to encourage angiogenesis, stem cell therapy is also being studied: autologous stem cell therapies aspirated from bone marrow mononuclear cells or endothelial progenitor cells and directly injected concentrated solutions of these cells back into the individual patient's ischaemic tissue. Early trials using this method have shown promise but much work remains before this can become recommended therapy.[129,130] Allogeneic stem cell therapies are being studied for this purpose as well.

CONCLUSIONS

PAD and CLTI remain under-diagnosed and under-treated. A diagnosis of PAD is an indicator of increased cardiovascular risk and as such risk factor modification can have a profound impact, for both the extremity and the cardiovascular system. The therapeutic approach to patients with PAD includes two aspects. The first is to address specific symptoms of any localisation and the risk related to a specific lesion. The second aspect of management in these patients is related to their increased cardiovascular risk factors. Optimal medical therapy includes mitigation of cardiovascular risk factors through a combination of pharmacological therapy, as well as non-pharmacological measures such as smoking cessation, healthy diet, weight loss and regular physical exercise. The pharmacological components of optimal medical management includes lipid-lowering agents, antihypertensives, antithrombotic drugs and optimising glucose control in diabetic patients.

Key points

- Asymptomatic and symptomatic patients with PAD are at high risk of cardiovascular events and will benefit from minimising risk factors.
- Best medical therapy includes pharmacological therapy with antihypertensives, lipid-lowering, antithrombotic agents, and glycaemic control in patients with diabetes, as well as non-pharmacological measures such as smoking cessation, healthy diet, weight loss and exercise.
- Supervised exercise should be available and offered to patients with intermittent claudication.
- There are effective behavioural and pharmacological interventions to assist in smoking cessation, which should be utilised for all patients with PAD.
- All patients with symptomatic PAD should be on a statin and antiplatelet agent, unless they have a strong contraindication for one of these medications.
- Every symptomatic PAD patient should be given long-term treatment with platelet aggregation inhibitors; clopidogrel may be preferred over aspirin.
- Dual therapy with low-dose rivaroxaban in addition to aspirin has recently been shown to decrease the risk for MACE in patients with atherosclerotic disease but is associated with an increased bleeding risk.
- The role of dual antiplatelet therapy in patients with asymptomatic PAD for secondary prevention of cardiovascular events is unclear and requires further investigation.
- Angiogenesis and stem cell therapies are exciting concept but require considerable further evaluation before they can be put into practice.

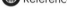 References available at http://ebooks.health.elsevier.com/

KEY REFERENCES

[5] Norgren L, Hiatt WR, Dormandy JA, et al. Inter-society consensus for the management of peripheral arterial disease (TASC II). J Vasc Surg 2007;45(Suppl. S):S5–67. PMID: 17223489

The majority of patients with PAD are thought to be asymptomatic. Out of those with symptoms, few with claudication go on to develop CLTI but risk factors for this include increased age, diabetes, smoking and lipid abnormalities. Exercise therapy in addition to control of risk factors has been proven to help improve symptomatic PAD.

[7] Selvin E, Erlinger TP. Prevalence of and risk factors for peripheral arterial disease in the United States: results from the national health and nutrition examination survey, 1999–2000. Circulation 2004;110(6):738–43. PMID: 15262830

Risk factors for PAD include increasing age, black race, current smoking, diabetes, hypercholesterolaemia and kidney disease.

[36] Rooke TW, Hirsch AT, Misra S, et al. 2011 ACCF/AHA Focused update of the guideline for the management of patients with peripheral artery disease (updating the 2005 guideline): a report of the American college of cardiology foundation/ American heart association task force on practice guidelines. J Am Coll Cardiol 2011;58(19):2020–45. PMID: 21963765

Ankle to brachial pressure index is an important diagnostic tool in high-risk populations and in those identified as having PAD every effort should be made to reduce risk factors for progression of disease, especially smoking cessation.

[46] Arya S, Khakharia A, Binney ZO, DeMartino RR, Brewster LP, Goodney PP, et al. Association of statin dose with amputation and survival in patients with peripheral artery disease. Circulation 2018;137(14):1435–46. PMCID: PMC5882502

The first population-based observational study to show that high-intensity statin use at the time of PAD diagnosis is associated with a significant reduction in limb loss and mortality in comparison with low-to-moderate-intensity statin users.

[76] Whelton PK, Carey RM, Aronow WS, Casey DE, Collins KJ, Dennison Himmelfarb C, et al. 2017 ACC/AHA/AAPA/ABC/ ACPM/AGS/APhA/ASH/ASPC/NMA/PCNA guideline for the prevention, detection, evaluation, and management of high blood pressure in adults: a report of the American college of cardiology/American heart association task force on clinical practice guidelines. J Am Coll Cardiol 2018;71(19):e127–248. PMID: 29146535

2017 ACC/AHA Clinical Practice Guidelines on the Management of Hypertension.

[87] CAPRIE Steering Committee. A randomised, blinded, trial of clopidogrel versus aspirin in patients at risk of ischaemic events (CAPRIE). CAPRIE Steering Committee. Lancet 1996;348(9038):1329–39. PMID: 8918275

Results from the multi-centre, double blind RCT demonstrating clopidogrel reduced the risk of cardiovascular events compared to aspirin without an increase in bleeding events.

[88] Aboyans V, Ricco J-B, Bartelink M-LEL, Björck M, Brodmann M, Cohnert T, ESC Scientific Document Group, et al. 2017 ESC guidelines on the diagnosis and treatment of peripheral arterial diseases, in collaboration with the European society for vascular surgery (ESVS): document covering atherosclerotic disease of extracranial carotid and vertebral, mesenteric, renal, upper and lower extremity arteries. endorsed by: the European stroke organization (ESO)the task force for the diagnosis and treatment of peripheral arterial diseases of the European society of cardiology (ESC) and of the European society for vascular surgery (ESVS). Eur Heart J 2018;39(9):763–816. PMID: 28886620

2017 European Society for Vascular Surgery Guidelines on the Diagnosis and Treatment of Peripheral Arterial Diseases.

[94] Anand SS, Bosch J, Eikelboom JW, Connolly SJ, Diaz R, Widimsky P, et al. Rivaroxaban with or without aspirin in patients with stable peripheral or carotid artery disease: an international, randomised, double-blind, placebo-controlled trial. Lancet 2018;391(10117):219–29. PMID: 29132880

Results from the multi-center, double-blind RCT the combination of low-dose rivaroxaban in addition to aspirin reduces thrombotic outcomes in patients with established atherosclerotic disease but is associated with a higher bleeding risk.

[95] Bonaca MP, Bauersachs RM, Anand SS, Debus ES, Nehler MR, Patel MR, et al. Rivaroxaban in peripheral artery disease after revascularization. N Engl J Med 2020;382(21):1994–2004. PMID: 32222135

Results from the VOYAGER-PAD trial showing dual therapy with low-dose rivaroxaban in addition to aspirin decreases risk for cardiovascular and ischemic limb events including amputation in patients undergoing lower extremity revascularization.

Intervention for chronic lower limb ischaemia

4

Nedal Katib | Ramon L. Varcoe

INTRODUCTION

Peripheral artery disease (PAD) is a process characterised by the formation of atheromatous plaque and calcification within the arteries of the lower extremity. Typically, this leads to luminal stenosis or occlusions of both large and small arteries. Patients who suffer from the condition may either be asymptomatic or complain of a broad variety of clinical symptoms ranging from calf claudication to ischaemic tissue loss. Interventional therapy for PAD has traditionally been reliant upon open vascular surgery, such as endarterectomy and bypass to achieve definitive revascularisation. However, since the advent of peripheral angioplasty in the mid-1960s, there has been a large increase in its use, driven in large part by technological advances in what we now know as the field of endovascular surgery. Herein we seek to outline the contemporary literature and recommend an evidence-based approach to revascularisation of patients with chronic lower extremity ischaemia.

PRESENTING SYMPTOMS

The spectrum of symptoms that may occur when lower extremity PAD becomes symptomatic range from intermittent claudication (IC), through to ischaemic rest pain, ulceration and gangrene.

IC is muscular discomfort in a particular compartment of the lower limb that occurs reproducibly upon exercise and is relieved after a short period of rest. It occurs when muscular oxygen demand increases above its limited metabolic supply. It most often affects the calf muscles but can also affect more proximal muscle groups such as the thigh, hip and buttock. It is typically described as cramp, ache, fatigue or a combination of the three, and is graded according to severity (Table 4.1). The decision to intervene is based upon an individualised patient assessment that considers severity of symptoms, quality of life (QoL), risk of intervention and predicted durability of treatment.

Chronic limb-threatening ischaemia (CLTI) is the chronic manifestation of an ischaemic process (>2 weeks) with symptoms that include rest pain, ulceration or gangrene. Whilst ulceration may be triggered by a non-ischaemic process such as trauma or neuropathy, a non-healing ulcer perpetuated by ischaemia is also considered CLTI. Ischaemic rest pain may be constant or nocturnal. It is typically present in the distal portion of the foot and often relieved by hanging the leg dependent. It should not be confused with neuropathic symptoms, which are common in diabetes mellitus. When gangrene occurs, it typically affects digits and pressure areas such as the heel. Often forming an eschar, it may remain dry or develop an underlying suppurative infection.

GLOBAL VASCULAR GUIDELINES ON THE MANAGEMENT OF CHRONIC LIMB-THREATENING ISCHEMIA

In 2019 the European Society of Vascular Surgery, Society for Vascular Surgery (SVS) and the World Federation of Vascular Societies published guidelines to address the growing prevalence of CLTI, with its associated morbidity, mortality, increased healthcare costs and variability of practice (further information in Chapter 2).[1] Key components of that document were the promotion of the term *CLTI* to replace critical limb ischaemia (CLI), as the authors felt the term *CLI* '…connotes specific hemodynamic thresholds and fails to recognise the full spectrum and inter-relatedness of components beyond ischaemia that contribute to major limb amputation…'. They also incorporated the SVS Lower Extremity Threatened Limb Classification System known as *WIfI* (*Wound Ischaemia foot Infection*) as part of disease staging, and the Global Limb Anatomic Staging System (GLASS) as a new anatomical system to facilitate clinical decision making in CLTI.

The WIfI classification system was designed as a pathophysiological grading tool, analogous to the TNM staging system for malignancy.[2] With four different grades for each of wound, infection and ischaemia there are 64 combinations and individual classes. Each class is placed into a particular clinical stage. To gauge the significance of those grades, an expert Delphi consensus panel was asked two questions regarding each combination (Fig. 4.1). The first question was 'what is the perceived risk of amputation, assuming medical therapy alone', then 'what is the perceived benefit from revascularisation'. Each response was allocated to one of four predictive clinical stages (very low risk– Clinical Stage 1, low risk-2, moderate risk-3 and high risk-4). A meta-analysis of predominantly retrospective and observational studies evaluated the prognostic value of WIfI, finding the likelihood of amputation in patients with CLTI increased with higher WIfI stage, recommending a more rigorous prospective evaluation.[3]

Current anatomical staging systems for PAD may be vague, lesion focussed and lack detail beyond the concept of 'in-line pulsatile flow to the foot'. GLASS attempts to stage the disease by incorporating a full spectrum of anatomies

Table 4.1 Classification of peripheral artery disease

Fontaine's classification		Rutherford-Becker classification	
Stage	Symptom	Category	Symptom
I	Asymptomatic	0	Asymptomatic
II	Intermittent claudication	1	Mild claudication
		2	Moderate claudication
		3	Severe claudication
III	Ischaemic rest pain	4	Ischaemic rest pain
IV	Ulceration or gangrene	5	Minor tissue loss
		6	Major tissue loss

a, Estimate risk of amputation at 1 year for each combination

	Ischemia – 0				Ischemia – 1				Ischemia – 2				Ischemia – 3			
W-0	VL	VL	L	M	VL	L	M	H	L	L	M	H	L	M	M	H
W-1	VL	VL	L	M	VL	L	M	H	L	M	H	H	M	M	H	H
W-2	L	L	M	H	M	M	H	H	M	H	H	H	H	H	H	H
W-3	M	M	H	H	H	H	H	H	H	H	H	H	H	H	H	H
	fI-0	fI-1	fI-2	fI-3	fI-0	fI-1	fI-2	fI-3	fI-0	fI-1	fI-2	fI-3	fI-0	fI-1	fI-2	fI-3

b, Estimate likelihood of benefit of/requirement for revascularization (assuming infection can be controlled first)

	Ischemia – 0				Ischemia – 1				Ischemia – 2				Ischemia – 3			
W-0	VL	VL	VL	VL	VL	L	L	M	L	L	M	M	M	H	H	H
W-1	VL	VL	VL	VL	L	M	M	M	M	H	H	H	H	H	H	H
W-2	VL	VL	VL	VL	M	M	H	H	H	H	H	H	H	H	H	H
W-3	VL	VL	VL	VL	M	M	M	H	H	H	H	H	H	H	H	H
	f-0	fI-1	fI-2	fI-3	fI-0	fI-1	fI-2	fI-3	fI-0	fI-1	fI-2	fI-3	fI-0	fI-1	fI-2	fI-3

fI, foot Infection; I, Ischemia; W, Wound.

Premises:

1. Increase in wound class increases risk of amputation (based on PEDIS, UT, and other wound classification systems)
2. PAD and infection are synergistic (Eurodiale); infected wound + PAD increases likelihood revascularization will be needed to heal wound
3. Infection 3 category (systemic/metabolic instability): moderate to high-risk of amputation regardless of other factors (validated IDSA guidelines)

Four classes: for each box, group combination into one of these four classes

Very low = VL = clinical stage 1
Low = L = clinical stage 2
Moderate = M = clinical stage 3
High = H = clinical stage 4

Clinical stage 5 would signify an unsalvageable foot

Figure 4.1 WIfI clinical stages: **(a)** and **(b)**, risk/benefit: clinical stages by expert consensus (This figure was published in Mills Sr JL, Conte MS, Armstrong DG, et al., Society for Vascular Surgery Lower Extremity Guidelines Committee. The society for vascular surgery lower extremity threatened limb classification system: risk stratification based on wound, ischemia, and foot infection [WIfI]. J Vasc Surg. 2014;59(1):220–34, Copyright Journal of Vascular Surgery [2014])

and calcification with the goal of facilitating evidence-based revascularisation outcomes. Described within the Global Vascular Guidelines after consensus was sought from an expert panel of that document's authors, it incorporates two novel concepts: The Target Arterial Path, defined as the physician preferred route for endovascular therapy and the estimated Limb-Based Patency (LBP). It focusses on infra-inguinal disease, with the aorto-iliac segment, common and deep femoral arteries considered the inflow. It is assumed that inflow disease is corrected before, or at the same time as, the infra-inguinal revascularisation. Infra-inguinal assessment is based on length of disease and extent of complete occlusions. There is a dichotomous calcification scale, whereby if there is >50% circumference of calcification, diffuse, bulky calcification or 'coral reef' plaque, the within-segment grade is increased by one numerical value. Once the grade for femoropopliteal (Fig. 4.2) and infra-popliteal (IP) (Fig 4.3) disease is determined (0–4) then staging can be performed based on the matrix grid provided (1–3). Staging allows for estimation of the peripheral endovascular intervention outcomes to be predicted, Immediate Technical Failure and 1-year LBP. Like WIfI, GLASS has also been validated and shows an association with treatment outcomes for CLTI.[4]

EXERCISE THERAPY

✅✅ There is a body of evidence to support the effectiveness of supervised exercise therapy (SET) for the resolution of IC symptoms[5] and multiple guidelines recommend its use as first-line therapy for IC.[6–8]

Such a programme must be supervised walking,[7–9] 30–60-minute treadmill walks per day, be associated with risk factor modification and best medical therapy (BMT) to be most effective. The patient is instructed to walk until they experience moderate claudication, stop until symptoms resolve, then repeat until the predetermined time period has elapsed. The speed, inclination and treadmill walking time are incrementally increased throughout the programme.

The CLEVER (Claudication: Exercise Versus Endoluminal Revascularization) study was a randomised, multicentre, clinical trial.[9] One-hundred and eleven participants with aorto-iliac occlusive disease were randomised to SET with BMT, endovascular revascularisation (ER) with BMT or general advice to exercise and BMT. SET consisted of a 26-week programme of 60-minute treadmill walking followed by telephone counselling to encourage ongoing exercise participation. After 18 months of follow-up, functional walking improvement and QoL were persistently improved in both the SET + BMT and ER + BMT groups. Those two groups could not be separated in their effectiveness, attesting to the value of each; and both of those strategies were superior to BMT with general advice to exercise.

In the CETAC study, 151 patients were randomised to either SET or ER for PAD of the aorto-iliac or femoropopliteal arterial segments and both groups received BMT.[10] SET consisted of a 24-week programme whereby participants walked for 30 minutes on a treadmill twice a week, were encouraged to walk for an additional 30 minutes three times per week at home and continue walking for at least 1 hour per day after the programme was complete. After a mean follow-up period of 7 years, both groups had significantly improved maximum walking distance, pain-free walking distance and QoL. There was no difference between the two groups in any of those outcome measures. This trial demonstrated the long-term effectiveness of SET as an alternative therapy, equivalent to ER.

Despite this compelling evidence to support the use of SET, ER is widely used in the treatment of patients with claudication. The reasons for this are multifactorial. First, ER offers a fast treatment with almost instant relief of symptoms. It is less labour-intensive than SET, which requires effort and

persistence. Moreover, SET is frequently unavailable or not reimbursed in countries with insurance-based health care, a fact that is disappointing given the additional benefits of exercise in obesity reduction, blood pressure control, lipid lowering and glucose control, over-and-above that of claudication treatment.

MEDICAL THERAPY

All patients with macroscopic arterial disease benefit from risk factor management. Optimal medical therapy should be instigated in conjunction with interventional therapy and continued long term to prevent secondary cardiovascular morbidity. Medical treatment for PAD, and risk factor modification have been comprehensively described in Chapter 3.

GLOBAL TRENDS TOWARD REVASCULARISATION TREATMENT

There are more than 200 million people living with PAD around the world and the incidence is increasing.[11,12] In high-income countries, there has been an increase in the proportion of patients undergoing ER procedures, with decreasing open-surgical revascularisation procedures, in-hospital mortality and major amputation.[12] Factors that may be driving this trend include the association of endovascular procedures with reduced in-hospital mortality, length-of-stay and cost when compared to surgical revascularisation.[12,13] However, a causal relationship linking the endovascular approach to reduced amputation and improved outcomes remains to be demonstrated.

A REGIONAL APPROACH TO INTERVENTION

AORTO-ILIAC OCCLUSIVE DISEASE

The aorto-iliac segment is a frequently diseased vascular territory, which may be found both in isolation (claudication) and in conjunction with multilevel, occlusive disease in CLTI. Isolated aorto-iliac revascularisation may be sufficient to address symptoms in patients who also have concomitant infra-inguinal disease, and it is often necessary to maximise inflow to maintain infra-inguinal revascularisation strategies. It is therefore recommended that all vascular specialists have a thorough knowledge of treatment options for aorto-iliac occlusive disease.

The open-surgery, gold-standard for the treatment of aorto-iliac occlusive disease is aorto-(bi)-femoral (ABF) or bi-iliac bypass, which has durable patency that remains unchallenged by all other peripheral bypass operations.[14] However, whilst those patency rates are excellent, one must also consider the risk of major complications, which may occur in up to a quarter of patients, sexual dysfunction in up to 40% and perioperative mortality rates as high as 5%.[14,15] It is this burden of risk, which has led some to question whether a first-line, endovascular approach is more appropriate for most patients with aorto-iliac disease.

FP Grade 0	Mild or no significant (<50%) disease	
FP Grade 1	• Total length SFA disease <1/3 (<10 cm) • May include single focal CTO (< 5 cm) as long as not flush occlusion • Popliteal artery with mild or no significant disease	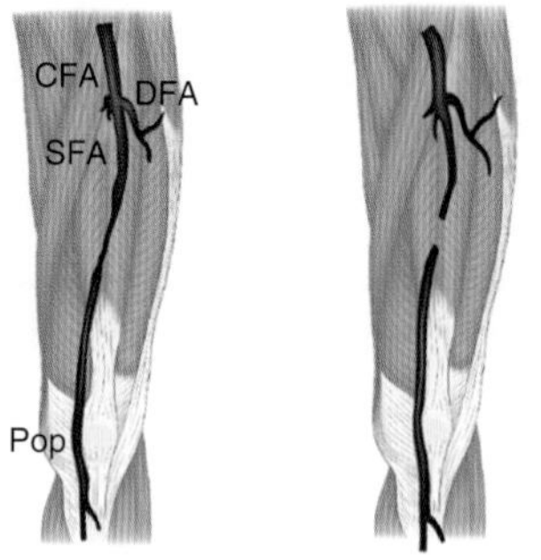
FP Grade 2	• Total length SFA disease 1/3-2/3 (10-20 cm) • May include CTO totaling < 1/3 (10 cm) but not flush occlusion • Focal popliteal artery stenosos <2 cm, not involving trifurcation	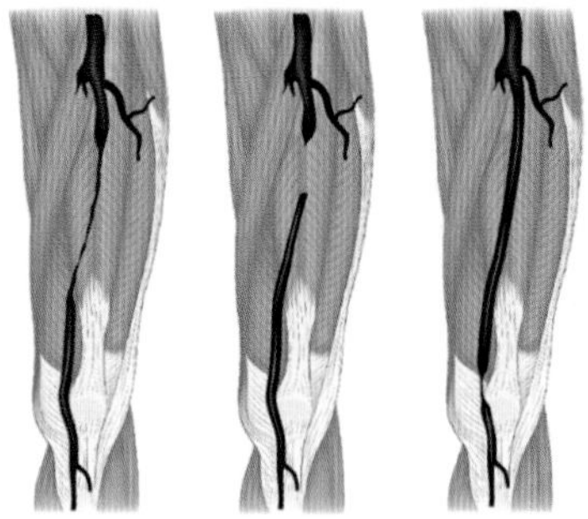
FP Grade 3	• Total length SFA disease > 2/3 (>20 cm) length • May include any flush occlusion < 20 cm or non-flush CTO 10-20 cm long • Short popliteal stenosis 2-5 cm, not involving trifurcation	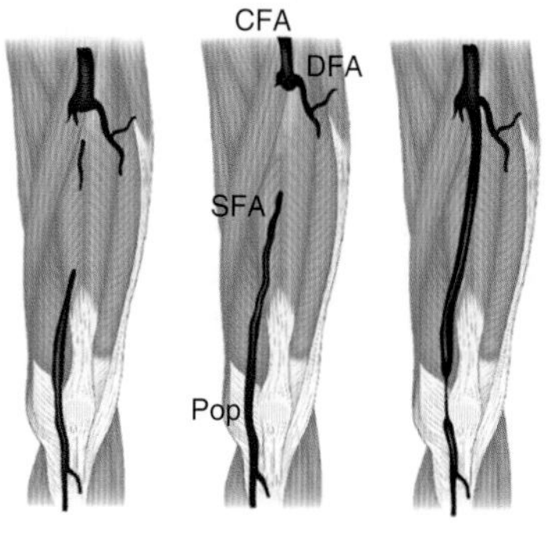
FP Grade 4	• Total length SFA occlusion > 20 cm • Popliteal disease > 5 cm or extending into trifurcation • Any popliteal CTO	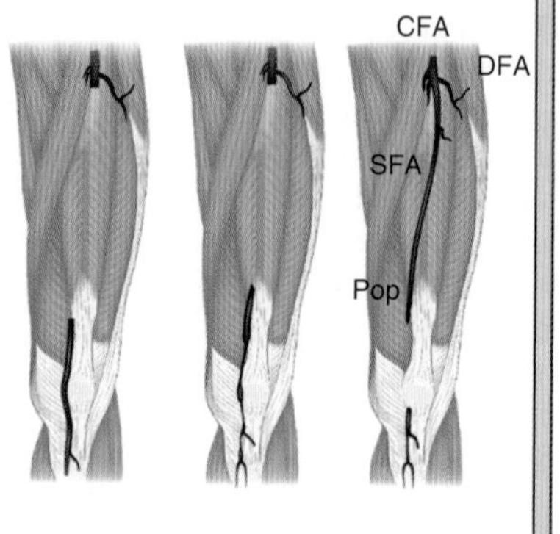

Figure 4.2 Femoropopliteal (FP) disease grading in Global Limb Anatomic Staging System (GLASS). Trifurcation is defined as the termination of the popliteal artery at the confluence of the anterior tibial (AT) artery and tibioperoneal trunk. *CFA*, Common femoral artery; *CTO*, chronic total occlusion; *DFA*, deep femoral artery; *Pop*, popliteal; *SFA*, superficial femoral artery. (This figure was published in Conte MS, Bradbury AW, Kolh P, et al. Global vascular guidelines on the management of chronic limb-threatening ischemia. Eur J Vasc Endovasc Surg. 2019;58(1):S1–09, Copyright Elsevier [(2019)])

IP Grade 0	• Mild or no significant disease in the primary target artery path
IP Grade 1	• Focal stenosis of tibial artery < 3cm
IP Grade 2	• Stenosis involving 1/3 total vessel length • May include focal CTO (<3 cm) • Not including TP trunk or tibial vessel origin
IP Grade 3	• Disease up to 2/3 vessel length • CTO up to1/3 length (may include tibial vessel orgin but not tibioperoneal trunk)
IP Grade 4	• Diffuse stenosis > 2/3 total vessel length • CTO > 1/3 vessel length (may include vessel origin) • Any CTO of tibioperoneal trunk if AT is not the target artery

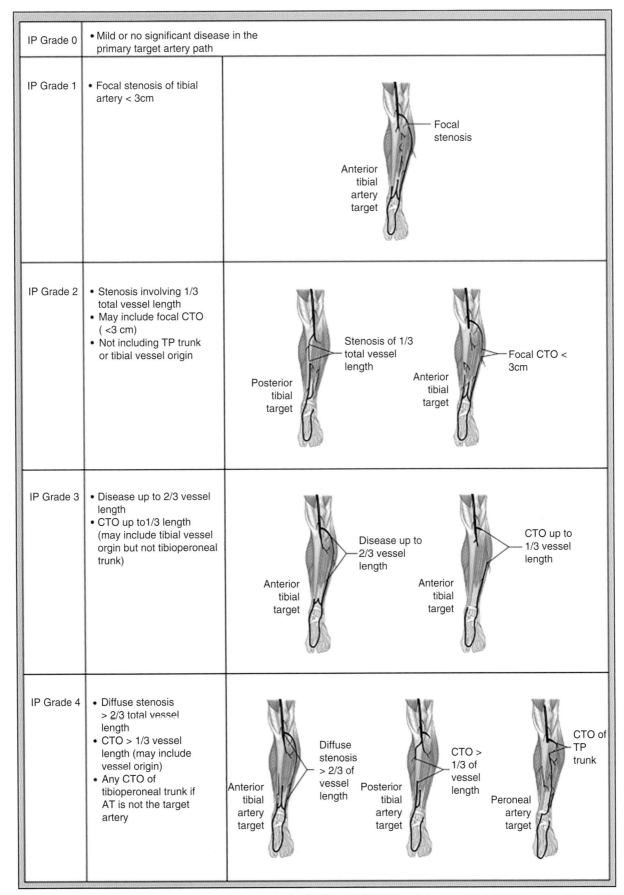

Figure 4.3 Infrapopliteal (IP) disease in Global Limb Anatomic Staging System (GLASS). *AT,* Anterior tibial; *CTO,* chronic total occlusion; *TP,* tibioperoneal. (This figure was published in Conte MS, Bradbury AW, Kolh P, et al. Global vascular guidelines on the management of chronic limb-threatening ischemia. Eur J Vasc Endovasc Surg. 2019;58(1):S1–09, Copyright Elsevier [2019]).)

REVASCULARISATION OF AORTO-ILIAC DISEASE

Percutaneous interventions have gained increasing popularity, driven by patient preference, enhanced safety and the increasingly complex patient comorbidities encountered in an ageing population. Moreover, minimally invasive procedures have demonstrated reduced length-of-stay requirements and intensive care utilisation, making them extremely attractive.

Whilst in the past it was common for endovascular therapies to face insurmountable technical challenges to wire passage and stent delivery during the treatment of extensive aorto-iliac disease, dedicated chronic-total-occlusion wires and catheters, bi-directional techniques and re-entry devices have contributed to very high technical success in contemporary experience.[8,16] This has made possible the percutaneous treatment of even the most extensive aorto-iliac occlusion for the skilled interventionist.

SURGICAL TREATMENT FOR AORTO-ILIAC DISEASE

Several open surgical options exist to revascularise the lower limbs in the presence of aorto-iliac occlusive disease. They include extra-anatomical bypass (femoro-femoral crossover and axillo-(bi)-femoral bypass), aortic endarterectomy and ABF bypass.

ABF bypass grafting has been performed since the advent of the synthetic aortic graft in the early1950s. The aorta may be approached from a trans- or retro-peritoneal route, and the bypass may be configured with either a proximal anastomosis that is end-to-end, or end-to-side. The latter configuration has the advantage of preserving flow to the distal inferior mesenteric, aberrant renal or internal iliac arteries; however, no patency advantage has been demonstrated with either technique and the decision as to which method is best remains contentious amongst vascular surgeons. An individual patient approach appears reasonable, dependent upon patient anatomy and disease morphology.

Patency rates with ABF are considered the gold standard for the treatment of aorto-iliac occlusive disease. A meta-analysis by De Vries et al. analysed 23 studies published between 1970 and 1996. Primary patency at 5 and 10 years was 91% and 86.8%, respectively, in those with claudication.[14] For those with CLI, the rates were slightly lower at 86.8% and 81.8%. However, despite those excellent surgical results, current practice in most units is to favour an endovascular-first approach for the majority of patients because of the relatively high perioperative risk. De Vries et al. found a combined 30-day mortality rate of 4.4%, which was higher in the older series (4.6% in studies published before 1975; 3.3% 1975–1996; $P = 0.01$). Furthermore, major morbidity rates were 19.7% (12.1% systemic complications; 7.6% local) and in series that looked specifically at sexual dysfunction, morbidity was noted in as many as 40%, with a combination of retrograde ejaculation and iatrogenic impotency.[15,17]

Extra-anatomic bypass is a less morbid operation than ABF, but it suffers from lower 5-year primary patency rates of 51% (range 44–79%) for axillo-uni-femoral, 71% (range 50–76%) for axillo-bi-femoral and 75% (range 55–92%) for femoro-femoral bypass.[8] For that reason, most vascular surgeons are likely to reserve those options for patients with severe comorbidities or a hostile abdomen where transperitoneal surgery is best avoided.

It should be noted that many of the studies included in the meta-analyses, which have evaluated open-surgical techniques for aorto-iliac occlusive disease are from an era when open surgery was used in the majority. Although outcomes from vascular surgery have generally improved over the years, care must be taken in their interpretation to consider that they are likely to have included patients with relatively minor disease who would be treated with angioplasty or stenting using current standards of practice. The inclusion of those relatively simple cases means that the patency and morbidity results from these studies may be skewed towards longevity and safety relative to the real-world application of ABF using present-day treatment algorithms.

PERCUTANEOUS TREATMENT FOR AORTO-ILIAC DISEASE

Patients often prefer minimally invasive therapeutic options, as they experience less pain, less operative risk and a faster return to normal activities. The TASC II document pooled results of 2222 iliac artery angioplasty procedures for both claudication (76%) and critical ischaemia (24%). They found a high technical success rate of 96% (range 90–99), as well as 1-, 3- and 5-year primary patency rates of 86% (range 81–94%), 82% (72–90%) and 71% (64–75%), respectively, demonstrating both the technical feasibility and durability of percutaneous transluminal angioplasty (PTA) for aorto-iliac occlusive disease.[8] In other contemporary findings from a large, single-centre study describing an experience with 505 aorto-iliac lesions treated with angioplasty ± stenting over a 9-year period, the authors found a technical success rate of 98%.[18] Eight-year primary and primary-assisted patency rates were 74% and 81%, respectively and safety was demonstrated with a 30-day mortality of 0.5%, comparing favourably to open surgery.

New techniques and technology have allowed us to treat ever more extensive patterns of disease, including long infra-renal aortic occlusions that extend into the iliac arteries (Fig. 4.4). These have traditionally been considered only suitable for open surgery. The most important technical aspect of treating advanced aorto-iliac occlusive disease proximal to the aortic bifurcation is the reliable passage of guidewire into the aortic true lumen from below. When the occlusion approaches the renal arteries, then accurate localisation of the true lumen entry point becomes particularly critical in order that stents can be deployed in the true lumen but as far distal to the renal arteries as possible. These two aspects of treatment are reliably achieved using a bi-directional approach (combined antegrade from an upper limb access and retrograde from a femoral access) and by using re-entry devices with fine, retractable needles that can accurately facilitate a point of re-entry.

PERCUTANEOUS VERSUS OPEN SURGERY FOR AORTO-ILIAC OCCLUSIVE DISEASE REVASCULARISATION

Whilst it is generally accepted that an endovascular-first approach should be the treatment of choice for those with less extensive disease (TASC A and B; for details of TASC classification see Chapter 2), there are few robust data with which to compare the two methods of revascularisation for more complex and extensive disease patterns. Current

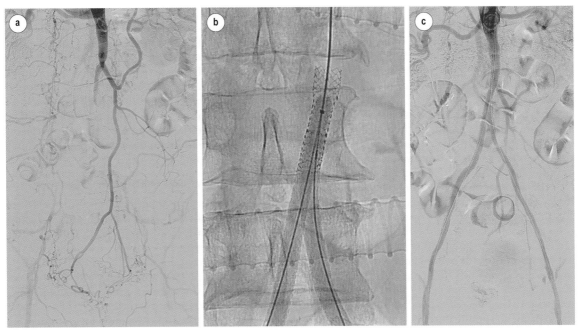

Figure 4.4 **(a)** Complete occlusion of the aorta (distal to the inferior mesenteric artery), common and external iliac arteries. **(b)** Post-dilatation after implantation of two self-expanding iliac stents within a single large balloon-expandable stent for the aorta. **(c)** Completion subtraction angiogram demonstrating unimpeded flow and complete revascularisation.

evidence is largely based on single-centre, retrospective studies with no large-scale, contemporary, randomised clinical trials to compare endovascular and open surgery for the treatment of TASC C and D aorto-iliac lesions. However, a contemporary meta-analysis has identified all studies that included TASC C and D disease between 1989 and 2010. Data were extracted for 1625 patients from all 28 studies that evaluated ER and 3733 patients from the 29 studies, which evaluated open bypass surgery. ER was found to be safer (complication rate 13.4% vs. 18.0%, P <0.001; 30-day mortality 0.7% vs. 2.6%, P <0.001) and incur a shorter length-of-stay (4 days vs. 13 days, P <0.001). The complications observed in the ER studies were more likely to be minor and self-limiting, such as haematoma and fever; whereas cardiac complications were frequent after bypass surgery, as were wound and graft infections. Findings favouring the more invasive procedure were that bypass surgery had increased primary patency rates at 1, 3 and 5 years of 94.8% versus 86.0%, 86.0% versus 80.0% and 82.7% versus 71.4%, respectively (all P <0.001), with a similar difference seen in secondary patency. It is apparent that ER is safer and less invasive, whilst surgery remains more durable. The published data reinforce the fact that both approaches are reasonable and should be considered a standard part of the armamentarium in the everyday clinical practice of patients with aorto-iliac disease. A reasonable approach is to apply the most appropriate form of treatment, matched to the individual patient's needs, disease morphology and risk factors. That may favour the durability of overall survival for the young, fit patient with claudication or a minimally invasive strategy for the elderly patient with tissue loss. Some argue that an endovascular-first approach to all patients remains reasonable as long as that procedure does not impact future surgical options.

ANGIOPLASTY VERSUS STENT VERSUS COVERED STENT

The Dutch Iliac Stent Trial randomised 279 patients with mostly stenotic disease to undergo either primary stent placement (n = 143) or PTA (n = 136) between 1993 and 1997.[19] At a mean follow-up of 6.3 and 5.7 years for the two groups respectively, there was no difference between the group who ultimately received stents versus those who underwent uncomplicated PTA. The group that fared best were those that underwent PTA and had bailout stenting. Those patients had superior preservation of symptomatic relief and long-term quality of life. No difference was observed between ankle-brachial pressure index (ABPI) or patency between any of the groups. The authors concluded that PTA with selective stenting strategy was the preferred method of iliac revascularisation.

The STAG trial was a contemporary, British, multicentre randomised controlled trial (RCT), which recruited 118 patients with iliac artery occlusions to undergo either PTA (n = 55) or primary iliac stenting (n = 57) (six were excluded because of protocol violations).[20] Primary stent placement resulted in increased technical success rates (98% vs. 84%; P = 0.007) and reduced major complication rates (5% vs. 20%; P = 0.010) compared with simple PTA. There was no difference in primary patency after a median follow-up period of 721 days and the authors concluded that primary stent placement was preferable to improve technical success and reduce complications.

Whilst there is no randomised trial that has compared self-expanding and balloon-expandable stents for the iliac artery, there are 24-month follow-up data from the BRAVISSIMO European prospective, multicentre registry.[21] That study enrolled 325 patients with aorto-iliac occlusive disease (n = 190, TASC A and B; n = 135 TASC C and D) and followed them with duplex ultrasound. They found similar primary patency rates of 88.0%, 88.5%, 91.9% and 84.8% for TASC A, B, C and D groups, respectively. There was a trend toward better patency for self-expanding stents (92.1%), compared with balloon expandable (85.2%) or a combination of both stent types (75.3%) ($P = 0.06$). These results suggest that more advanced disease may also be treated with endovascular intervention and that both stent types are reasonable to use in the aorto-iliac segment. However, when stenting the iliac arteries, it is worthwhile to consider the common and external iliac segments as separate regions with individual characteristics that favour different stent types. The common iliac artery is well suited to a balloon-expandable stent, which has placement accuracy and increased radial strength to overcome the calcification that is common in this region. Typically, disease involving the aortic bifurcation will be treated with bilateral stents placed in a 'kissing' configuration to reduce the risk of plaque-shift compromising the contralateral flow lumen. The external iliac artery is exposed to increased range of movement and mechanical strain upon hip flexion, which may benefit from a more flexible, self-expanding stent. The external iliac is also prone to rupture during dilatation, which may lead to sudden, catastrophic blood loss. This should always be considered, and a range of covered stents kept available to expeditiously deal with such events.

Covered stents may also be used as primary therapy in the iliac arteries because of their known property of in-stent restenosis reduction. COBEST (Covered versus Balloon Expandable Stent Trial) was an Australian, multicentre trial, which enrolled 125 patients with iliac occlusive disease (TASC B–D) and randomised them to treatment with a PTFE-covered (Advanta V12; Atrium) or a bare-metal stent (BMS; both self-expanding and balloon-expandable varieties were used) chosen at the operator's discretion.[22] The long-term results showed a significantly higher patency for covered stents compared to bare metal stents at 5 years (74.7% vs. 62.5%; $P = 0.01$). Subgroup analysis after 5 years found better patency of the TASC C and D lesions treated with covered stents (hazard ratio [HR], 8.64; 95% confidence interval [CI], 54.25–75.75; $P = 0.003$) along with a survival benefit compared to BMS. There was no such patency difference observed in the TASC B subgroup.[23]

✅ The COBEST trial results suggested that covered stents may confer protection from restenosis and should be considered in more severe patterns of aorto-iliac occlusive disease.

COMMON FEMORAL ARTERY DISEASE

Common femoral artery (CFA) disease has continued to be treated predominantly by open surgery. This is partly because of the nature of the disease as well as the technical difficulties with using stents in this region.

The CFA is prone to the development of eccentric and calcified atheromatous plaque with a predilection for the posterior artery wall (Fig. 4.5). Upon handling, the plaque is often friable and it frequently involves the bifurcation, proximal superficial femoral (SFA) and profunda femoris arteries. Whilst PTA can be effective in treating CFA disease, there is a risk of embolisation and if stents are required,

there is not a good solution for dealing with the bifurcation. Furthermore, it is a commonly held belief that the CFA is a flexion point that puts stents at risk of fracture, and that following implantation, the blood vessel cannot be used as an access site for future arterial access. Whilst neither of these points are entirely true, with the majority of vessel flexion taking place through the distal external iliac artery[24] and sheath insertion through well-incorporated self-expanding stents, a simple, safe manoeuvre, it helps explain the general reluctance to use endovascular techniques in this short arterial segment.

COMMON FEMORAL ENDARTERECTOMY

The CFA is located superficially within the femoral triangle and is easily accessed through surgical exposure under either local or general anaesthesia. Common femoral endarterectomy (CFE) can be extended proximally into the distal external iliac artery or distally into the profunda femoris and SFA. The longitudinal arteriotomy is commonly patched using the adjacent great saphenous vein, synthetic material (polytetrafluoroethylene [PTFE] or polyethylene terephthalate [Dacron]) or even an occluded segment of SFA, which can be resected, endarterectomised and used as patch material. Whilst that manoeuvre may be used to avoid the risk of infection associated with synthetic material, it prevents the option of future endovascular recanalisation of the occluded SFA and is therefore not recommended.

CFE is generally considered a safe surgical procedure; however, most published literature is based on single-centre case series of fewer than 100 patients. One exception is a large North American study that retrospectively reviewed admission and 30-day outcomes data of 1843 patients, which was recorded prospectively in the American College of Surgeons National Surgical Quality Improvement Program database.[25] That study found 30-day mortality to be 3.4%, wound complications 8.4% (86% were after discharge) and return to the operating theatre in 10%, indicating that CFE may not be as benign as previously thought. There remains little doubt that the procedure has excellent durability. In one single-centre study, 121 CFEs were performed over 8 years. They obtained complete follow-up (mean 4.2 years) in 111 patients (115 limbs). The 7-year primary patency, assisted primary patency and limb salvage rates were 96%, 100% and 100%, respectively; whilst freedom from further revascularisation and survival rates were 79% and 80%, respectively.[26] Another contemporary study, again from a single centre, demonstrated 1- and 5-year primary patency of 93% and 91%, respectively, in 65 CFE in 58 patients.[27]

In contemporary practice, CFE may be combined with an endovascular procedure to revascularize occlusive disease of the inflow or outflow arteries (Fig. 4.6). These so-called 'hybrid' procedures offer a durable solution for the CFA with fewer incisions to avoid long wounds, lymphatic disruption and the need to find long lengths of venous conduit.

Profundaplasty

Endarterectomy and patch repair of the profunda femoris artery (profundaplasty) may be performed in isolation to improve lower extremity perfusion, or as an adjunct during an inflow (aorto-femoral) or outflow (femoropopliteal/tibial) bypass procedure. Under those circumstances, it may be convenient to use the profunda femoris as the location of

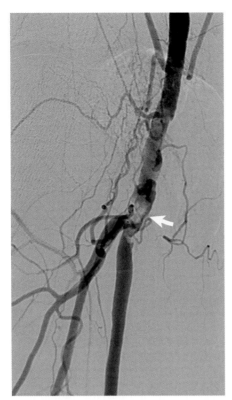

Figure 4.5 Typically, atherosclerotic disease found in the common femoral artery is calcified and eccentric (*arrow*). It frequently involves the origins of both superficial femoral and profunda femoris arteries, making femoral endarterectomy preferable to percutaneous transluminal angioplasty and stent implantation.

the proximal/distal anastomosis or extend the hood of the graft from the common femoral artery into the profunda artery. Profundaplasty, in isolation, has value in improving direct perfusion to the thigh and indirect to the calf/foot via geniculate collaterals. It may reduce the severity of claudication and ischaemic rest pain but is unlikely to result in wound healing in cases of ulceration or gangrene.

PERCUTANEOUS TREATMENT FOR THE COMMON FEMORAL ARTERY

There are only very few reports in the literature of endovascular treatment for isolated common femoral disease, with most reporting good outcomes in small selected patient cohorts. However, there is one large, prospective multicentre study with published experience using PTA alone, provisional stenting and atherectomy with PTA in 167 patients.[28] Over a 7-year period, they treated 114, 15 and 38 patients in each of those groups, respectively. The entire cohort underwent a mean follow-up period of 42.5 months. Twelve-month primary patencies were reported as 78.4% for PTA alone, 100% for provisional stenting and 94.5% for atherectomy with PTA; with only 3% suffering major complications and 0.6% perioperative death. They concluded that percutaneous CFA interventions are safe and effective in selected patients.

The Endovascular Versus Open Repair of the Common Femoral Artery trial (NCT01353651) was a 117-subject, French, multicentre RCT designed to compare CFE with direct stenting for the CFA. Results published in 2017 found that stenting was safer, with a 1-month combined endpoint of mortality and/or major morbidity rate of 12.5% versus 26% (*P* = 0.05) and a shorter length of hospital stay (3.2 vs. 6.3 days; *P*<0.0001). At 2-years of follow-up primary patency,

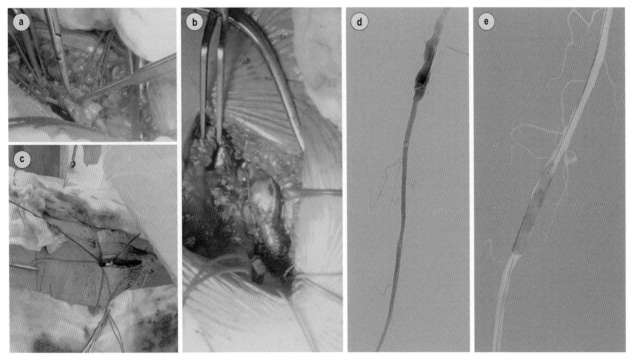

Figure 4.6 A hybrid procedure may involve common femoral endarterectomy followed by an endovascular intervention through that exposed artery or its patch repair. **(a)** Posterior wall plaque being removed during common femoral endarterectomy. **(b)** Arterial repair with a saphenous vein patch. **(c)** A sheath is introduced after direct patch puncture under fluoroscopic guidance. **(d)** Subtraction angiography with injection of contrast through the sheath. **(e)** Percutaneous transluminal angioplasty of an atherosclerotic lesion at the adductor canal.

freedom from TLR and overall survival rates were statistically indistinguishable between the two groups. Suggesting that there is a role for the less invasive treatment, particularly in the medically comorbid.[28a]

In a meta-analysis (28 studies; 2914 limbs) comparing CFE and endovascular therapy with routine or selective stenting of the CFA, the authors observed a primary patency rate of 84% (95% CI, 75–92%) for routine stenting, 78% (95% CI, 69–85%) for selective stenting and 93% (95% CI, 90–96%) for CFE. There was no difference in long-term patency rates between routine stenting and CFE but a significantly higher local complication rate with surgery 22% (95% CI, 14–32%) versus 5% (95% CI, 2–10%). Mortality was also higher for CFE, 23.1% (95% CI, 14–33%) versus 5.3% (95% CI, 1–11%) for routine stenting, reinforcing that the endovascular approach is associated with fewer complications.[29]

SUPERFICIAL FEMORAL ARTERY DISEASE

The SFA extends from the CFA bifurcation to the adductor hiatus. It runs through the muscular borders of the adductor canal and comes under a great deal of mechanical strain (forces including flexion, torsion, compression and elongation) during hip and knee flexion.[30] This results in the development of dense atherosclerosis, particularly in smokers, with stenosis and heavy calcification a common feature. It also poses a mechanical challenge to the implantation of permanent metallic devices, such as stents that need to be resistant to such forces over time.

SURGICAL BYPASS

Surgical bypass can be performed using synthetic material (PTFE or Dacron) or autogenous vein. To maximise patency, proximal anastomosis at a site with adequate inflow should be undertaken. This would typically be the CFA, but may be the SFA or profunda femoris artery depending on the pattern of disease and length of available conduit. The distal anastomosis would be to the most proximal vessel sufficiently free of disease to suture, which can provide at least one in-line blood vessel to the foot, although bypass to a blind segment of popliteal artery ('isolated popliteal segment') is well described. The most common distal anastomotic sites are the above- and below-knee popliteal arteries. Anastomosis to the above-knee popliteal artery is now infrequent given these are usually patients with claudication (rather than having more extensive disease and CLTI) and are treatable by endovascular means if necessary. The crural vessels may also be used for the distal anastomosis. They are accessible throughout their lengths with varying approaches and degrees of technical difficulty. The choice of crural vessel to use is based on that which is least diseased, and which provides continuous run-off to the foot. The quality of the outflow system is an important determinant of graft patency.

The great saphenous vein is the preferred conduit and may be used in situ after valvotomy or be reversed. There is no difference in patency between in situ and reversed grafts,[31] but in situ grafts provide an appropriately small distal segment for use in tibial bypass and therefore may be preferred at the ankle. Vein may be harvested in one single incision or by leaving skin bridges to better approximate the wound and relieve tension. It may then be tunnelled in an anatomical or subcutaneous plane to facilitate future surgical access for patch graft repair. No patency advantage has been demonstrated for any of these techniques over another. If ipsilateral great saphenous is not available then contralateral great saphenous, spliced small saphenous, arm vein or synthetic material should be used in that order.[32] Conduit should preferably be a single graft but splicing and/or repair of varicose segments is sometimes required. Synthetic graft should be used as a last option, and has very poor patency rates below the knee. If a tibial anastomosis is to be performed with synthetic material, a vein cuff configured as a Miller cuff, Taylor patch or St Mary's boot is generally recommended to improve patency through minimising compliance mismatch, reducing mechanical injury and expanding the distal anastomosis to lessen the impact of perianastomotic intimal hyperplasia.[32] There is no short-term difference in patency rates between PTFE and Dacron,[31] but long-term patency may be superior with the latter.[32,33]

The patency of surgical bypass has traditionally been evaluated using a combination of ankle–brachial index, to compare with the preoperative value, history of symptom return, clinical examination and occasionally, duplex ultrasound to check for flow within the graft.

The PREVENT III trial is the largest prospective, randomised, double-blind, multicentre trial to have performed an objective evaluation of patency rates for venous bypass surgery in patients with CLI.[34] Some 1404 subjects were enrolled to determine whether a novel molecular therapy agent (edifoglide) was useful in the prevention of vein graft failure. Whilst no difference was detected as a result of the drug, the dataset serves as a useful cohort to determine the patency rates of vein bypass. Binary restenosis was defined as >70% on angiography, >50% with recurrent symptoms, ABPI <0.4, toe pressure <30 mmHg or duplex ultrasound stenosis with a peak systolic velocity ratio of >3.0 or velocity >300 cm/s; less sensitive standards compared with those used to evaluate endovascular therapy patency in contemporary trials (>50% on angiography or peak systolic ratio >2.0–2.5). Twelve-month graft primary patency, limb salvage and patient survival rates were 61%, 88% and 84%, respectively. There was no difference in patency when vein bypass was performed at a distal anastomotic site above or below the knee. This trial gives us a well-defined and rigorously adjudicated measure of patency with which to compare other methods of SFA revascularisation in patients with CLI.

✔ Bypass graft surveillance programmes with duplex ultrasound have been used to detect patency-threatening lesions before complete thrombosis. This is thought to be worthwhile as these lesions are common and may often be asymptomatic before complete graft occlusion. Several studies have demonstrated a patency advantage with intense duplex surveillance over the first 2 years, the period where significant intimal proliferation is most common.[35,36] However, there is conflicting evidence, with a large RCT showing that duplex surveillance after venous femoral distal bypass grafts leads to no significant clinical benefit or QoL improvement at 18 months.[37] Most guidelines recommend at least 2 years of formal, structured, combined clinical and ultrasound surveillance for vein bypass grafts.[8,38] This is not true for synthetic bypass, where patency failure is less likely to be preceded by a detectable stenotic lesion.

PERCUTANEOUS TREATMENT FOR THE SUPERFICIAL FEMORAL ARTERY

Since the first PTA in 1964, there has been an ever-expanding number of endovascular options developed to treat occlusive disease of the SFA. Angioplasty itself has become more sophisticated and its technique has matured. There has been extensive development in the field of stents, stent grafts, atherectomy and drug-coating technology. However, evidence of effectiveness has often lagged behind the rapid pace of technological evolution. When comparative trials have been performed, they have usually included a high proportion of claudicants with short to moderate length, single-level disease, and most have compared the investigational technology to conventional balloon angioplasty. These trials have largely focused on angiographic outcomes and not patient-centred measures.

Nitinol self-expanding stents

✔ ✔ Nitinol self-expanding stents have superior effectiveness to PTA. A contemporary meta-analysis accumulated results from 17 randomised clinical trials (627 subjects), which used either primary nitinol stenting or PTA for symptomatic femoropopliteal occlusive disease (mean length 74.6 mm nitinol stent group, 66.7 mm PTA group).[39] They found that the nitinol stent group had higher rates of technical success (95.8% vs. 64.2%, P <0.001), and at 12-month follow-up lower rates of both target lesion revascularisation (TLR) (odds ratio [OR], 2.47; 95% CI, 0.72–8.49, P = 0.065), a subjective endpoint that may be susceptible to bias if not properly defined, and binary restenosis (OR, 3.02; 95% CI, 1.3–6.71, P <0.001), with similar safety outcomes. Whilst lower rates of restenosis have been demonstrated, the neointimal proliferation that does form within these permanent metallic implants is a bulky lesion that poses a particular challenge to future attempts at endovascular intervention, which may be difficult to cross and frequently recoil after angioplasty. It is for this reason that many vascular specialists have explored alternative technologies.

Stent grafts

Stent grafts covered in PTFE offer a theoretical advantage over uncovered stents. The PTFE acts as a barrier to neointimal migration and proliferation, which can then only compromise the lumen at the proximal and distal edges of the stent (edge-restenosis). The VIBRANT trial randomised 148 subjects with symptomatic and complex (TASC C and D) SFA disease to a bare-metal, nitinol stent or Viabahn stent graft at 19 US centres.[40] Although this differing pattern of edge-restenosis was observed, there was no difference in primary patency rates over a follow-up period of 3 years. Given that stent grafts are costly and cover collaterals, which may be important if future patency is lost, their use is difficult to justify as part of routine practice.

Atherectomy

Atherectomy is another technology that has theoretical advantages over stenting. It debulks the atheromatous plaque and leaves behind no permanent implant. However, it may pose a risk of distal embolisation and there are concerns about its potential to stimulate restenosis through aggressive vessel wall injury. Whilst no randomised, comparative data exist, the DEFINITIVE LE study was a large, prospective, multicentre, single arm trial, which demonstrated the effectiveness of directional atherectomy through satisfactory 12-month primary-patency rates with a low incidence of perforation and distal embolisation.[41]

Drug-coated balloon angioplasty

✔ ✔ Angioplasty balloons coated with the antiproliferative drug paclitaxel (DCB) offer a novel method of revascularisation and drug delivery, which also leaves behind no permanent metallic implant and has the potential to be combined with other therapies, such as atherectomy and stenting. A 2016 meta-analysis examined data from eight multicentre RCTs, which each compared DCB to PTA for stenotic femoropopliteal lesions.[42] These studies each assessed short-to-moderate-length lesions, ranging in length between 4.3 cm and 8.9 cm, with proportion of total occlusions ranging from 26–100%. The meta-analysis found that paclitaxel-coated balloons were superior to PTA in reducing TLR at 12 months, an effect, which persisted during longer follow-up. However, there was some evidence of differential efficacy, with not all paclitaxel-coated balloons having as pronounced an anti-restenotic effect. It is likely that this relates to the differing excipient (spacer) molecule, which plays a major role in determining efficiency of drug transfer and the deposition of drug reservoirs into the arterial wall. It may also be related to the different formulation (crystalline or amorphous) or concentration of paclitaxel, which ranges between 2.0 and 3.5 μg/mm[42] in commercially available balloon catheters, as well as the stability of the drug coating as it traverses the haemostatic sheath and target arteries.

Drug-eluting stents

✓✓ Nitinol, paclitaxel-eluting, self-expanding stents (DES) have demonstrated efficacy in the SFA, superior to both PTA and BMS. The ZILVER PTX trial randomised subjects with symptomatic femoropopliteal disease (91% claudicants) to DES (n = 236) or PTA (n = 238).[43] Of those in the PTA arm who required a bailout stent, a secondary randomisation took place to DES (n = 61) or BMS (n = 59). After 5 years, the DES was superior to PTA in freedom from persistent or worsening symptoms of ischaemia (79.8% vs. 59.3%, P <0.01), primary patency (66.4% vs. 43.4%, P <0.01), and freedom from TLR (83.1% vs. 67.6%, P <0.01). Similarly, clinical benefit (81.8% vs. 63.8%, P = 0.02), patency (72.4% vs. 53.0%, P = 0.03), and freedom from TLR (84.9% vs. 71.6%, P = 0.06) with provisional DES were improved over provisional BMS. The IMPERIAL trial was a large multicenter, non-inferiority RCT conducted over 65 centres in Austria, Belgium, Canada, Germany, Japan, New Zealand, and the USA.[44] Patients were randomly assigned (2:1) to receive treatment with Eluvia (a newer generation of paclitaxel and polymer-coated DES) or Zilver PTX. Non-inferiority was shown for both efficacy and safety endpoints at 12 months: primary patency was 86.8% (231/266) in the Eluvia group and 81.5% (106/130) in the Zilver PTX group (difference 5.3%; P <0.0001), suggesting that both DES are effective at providing mid-term patency and reasonable options for claudicants with femoropopliteal disease.

The femoropopliteal area is becoming increasingly crowded with new technology; however, studies comparing the latest devices are lagging well behind the expanding therapeutic arsenal. BASIL (Bypass vs. Angioplasty in Severe Ischaemia of the Leg)-3 is a randomised, pragmatic, multicentre, three-arm, open-label trial of alternative revascularisation strategies, designed to evaluate the clinical benefit and cost-effectiveness of DCB, DES and plain balloon angioplasty with bailout BMS revascularisation for severe limb ischaemia secondary to femoropopliteal disease. It is aiming to recruit 861 subjects from approximately 60 vascular centres in England, Wales, Scotland and other European Union states. More comparative trials such as these are expected to follow.

A meta-analysis was published in 2018, which brought into question the safety of the anti-proliferative drug paclitaxel. It specifically investigated all-cause mortality in patients with claudication (89%) undergoing paclitaxel-coated balloon angioplasty in the femoropopliteal arterial segment (28 RCTs; 4663 patients). At 1 year all-cause mortality was similar between paclitaxel-coated devices and control arms (2.3% vs. 2.3%). At 2 years (12 RCTs; 2316 patients) mortality was significantly increased in the paclitaxel arm (7.2% vs. 3.8% crude risk of death; risk ratio, 1.68; 95% CI, 1.15–2.47; —number-needed-to-harm, 29 patients [95% CI, 19–59]). At follow-up of 4 to 5 years (3 RCTs with 863 cases) that risk increased further (14.7% vs. 8.1% crude risk of death; risk ratio, 1.93; 95% CI, 1.27–2.93; with a number-needed-to-harm of 14 patients [95% CI, 9–32]).[45] However, a subsequent meta-analysis evaluated all-cause death in patients with CLTI demonstrating no difference between paclitaxel-coated devices compared to uncoated controls in 11 RCTs with a mean follow-up of 25.6 months (18.6% paclitaxel vs. 19.9% control groups relative risk, 0.93; 95% CI, 0.78–1.12, P = 0.45.[46] In response to those safety concerns, the SWEDEPAD trial published interim results looking at safety. SWEDEPAD is a multicentre, randomised, open-label, registry-based clinical trial. At the time of the analysis, 2289 patients had been randomly assigned to treatment with drug-coated devices (1149 patients) or treatment with uncoated devices (1140 patients). There was no mortality difference observed in the paclitaxel coated or control arms during 1 to 4 years of follow-up.[47] There is ongoing research underway to continue to investigate this safety concern, however, most regulatory bodies have allowed ongoing use of these devices until more information is available.

SURGICAL BYPASS VERSUS PERCUTANEOUS INTERVENTION

Direct comparisons of surgical bypass and ER methods are very much needed; however, they are limited because of variations in vascular anatomy, extent of disease and indications for treatment.

The BASIL trial was a randomised controlled trial designed to compare infra-inguinal vein bypass with PTA for patients with severe limb ischaemia and was published in 2005.[13] They found broadly similar amputation-free survival (AFS) and overall survival rates during the first 2 years of follow-up. A subsequent analysis showed that there was an increase in overall survival for the bypass group beyond 2 years of follow-up. Conversely, endovascular therapy was found to be safer with equivalent QoL outcomes and was significantly less costly. In that trial, the endovascular therapy arm did not use stents, drug-eluting devices or atherectomy; adjunctive procedures that are now commonplace and known to improve patency rates and add cost compared with PTA alone.

✓ In a meta-analysis, which included 23 unique studies (12 779 patients) that evaluated the comparative effectiveness of endovascular and surgical revascularisation between 1995 and 2012 the authors commented on the dearth of high-quality evidence.[48] There was only one directly comparative RCT. Their analysis of these mostly observational studies found no difference in all-cause mortality, lower extremity amputation or AFS between the two forms of treatment. Rates of primary patency favoured ER at 1 year (OR 0.63, 0.46–0.86), and secondary patency at both 1 year (OR 0.57, 0.40–0.82) and 2–3 years (OR 0.49, 0.28–0.85).

The Best Endovascular versus Best Surgical Therapy in Patients with Critical Limb Ischemia (BEST-CLI) trial (NCT02060630) expects to enrol 2100 participants over 120 North American and other centres internationally, with the intent to randomise 1:1 to open surgery with venous conduit or best contemporary endovascular treatment. Enrolment is ongoing, having surpassed 1843 enrolled subjects in late 2019. The ZILVERPASS randomised trial (NCT01952457), evaluated 220 patients with extensive and symptomatic SFA disease, comparing treatment with a paclitaxel DES to prosthetic bypass. It found similar 12-month patency rates (74.5%; 95% CI, 66.3–82.7 for Zilver PTX stents and 72.5%; 95% CI, 63.7–81.3 for prosthetic bypass). However, the 30-day complication rate was significantly lower in the Zilver PTX group (4.4% vs. 11.3% P = 0.0004) as was the procedural time and hospital stay.[49]

POPLITEAL ARTERY DISEASE

The popliteal artery is one of the most challenging infra-inguinal vessels to treat with endovascular means and warrants individual consideration beyond that of the SFA. Coursing between the adductor hiatus and the origin of the anterior tibial artery, it suffers repeated biomechanical stresses during knee flexion and has a tapering diameter, which provides sizing challenges for most current generation implantable devices.[50] Management may be challenging, and with few randomised trials dedicated to answering questions of technical success and durability, the correct approach remains contentious. The popliteal artery is also the location for several non-atherosclerotic disease processes such as aneurysm, cystic adventitia disease and popliteal entrapment, which may occasionally make accurate diagnosis a challenge and should be considered in younger patients with few vascular risk factors.

PERCUTANEOUS TREATMENT FOR THE POPLITEAL ARTERY

Due to the repetitive and extreme physical forces that exist on devices implanted into the popliteal artery, it has been attractive for interventionists to consider options that leave behind no permanent implant. In the past, PTA has played a primary strategic role with early generation stents thought to be at high risk of fracture and technical failure.

The TASC II guidelines recommended PTA for patients with stenoses or occlusions up to 15 cm in length of both the superficial femoral and popliteal arteries, if the infrageniculate popliteal artery or trifurcation are not involved.[8] Despite these recommendations, there are few studies dedicated to assessing the performance of PTA in the popliteal artery. What scientific reports are available reveal generally disappointing patency rates, inferior to that seen in the superficial femoral artery and as low as 30–45% at 12 months.[51] This has led many vascular specialists to seek more durable solutions for PAD of the popliteal artery.

Atherectomy

Directional atherectomy may be used for debulking atheroma from the popliteal artery, but it has been rarely assessed in clinical studies. In a subset analysis of the DEFINITIVE LE study, 162 target lesions in 158 subjects with short popliteal artery lesions (mean length 5.8 cm) were assessed after 1 year. They found a promising 80.3% core-lab-adjudicated, duplex and angiography-assessed primary patency with a low 3.7% bailout stenting rate.[52] It may be that atherectomy has a role in the popliteal artery, particularly in debulking heavily calcified atheroma, which may be otherwise resistant to angioplasty or stenting.

Nitinol, self-expanding stents

✓ The ETAP (Endovascular Treatment of Atherosclerotic Popliteal Artery Lesion-Balloon Angioplasty Versus Primary Stenting) trial is the only RCT to have addressed endovascular treatment for the popliteal artery specifically.[51] It was a prospective, multicentre trial conducted on single, de novo, popliteal artery lesions throughout nine European centres. Lesions were not included if they involved the SFA or extended to the crural arteries. Two hundred and forty-six subjects were randomised to either nitinol stent placement (n = 127) or PTA (n = 119) and evaluated with colour duplex ultrasound at 6 and 12 months. Twelve-month primary patency was significantly higher in the nitinol stent group compared to PTA (67.4% vs. 44.9%; P = 0.002) and clinically driven TLR was significantly lower (14.7% vs. 44.1%; P = 0.0001). This difference was solely accounted for by a 25.2% acute failure rate in the PTA group because of either residual stenosis >30% or a flow-limiting dissection that did not resolve after prolonged balloon dilatation. In a secondary analysis where provisional bailout stenting was not considered loss of patency and TLR, no difference was observed between the groups at 12 months. The authors concluded that primary PTA with provisional bailout stenting for short lesions of the popliteal artery is a reasonable strategy. The 2-year technical and clinical results were also published with 183 patients (89 stent and 94 PTA) available for analysis. Primary patency rate was significantly higher in the stent group (64.2%) than for PTA (31.3%, P = 0.0001) with a provisional stent placement considered a TLR (and loss of primary patency) and the authors concluded a shift towards primary stenting versus provisional stenting.[53] These results suggest patency to be poor with both PTA and stenting in the isolated popliteal lesion suggesting that surgery or newer generation endovascular devices warrant increased consideration.

Novel devices for the popliteal artery

There are several new devices with early, observational data to support their use in the popliteal artery. These include DCB, the BioMimics 3D (Veryan, West Sussex, UK), a nitinol stent with unique three-dimensional helical geometry and swirling flow properties and the Supera stent (Abbott Vascular, Santa Clara, CA, USA) made from six nitinol wires interwoven around a duly-sized mandrill. The results from the prospective, single arm MIMICS-2 trial investigating the BioMimics 3D stent (NCT02400905) have been promising with 12-month primary stent patency of 73.1% (95% CI, 67.3–78.2) and a 30-day freedom from major adverse event of 99.6% (95% CI, 97.7–100).[54] The Supera stent is extremely flexible, fracture- and kink-resistant with high-resistive radial strength properties, which make it ideal for use in the popliteal artery. The largest of these observational, single-centre studies was a retrospective review of 101 patients who had Supera stents placed in the popliteal artery for both de novo atherosclerotic disease and restenosis.[55] With a mean lesion length of 58.4 mm, they found impressive primary and secondary patencies of 94.6%/97.9% at 6 months and 87.7%/96.5% at 12 months, respectively.

Whilst much research has been conducted with a focus on PAD of the SFA, the popliteal artery is often ignored or included in smaller numbers within those SFA trials. PTA remains the cornerstone for endovascular treatment; however, there are a host of new devices broadly suited to the popliteal territory. Whilst results from registry data evaluating new stent technology in the popliteal artery are encouraging, further randomised trials are necessary to confirm their safety and long-term durability.

INFRA-POPLITEAL ARTERY DISEASE

Intervention for occlusive disease of the IP arteries is performed almost exclusively for CLTI. Therefore, there is no evidence by which to recommend IP intervention for patients with claudication. The practice of treating IP arteries to improve patency after a more proximal intervention (surgical or endovascular), whilst intuitive, also lacks supportive evidence.

There are several revascularisation options to achieve in-line blood flow to the periphery to facilitate wound healing or pain relief in the patient with CLTI. These include a variety of different percutaneous interventions, including balloon angioplasty with uncoated or DCB, cutting balloons, cryoplasty, atherectomy, laser atherectomy, stenting with bare-metal, bioresorbable or DES, as well as surgical bypass. Many of these endovascular technologies suffer from poor-quality, retrospective datasets to support their use. Relatively few have sufficient supporting evidence to withstand evidence-led, scientific interrogation.

SURGICAL BYPASS FOR INFRA-POPLITEAL DISEASE

✔ There is an extensive body of literature to attest to the efficacy of lower extremity bypass to treat occlusive IP disease.[56] In these smaller distal vessels, venous conduit is preferred. This is normally great saphenous vein in an in situ or reversed configuration; however, spliced small saphenous and arm vein may be used. Synthetic grafts with a vein cuff have also been used in the past, with inferior results. As with bypass for femoropopliteal lesions, the proximal anastomosis site may vary depending on the extent of disease. Whilst bypass from the CFA may be performed, the proximal anastomosis can also be taken from a more distal location, such as the SFA or popliteal artery, which may reduce the length of conduit required. The distal anastomosis can be to any of the crural arteries, or indeed to the proximal pedal arteries themselves. If the surgery is distal to the proximal thigh, the use of a pneumatic tourniquet may avoid clamping of the tibial arteries, which are often small and calcified.

There are no large RCTs that have evaluated surgical bypass in isolated IP disease; however, both the BASIL and PREVENT III trials included a significant proportion of subjects with disease in that location, with the tibial or pedal arteries the site of distal anastomosis in 31% and 65% of

participants in those two trials, respectively.[13,34] In PREVENT III, 12-month primary patency, limb salvage and patient survival were 61%, 88% and 84%, respectively, with no observed difference for bypass above or below the knee. In BASIL, 12-month AFS was 68%, and overall survival 71%; patency was not evaluated. Major morbidity in those two trials is particularly relevant, with 30-day mortality 5.5% and 2.7%, myocardial infarction 7% and 4.7%, stroke 1.5% and 1.4% and wound complications seen in 22% and 4.8% of subjects in BASIL and PREVENT II, respectively. These results clearly demonstrate that bypass surgery in patients with CLI carries a significant risk. In a meta-analysis of autologous, popliteal-to-distal bypass grafts from 31 published series between 1981 and 2004, the authors found 1-, 3- and 5-year primary patency of 81.5%/72.3%/63.1%, secondary patency 85.9%/76.7%/70.7% and limb salvage rates of 88.5%/82.3%/77.7%, respectively.[56] This demonstrates the durability and limb preservation efficacy of a good-quality, IP, venous bypass graft.

PERCUTANEOUS TREATMENT FOR INFRA-POPLITEAL DISEASE

The use of endovascular techniques for the treatment of occlusive IP disease has gained widespread acceptance and is now undertaken by many as the first-line treatment for patients with CLI. In the past, tibial artery intervention was plagued by low rates of immediate technical success. This was caused by a paucity of dedicated endovascular devices and purpose-built guidewires, as well as rudimentary technique. There has been a rapid increase in the availability of dedicated guidewires designed to cross chronic total occlusions, support catheters, angioplasty balloons and re-entry devices, which have steadily increased those rates of success. Moreover, advanced refinements of technique to perfect the bi-directional approach with retrograde (pedal/tibial) access, introduce coronary techniques such as controlled antegrade–retrograde subintimal tracking (CART), reverse CART (where an inflated balloon creates a target space for the opposite wire), and the double balloon technique (where overlapping balloons are positioned from antegrade and retrograde before simultaneous inflation to connect bi-directional subintimal guidewires) have concurrently laid the foundation for success. As a result, most contemporary series now have technical success rates in the high 90% range.[57]

Percutaneous transluminal angioplasty

✔ There are many case series reporting outcomes of PTA performed to the crural arteries. Romiti et al. performed a meta-analysis comparing 30 published articles reporting outcomes of 2693 crural artery PTAs from 1990–2006.[58] They found an immediate technical success rate of 89%, 1- and 3-year primary patency of 58.1% and 48.6% and secondary patency rates of 68.2% and 62.9%, respectively. Despite those rates of success and patency, which are poor by today's standards, limb salvage rates remained acceptable at 86% and 82.4% after 1 and 3 years. Furthermore, those limb salvage rates were comparable with another meta-analysis conducted to evaluate results of distal bypass surgery over that same period.[56]

Drug-coated balloon angioplasty

A large number of retrospective studies and small, single-centre, randomised trials emerged between 2010 and 2013, with results that suggested DCB may have the potential to limit restenosis and improve patency for angioplasty to the arteries below the knee.[59–61] However, following that period the IN.PACT Deep trial published results from 358 patients with IP lesions who were randomised 2:1 to DCB or PTA.[62] This large, multicentre study was well adjudicated, using independent, blinded core labs and a clinical events committee. At 12 months, they found no difference in late lumen loss (LLL; 0.61 mm vs. 0.62 mm; $P = 0.95$), or clinically driven TLR rates (17.7% vs. 15.8%; $P = 0.66$). There was also a trend toward higher amputation rates in the DCB arm compared to PTA (8.8% vs. 3.6%; $P = 0.08$), which did not reach statistical significance. This led to a complete withdrawal of the device and a root cause analysis, performed to determine the reasons for its failure. This result leaves us uncertain as to whether DCB technology has any benefit over PTA and some have questioned its safety in patients with CLI.

A 2020 meta-analysis included 10 studies (1593 patients), which were graded as moderate to low quality.[63] Twelve-month outcomes for DCB versus PTA were limb salvage rate, 94.0% versus 95.7% (OR, 0.92; 95% CI, 0.39–2.21); and survival rate, 89.8% versus 92.9% (OR, 0.69; 95% CI, 0.39–1.21). Twelve-month outcomes for PTA versus DCB were restenosis rate, 62.0% versus 32.9% (OR, 2.87; 95% CI, 0.83–9.92); and TLR rate, 27.8% versus 14.0% (OR, 2.76; 95% CI, 0.90–8.48). Twelve-month AFS rate for DCB versus PTA; 82.5% versus 88.7% (OR, 0.79; 95% CI, 0.23–2.75). Although there were trends toward reduced rates of restenosis and TLR with DCB, no statistically significant differences were found in any of those outcome measures. However, since that time data from several other RCTs have become available.

The IN.PACT BTK RCT (NCT02963649) investigating safety and efficacy of the paclitaxel Drug-eluting balloon IN.PACT 014 versus PTA below the knee, began recruiting in 2016 with a primary outcome of LLL at 9 months. Their results were presented in late 2020, demonstrating no difference in primary safety or efficacy endpoints between DCB and PTA.

The Lutonix BTK trial (NCT01870401) completed its recruitment of 442 patients across 51 sites throughout the USA, Europe, Canada, Japan and Australia in 2019. Their 6-month follow-up published data showed freedom from lower limb major amputation to be non-inferior in the DCB group (99.3%) versus PTA (99.4%; non-inferiority $P<0.001$) and Kaplan–Meier analyses demonstrated superior patency for DCB in both the overall intention-to treat (ITT) and proximal-segment groups.[64] However, their 12-month results presented in January 2021 showed those Kaplan–Meier patency curves converge and become statistically indistinguishable.

Despite those two negative trials, results from the ACoART II-BTK trial were more promising. This prospective, multicenter, randomised study (NCT02137577) enrolled 120 patients and randomly assigned them to angioplasty with either paclitaxel DCB ($n = 61$) or conventional PTA ($n = 59$). Primary patency at 6 months was 75.0% in the DCB and 28.3% in the control groups ($P<0.001$), while LLL was 0.43±0.62 mm for DCBs versus 0.99±0.55 mm for

control ($P<0.001$). Freedom from CD-TLR at 12 months was 91.5% in the DCB group versus 76.8% in the controls ($P=0.03$); there was no significant difference in mortality (1.7% DCB vs. 3.6% controls; $P=0.53$).[65] This suggests there may still be a role for certain paclitaxel DCB in the IP circulation but further effectiveness data is needed to support their use. It is noteworthy that several DCBs with sirolimus coating are currently undergoing early clinical trials with some proponents believing this may be a more effective antiproliferative agent for arteries below the knee based on the success of limus coated stents in that region.

Bare-metal stents

Even though simple angioplasty has become technically achievable, in the majority of patients it remains relatively common to achieve a suboptimal outcome with PTA alone. The goal of stenting has been to treat an unsatisfactory result because of elastic recoil, residual stenosis, flow-limiting dissection or perforation.

A single RCT has compared a variety of BMS (balloon- and self-expanding) to PTA in 38 limbs. In this small and under-powered study, there was no statistical advantage to BMS over PTA in survival (74.7% vs. 69.3%), limb salvage (91.7% vs. 90%), primary (56% vs. 66%) or secondary (64% vs. 79.5%) patency rates after 12 months.[66] In a 2009 systematic review, 18 non-randomised studies comprising 640 patients who had infra-genicular stent implantation at experienced centres had data pooled.[67] Of those, 232 had balloon-expandable BMS, 116 self-expanding BMS, 272 balloon expandable DES and 20 bioresorbable stents. They found that bailout stenting after unsatisfactory PTA in this region derived satisfactory angiographic results but no patency advantage. Balloon- and self-expanding stent types were unable to be separated in terms of primary patency (73% vs. 79%; $P = 0.18$) and clinical outcomes (TLR 18% vs. 6%, $P = 1.0$; limb salvage 98% vs. 96%, $P = 1.0$) after a median follow-up of 12 months.

It is apparent that BMS are effective at treating residual stenosis, elastic recoil and dissection after PTA, thus improving the immediate technical result, but they are not able to achieve improved long-term patency as they also suffer from significant restenosis.

Drug-eluting stents

✓✓ DES are known to reduce the neointimal proliferation response to vascular wall injury, which in turn leads to reduction in the luminal area (negative remodelling), recurrent stenosis and loss of patency. In contrast to the low-level evidence, which exists for the use of other endovascular technologies below the knee, the use of coronary DES is supported by results from four RCTs[68–71] (Table 4.2) and four meta-analyses.[72–75]

The YUKON-BTK trial was the first to publish, after randomising 161 patients with CLI (47%) and IC (53%) to treatment with a polymer-free, 2% sirolimus-coated stent or the same stent uncoated.[69] The DES achieved a superior primary patency at the 12-month follow-up of 80.6% versus 55.6% for the BMS ($P = 0.004$). TLR was also improved upon with the use of the DES (9.7% vs. 17.5%; $P = 0.29$) but not significantly so. At a longer

Table 4.2   Randomised controlled trials that have evaluated drug-eluting stents in the infra-popliteal circulation

Trial	Year	Study design		Patients (n)	Mean lesion length (mm)	Endpoints
YUKON-BTK (Rastan et al.[69])	2011 and 2012	RCT	Sirolimus-eluting stent (polymer free) vs. Bare-metal stent	161 (75 CLI; 86 IC)	31	Primary patency (12 month); 81% vs. 56% (P = 0.004) Secondary patency (12 month); 92% vs. 71% (P = 0.005) TLR (12 month); 9.7% vs. 17.5% (P = 0.29) Limb salvage in CLI (2.8 y); 97.4% vs. 87.1% (P = 0.10) Freedom from amputation, TVR, AMI and death (2.8 y) 65.8 vs. 44.6% (P = 0.02)
DESTINY (Bosiers et al.[68])	2012	RCT	Everolimus-eluting stent vs. Bare-metal stent	140 (all CLI)	17	Primary patency (12 month); 85% vs. 54% (P = 0.0001) LLL (12 month); 0.78 mm vs. 1.41 mm (P = 0.001) TLR (12 month); 8% vs. 35% (P = 0.005) Limb salvage (12 month); 99% vs. 97% (NS) Death (12 month); 18% vs. 16% (P = 0.06)
ACHILLES (Scheinert et al.[70])	2012	RCT	Sirolimus-eluting stent vs. Angioplasty	200 (CLI and IC)	27	Primary patency (12 month); 78 vs. 58% (P = 0.019) TLR (12 month); 10% vs. 17% (P = 0.257) Limb salvage (12 month); 86% vs. 80% (P = 0.3) Death; 10% vs. 12% (P = 0.82)
IDEAS (Siablis et al.[71])	2014	RCT	Zotarolimus-, sirolimus- or everolimus-eluting stents vs. Paclitaxel-coated balloon	50 (CLI and IC)	148/127	Binary restenosis (6 month); 28% vs. 57.9% (P = 0.0457) TLR (6 month); 7.7% vs. 13.6% (P = 0.65)

AMI, Acute myocardial infarction; *CLI*, critical limb ischaemia; *IC*, intermittent claudication; *LLL*, late lumen loss; *NS*, not significant; *RCT*, randomised controlled trial; *TLR*, target lesion revascularisation; *TVR*, target vessel revascularisation.

follow-up of mean 2.8 years, limb salvage was higher in the CLI patients; however, this was not statistically significant (97.4% vs. 87.1%; P = 0.10); the primary endpoint of freedom from amputation, TVR, acute myocardial infarction (AMI) and death found in favour of the DES (65.8% vs. 44.6%; P = 0.02).

Following that study, the DESTINY trial randomised 140 CLI patients to primary treatment with an everolimus eluting stent or BMS comparator.[68] At the 12-month follow-up, primary patency was higher in the DES group (85.2% vs. 54.4%; P = 0.0001), and LLL was significantly lower (0.78 mm vs. 1.41 mm; P = 0.001), as was TLR (8%

vs. 35%; P = 0.005). Once again, these results are in favour of the DES.

The ACHILLES (Angioplasty and DES in the Treatment of Subjects with Ischemic Infrapopliteal Arterial Disease) trial randomised 200 patients with CLI and occlusive tibial disease (<120 mm; mean length 27 mm) to treatment with a sirolimus-eluting stent or standard PTA.[70] The primary endpoint was 12-month, in-segment, binary restenosis determined by quantitative angiography, which once again found in favour of the DES (22.4% vs. 41.9%; P = 0.019). This result was even more pronounced when diabetic patients were analysed separately (17.6% vs. 53.2%; $P <0.001$), however, there was no significant difference seen in clinically driven TLR (10% vs. 16.5%; $P = 0.257$) or limb salvage (86.2% vs. 80%; $P = 0.3$), reflecting the multiple factors that impact those endpoints.

The IDEAS trial compared paclitaxel DCB with DES (zotarolimus-, sirolimus- or everolimus-eluting stents) for longer lesions (>70 mm), in patients of Rutherford category 3 to 6.[71] Randomisation took place over 52 limbs in 50 patients and found that the 6-month angiographic restenosis rate was lower in the DES group (28% vs. 57.9%; $P = 0.046$). There were no differences observed in clinically driven TLR, major amputation or survival rates.

The PADI trial randomised 137 patients across three centres in the Netherlands, to PTA and BMS versus DES (paclitaxel-eluting stainless steel coronary stents) published their 5-year follow-up showing that AFS rates were significantly higher in the DES group compared to PTA-BMS (31.8% vs. 20.4% $P = 0.041$). Although this is only one study these unique long-term results do emphasise the potential in below the knee drug-coated technology.[76]

Finally a systematic review and meta-analysis (7 studies; 801 patients, 329 DES, 409 control) of RCTs to have evaluated the use of DES in IP arteries after median follow-up of 12 months demonstrated improved primary patency (OR, 3.49; 95% CI, 2.38–5.12; $P=<0.00001$), freedom from TLR (OR, 2.19; 95% CI, 1.3–3.69; $P = 0.003$), major amputation (OR, 0.56; 95% CI, 0.31–0.99; $P= 0.049$) and improvement in Rutherford Class (OR, 1.62; 95% CI, 1.01–2.59; $P= 0.046$) in favour of DES, but no effect on mortality (OR, 1.05; 95% CI, 0.68–1.62; $P= 0.91$) compared to controls.[77]

✔✔ Together these studies demonstrate a consistent 12-month primary patency result with DES for short lesions below the knee, clearly superior to standard therapy of PTA or BMS. Furthermore, the IDEAS trial result suggests that DES may have advantages over DCB, both in terms of immediate angiographic results and mid-term patency.

CHOICE OF REVASCULARISATION METHOD FOR THE INFRA-POPLITEAL ARTERIES

There is currently no published RCT dedicated to determining the superiority of open surgery or endovascular treatment for IP disease. However, BASIL 2 is a multicentre RCT (ISRCTN:27728689) designed to find out if a 'vein bypass-first' or a 'best endovascular-first' revascularisation strategy derives superior clinical outcomes and cost-effectiveness for the treatment of patients with severe limb ischaemia. It has currently ended its recruitment of 345 patients (88.7% of its 389 target) from England, Scotland, Wales, Denmark and Sweden, who will be followed over a 3-year period. Patients will be randomised 1:1, to have either vein bypass or endovascular intervention as their first treatment. They will be followed up for an average of just over 3 years following intervention. This trial should provide valuable insights into the differing treatment options for this challenging region.

THE ANGIOSOME CONCEPT

✔ The angiosome concept is that each foot is divided into distinct blocks of tissue fed by source arteries that interconnect through functional arterio-arterial communications (Fig. 4.7). When tissue loss occurs because of CLTI, proponents of the concept suggest that performing a direct revascularisation procedure to the source artery may lead to superior rates of tissue healing and limb salvage compared with indirect revascularisation.

There are no randomised studies, which have compared direct to indirect revascularisation. However, a 2015 meta-analysis identified nine non-randomised studies, three of which used comparative analysis techniques to compare the two strategies.[78] The authors evaluated 779 lower limbs and found that direct revascularisation significantly improved the overall survival of limbs (HR, 0.61; 95% CI, 0.46–0.80;

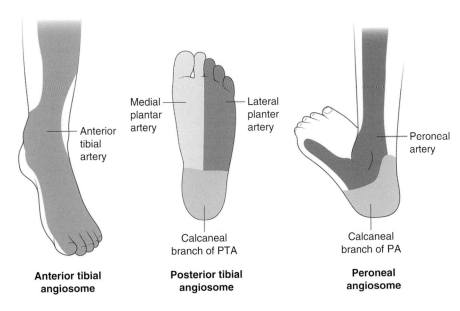

Anterior tibial angiosome   **Posterior tibial angiosome**   **Peroneal angiosome**

Figure 4.7 The six angiosomes of the foot and calf, arising from the three crural arteries. The anterior tibial artery supplies the anterior calf and then crosses the ankle as the dorsalis pedis artery, which supplies the dorsum of the foot. The posterior tibial artery (PTA) supplies the posterior calf then goes on to supply the plantar surface of the foot, toes and web spaces after splitting into medial and lateral plantar arteries. It also gives off a calcaneal branch, which supplies the medial aspect of the heel. The peroneal artery (PA) supplies the lateral aspect of the calf and ankle. It also has a calcaneal branch that supplies the lateral aspect of the heel. It is noteworthy that the heel has dual supply with crossover between the calcaneal branches of the posterior tibial artery and peroneal artery.

P <0.001) and time to wound healing (HR, 1.38; 95% CI, 1.13–1.69; *P* = 0.002). Insufficient data were available to compare mortality rates. The authors concluded that based on these data, direct revascularisation was preferred and that a randomised controlled study was necessary to confirm the results and eliminate bias.

Whilst the angiosome concept is a useful method of considering the vascular supply of the foot, the reality is that anomalous variation in the IP vascular circulation is common and occlusive disease within the pedal arch may make the revascularisation of a non-angiosomal artery more effective at optimising perfusion to the region of tissue loss. We advocate a dedicated foot angiogram in orthogonal planes to determine the preferred target vessel for revascularisation as a practical approach before tibial interventions, both surgical and endovascular.

PRIMARY AMPUTATION

Despite a movement towards aggressive revascularisation and limb-salvage 'centres of excellence', major amputations are still performed for a variety of indications. These include extensive pedal gangrene, overwhelming sepsis arising from the foot, exhausted treatment options for CLI, late presentation of acute limb ischaemia and non-ambulatory status. The most common cause is chronic CLI with no option left for revascularisation. This is often exacerbated by late referral to a specialist centre.

Major amputation incurs a considerable survival penalty, with mortality rates of approximately one-third at 12 months, 50% at 24 months and almost 75% at 5 years.[79] It also carries a significant financial burden, of more than $US 500 000 per amputation[80] – a lifetime healthcare cost, which is borne by the community. It therefore remains preferable to salvage a limb wherever feasible and reserve major amputation for when extensive gangrene has devitalised the weight-bearing surface of the foot beyond salvage.

Key points

- Best medical therapy is mandatory, and supervised exercise programmes should be considered for initial treatment in patients with claudication. Exercise programmes are underused, as they take time, persistence and are often underresourced by healthcare providers.
- There is a global trend towards an endovascular-first approach to revascularisation, but few robust data support this approach, other than demonstrating its safety compared with open surgery.
- Extensive aorto-iliac occlusive disease can now be safely treated with endovascular techniques, which have acceptable mid- to long-term patency.
- Iliac occlusions should be treated with primary stenting, with the use of covered stents determined by the extent of disease and other individual factors.
- Supra-inguinal surgery remains a useful treatment option with durable patency; however, the high risk of major complications makes it most suitable for patients with few comorbidities.
- Autologous vein remains the conduit of choice particularly for a distal anastomosis at the IP level.
- There are a multitude of technologies available for the percutaneous treatment of disease within the femoropopliteal segment; however, most comparative trials have used the historical treatment of PTA as a control rather than comparing with an endovascular gold standard.
- Stents and angioplasty balloons coated with the antiproliferative drug paclitaxel show promise in the femoropopliteal region. A recent concern over safety in patients with claudication has raised concern and driven a great deal of contention. Ongoing clinical trial data are continuing to monitor this situation.
- Advancements have been made in the endovascular treatment of IP disease, both with regards to increased technical success rates and durable patency in short- to moderatelength lesions; however, long lesions continue to demonstrate poor patency.
- DES appear more durable than other forms of endovascular therapy for short- to moderate-length lesions below the knee.
- The angiosome concept of direct revascularisation for tissue loss in CLTI has promise; however, further evidence is required.
- Primary amputation has a diminishing role in the treatment of CLTI with the expansion of techniques now available to revascularize even the most challenging of patients and disease processes.

 References available at http://ebooks.health.elsevier.com/

KEY REFERENCES

[8] Norgren L, Hiatt WR, Dormandy JA, et al. Inter-Society Consensus for the management of peripheral arterial disease (TASC II). J Vasc Surg 2007;45(Suppl. S):S5–67. PMID: 17223489.
   Comprehensive guidelines for the treatment of peripheral arterial disease.

[9] Murphy TP, Cutlip DE, Regensteiner JG, et al. Supervised exercise, stent revascularization, or medical therapy for claudication due to aortoiliac peripheral artery disease: the CLEVER study. J Am Coll Cardiol 2015;65(10):999–1009. PMID: 25766947.
   An RCT of patients with aorto-iliac occlusive disease comparing a structured exercise programme with endovascular revascularisation. Functional walking improvement and QoL were improved in both and the two groups could not be separated in their effectiveness.

[10] Fakhry F, Rouwet E, Den Hoed P, et al. Long–term clinical effectiveness of supervised exercise therapy versus endovascular revascularization for intermittent claudication from a randomized clinical trial. Br J Surg 2013;100(9):1164–71. PMID: 23842830.
   A RCT comparing structured exercise with endovascular therapy for aorto-iliac or femoropopliteal disease.

[13] Bradbury A, Ruckley C, Fowkes F, et al. Bypass versus angioplasty in severe ischaemia of the leg (BASIL): multicentre, randomised controlled trial. Lancet 2005;366(9501):1925–34. PMID: 16325694.
   Whilst now representing a historical period, the BASIL trial remains the only RCT to have made a direct comparison between open and ER for the treatment of patients with severe limb ischaemia. They found equivalence in amputation-free and overall survival between the two techniques over the first 2 years; however, a late overall survival advantage was seen in the open surgery arm for those who survived beyond that time.

[19] Klein WM, Graaf Y, Seegers J, et al. Dutch iliac stent trial: long-term results in patients randomized for primary or selective stent placement 1. Radiology 2006;238(2):734–44. PMID: 16371580.
This randomised trial compared primary stent placement or PTA for aorto-iliac occlusive disease (1993–1997). There was no difference between the group who ultimately received stents versus those who underwent uncomplicated PTA.

[20] Goode S, Cleveland T, Gaines P. Randomized clinical trial of stents versus angioplasty for the treatment of iliac artery occlusions (STAG trial). Br J Surg 2013;100(9):1148–53. PMID: 23842828.
A multicentre randomised controlled trial where 118 patients with iliac artery occlusions underwent either PTA or primary iliac stenting. They found that primary stent placement resulted in increased technical success rates and reduced major complication rates compared with simple PTA, with no difference in primary patency at mid-term follow-up.

[22] Mwipatayi BP, Thomas S, Wong J, et al. A comparison of covered vs bare expandable stents for the treatment of aortoiliac occlusive disease. J Vasc Surg 2011;54(6):1561–70.e1.PMID: 21906903.
A multicentre, randomised trial comparing PTFE-covered- or bare-metal stents for the treatment of aorto-iliac occlusive disease. They found a patency advantage to the TASC C and D lesions treated with covered stents, with no such difference observed in the TASC B subgroup.

[34] Conte MS, Bandyk DF, Clowes AW, et al. Results of PREVENT III: a multicenter, randomized trial of edifoligide for the prevention of vein graft failure in lower extremity bypass surgery. J Vasc Surg 2006;43(4):742–51.e1. PMID: 16616230.
The largest prospective, randomised, double-blind, multicentre trial to have performed a rigorous, objective evaluation of patency rates for venous bypass surgery in patients with CLI. They found a 12-month graft primary patency rate of 61%, with no difference when the bypass was performed at a distal anastomotic site above or below the knee.

[38] Anderson JL, Halperin JL, Albert N, et al. Management of patients with peripheral artery disease (compilation of 2005 and 2011 ACCF/AHA guideline recommendations) a report of the American College of Cardiology Foundation/American Heart Association Task Force on Practice guidelines. J Am Coll Cardiol 2013;61(14):1555–70. PMID: 23473760.
Comprehensive guidelines for the treatment of peripheral arterial disease.

[39] Acin F, De Haro J, Bleda S, et al. Primary nitinol stenting in femoropopliteal occlusive disease: a meta-analysis of randomized controlled trials. J Endovasc Ther 2012;19(5):585–95. PMID: 23046322.
A meta-analysis with results from 17 randomised clinical trials, which used either primary nitinol stenting or PTA for symptomatic femoropopliteal occlusive disease. They found that the nitinol stent group had higher rates of technical success, and at 12-month follow-up lower rates of both TLR and binary restenosis, with similar safety outcomes.

[42] Giacoppo D, Cassese S, Harada Y, et al. Drug-coated balloon versus plain balloon angioplasty for the treatment of femoropopliteal artery disease: an updated systematic review and meta-analysis of randomized clinical trials. JACC: Cardiovasc Interv. 2016;9(16):1731–42. PMID: 27539695.
A meta-analysis of data from eight multicentre, randomised controlled trials, which compared DCB to PTA for femoropopliteal lesions. They found that paclitaxel-coated balloons were superior to PTA in reducing TLR over mid- to long-term follow-up.

[43] Dake MD, Ansel GM, Jaff MR, et al. Durable clinical effectiveness with paclitaxel-eluting stents in the femoropopliteal artery 5-year results of the Zilver PTX randomized trial. Circulation 2016;133(15):1472–83. PMID: 26969758.
This RCT randomised patients with symptomatic femoropopliteal disease to DES or PTA, and then performed a secondary randomisation between DES and BMS for those that failed PTA. After 5 years, DES was superior to PTA in freedom from persistent or worsening symptoms of ischaemia, primary patency, and freedom from TLR. Provisional DES also had superior clinical and patency outcomes over provisional BMS.

[51] Rastan A, Krankenberg H, Baumgartner I, et al. Stent placement versus balloon angioplasty for the treatment of obstructive lesions of the popliteal artery: a prospective, multicenter, randomized trial. Circulation 2013;127(25):2535–41. PMID: 23694965.
A prospective, multicentre trial conducted on isolated popliteal artery lesions. They randomised subjects to either nitinol stent placement or PTA. Twelve-month primary patency was significantly higher in the nitinol

stent group compared to PTA and clinically driven TLR was significantly lower; however, this difference was solely accounted for by a 25.2% acute failure rate in the PTA group. The authors concluded that primary PTA with provisional bailout stenting for short lesions of the popliteal artery is a reasonable strategy.

[56] Albers M, Romiti M, Pereira C, et al. Meta-analysis of allograft bypass grafting to infrapopliteal arteries. Eur J Vasc Endovasc Surg 2004;28(5):462–72. PMID: 15465366.
A meta-analysis of autologous, popliteal-to-distal bypass grafts from 31 published series between 1981 and 2004 found excellent 5-year patency and limb salvage rates. Demonstrating the durability and limb preservation efficacy of autogenous, infrapopliteal bypass graft.

[62] Zeller T, Baumgartner I, Scheinert D, et al. Drug-eluting balloon versus standard balloon angioplasty for infrapopliteal arterial revascularization in critical limb ischemia: 12-month results from the IN.PACT DEEP randomized trial. J Am Coll Cardiol 2014;64(15):1568–76. PMID: 25301459.
This large, well-adjudicated RCT evaluated patients with infrapopliteal lesions randomising 2:1 to DCB or PTA. At 12 months, they found no difference in LLL or clinically driven TLR rates, with a trend toward higher amputation rates in the DCB arm compared to PTA.

[67] Biondi-Zoccai GG, Sangiorgi G, Lotrionte M, et al. Infra-genicular stent implantation for below-the-knee atherosclerotic disease: clinical evidence from an international collaborative meta-analysis on 640 patients. J Endovasc Ther 2009;16(3):251–60. PMID: 19642789.
A systematic review, combining 18 non-randomised studies, which evaluated patients who had infra-genicular stent implantation. They found that bailout stenting after unsatisfactory PTA in this region derived satisfactory angiographic results but no patency advantage over simple angioplasty.

68. Bosiers M, Scheinert D, Peeters P, et al. Randomized comparison of everolimus-eluting versus bare-metal stents in patients with critical limb ischemia and infra-popliteal arterial occlusive disease. J Vasc Surg 2012;55(2):390–8. PMID: 22169682.
The DESTINY RCT randomised patients with infra-popliteal disease to primary treatment with an everolimus-eluting stent or BMS comparator. At the 12-month follow-up primary patency was higher in the DES group, and late lumen loss and TLR significantly lower.

[69] Rastan A, Brechtel K, Krankenberg H, et al. Sirolimus-eluting stents for treatment of infra-popliteal arteries reduce clinical event rate compared to bare-metal stents: long-term results from a randomized trial. J Am Coll Cardiol 2012;60(7):587–91. PMID: 22878166.
The YUKON-BTK trial was the first RCT to publish a comparison between DES and BMS in the infra-popliteal circulation. The DES achieved a superior primary patency at 12 months. TLR was also improved with the use of the DES but not significantly so. At a longer follow-up of 2.8 years the primary endpoint of freedom from amputation, TVR, AMI and death also found in favour of the DES.

[70] Scheinert D, Katsanos K, Zeller T, et al. A prospective randomized multicenter comparison of balloon angioplasty and infrapopliteal stenting with the sirolimus-eluting stent in patients with ischemic peripheral arterial disease: 1-year results from the ACHILLES trial. J Am Coll Cardiol 2012;60(22):2290–5. PMID: 23194941.
This RCT randomised patients with CLI and occlusive tibial disease to treatment with a DES or standard PTA. The primary endpoint was 12-month, in-segment, binary restenosis determined by quantitative angiography, which once again found in favour of the DES. However, there was no significant difference seen in clinically driven TLR or limb salvage, reflecting the multiple factors, which impact those endpoints.

[78] Huang T-Y, Huang T-S, Wang Y-C, et al. Direct revascularization with the angiosome concept for lower limb ischemia: a systematic review and meta-analysis. Medicine 2015;94(34). PMID: 26313800.
A meta-analysis of nine non-randomised studies, three of which used comparative analysis techniques to compare direct (angiosomal) and indirect revascularisation strategies for patients with CLI. The authors found that direct revascularisation significantly improved the overall survival of limbs and time to wound healing, concluding that it was preferred and that a randomised controlled study was necessary to confirm the results.

5 The diabetic foot

Fran Game | David Russell

INTRODUCTION

Foot problems are one of the most common complications of diabetes, with 15% of patients developing a foot ulcer in their lifetime.[1] They account for more hospital admissions than other complications of diabetes[2] and are associated with high mortality, worse than many common forms of cancer.[3]

The term *diabetic foot disease* actually encompasses a number of different conditions, including peripheral sensory neuropathy and/or neuropathic pain, peripheral artery disease (PAD), ulceration, infection including osteomyelitis and Charcot neuroarthropathy. Unfortunately, people with diabetes are still eight to 24 times more likely than those without diabetes to undergo a lower limb amputation.[4] It is thought that around 85% of those amputations could be avoided by early detection and involvement of a specialist foot team, as the majority of amputations are preceded by ulceration.[5]

EPIDEMIOLOGY

The estimated global prevalence of diabetes in 2019 was approximately 463 million adults and by 2045, this is estimated to rise to 700 million,[6] and, as a consequence, the burden of foot ulceration is also likely to increase. In 2002 in a study from the north-west of England, the annual incidence of foot ulceration was reported to be 2.2% among 10 000 community-based patients with type 2 diabetes,[7] a similar incidence to an earlier US study.[8]

The main risk factors for the development of foot ulcers in diabetes are peripheral neuropathy and PAD, either alone or in combination with deformity.[5] In the UK, new Public Health England data show that the annual number of diabetes-related amputations in England is now over 7000 a year[9] and it is now estimated that every 27 seconds, a leg is lost to diabetes somewhere in the world.[10]

DEVELOPMENT OF FOOT ULCERATION

DIABETIC PERIPHERAL NEUROPATHIES

The prevalence of diabetic peripheral sensory neuropathy (DPSN) is approximately 30% in hospitalised diabetes patients and 20–30% in community-based patients.[11] It is now increasingly accepted that it is one of the earliest complications to develop in diabetes, often developing in those with prediabetes.[12] The main clinical features of DPSN include symmetrical, predominantly sensory deficits in the distal lower extremities, and neuropathic pain.[13] The development of neuropathy is linked to the duration of diabetes and poor glycaemic control over many years[13] as well as height, hypertension, dyslipidaemia, obesity and possibly smoking.[14] Annual foot examination is recommended to identify DPSN as it is a risk factor for ulceration in all patients with diabetes, and appropriate regular foot review should be instituted depending on the result.[5]

Not every patient with sensory diabetic neuropathy will describe symptoms of painful peripheral neuropathy (PPN). Although the two conditions may coexist, this is not inevitable, with one study showing painful symptoms occurring in 26% of patients without neuropathy (Neuropathy Disability Score [NDS] ≤2) and 60% of patients with severe neuropathy (NDS >8).[15] The symptoms of PPN can be extremely disturbing, and include symptoms such as burning, altered temperature perception, paraesthesia or allodynia (touch perceived as a painful stimulus), or numbness or deadness in the limb. Symptoms of neuropathy can be differentiated from pain caused by arterial disease by the nocturnal exacerbations, lack of relationship to exercise and location of symptoms, although this is not always straightforward.

Coexistent autonomic neuropathy causes a reduction in sweating in the skin and open arteriovenous shunts.[16] Although this appears to increase blood flow to the limb, with easily bounding pulses, the consequence of the shunting of blood away from skin capillaries results in functional local skin ischaemia. The neuropathic foot therefore appears warm with bounding pulses but has dry, often cracked, skin.

Motor neuropathy mainly affects the intrinsic muscles of the foot, causing wasting (guttering between the metatarsals) and altered foot shape, with clawed toes and prominent metatarsal heads (Fig. 5.1). The subsequent deformity, particularly in conjunction with DPSN, may lead to unnoticed trauma from ill-fitting footwear. Neuropathy is responsible for a high proportion of foot ulcers. In the Eurodiale study, which looked at 1232 patients across 14 European centres, peripheral neuropathy was present in 86% of patients undergoing treatment for foot ulcers.[17]

DIAGNOSIS OF NEUROPATHY

The diagnosis of DPSN, particularly for the assessment of foot ulceration risk, is usually done by clinical examination, which reveals a 'stocking' distribution of sensory loss to one or more of pain, pressure, temperature and vibration modalities. Quantitative sensory testing can be performed for

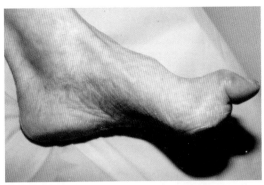

Figure 5.1 Typical appearance of a neuropathic foot, with clawed toes, dry skin, callouses and prominent metatarsal heads.

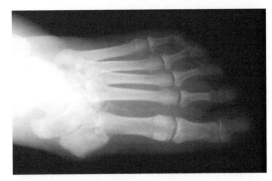

Figure 5.2 Calcification of the foot arteries in a patient with diabetes and neuropathy. This may falsely elevate Doppler pressures even within the normal range.

perception of vibration, pressure and temperature thresholds, but the perception of pressure threshold is the simplest and most commonly used in clinical practice. A nylon monofilament is used; by pressing against the skin until it buckles by about 1 cm, a load of 10 g of pressure can be accurately applied. Patients unable to feel this at a number of pre-specified sites of the foot are at approximately four-fold increased risk of ulceration.[7] This test can be simplified further by using the Ipswich Touch test,[18] a test with a good sensitivity and specificity compared with the monofilament and dispensing with the requirement for specific equipment.

PERIPHERAL ARTERY DISEASE

Atherosclerotic vascular disease is probably present in all patients with a long-standing history of diabetes.[19]

The distribution of vascular disease in the lower limb is thought to be different in patients with diabetes, with more frequent involvement of vessels below the knee. One study of patients referred for angiography showed no difference in proximal disease (iliac, femoropopliteal vessels) but distal disease (calf vessels) was twice as high in patients with diabetes as those without.[19] In clinical practice, it is not uncommon to see patients with extensive PAD of the posterior and anterior tibial arteries. Long calcified occlusions of these vessels are typical. There is frequently relative sparing of the peroneal artery and digital vessels. The distribution of disease has important consequences for revascularisation strategies. Bypasses are often required into the foot and angioplasty may be difficult because of the long length of occlusion and calcified nature of the atherosclerotic plaques.

Patients with diabetes and PAD may present with intermittent claudication; however, because of coexistent sensory peripheral neuropathy, the symptoms of vascular disease are frequently absent. The first clinical presentation may unfortunately therefore be foot ulceration.

Peripheral neuropathy, and other comorbidities, have an influence on the results of investigations recommended to investigate PAD and the choice of investigation will also differ depending on the clinical scenario. The International Working group of the Diabetic Foot (IWGDF) suggests that all patients' feet are examined at least annually for the presence of PAD and that at a minimum, this should include taking a relevant history and manually palpating foot pulses.[20] If however, the person with diabetes has a foot ulcer, the

IWGDF recommends that pedal Doppler arterial waveforms in combination with ankle systolic pressure and systolic ankle brachial index (ABI) or toe systolic pressure and toe brachial index (TBI) measurement are done. This is because the presence of pedal pulses on clinical examination does not reliably exclude PAD in a person with diabetes.[20] It is recognised however, that no single test has been shown to be optimal to exclude PAD, and there is no definite threshold value above which PAD can reliably be excluded. However, PAD is a less likely diagnosis in the presence of ABI, 0.9–1.3; TBI ≥0.75; and triphasic pedal Doppler waveforms. The suboptimal performance of these bedside tests may relate to the frequent presence of arterial calcification secondary to peripheral neuropathy and/or chronic kidney disease, which will falsely elevate the measurement even within the normal range[21] (Fig. 5.2). Transcutaneous oxygen tension (measured by an electrode placed on the foot) accurately reflects skin oxygenation and has been used to determine the severity of ischaemia and the likelihood that an ischaemic ulcer will heal; however, as the result depends on the assumption of capillary dilatation when the sensor is heated to a pre-specified temperature, then once again the presence of neuropathy may affect the result as capillary dilatation may be altered in the presence of autonomic neuropathy.[21]

BIOMECHANICAL ASPECTS

The most important cause of foot ulceration is loss of protective pain sensation, permitting 'painless' repetitive trauma and tissue injury particularly in those with deformity. Pedal plantar pressures can be measured by a number of methods, both dynamic and static. Patients with peripheral neuropathy and particularly patients with foot ulcers have high plantar pressures, although high pressures alone in the absence of insensitivity do not lead to ulceration. Frykberg et al.[22] used an F-scan pressure mat system and identified patients at risk of ulceration with foot pressures >6 kg/cm^2. Stacpoole-Shea et al.[23] studied an in-shoe pressure analysis system and demonstrated its ability to predict potential sites for foot ulceration with a sensitivity of 83% and a specificity of 69%.

Neuropathy and altered proprioception, and small-muscle wasting can, in themselves, lead to alteration of the foot architecture and shape, resulting in clawing of the toes, prominent metatarsal heads and a high arch, resulting in foot pressure changes.[24] To some extent, this can be reviewed clinically and raises suggestions as to where ulcers are likely to occur on the foot. The more severe deformities associated with Charcot neuroarthropathy, with joint dislocation and bony deformities, can also result in increased foot pressures and subsequent ulceration.

Limited joint mobility is a further contributing factor to elevated plantar pressures. Chronic hyperglycaemia results in glycosylation of proteins and, when collagen is involved, the collagen bundles become thickened and cross-linked. This alters the mechanics of walking and is strongly associated with high plantar pressures.[25]

Neuropathy alone does not usually lead to spontaneous ulceration, the precipitating factor commonly being from some traumatic event, including rubbing from inappropriate or ill-fitting footwear. In the North West diabetes study,[7] approximately half the ulcers were precipitated by problems with footwear. The presence of callus (produced in response to pressure) may exacerbate the problem by increasing pressure further.[26] Removal of callus significantly reduces foot pressures,[27] and should be done regularly by an experienced podiatrist.

Although measurement of foot pressures can predict risk of ulceration with a degree of accuracy, it requires equipment that may not be available in all centres. Good clinical examination that inspects foot shape and identifies the presence of callus can provide very valuable information. In particular, the presence of haemorrhage into callus is a pre-ulcerative phenomenon and requires urgent attention. Footwear, and the wear pattern of the footwear, should also be inspected as part of this assessment.[5]

OTHER RISK FACTORS

Impaired vision and immobility make it difficult for patients to inspect and care for their feet on a daily basis as recommended in most guidelines and are therefore additional risk factors. By far and away the most important additional risk factor, however, is end-stage renal disease, particularly if the patient is receiving renal replacement therapy (RRT). The development of foot ulcers increases exponentially in the first year after the onset of RRT.[28,29] It is not clear exactly why this is, although a small study has noted a marked drop in the transcutaneous pressure of oxygen (TcPO$_2$) throughout and for at least 4 hours after a standard haemodialysis session.[30] In addition, there may be a risk to patients' heels from being stationary for prolonged periods of time during RRT and greater risks from shoe rubbing given the variation in peripheral oedema, which may occur between dialysis sessions. Recent guidance has emphasised the need for extra podiatric input to this extremely high-risk group.[31]

MANAGEMENT

The management of diabetic foot problems requires input from a number of different healthcare professionals, and evidence strongly suggests that specialist diabetic foot clinics can significantly reduce ulceration and amputation rates. One retrospective study showed an approximate 75% reduction in major amputation after introduction of a multidisciplinary foot team (MDFT).[32]

National Institute for Health and Care Excellence (NICE) Guidelines 2015 have suggested that the MDFT should

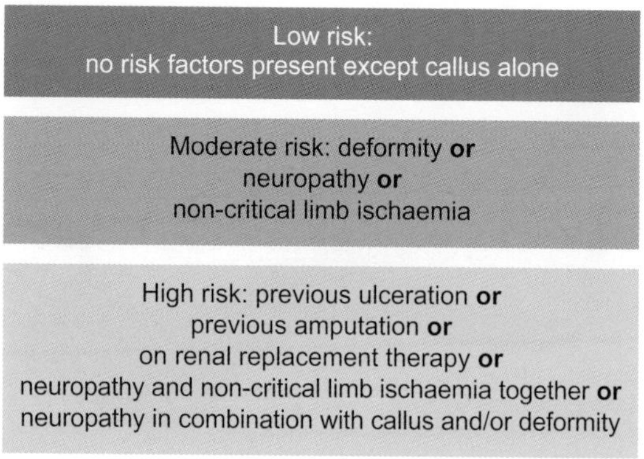

Figure 5.3 Risk classification for the development of diabetic foot ulceration.

consist of specialists with skills in the following areas for optimal patient care:[5]

- Diabetology
- Podiatry
- Diabetes specialist nursing
- Vascular surgery
- Microbiology
- Orthopaedic surgery
- Biomechanics and orthoses
- Interventional radiology
- Casting
- Wound care.

THE 'AT-RISK' FOOT

NICE recommends[5] that the identification of patients at risk of foot ulceration should be done on an annual basis for all patients with diabetes. Screening does not require expensive equipment and testing can be done in an ordinary clinic setting. In addition to 10-g monofilament testing and palpation of pulses, as described earlier, skin should be checked for the dryness and cracking associated with autonomic neuropathy, any signs of tinea pedis, which may cause fissuring between the toes, and shoes should be examined. Symptoms of neuropathic pain (burning, paraesthesia, etc.) should be actively sought.

Risk status – low, moderate or high (Fig. 5.3) – should be ascertained,[5] the patient advised of this, and any necessary care of their feet explained along with the requirement for follow-up in a foot protection service.

Patients also need to know how to gain rapid access to advice and treatment from the footcare team, and in the event of a new foot ulcer, urgent referral to a multidisciplinary team should be made within 24 hours.[5]

Regular podiatry is needed for most at-risk patients. Callus needs to be debrided regularly; although it develops in response to pressure and friction, its removal can reduce pressure, as stated previously. Callus can sometimes hide ulceration, which will only be revealed when the callus is removed. Without removal, infection and abscess formation are more likely, but it is important to explain to the patient that the podiatrist has not caused the underlying ulcer revealed when the callus is removed. The presence of callus should always prompt a search for its cause, and shoe modification may be necessary.

	Score = 0	Score = 1
Site	Forefoot	Midfoot, hindfoot
Ischaemia	At least one pulse palpable	Clinical evidence of reduced pedal blood flow
Neuropathy	Protective sensation intact	Protective sensation lost
Bacterial infection	None	Present
Area	< 1 cm^2	$\geq$ 1 cm^2
Depth	Ulcer confined to skin and subcutaneous tissue	Ulcer reaching muscle, tendon or deeper

Figure 5.4 The SINBAD classification.

The surgical correction of specific foot deformities is sometimes necessary to prevent ulceration. This should be done only after confirming that there is good peripheral circulation, and it is important to remember that correction of foot deformities may create pressure problems elsewhere; for example, correction of a hallux valgus may leave a rigid hallux with resultant high plantar pressures on the plantar aspect of the hallux. Correction of deformity is usually only performed in patients with a history of ulceration, rather than for primary prevention.

ULCER MANAGEMENT

All patients with diabetes presenting with foot ulcers need a full examination of the foot, including peripheral sensation and circulation to classify and understand the main aetiology of the ulcer. They also need assessment of footwear and deformities. Being very simplistic, ulcers can be classified by their dominant aetiology into neuropathic or ischaemic.

A number of classification and scoring systems have been published but none has been universally accepted,[33] few have been fully validated outside the population from which they were drawn, and none have been validated to predict individual patient outcomes. The ideal classification system would include patient, limb and ulcer factors known to affect healing, but the components and complexity of a classification reflects the purpose for which it is being designed, for example, research, audit or clinical prognosis.[34]

SINBAD[35] (Fig. 5.4) was designed for the purposes of audit and is used in the UK National Diabetes Foot Care Audit.[36] It is a simple, quick classification, which has been validated across continents for ulcer healing and amputation prediction with good reliability. The IWGDF have recommended SINBAD for communication among health professionals and for audit of outcome between populations.[34]

The Wound, ischaemia and Foot Infection[37] (Fig. 5.5) uses a combination of wound characteristics, perfusion assessment, and presence and severity of infection to predict a 1-year risk of amputation and benefit of revascularisation (see Chapter 2). It has been well validated in chronic limb-threatening ischaemia cohorts including patients with diabetes, but less well in diabetic foot ulcer specific cohorts. Whilst it requires performance of ankle-brachial pressure index, toe pressure or transcutaneous oxygen assessment of perfusion, and thus is limited in a primary care setting, it can be helpful in aiding decisions on revascularisation in a specialist vascular or diabetic foot clinic setting. Its use is recommended by both the IWGDF for diabetic foot ulcers, and the Global Vascular Guidelines in the wider context of chronic limb-threatening ischaemia.[34,38]

NEUROPATHIC ULCERS

Typically, the foot is warm and well perfused, with bounding pulses and distended veins. The ulcer is usually at the site of repetitive trauma and, as ulcers are most commonly caused by a shoe rub, on the dorsum of the toes or a high-pressure area under the metatarsal heads. Due to dense sensory neuropathy, a patient may walk on a foreign body for hours or even days without realising it, for example, a nail through the sole of a shoe, or an old dressing or sock stuffed in the end of a shoe, and these may easily cause quite significant ulcers before the patient is aware.

The key to management of neuropathic ulcers is pressure relief or offloading.[39] With shoe-induced ulcers, new footwear must be provided to prevent future ulcers in the longer term. Merely providing the shoes may not be enough; patients often fail to wear the shoes because of appearance, or a belief that they are only to be used outside the home, and so continued support must be provided to encourage the patient to carry on with this form of therapy.

To relieve sufficient pressure from a plantar ulcer to allow it to heal, however, shoes are insufficient, and a more aggressive approach is required. Bed rest is simple, but expensive in hospital and difficult to enforce in a patient who feels well and is pain free, so ambulatory methods have been designed. The total contact cast was originally used for patients with neuropathic ulcers caused by leprosy and modified for use in patients with diabetic neuropathic ulcers. The cast extends from below the knee and encases the whole foot and works by transferring load from the forefoot to the heel, and directly to the leg via the cast wall, as well as reducing oedema and shear forces. Excellent healing rates have been described in randomised controlled trials[40] compared with other forms of offloading if the ulcers are on the plantar forefoot; the results for heel ulcers have been less impressive.[41] The main disadvantage is that it is labour-intensive and requires a high level of skill. It may need frequent changes, and signs of wound infection or new ulceration secondary to the cast may not be seen. A number of commercially produced pressure-relieving boots are now available, with proven capacity to reduce pressure. However, since these alternative devices are removable, patients may take them off whilst at home, and therefore impede further healing. These can be made non-removable by wrapping the removable cast with fibreglass casing material or using

Score	Wound	Ischaemia	Infection (IDSA/IWGDF)
0	No ulcer; no gangrene	Toe pressure(TP)/TcPO$_2$ ≥60mmHg Ankle pressure >100mmHg ABI ≥0.80	Uninfected
1	Small shallow ulcer; or gangrene limited to distal phalanx	TP/TcPO$_2$ 40-59mmHg Ankle pressure 70-100mmHg ABI 0.6-0.79	Mild infection
2	Deep ulcer not involving heel; shallow heel ulcer; or gangrene limited to toes	TP/TcPO$_2$ 30-39mmHg Ankle pressure 50-70mmHg ABI 0.4-0.59	Moderate infection
3	Extensive deep ulcer involving forefoot +/- midfoot; full thickness heel ulcer; or extensive gangrene	TP/TcPO$_2$ <30mmHg Ankle pressure <50mmHg ABI ≤0.39	Severe infection

a. Estimate risk of amputation at 1 year

	Ischaemia - 0				Ischaemia - 1					Ischaemia - 2				Ischaemia - 3			
W-0	VL	VL	L	M	VL	L	M	H		L	L	M	H	L	M	M	H
W-1	VL	VL	L	M	VL	L	M	H		L	M	H	H	M	M	H	H
W-2	L	L	M	H	M	M	H	H		M	H	H	H	H	H	H	H
W-3	M	M	H	H	H	H	H	H		H	H	H	H	H	H	H	H
	fl-0	fl-1	fl-2	fl-3	fl-0	fl-1	fl-2	fl-3		fl-0	fl-1	fl-2	fl-3	fl-0	fl-1	fl-2	fl-3

a. Estimate likelihood of benefit of / requirement for revascularisation (assuming infection can be controlled first)

	Ischaemia - 0				Ischaemia - 1					Ischaemia - 2				Ischaemia - 3			
W-0	VL	VL	VL	VL	VL	L	L	M		L	L	M	M	M	H	H	H
W-1	VL	VL	VL	VL	L	L	M	M		M	H	H	H	H	H	H	H
W-2	VL	VL	VL	VL	M	M	H	H		H	H	H	H	H	H	H	H
W-3	VL	VL	VL	VL	M	M	M	H		H	H	H	H	H	H	H	H
	fl-0	fl-1	fl-2	fl-3	fl-0	fl-1	fl-2	fl-3		fl-0	fl-1	fl-2	fl-3	fl-0	fl-1	fl-2	fl-3

Four classes: for each box, group combination into one of these four classes
Very low = VL = clinical stage 1
Low = L = clinical stage 2
Moderate = M = clinical stage 3
High = H = clinical stage 4

Figure 5.5 The Wound, Ischaemia and Foot Infection (WIfI) classification.

Clinical manifestations of infection	Infection severity
Wound lacking purulence or any manifestation of inflammation	Uninfected
Presence of ≥ 2 manifestations of inflammation (purulence, or erythema, pain, tenderness, warmth, or induration), but any cellulitis/erythema extends ≤ 2 cm around the ulcer, and infection is limited to the skin or superficial subcutaneous tissues; no other local complications of systemic illness	Mild
Infection (as above) in a patient who is systemically well and metabolically stable but who has ≥ 1 of the following characteristics: cellulitis extending > 2 cm, lymphangitic streaking, spread beneath the superficial fascia, deep tissue abscess, gangrene and involvement of muscle, tendon, joint or bone	Moderate
Infection in a patient with systemic toxicity or metabolic instability (e.g. fever, chills, tachycardia, hypotension, confusion, vomiting, leukocytosis, acidosis, severe hyperglycaemia or azotaemia)	Severe

Figure 5.6 The Infectious Disease Society of America/International Working group of the Diabetic Foot (IDSA/IWGDF) classification of diabetic foot infection. *ABI*, Ankle–brachial index; *TcPO$_2$*, transcutaneous pressure of oxygen.

plastic tags. Evidence suggests that healing with this form of offloading is almost on a par with total contact casting.[42]

The second important element of management of neuropathic ulcers is debridement of callus. Wounds heal from the margins and callus prevents the migration of epidermal cells from the wound margin and encourages and masks wound infection. Debridement of callus and necrotic tissue may be required as often as weekly, and continued presence or rapid re-accumulation of callus should prompt a review of the pressure relief used.

ISCHAEMIC AND NEUROISCHAEMIC ULCERS

Purely ischaemic ulcers are relatively rare and most are, in fact, neuroischaemic as the majority of patients have neuropathy.[36] Typical sites include the toes, heel and medial aspect of the first metatarsal head. Callus is usually absent, and the ulcer is often surrounded by a rim of ischaemia and may have a necrotic centre. The presence of pain depends on the degree of neuropathy. Ulceration is often precipitated by minor trauma; again, the most common culprit is ill-fitting shoes. Prompt vascular assessment is crucial. Revascularisation should be performed whenever possible, both for ulcer healing (ischaemic and neuroischaemic ulcers only rarely heal without improvements in blood flow) and to prevent future ulceration.

Gangrene and amputation are among the most feared complications of diabetes. Although gangrene may complicate neuropathic ulceration (microorganisms in infected digital ulcers may produce necrotising toxins, which lead to thrombotic occlusion of digital arteries and subsequent gangrene), it usually only occurs when significant vascular disease is present.

INFECTION

Infection in diabetic foot ulcers can vary from superficial cellulitis to deeper infection of the soft tissues and bones. All ulcers are colonised with bacteria but when a species invades and there is a local response to this then it is said that the ulcer is infected. The distinction between colonisation and infection cannot be made with microbiological investigations,[43] and must be made by assessment of the clinical signs. Infection can be classified as mild, moderate or severe[43] depending on the degree of erythema or the development of systemic symptoms (severe) (Fig. 5.6). Treatment decisions, particularly the choice of antibiotics, will vary depending on the severity of the infection and particularly whether bone infection is suspected.[43] Mild infection in superficial ulcers is usually caused by Gram-positive organisms such as *Staphylococcus aureus* or streptococcal species. Deeper ulcers or ischaemic ulcers, or an ulcer that has been present for a longer period of time, may be colonised with more Gram-negatives and/or anaerobic organisms and antibiotic protocols should reflect this.[43] Microbiological sampling should be done before antibiotic therapy is instituted and ideally should consist of tissue rather than surface swabs, which may just grow colonisers rather than invading pathogens.[44] Newer molecular biological techniques may in future overcome the problem of fastidious organisms failing to grow in standard culture, but the role of these techniques in routine practice has not yet been fully evaluated.[45]

Osteomyelitis is an important predisposing factor for amputation, and occurs in about 20% of patients with diabetes and a foot ulcer[45] and should be suspected in any deep infected ulcer, particularly if bone is palpable.[43] The use of the simple clinical test 'the probe to bone test' (the ability to probe to bone with a blunt instrument at the base of the ulcer) in diagnosing osteomyelitis has been controversial. Latest guidance suggests that in the presence of an infected ulcer, the ability to probe to bone can support the diagnosis of osteomyelitis, whilst the inability to probe to bone in a clinically uninfected ulcer can virtually rule out the diagnosis.[43]

Plain radiography is often used as the first-line test when osteomyelitis is suspected, but the characteristic changes of bone destruction (Fig. 5.7) can take 2 weeks or longer to develop and do not occur until 30–50% of the bone has been destroyed.[46]

Recent guidelines from the IWGDF,[42] suggest that if a plain radiograph (X-ray) does show osteomyelitis then no further imaging of the foot to establish the diagnosis is required. However, if the diagnosis remains in doubt, advanced imaging such magnetic resonance imaging (MRI)

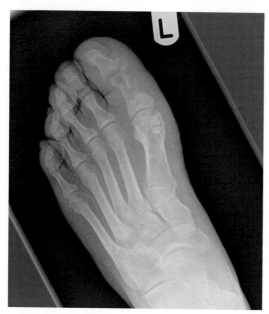

Figure 5.7   Osteomyelitis of the hallux in a patient with diabetes.

scan, 18F-fluorodeoxyglucose-positron emission tomography/computed tomography (CT) or leukocyte scintigraphy (with or without CT) may be helpful. MRI can show marrow oedema before cortical bone loss occurs, although there may be difficulty differentiating osteomyelitis from Charcot neuroarthropathy, particularly where the two coexist.

Antibiotics are only required for clinically infected wounds or osteomyelitis. They do not aid wound healing per se. When choosing an antibiotic regimen, the severity of infection and whether osteomyelitis is suspected are important, as well as the spectrum of antibiotic activity, the intended duration of treatment, local policy and patients' other comorbidities, particularly renal disease. Mild infections can often be treated with relatively narrow-spectrum antibiotics with coverage against Gram-positive cocci, for example, oral flucloxacillin or a tetracycline. Ciprofloxacin or co-amoxiclav can be used if Gram-negative infection is suspected, although the potential for these particular antibiotics to be implicated in *Clostridium difficile* diarrhoea should be considered.

There are a number of other factors that must be addressed to ensure healing of an infected foot wound. Attention must be paid to the patient's general medical condition, and it is important to correct any accompanying hyperglycaemia, renal failure or electrolyte disturbance. Regular debridement is important to remove necrotic or devitalised tissue and pus should be drained and the foot offloaded. The principles of dressing a healing wound include keeping it moist, managing exudate and protecting the surrounding intact skin.[27] Limb-threatening infections require urgent hospitalisation, bed rest, relevant surgical debridement and broad-spectrum antibiotics.

SURGICAL MANAGEMENT OF DIABETIC FOOT INFECTION

FOOT ANATOMY AND BIOMECHANICS

The foot needs to be versatile in providing absorption of energy on heel strike, adapting to uneven surfaces through the gait cycle, yet acting as a rigid lever for propulsion.

During the gait cycle, there is initial contact of the foot on the lateral aspect of the heel during heel strike. Weight is then transferred across to the first metatarsal and hallux for propulsion and push off. The change from supination to pronation of the foot over the gait cycle accounts for the change in biomechanical properties from shock absorbing and adaptable, to a rigid platform.

Any surgical debridement or minor amputation affects the biomechanics of the foot, with consequent risk of transfer ulceration. Hallux amputation leads to loss of buttress for rotation of the first metatarsal head, reducing its weight bearing ability and transferring weight to the second toe and metatarsal, with risk of stress fractures. This is exacerbated by amputations involving the first metatarsal whilst preservation of the first 1 cm of proximal phalanx will preserve the Windlass mechanism and minimise the consequences. Almost 20% of patients will have a further amputation in the 24 months following a hallux amputation, with the level relatively evenly spread between further toes, transmetatarsal and major amputation.[47] Amputation of lesser digits have fewer consequences, but loss of buttress effect leads to lateral toe drift and hallux valgus. This can be minimised by the use of toe fillers. The axis of the first and fifth metatarsals are independent whilst the second to fourth metatarsals act as a functional unit. The metatarsal heads are connected by the intermetatarsal ligaments. Loss of the fifth metatarsal carries similar risks to loss of the first metatarsal with additional stresses on the neighbouring fourth metatarsal head and transfer ulceration. Loss of two central rays also increases residual metatarsal head pressures, leading to the concept of 'too few toe syndrome', and the suggestion that a transmetatarsal amputation may have a better biomechanical outcome.[48] The peroneus brevis tendon attaches to the base of the fifth metatarsal and loss of this segment of bone therefore leads to equinovarus deformity of the foot and poor function. If the fifth metatarsal styloid cannot be preserved, then splitting of the tibialis anterior tendon to rebalance the foot should be performed.

SURGICAL APPROACH FOR ACUTE DIABETIC FOOT SEPSIS

Purulent sepsis in the diabetic foot is a surgical emergency. The inflammatory response may lead to compartment syndrome within one of the four plantar compartments of the foot, leading to tissue destruction and propagation of sepsis up the tendon sheaths, which provide the path of least resistance. Clinical features of fluctuance, deep plantar tenderness, pus following debridement of unhealthy tissue, remote wound sinuses and soft tissue gas on plain X-ray are all suggestive of purulence requiring urgent drainage.

Patients with severe sepsis require fluid resuscitation, intravenous insulin regimes and broad-spectrum antibiotics, ideally after an initial sample of pus or tissue has been collected for microbiology. If there is to be any delay in access to an operating theatre, then incising any non-viable skin and deep fascia to decompress the compartment may help to prevent ongoing deep tissue destruction.

The Loeffler-Ballard incision (Fig. 5.8) extends from any interdigital space proximally along the line of the flexor tendons, extending up into the calf if necessary.[49] It allows access to all four plantar compartments whilst preserving healthy soft tissue and bone for reconstruction options. All unhealthy

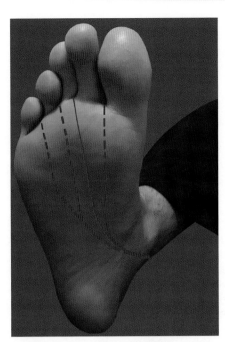

Figure 5.8   Loeffler-Ballard incision for drainage of plantar foot sepsis.

tissue should be debrided, including tissue with thrombosed vessels, using serial slices until a healthy margin is achieved. It is the authors practice to take clean soft tissue and bone samples post-debridement and lavage to guide the need for, and duration of antibiotics post-operatively, with weak evidence that untreated residual osteomyelitis increases the risk of wound healing complications.[42] These wounds may require serial debridement before closure/reconstruction, and urgent arterial imaging and revascularisation for any ischaemic element. It is helpful to consider the end goal at the time of debridement: is this the definitive procedure, or can future soft tissue reconstructive options using split skin graft, local rotation flaps, dermal substitutes or free flaps be used (Fig. 5.9). There is some evidence to suggest that outcomes are improved in wounds left to heal by secondary intention with the use of post-operative negative pressure wound therapy.[50] Offloading forms a crucial component of post-operative care and needs to be optimised for both ambulation and in bed.

Amputation of digits is common for necrosis or osteomyelitis of the toes. There is no established perfusion cut-off for healing of minor amputations, but a toe pressure >50 mmHg is reassuring,[20] Either anterior and posterior flaps, or a racquet head incision can be safely used, and for sepsis, it is usual to perform the amputation at a level including at least one joint proximal to the known level of sepsis. The wound may either be tacked closed with interrupted sutures or left open and loosely packed.

Ray amputation is commonly performed for sepsis of the metatarsal head with a racquet head incision that can be extended either into a Loeffler-Ballard plantar incision for plantar sepsis, or dorsally over the metatarsal of interest if the sepsis is localised to the metatarsal head. Dividing the bone with a power saw allows an angled cut with a longer length on the dorsal edge, leaving a more oblique angle on the residual weight-bearing aspect of the bone. Dividing a central metatarsal in the proximal third allows better approximation of adjacent rays during healing.

Transmetatarsal amputation was first popularised by McKittrick for forefoot gangrene[51] but is now more commonly performed for sepsis. This is optimally performed using a long posterior flap, but may use anterior and posterior flaps. The bones should be divided to maintain the natural metatarsal parabola, with the second metatarsal being the longest. The consequence of division of the extensor tendons is unopposed plantar flexion via the flexor tendons and Achilles tendon, leading to equinovarus deformity of the residuum and a high incidence of ulceration on the plantar aspect of the residual fifth metatarsal. Several techniques have been used to minimise this, with concomitant percutaneous Achilles tendon lengthening and tendon rebalancing being most popular but with limited evidence of efficacy in reduction in ulcer incidence.[52]

TOPICAL WOUND HEALING AGENTS

There are now innumerable topical agents, applications and dressings that are marketed to accelerate wound healing in the diabetic foot. Few of these have been subject to rigorous controlled trials, which prove their efficacy and/or cost-effectiveness, and of those that have, the evidence to suggest benefit is poor.[50] Their availability should not obscure the fact that most ulcers respond to simple care, comprising pressure relief, debridement and control of infection, and must not be seen as a replacement, but as an addition to good wound care.

MEDICAL PROBLEMS ON THE SURGICAL WARD

Patients with diabetes on the vascular surgical ward will often have multiple comorbidities and other complications related to their diabetes. Apart from peripheral neuropathy and PAD, they may have evidence of ischaemic heart disease, diabetic nephropathy and autonomic neuropathy, all of which can affect their eventual outcomes. These comorbid conditions need to be considered and addressed – for example, patients with significant renal impairment may need a renal review before any procedures, particularly angiography with contrast media, as this carries a risk of worsening renal function. Metformin must be stopped for 48 hours following elective angiography in those with chronic kidney disease stage ≤3 because of a risk of worsening renal failure and consequent lactic acidosis. Coronary artery disease and cardiac autonomic neuropathy increase the risk of intraoperative cardiac events and should be addressed before surgery. The hormonal and metabolic changes associated with surgery create a particular problem in diabetes, and intravenous insulin infusions (with dextrose and potassium) are usually needed for the perioperative period, unless the duration of anaesthesia is short (<45 minutes) and the patient is not usually on insulin.

Patients with neuropathy are at great risk of developing heel ulcers whilst lying immobile in bed for several days.[53] These can be difficult to heal, are entirely preventable and medicolegally indefensible. The simple provision of foam or padded heel protectors is often all that is needed to relieve pressure on the heels whilst the patient is in bed and should be routine in patients at risk.

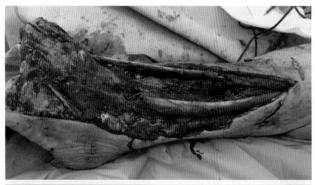

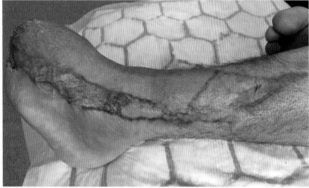

Figure 5.9 Latissimus Dorsi myocutaneous flap reconstruction of severe diabetic foot sepsis and fasciitis into lower leg.

CHARCOT NEURO-OSTEOARTHROPATHY

Charcot neuro-osteoarthropathy (the Charcot foot) is a complication of neuropathy characterised by inflammation, bone and joint destruction, fragmentation and remodelling.[54] It can be one of the most devastating foot complications of diabetes, and was first described as a complication of tabes dorsalis. It can develop in any joint, and has been reported in most sensory neuropathies, but diabetes is now the commonest cause. The exact prevalence is unknown and estimates vary from 0.04/1000 patients with diabetes[55] to about 3/1000 patients[56] and was present in 1% of those patients registered with ulcers in the UK national diabetes footcare audit.[36] Charcot foot can be triggered by trauma to the foot (of which the patient may be unaware as they have sensory neuropathy), including surgical interventions or preceding ulceration and/or infection trauma of the foot.[57] In the early stages, the foot becomes swollen, warm and erythematous, and may be incorrectly diagnosed as a sprain, gout, cellulitis or deep vein thrombosis. If not treated promptly, osteolysis and osteopenia can occur; ligaments can become lax and gradual remodelling of the foot occurs, with chronic deformity and fusion of the bones in abnormal positions.

Most textbooks describe this as a painless condition, but there is frequently some discomfort, although usually not enough to prevent walking. The presentation may be several weeks after the onset of symptoms and, because of the lack of significant pain, plain radiographs are not always performed. Plain radiography may be sufficient to make the diagnosis once fracturing/dislocations have occurred but

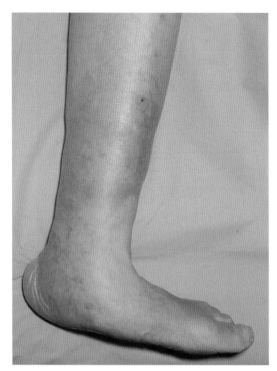

Figure 5.10 'Rocker bottom foot' associated with Charcot foot.

in the early stages when the architecture of the foot is still preserved (and it is preferable to make the diagnosis at this stage) then MRI can be used to demonstrate marrow oedema.[54] Treatment is aimed at minimising weight-bearing to reduce potential bone and joint destruction and reduce the inflammatory phase. The midfoot is the commonest site of Charcot neuroarthropathy[57] and, when affected, can result in midfoot collapse, with a plantar bony prominence and 'rocker-bottom deformity', which has a very high risk of ulceration (Fig. 5.10). The mainstay of treatment is rest and immobilisation, usually in a total contact cast, which may need to be continued for many months until disease activity has subsided. In one UK study, the median time in offloading before the patient was fully able to mobilise in orthotic or other footwear was 10 months.[57] Disease activity is usually judged by measuring the temperature of the skin with an infrared thermometer and comparison with the contralateral (non-affected foot). A 2°C difference is often quoted as being significant, although the evidence behind this is weak.[54] Once the temperature difference is <2°C then the patient can be weaned out of offloading devices/casts into orthotic footwear manufactured to fit any deformity.

Trials of bisphosphonates have been undertaken in the past in an attempt to improve the outcome of the disease. A recent systematic review concluded, however, that there is no evidence to support their use in this disease process.[58]

If the Charcot is in the fore- or mid-foot then surgery is usually avoided in the active stage, because of the gross oedema of the involved bone, and the risk that it (like trauma) will trigger further bone resorption. In the hindfoot/ankle immediate surgery may be necessary, however, to stabilise the joint.[55] However, corrective surgery may also be useful at a later stage to remove bony prominences, which may increase risk of ulceration.

Key points

- The management of the diabetic foot is challenging and requires a multidisciplinary approach, ideally coordinated by a specialised clinic.
- Identification of at-risk patients requires screening that must be both comprehensive and regular, supported by appropriately trained staff.
- If ulcers develop, early aggressive management can achieve good results with a significant reduction of both amputation and re-ulceration rates.
- Future research may ultimately enable the prevention of foot ulcers and predisposing factors that lead to ulceration and may demonstrate superior ways of healing ulcers. However, the dissemination of current 'best practice' should have the greatest impact on the outlook for this condition.

🌐 References available at http://ebooks.health.elsevier.com/

KEY REFERENCES

[17] Prompers L, Huijberts M, Apelqvist J, et al. High prevalence of ischaemia, infection and serious comorbidity in patients with diabetic foot disease in Europe. Baseline results from the Eurodiale study. Diabetologia 2007;50:18–25. PMID: 17093942.

   A A large multicentre study looking at the outcomes of 1232 patients from 14 large European centres.

[27] Schaper NC, Van Netten JJ, Apelqvist J, et al. International Working Group on the Diabetic Foot (IWGDF). Practical Guidelines on the prevention and management of diabetic foot disease (IWGDF 2019 update). Diabetes Metab Res Rev 2020;36(S1):e3266.

   First of a series of guideline papers from the International Working Group of the Diabetic Foot, based on systematic reviews.

[43] Lipsky BA, Senneville E, Abbas ZG, et al. Guidelines on the diagnosis and treatment of foot infection in persons with diabetes (IWGDF 2019 update). Diabetes Metab Res Rev 2020;36(S1):e3280.

   Guidelines on the management of infection in the diabetic foot based on a systematic review.

[54] Rogers LC, Frykberg RG, Armstrong DG, et al. The Charcot foot in diabetes. Diabetes Care 2011;34(9):2123–9. PMID: 21868781.

   Review of diagnosis and management of the Charcot foot in diabetes.

6 Amputation, rehabilitation and prosthetic developments

Shigong Guo

INTRODUCTION

Amputation is defined as the partial or complete removal of a limb or extremity arising from surgery, underlying disease or trauma.[1] Minor amputations are those performed in the foot and major amputations are those above the level of the ankle.

Over 90% of major leg amputations carried out in England are attributed to peripheral arterial disease (PAD)[2] with similar rates in the United States.[3] Therefore the vascular surgeon and surgeon-in-training must be familiar with the pre-, peri- and post-operative management of the amputee patient in terms of not only the amputation itself but also prosthetic management and rehabilitation.

Traditionally, amputation was considered a 'nadir' or 'failure' in vascular surgery[4,5] when revascularisation has failed or the limb is deemed unsalvageable. However, it is increasingly recognised that surgical amputation is the first step in the vascular patient's rehabilitation process,[6] especially in terms of pain relief, removal of necrotic, ischaemic or infected tissue and improvement in quality of life (QoL), irrespective of whether the patient is a prospective prosthetic limb user or not.

Amputation management should start before the amputation itself and continue into the community. Specialist and holistic assessment of the patient leading to careful pre-operative planning, selection of the amputation level, good surgical technique and optimal post-operative management are all vital in the initial stages of amputee rehabilitation. Subsequent stages involve post-operative early rehabilitation, including wound management, the use of early walking aids, wheelchair and home assessments, prosthetic limb fitting (where appropriate), and continuing long-term follow-up and support to patients and their families in the community.

This chapter focuses on the rehabilitation of adult patients undergoing lower extremity amputation caused by PAD and or diabetes although its general principles can also be applied to non-vascular amputations such as those caused by trauma, infection, frostbite or neoplasm.

EPIDEMIOLOGY

In the United States, there are an estimated 2 million amputees with this figure forecasted to double by 2050.[7] The incidence of all amputations is estimated to be over 150 000 per year in the USA.[8]

Major amputations are a common operation in Europe and the numbers are well recorded in routinely collected data. In 2014 16 645 major amputations were performed in Germany[9] and 25 312 amputations over a 6-year period in England.[2]

In higher-income Western countries, the overwhelming majority (>80%) of lower extremity amputations are resulting from PAD,[28] whereas in lower-income countries the most common reason for amputation is trauma.[10]

Amputation carries a significant financial burden with annual costs in the United States alone reaching US$ 4.3 billion.[8]

There is a strong association between PAD and diabetes mellitus in terms of the risk of amputation. Approximately one-third of amputees have diabetes mellitus in the United Kingdom.[11] This figure rises to 50% in Australia[12] and 70% in Germany.[13] In men with PAD, the presence of diabetes mellitus alongside PAD confers a significant amputation risk.[14]

A systematic review in 2011 of 57 studies reported a marked difference in the incidence of amputation globally. Rates were highest in the United States (9600 per 100 000 population in the US state of Louisiana) followed by Northern Europe, and lowest in Taiwan, Japan and Spain (1.5 per 100 000 population).[15] In the United States, there are also significant ethnic and racial variations with African Americans twice as likely to undergo amputation compared to White Americans.[16] However, the causes of this variation are unclear, especially as similar disparities amongst Black and White populations are not found in other countries such as the United Kingdom.[17]

The UK Limbless Statistics report last published in 2012 showed that a total of 5906 new referrals to amputee rehabilitation centres were made for the preceding 1 year, with lower extremity amputations accounting for 91% of referrals and 'dysvascularity' (a term that suggests an amputation is the result of inadequate blood supply and usually associated with the complications of PAD and/or diabetes) as the most common cause of amputation. In this lower extremity group, half underwent an amputation at a transtibial level and 34% at transfemoral level. The sex breakdown of new referrals has remained consistent, with female referrals accounting for 30% of all new referrals with an average age of 68 years (65 years for men).[18]

There is increasing evidence that the impact of modern vascular surgery may have resulted in a reduction in the incidence of amputation. A 2018 British study of 103 934 patients with PAD who underwent revascularisation showed that there was a marked reduction in the estimated 1-year risk of major amputation from 5.7–3.9%.[19]

Similar trends have also been observed in the United States, where national billing data have revealed a 45% reduction in the rate of lower extremity amputations during the period 1996 to 2011 associated with a quadrupling in the number of therapeutic endovascular interventions.[20]

Survival rates after an amputation depend upon the cause of the amputation rather than the amputation itself. Patients who have amputations following trauma tend to have good long-term outcomes in terms of QoL and survival.[21] However, those who undergo amputation because of dysvascularity face a significantly worse prognosis. A 2020 systematic review and meta-analysis of 61 studies comprising a total of 36 037 patients from 17 countries and regions, and showed that patients who had amputations because of dysvascularity (including associated diabetes mellitus) faced pooled mortality rates of 33.7% at 1-year post-amputation, and rising steadily to 80% at 10-years follow-up.[22]

Following an initial major leg amputation caused by dysvascularity, amputees who also had diabetes were 2.8 times more likely to undergo an *additional* major amputation of the contralateral leg, compared to those without diabetes.[23]

INDICATIONS FOR AMPUTATION

The clinical decision to perform amputation can appear straightforward when there is extensive tissue loss resulting in non-functioning limb. In other situations, the decision to amputate may not be so straightforward and the role of amputation in the management of chronic limb-threatening limb ischaemia (CLTI) remains controversial.

The Trans-Atlantic Inter-Society Consensus for the Management of Peripheral Arterial Disease (TASC II) recommends that if revascularisation is unlikely to be successful and the patient suffers intolerable pain or has a spreading infection, then primary amputation should be considered.[24] This approach is supported by the literature in that it appears to be the most viable outcome in terms of QoL[25] and cost-effectiveness.[26]

TASC II also recommended that non-ambulatory elderly patients presenting with CLTI should be considered for primary amputation, especially if they have flexion contractures.[24] The reasoning is that where patients with CLTI also have co-existing disabilities or co-morbidities that would render them unable to make use of a salvageable limb, then primary amputation with appropriate rehabilitation offers the best option (even if the patient is unlikely to be a prosthetic limb user). Further examples of such patients include those with severe dementia, dense hemiplegia or spinal paralysis, severe arthritis and severe cardiorespiratory disease. Fig. 6.1 is an algorithm on the TASC II recommendations on the management of CLTI.

AMPUTATION LEVEL

Selection of the anatomical level of amputation depends on the potential for surgical wound healing and rehabilitation as well as prosthetic considerations. The potential for rehabilitation and setting of likely goals can only be determined through a holistic assessment of the patient by the multidisciplinary specialist amputee rehabilitation team. This assessment should include co-morbidities and disabilities, cognitive state and motivation, likely discharge destination, patient's occupation, lifestyle and support network, as well as their aspirations and wishes.

In general terms, the more proximal the level of amputation, the more difficult it will be for the patient to achieve independent ambulation with a prosthetic limb, especially if functional native joints such as the knee are lost.

The most common amputation levels in CLTI are transtibial, transfemoral, knee disarticulation and Gritti–Stokes amputation. Using an anatomical approach, this section will cover the main amputation levels along the lower extremity from distal to proximal, before summarising on amputation level selection.

MINOR AMPUTATIONS

Minor amputations that are distal to the ankle joint require an abundant blood supply to heal. Unless the foot can be successfully revascularised, wounds following local amputation of single or multiple digits are generally difficult to heal.[27,28]

✔ Minor amputations should generally be avoided unless the foot can be successfully revascularised.[27,28]

RAY AMPUTATION

Ray amputation, which involves removal of the toe and partial removal of the metatarsal can be considered in forefoot ischaemia and can ensure a more adequate surgical debridement of the infected or necrotic margins.[29] In 2014 a single centre study, carried out in Singapore, of 150 patients with diabetes with infection or gangrene of the forefoot who underwent ray amputation found that 71% had healed without complication at 1-year follow-up.[30] However, a systematic review carried out in 2012, of 435 partial first ray amputations revealed that a fifth of these patients required more proximal re-amputation within 26 months.[31]

TRANSMETATARSAL AMPUTATION

Transmetatarsal amputations (TMA), if technically feasible with or without revascularisation, also produce satisfactory results in forefoot ischaemia.

Intra-operatively, soft tissue should be preserved as much as possible, and consideration is given to leaving the flaps open with delayed closure, as infection and gangrene of the flaps may occur if primary closure is attempted.

A single centre study in Italy from 2016, explored the effects of TMA *with* revascularisation in 206 patients with diabetes with forefoot infection and gangrene. The authors found that on discharge from hospital, 38% of these patients were ambulating independently, 43% with assistance and 60% were directly discharged home. At 1-year follow-up, the percentage of patients ambulating independently had risen to 77% and 81% of patients were living at home.[32]

A more recent Chinese study from 2019 explored the effects of TMA on 97 patients with diabetes with forefoot gangrene who were *unsuitable* for revascularisation. The authors

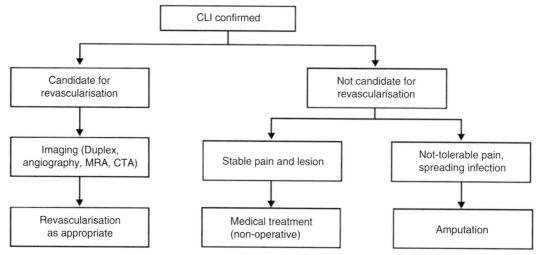

Figure 6.1 Algorithm for management of a patient with critical limb ischemia. *CLI*, Critical limb ischemia; *CTA*, computed tomographic angiography; *MRA*, magnetic resonance angiography. (From Norgren L, Hiatt WR, et al. Inter-Society Consensus for the Management of Peripheral Arterial Disease (TASC II). Eur J Vasc Endovasc Surg. 2007;33(40). Copyright 2006 by Elsevier Ltd. Reproduced with permission.)

found that 64.9% of these patients had their wound completely healed after a median of 8 months.[33]

MIDFOOT AMPUTATIONS

Amputations of the midfoot include Lisfranc and Chopart amputations. A Lisfranc separates all five metatarsals from the cuboid and their respective cuneiforms, whereas a Chopart amputation removes more of the midfoot and separates the talonavicular and calcaneocuboid joints.[34]

Midfoot amputations have a significant risk of postoperative equinovarus deformity caused by detaching the insertions of peroneal longus, brevis and tibialis anterior as part of the amputation surgery, which in turn leads to unopposed plantarflexion by the gastrocsoleus complex.[34] If midfoot amputations are absolutely necessary, the surgeon should consider inter-operative rebalancing techniques such as Achilles tenotomy, tibialis anterior or extensor digitorum transfer to the talus or even ankle arthrodesis.

Prosthetic options with these amputations are limited and midfoot amputations also have high rates of subsequent proximal revision amputations (i.e., 'salami-slicing surgery').[35]

✔ Amputations of the midfoot are not usually recommended in CLTI.[34,35]

SYME AMPUTATION

A Syme amputation involves disarticulation of the ankle joint, removal of both malleoli and securing a long posterior flap containing the heel pad to the anterior tibia[36] to facilitate intermittent weight-bearing. It can be used to successfully treat forefoot gangrene, especially in diabetic patients with dysvascularity. Viability of the posterior flap and heel pad is heavily dependent on the patency of the posterior tibial artery. Thus an ankle-brachial index of less than 0.5 is generally considered to be a contraindication to a Syme amputation.[37]

As the heel pad allows for intermittent weight-bearing, the residual limb in a Syme amputation can be walked on for very short distances without a prosthetic limb (such as when ambulating from the bedroom to the toilet).

Compared to a transtibial amputation (TTA), a Syme amputation offers reduced energy expenditure when ambulating,[38] greater gait stability and thus requires less physiotherapy and gait retraining.[39] However, breakdown and migration of the posterior flap and heel pad may occur if a prosthesis is used regularly. Prosthetic options are also limited with a Syme amputation and there are considerable difficulties in prosthetic fitting as the prosthesis would inevitability be bulky to encompass the bulbous residual limb,[40] which may also impede the contralateral limb when walking.

✔ Syme amputations are not usually recommended in CLTI, especially if the patient is a potential regular prosthetic limb user.[40]

TRANSTIBIAL AMPUTATION AND TRANSFEMORAL AMPUTATION

Approximately half of all referrals to amputee rehabilitation centres in the United Kingdom involve TTAs making it the most common amputation level. The second most common level was transfemoral amputation (TFA) at 34%.[18]

Preservation of the native functioning knee joint has tremendous advantages in terms of mobility with a prosthetic limb.

Compared to independently mobile non-amputees, the energy cost of walking with a prosthetic limb in dysvascular amputees who have undergone a unilateral TTA is increased by 40%, whilst in unilateral transfemoral amputees by 120%.[41] This energy cost can increase to 280% in bilateral transfemoral amputees when mobilising with two prosthetic limbs.[42] The increased energy demands invariably affect an amputee's ability to use a prosthetic limb with approximately 74% of bilateral amputees not being able to walk with prosthetic limbs 5 years following surgery.[43]

In 2013 a Dutch longitudinal study of 82 patients exploring QoL following lower extremity amputation and found that amputation level was a key factor in determining QoL. Using the RAND-36 questionnaire, the authors noted that transtibial amputees reported better QoL scores compared to transfemoral amputees within the 18 months following an amputation. This was because of a better walking ability leading to greater social participation amongst patients who had a TTA.[44]

A previous British observational study from 2003, of 281 unilateral lower extremity amputees, found that amongst older (>50 years old) amputees, approximately 50% and 60% of transtibial amputees were ambulating independently in the community or at home, respectively 1-year following surgery. Whereas for transfemoral amputees, the respective figures were much lower at 25% and 50%.[45]

✓✓ The native knee joint should be preserved where possible to facilitate rehabilitation and ambulation with a prosthetic limb.[44,45]

THROUGH-KNEE AMPUTATION: KNEE DISARTICULATION AND GRITTI–STOKES

Traditionally, through-knee amputation was only considered in those patients who were deemed incapable of walking. The often-quoted Lower Extremity Assessment Project (LEAP) study showed worse outcomes in *trauma* patients who had knee disarticulation compared to transtibial and TFAs, slower walking speeds and greater difficulty walking on uneven ground or outdoors in bad weather.[46]

However, more recent studies have suggested no significant differences in post-operative complications or functional outcomes in terms of mobility, activities of daily living, QoL or pain between knee disarticulation and transfemoral amputees in both vascular and trauma patients.[47–49]

With through-knee amputations, the longer lever-arm of the residual limb assists transfers, sitting balance and maintains hip adductor muscle attachment and distal proprioception.[50,51]

The conventional through-knee amputation (i.e., knee disarticulation) may cause problems related to the leakage of synovial fluid, bulbous femoral condyles and the retained patella, which could potentially cause difficulties with prosthetic socket fitting if the patient becomes ambulatory later on. The Gritti–Stokes amputation theoretically avoids these problems by resecting the bone at the supra-condylar femoral level, enucleating the patella and anchoring it to the distal femur as an end-cap (Fig. 6.2). However excision of femoral condyles could adversely affect the suspension and rotational stability of the applied prosthesis. Enucleating the patella and anchoring it to the distal femur has been associated with femora-patellar non-union and mal-union. In a Gritti-Stokes amputation, the load bearing axis lies posterior to the residual limb. This could to lead to greater mechanical stress on the femur, which in turn could adversely effect ambulation with a prosthetic limb.[51,52,53] Therefore, caution is strongly advised when considering Gritti-Stokes amputation in ambulatory patients.[54]

Due to a longer femoral component and lowered prosthetic knee centre, as well as limited availability of stance and swing phase control mechanisms in the prosthetic knee joint at this level, prosthetic limb fitting can be technically challenging in through-knee amputees.

HIP DISARTICULATION AND HEMIPELVECTOMY

Hip disarticulation and hemipelvectomy are rare procedures in patients with PAD. They comprise approximately 1% of all lower extremity amputees presenting to UK amputee rehabilitation centres.[18] The majority of these procedures are carried out for neoplasm (usually sarcoma) followed by infection[55] and major trauma,[56] rather than dysvascularity.

The complex neurovascular and visceral anatomy of the pelvic region and relative rarity of these procedures present significant technical, surgical and rehabilitative challenges. With intra-operative blood loss in hemipelvectomy averaging 3 litres and peri-operative mortality as high as 44%, both these operations should be considered as amputations of last resort.[55] Of the survivors, with an integrated multidisciplinary rehabilitative approach, approximately 43% can eventually use a prosthetic limb following either surgery.[57]

PRINCIPLES IN AMPUTATION LEVEL SELECTION

The selection of the amputation level in major lower extremity amputation can be multifactorial and complicated. Thus, it should be decided on after careful multidisciplinary assessment and discussion between the surgical and rehabilitation teams. However, there are general rehabilitation principles that should be taken into consideration by the vascular surgeon when making this decision, as outlined below. Fig. 6.3 illustrates this decision-making process via an algorithm.

1. Preserve the native functional knee joint if possible

   Preserving the native knee joint is the key factor in reducing the energy and metabolic cost when using a prosthetic limb. This should be considered whenever possible, especially if it is anticipated that the patient has the potential to transfer (e.g., from bed to chair) or walk with a prosthetic limb.

2. In non-ambulatory patients, consider knee disarticulation or Gritti–Stokes amputation

   In patients who are bed- or chair-bound, a TTA residual limb risks non-healing and may also lead to flexion contractures of the hip and knee joints and thus impeding patient transfers. A knee disarticulation or Gritti–Stokes amputation can avoid these aforementioned complications. These two amputations are also preferable to TFA as they provide longer lever-arms and larger residual limb surface areas, which are more conducive to transferring and promote wheelchair mobility by providing a more stable counterbalance.[50,51]

3. TFAs should be considered in fixed knee flexion of ≥30 degrees and/or severe knee arthropathy.

   A fixed knee flexion deformity of more than 15% can reduce foot clearance during the swing phase, which may impede walking[58] and can lead to quadriceps fatigue and anterior knee pain.[59] Usually, a flexion contracture of 30 degrees is considered the maximum limit for transtibial prosthetic limb fitting.[60] In addition, severe knee arthropathy can also impede walking. Therefore in these two circumstances, a more proximal amputation should be considered.

4. In ambulatory patients who cannot have a TTA, a TFA is the next best option.

   In patients where a TTA is not possible but the patient has the potential to walk, a TFA is preferred rather than knee disarticulation or Gritti–Stokes amputation. This is because of problems of prosthetic fitting, which may compromise cosmetic appearance and function.

Cosmesis is affected because the prosthetic knee joint extends beyond the length of the femur. Therefore for patients with a through-knee amputation, the femoral component is longer. Functionally, this may mean that sitting in small spaces is more cumbersome or restricted because of this increased length. Conversely, some studies have demonstrated better functional outcomes in patients with a knee disarticulation. This is explained by the longer lever-arm and the fact that the adductor muscles of the hip are preserved in a knee disarticulation. Both of these factors improve the thigh motion for ambulation, decreases energy expenditure and help maintain distal proprioception, which helps facilitate walking with a prosthetic limb.[50,51]

SURGICAL CONSIDERATIONS

A UK National Confidential Enquiry into Patient Outcome and Deaths (NCEPOD) in 2014 revealed that only 44% of patients undergoing amputations for dysvascularity were assessed as having received a good level of care. The

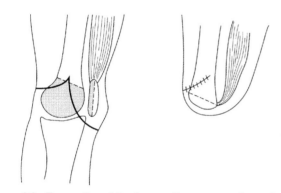

Figure 6.2 Transection of the femur with reverse angle results in a more stable attachment of the patella in the Gritti–Stokes amputation.

enquiry also reported that half of the patients lacked multidisciplinary involvement in their care as well as a clear patient pathway. The enquiry suggested that its findings may explain the marked discrepancy between mortality rates for amputation in patients with dysvascularity between the United Kingdom and the United States (12.4% vs. 9.6%, respectively).[61]

Therefore a multidisciplinary team (MDT) should be involved in the early stages of planning care for amputees with access to other medical and surgical specialities and allied health professionals, both pre- and post-amputation. In light of the significant risks of morbidities and mortalities, all amputations should be performed by experienced surgeons at consultant level and should not be delegated to unsupervised and inexperienced trainees.

Specific surgical considerations for transfemoral, transtibial and foot amputations will be covered later on in this section.

To enhance post-operative rehabilitation and facilitate limb sitting, the following general surgical principles should be followed:

- Tissues must be handled meticulously with care and strict haemostatic control
- A thigh tourniquet should be considered to reduce significant blood loss and transfusion requirements as well as ensure a bloodless operative field for the surgeon[62,63]
- Bony prominences around cut bone should be removed, the edges should be smoothed off and bevelled
- To reduce painful neuroma formation, nerves should be cut under tension, proximal to the bone edge in a scarfree environment and large nerves should be ligated when near an associated vessel
- To reduce arteriovenous fistula or aneurysm formation, larger arteries and veins should be individually dissected and ligated
- Skin and muscle flaps should be oversized initially and then shaped and trimmed as appropriate

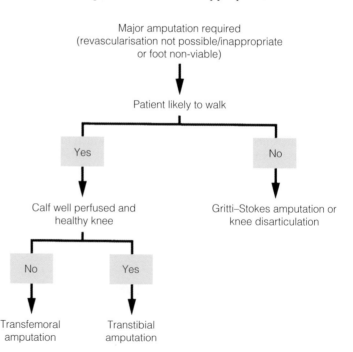

Figure 6.3 Algorithm for major amputation level selection.

- There should be good-quality sensate skin coverage of stump without any tension
- Muscle flaps should be anchored over the bone edge by myodesis, a long posterior flap sutured anteriorly or a balanced myoplasty[64]
- Skin and muscle flaps should be trimmed, fashioned and shaped to prevent 'dog-ears', redundant tissue or a bulbous stump
- Closure should be in layered with meticulous suturing technique. The skin should be closed with sutures rather than clips to reduce post-operative wound infection[65]

TRANSFEMORAL AMPUTATION

The ideal transection of the femur is 12 cm (10–15 cm acceptable) above the native knee joint, which is measured from the medial joint line. This length allows enough clearance for incorporating a prosthetic limb, and avoids using a lowered prosthetic knee centre, which gives an unacceptable cosmetic and functional disability when walking. The exact level of the bone cut will depend on the thickness of the thigh muscles and subcutaneous tissue. In morbidly obese patients with excessive soft tissue coverage, a through-knee amputation should be considered instead.

It is important to ensure adequate myoplastic coverage over the cut femur to reduce pain and discomfort as well as to allow muscle balancing of the hip adductors to abductors and rectus femoris to hamstrings.[66]

If muscle quality is adequate, adductor myodesis should be considered. The procedure, which involves anchoring of muscle to bone (i.e., the femur) via drill holes, reduces the risk of muscle slippage and overhang, creates a dynamic muscle balance, removes tension from the anterior myocutaneous flap, and provides a soft tissue envelope to facilitate limb fitting.

Similarly, a quadriceps myodesis should be considered, which can either be secured to the adductor flap or the posterior femur.[67]

The myoplasty and myodeses should be performed with the hip joint in neutral (in the sagittal plane) and the naturally adducted position of 5-10°. This prevents both hip flexion and abduction contractures[68] and is ideal for prosthetic function.

TRANSTIBIAL AMPUTATION

The ideal bone transection of the tibia is 12–15 cm below the native knee joint (measured from the medial joint line). The fibula should be divided around 1.5 cm proximal to the level of the tibial section. A short bevel and rounding off the sharp corners of the tibia must be undertaken to reduce pain and facilitate fitting.

With residual limbs less than 8–9 cm, the surgeon should consider performing a total fibulectomy and peroneal nerve resection.[69] This ensures an adequate lever-arm and enough ground clearance to fit a prosthetic limb. If the residual limb is likely to be even shorter, a TTA should not be performed, and the surgeon should consider through-knee or TFA instead.

Where possible, the skew flap should be considered in place of the traditional Burgess long posterior flap.

With a Burgess long posterior flap, the residual limb tends to change into a bulbous shape and 'dog ears' tend to develop at the far edges of the wound, which impedes prosthetic limb fitting. Moreover, as the gastrocnemius tendon and the deep fascia are brought forward and anchored to the fascia and periosteum anteriorly, this means that flap coverage over the anterior tibia is vulnerable. The line of skin closure is also placed directly in front of the bevelled anterior border of the tibia. This approach does not adhere to the optimal local blood supply to the skin and makes the wound susceptible to breakdown.[70]

Conversely, the skewed skin flaps are based on the arteries that run along the same course as the great and small saphenous veins, which provide the main blood supply to the skin. This theoretically means that there is greater vascularity around the anteromedial and posterolateral aspects of the proximal tibia.

Fig. 6.4 illustrates the surgical stages of a skew flap: (a) Following the creation of anteromedial and posterolateral fasciocutaneous flaps, the gastrocnemius muscle (with deep fascia attached) is narrowed; (b) the gastrocnemius muscle flap is lifted anterodistally, and (c) anchored to the deep fascia and periosteum of the anterior tibia; (d) the anteromedial and posterolateral fasciocutaneous flaps are closed in an oblique direction over a suction drain. The ensures that the suture line is placed away from the cut bone.

This technique promotes wound healing by minimising disruption to the blood supply and oxygenation[71] of the skin as well as avoiding a vulnerable scar line under tension. It also avoids 'dog ears' and a bulbous residual limb shape and thus facilitates early rehabilitation and limb fitting[72] (Fig. 6.5).

The Burgess long posterior flap is a useful alternative where skew flaps might be compromised by the medial skin incision of a failed femorodistal bypass graft or following fasciotomies (Fig. 6.6). When undertaking a long posterior flap, the skin flaps should be marked using the 'rule of thirds'. The anterior incision should be two-thirds of the total leg circumference and the posterior incision should be one-third of the total circumference. The posterior flap should be distal to the musculotendinous junction of the gastrocnemius and approximately one-and-a-half times longer than the anterior flap to allow for sufficient closure (Fig. 6.7). A Cochrane review analysed the outcomes of three randomised clinical trials of skew flaps and traditional long posterior flaps and was unable to determine that one technique was better than the other.[73]

✓✓ Skew flaps have some theoretical advantages compared to the traditional Burgess long posterior flap but reported outcomes in the literature appear similar.

For patients undergoing TTA, an Ertl osteomyoplastic procedure should be considered, which is the creation of a bone bridge connecting the cut tibia and fibula to support end-weight–bearing onto a prosthetic limb. The modified Ertl technique uses a fibular strut graft, which can be fixed to the tibia and fibula with cortical screws, fibre wire suture with end buttons, or heavy non-absorbable suture (Fig. 6.8).

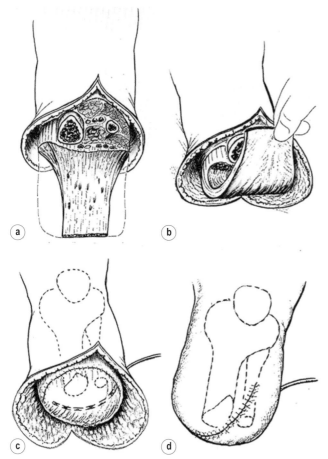

Figure 6.4 Skew flap stages. (Modified from Robinson K. Vascular surgical techniques. Philadelphia: WB Saunders, 1989.)

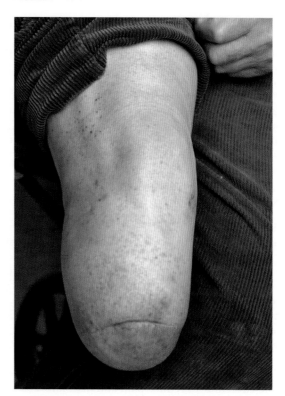

Figure 6.6 Healed Burgess long posterior flap in a transtibial amputee.

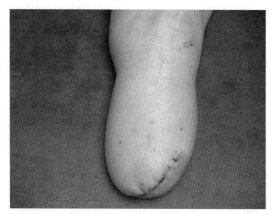

Figure 6.5 Skew flap at 2-weeks post-transtibial amputation showing a well-shaped residual limb and satisfactory wound healing, suitable for early limb fitting.

FOOT AMPUTATIONS

Digital amputation is most commonly performed in vascular patients with diabetes because of their susceptibility to infection. Digital amputation without sufficient perfusion into the foot means the wound is unlikely to heal. Toes with partial dry gangrene should be managed non-operatively. Digital amputation is best performed through the base of

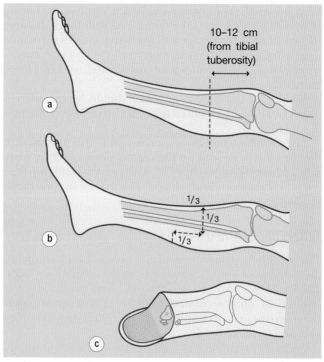

Figure 6.7 Marking the flaps for a Burgess long posterior flap transtibial amputation using the 'rule of thirds'. (From Marshall C, Barakat T and Stansby G. Amputation and rehabilitation. Surgery. 2016;34(4):188–91. Copyright 2016 by Elsevier Ltd. Reproduced with permission)

the proximal phalanx. In the great toe, this approach preserves the insertions of the flexor hallucis brevis, sesamoids and plantar fascia, which maintains gait stability during terminal stance,[74] reduces load transfer to the lesser toes and

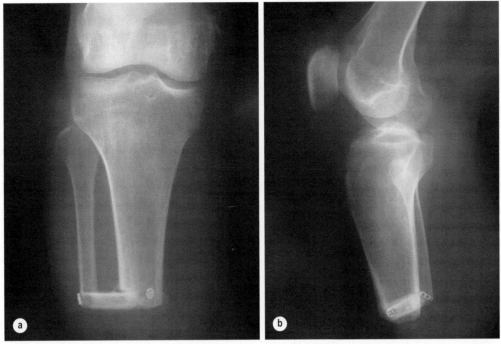

Figure 6.8 (a) Anteroposterior and (b) lateral x-rays of a modified Ertl procedure fixed using the TightRope device, at 3-months post-surgery. (From by Deol PS, Lee TH, et al. Evolution and modification of the Ertl osteomyoplastic transtibial amputation. Oper Tech Orthop. 2008;18(4):293–8. Copyright 2008 by Elsevier Ltd. Reproduced with permission)

associated pressure ulceration. In a second toe amputation, this approach helps maintain the position of the adjacent great toe, prevent hallux valgus and associated pressure ulceration.[75]

Although primary closure with a flap (e.g., plantar based flap) is possible, the flap is at risk dehiscence because of dysvascularity and potential tension, and so it is preferable to leave the wound open to heal by secondary intention.

When infection extends beyond the proximal phalanx, a 'ray amputation' is indicated. After excision of the affected toes, the line of excision is moved proximally through the infected tissue until healthy tissue is reached. The underlying metatarsal head is excised and the wound left open like a 'fish mouth'. Infection of the first or fifth metatarsophalangeal joint requires a 'tennis-racquet' incision; the handle of the racquet can usually be closed after excision of the metatarsal head. If osteomyelitis is present, a sample of the excised and retained bone should be sent for microbiological culture as the organisms causing the osteomyelitis are often different from those in the ulcer.

First ray amputations disrupt the medial column, which can lead to instability and loss of 'push-off' or propulsion, especially at a higher cadence. Thus it should be performed only after careful discussion with the MDT. The removal of a single ray in the middle of the foot (i.e., the second, third or fourth) gives a chevron-shaped wedge, maintaining good function and stability. However, because of the resultant narrow forefoot, shoe-fitting can be challenging, and forefoot equinus can also develop.[76]

A TMA can be useful when all the toes are gangrenous but when the plantar skin is still viable. An incision is made dorsally at mid-metatarsal level with a long plantar flap and bone transection through the metatarsal bases. Soft tissue should be preserved as much as possible,

and consideration given to leaving the flaps open with delayed closure, to reduce the risks of infection and gangrene. Negative pressure wound therapy may facilitate the healing of such open wound foot amputations. Due to the unopposed action of gastrocnemius, tibialis anterior and posterior and deficiencies of the extensor musculature and tendons, a TMA risks the development of equinovarus deformity and so a concomitant tendo-achilles lengthening may be considered to prevent this from happening.[77]

AMPUTEE REHABILITATION

The process of rehabilitation for vascular amputees, who are usually elderly and often have several other co-morbidities and disabilities, can pose a considerable challenge. An MDT approach to rehabilitation throughout the inpatient and amputee care pathway has now become the standard within the United Kingdom. The core members of the MDT should include a vascular surgeon, rehabilitation physician, specialist nurses, prosthetist, occupational therapist, physiotherapist, amputee psychologist/counsellor and wheelchair services. The availability of a social worker, community nurse, orthotist and amputee patient-volunteer can also be valuable to the patient's rehabilitation process.

The British Society of Physical & Rehabilitation Medicine (BSPRM) Amputee and Prosthetic Rehabilitation guidelines recommend that the operating surgeon should consult with the Rehabilitation Medicine physician to determine the most appropriate level of amputation and surgical technique to form a residual limb capable of comfortable load-bearing and ambulation in a prosthetic socket without breakdown.[78]

PRE-AMPUTATION CONSULTATION AND PLANNING

Where possible, a pre-amputation consultation by the amputee rehabilitation team should be carried out for every patient awaiting an amputation. This is both recommended in guidelines issued by the BSRM[78] and the Vascular Society for Great Britain and Ireland.[79] The pre-amputation consultation should involve an initial assessment and preparation of the patient for the likely rehabilitation programme to be implemented. This consultation should allow the patient to see and feel examples of prosthetic limbs that are appropriate, help the patient instil realistic expectations of their goals and outcomes, and address any specific questions or anxieties. This consultation also allows advice by the rehabilitation team regarding amputation level and ideal length of the residuum, pre- and post-amputation pain management. Objective clinical assessment tools used at this review can include the Trinity Amputation and Prosthesis Experience Scale, Amputee Mobility Predictor and Medicare Functional Classification Levels (also known as *K levels*) (Table 6.1). It is important to note that not all patients referred for a pre-amputation consultation are suitable for a prosthetic limb and where appropriate, other rehabilitation options should be discussed with the patient.

After the assessment, a rehabilitation therapy plan should be made and should commence pre-operatively before hospital admission.[78]

The rehabilitation therapy team should also review the patient's home environment, in terms of the need for adaptive equipment, wheelchairs, specialist seating and environmental changes (e.g., downstairs sleeping arrangements). This home review will also facilitate timely discharge planning from the hospital post-surgery.

RESIDUAL LIMB MANAGEMENT

Dressing selection post-amputation remains a topic of debate. Traditionally, soft dressings or bandages, which did not address post-operative oedema, were used in the United Kingdom. Newer studies have suggested that rigid dressings (vacuum-formed, pneumatic or Plaster of Paris) not only reduce post-operative oedema but may also reduce pain, the occurrence of knee contracture in transtibial amputees as well as providing wound protection. This can facilitate early residuum maturation leading to early mobilisation and rehabilitation with a prosthesis, which in turn shortens hospital length of stay.[80–82]

Amputee rehabilitation guidelines from both the BSRM and the British Association of Chartered Physiotherapists in Amputee Rehabilitation (BACPAR) recommend the use of rigid dressings where possible.[78,83] However, vigilant nursing care, with regular dressing changes, should be taken to avoid potential complications such as excessive pressure on the wound leading to necrosis.[78,84]

A recent 2019 Cochrane review of nine randomised controlled trial involving 436 transtibial amputees did not find any conclusive difference in the aforementioned outcomes between soft and rigid dressings, and therefore clinician discretion and judgement should be exercised on a case-by-case basis.[85]

Table 6.1 Definitions for the Medicare functional classification levels (K levels)

K-Level 0	Does not have the ability or potential to ambulate or transfer safely with or without assistance, and a prosthesis does not enhance quality of life or mobility.
K-Level 1	Has the ability or potential to use a prosthesis for transfers or ambulation in level surfaces at a fixed cadence. Typical of the limited and unlimited household ambulator.
K-Level 2	Has the ability or potential for ambulation with the ability to transverse low-level environmental barriers such as curbs, stairs or uneven surfaces. Typical of the limited community ambulator.
K-Level 3	Has the ability or potential for ambulation with variable cadence. Typical of the community ambulator who has the ability to transverse most environmental barriers and may have vocational, therapeutic or exercise activity that demands prosthetic use beyond simple locomotion.
K-Level 4	Has the ability or potential for prosthetic ambulation that exceeds basic ambulation skills, exhibiting high impact, stress or energy levels. Typical of the prosthetic demands of the child, active adult or athlete.

From Gailey RS, Roach KE, et al. The amputee mobility predictor: an instrument to assess determinants of the lower-limb amputee's ability to ambulate. Arch Phys Med Rehabil. 2002;83(5):613–7. Copyright 2002 by Elsevier Ltd. Reproduced with permission

If using a traditional soft dressing that is non-adhesive, an elasticated tubular bandage can be placed on the residuum to hold these dressings in place. Tight bandaging around the residual limb should be avoided in vascular amputees as it can impair tissue perfusion and healing (e.g., Tubifast® is preferred to Tubigrip® as the latter can be too tight[78]). Alternatively, an adhesive clear-plastic film dressing can allow easier and regular wound inspection, especially before and after application of walking aids.

If the wound is healed or healing satisfactorily, then elasticated compression shrinker socks (e.g., Juzo®) can be applied to the residual limb (Fig. 6.9). Shrinker socks can further reduce oedema, protect the wound and facilitate residuum maturation and thus early prosthetic socking fitting.[86]

Residual limb supports should be fitted to the patient's wheelchair so that the residuum can be kept elevated to reduce oedema and prevent knee flexion contractures (in TTAs). In vascular patients, especially with diabetic foot disease, specialist footwear is recommended to protect the contralateral foot from skin or tissue damage, when ambulating or transferring. Pressure-relief ankle-foot orthoses are effective for this purpose[87] and also relieve pressure on the heel when the patient is supine.

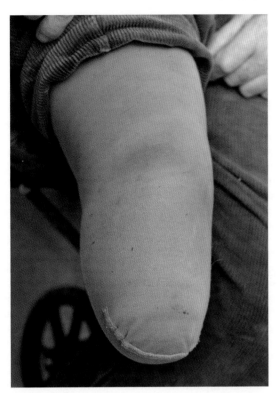

Figure 6.9 A stump shrinker sock applied over a transtibial amputation residual limb.

PAIN MANAGEMENT

Pain after an amputation can occur in up to 80% of patients.[88] It is often challenging to treat with a fluctuating natural history and various treatment methods proposed. Pain management is dependent on the type of pain experienced. Amputee pain can be divided into post-operative pain, acute and chronic residual limb pain, and phantom limb pain (PLP), with varying degrees of overlap. A multimodal approach is often needed to manage post-amputation pain effectively[89] and early involvement of the pain management team is recommended.

POST-OPERATIVE PAIN

Regional anaesthesia has been proposed as the 'gold standard' for the management of post-operative pain following amputation.[90] This can be achieved using perineural catheters (PNCs).

Intra-operatively, PNCs are placed along the transected sciatic nerve for TFAs or tibial nerve for TTAs. They can be used to provide continuous local anaesthetic infusion in the post-operative period. The catheter remains in place for a minimum of 3 days. A systematic review and meta-analysis of seven studies comprising 416 patients undergoing major lower-extremity amputation concluded that PNC placement, on average, halved post-operative opioid consumption, but interestingly did not significantly affect patient's subjectively reported pain scores.[91]

✔ PNCs should be considered to improve post-operative pain management following amputation.[91]

ACUTE RESIDUAL LIMB PAIN

In the first few weeks post-operatively, residual limb pain (also known as stump pain) is predominantly pain from the surgical site and wound. This pain is sharp, aching and severe, and is confined to the surgical site itself. It is a mixture of nociceptive and neuropathic pain, caused by the extensive tissue trauma and direct neural injury from the amputation.[90] Acute neuropathic residual limb pain can be managed with PNCs. However, acute nociceptive pain should be managed through a graded approach using the World Health Organisation analgesic ladder (e.g., paracetamol/non-steroidal anti-inflammatory drugs [NSAIDs], weak opioids, strong opioids).[92] In severe cases of acute residual limb pain, strong opioids (e.g., morphine) delivered via patient-controlled analgesia (PCA) may be required for a limited period post-operatively. Ketamine may also be used as a short-term adjuvant.[90]

CHRONIC RESIDUAL LIMB PAIN

Acute residual limb pain is expected to resolve after a few weeks post-amputation. However, at least 10% of these patients go on to experience chronic residual limb pain.[93] The causes of chronic limb pain are listed in Table 6.2. The three most pertinent causes discussed in this section are infection (including osteomyelitis), neuroma and heterotropic ossification.

INFECTION

Infection is more common in vascular amputees especially those with diabetes. Infections can include cellulitis, abscess or osteomyelitis, which can all present as a painful residual limb. Therefore the clinician must exercise a high index of suspicion for infection when assessing a painful residual limb. Early diagnosis and treatment are essential to prevent the spreading of infection and development of sepsis. Clinical signs include swelling, redness, purulent discharge and wound dehiscence. Haematological investigations include white cell count, inflammatory markers and blood cultures. A wound swab should also be taken for microbiological culture and sensitivities. Imaging can include plain x-rays, magnetic resonance imaging (MRI) or bone scan. In cases of osteomyelitis, early involvement of the bone infection team is advised. Long-term antibiotic treatment is often indicated along with surgical debridement. If this is unsuccessful, revision of the residual limb to a more proximal amputation level may be required.[90]

NEUROMA

After a nerve has been transected, an intense immune cell–mediated inflammatory reaction can occur. Trying to maintain the congruity of the cut axon, Schwann cells stimulate new growth of adjacent axons that grow in multiple directions to try to overcome the defect, which can form a bulbous entanglement at the cut end of the nerve (i.e., neuroma).[94] Neuromas have altered sodium channel function with reduced activation thresholds and spontaneous discharges. This leads not only to hypersensitivity but also spontaneous pain in the residual limb around the area of

Table 6.2   Causes of chronic residual limb pain

Causes of chronic residual limb pain
Infection (including osteomyelitis)
Neuroma
Heterotropic ossification
Wound dehiscence
Arterial insufficiency (impaired perfusion)
Bone spur
Haematoma
Insufficient myoplasty covering
Poorly fitting prosthetic limb

Adapted from by Neil MJE. Pain after amputation. BJA Educ. 2016;16(3):107–12. Copyright 2015 by Elsevier Ltd. Reproduced with permission

the neuroma. There is a close association between residual limb neuroma pain and PLP.[90]

Neuromas take time to form and so are not usually a cause of acute residual limb pain. Clinical features include focalised pain in an area of the residual limb, unprovoked pain, and localised sensory changes. Treatment options overlap with PLP, however, more specific treatments for neuroma-associated pain include neurolysis by alcohol, phenol or botulinum toxin, radiofrequency ablation, local anaesthetic/steroid injections and surgical interventions such as targeted muscle reinnervation.[95] Simple surgical resection of the neuroma should be avoided where possible, because of high recurrence rates and scar tissue formation. This in turn can worsen the pain and adversely affect prosthetic limb fitting and ambulation.[94]

HETEROTOPIC OSSIFICATION

Heterotopic ossification (HO) is the pathological formation of bone in tissues that are not normally osseous[96] and is usually triggered by severe trauma. It is traditionally associated with soldiers who have suffered blast injury amputations in combat.[97] However, in the civilian population, HO can also occur in vascular amputees because of the traumatic effect of the amputation surgery itself. Amongst civilian amputees, there is no significant difference between the aetiology of the amputation and the occurrence of HO.[98] Severe traumatic tissue injury leads to an influx of inflammatory cells and the subsequent downstream signalling sequelae among resident cells of mesenchymal origin. This downstream signalling inappropriately activates osteogenic or osteochondrogenic proliferation in extra-osseous sites.[99] The presence of concomitant traumatic brain injury or spinal cord injury increases the risk of HO.[100] Depending on the site of bone formation, HO can cause significant pain and reduce range of motion, which can interfere with prosthetic limb fitting and ambulation. Diagnosis is through clinical assessment, blood tests (elevated alkaline phosphatase) and plain x-rays (Fig. 6.10). Prophylactic treatment includes NSAIDS (e.g., indomethacin) and peri-operative radiotherapy. The use of bisphosphonates as prophylactic treatment is controversial with some studies suggesting that the anti-resorptive effects of bisphosphonates may conversely increase the risk of HO rather than reducing it.[99] Therapeutic options are limited

mainly to surgical excision, which carries inherent risks of recurrence.

PHANTOM LIMB PAIN

PLP can be defined as the perception of pain or discomfort in a limb that no longer exists.[101] It can occur in up to 80% of amputees. Of those patients affected, 75% develop PLP within the first week after amputation[90] with a second peak at 2-years post-surgery.[102] It is generally considered a type of neuropathic pain.[103] Its exact mechanism is not fully understood, however, it is thought to result from heightened neural activity and neural reorganisation in the peripheral nerves, spinal cord and brain following an amputation. There is also thought to be a psychogenic component with anxiety and depression associated with PLP.[101] The risks factors for PLP are illustrated in Table 6.3.

Pharmacological treatment of PLP includes simple analgesics (paracetamol, NSAIDs), antidepressants (e.g., amitriptyline, duloxetine), anticonvulsants (gabapentin, pregabalin), topical analgesics (e.g., capsaicin), NMDA receptor antagonists (e.g., ketamine), local anaesthetic myofascial injections to the contralateral limb and intra-cutaneous botulinum toxin injections around the residual limb,[101] continuous peripheral nerve blocks (e.g., to the sciatic nerve)[104] and lumbar sympathetic blocks.[105] Although some studies have suggested the effectiveness of opioids in the treatment of PLP,[106,107] opioids should be used with caution (and only for a limited period), because of risks of dependence, tolerance and drowsiness.

Non-pharmacological treatment of PLP includes transcutaneous electrical nerve stimulation (TENS), spinal cord stimulation,[108] peripheral nerve stimulation, graded motor imagery (left/right discrimination, explicit motor imagery, mirror therapy),[109] target muscle re-innervation,[110] virtual and argument reality,[111] biofeedback[112] and acupuncture.[113]

However, the evidence for the effectiveness of these treatments is variable. A Cochrane review in 2016, found there was inconclusive evidence with regards to the efficacy of seven common pharmacological treatments for PLP.[114] A separate Cochrane review conducted a year earlier, found similar inconclusive evidence with regards to the effectiveness of TENS in treating PLP.[115] Another systematic review conducted in 2017, of 86 papers covering 38 pharmacological and non-pharmacological treatments for PLP was again inconclusive with low levels of evidence.[116]

✔ Early involvement by the specialist pain management team is recommended and a multimodal approach is advised when managing pain in the person who has undergone amputation.

EARLY POST-OPERATIVE REHABILITATION

The occupational therapist and physiotherapist should work closely together to ensure an effective and timely post-operative rehabilitation programme. On the first day post-amputation, the physiotherapist usually reviews the patient on the surgical ward and will commence a programme of

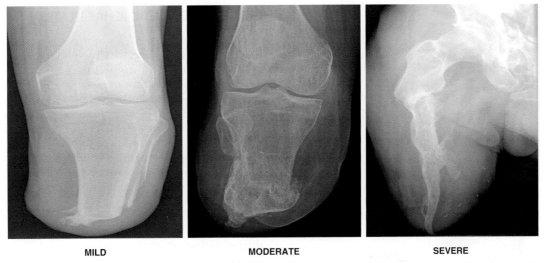

MILD   **MODERATE**   **SEVERE**

Figure 6.10   Anteroposterior x-rays of mild, moderate and severe heterotopic ossification in civilian amputees. (From Matsumoto ME, Khan M, et al. Heterotropic ossification in civilians with lower-limb amputations. Arch Phys Med Rehabil. 2012;95(9):1710–3. Copyright 2014 by Elsevier Ltd. Reproduced with permission)

Table 6.3   Risk factors for phantom limb pain
Female sex
Upper extremity amputation
Presence of pre-amputation pain
Residual limb pain
Time after amputation (first week or second year)
From Subedi B and Grossberg GT. Phantom limb pain: mechanisms and treatment approaches. Pain Res Treat. 2011; 864605. Published by Hindawi journals. Reproduced with permission under Creative Commons Attribution Licence.

bed mobility, joint movements, transfers techniques from bed to chair and wheelchair mobility. Residual limb exercises, exercises for the contralateral lower limb and upper limbs, muscle strengthening, maintaining range of movements of the proximal joints, sitting balance and improvement of general cardiovascular fitness will all be incorporated into the programme. The frequency and intensity of the programme will depend on the amputee's general condition, frailty and pain control. Each patient will be assessed for an appropriate wheelchair and cushion and taught the necessary skills for independent wheelchair use, as early as possible, to facilitate discharge. Discharge from the surgical ward is usually to the patient's residence following a home assessment by the occupational therapist, however, in complex cases such as those with multiple limb loss, the patient may benefit from being transferred to an inpatient amputee rehabilitation centre (where available).[78] After 1 week of assessments and therapy post-amputation, the rehabilitation team is usually able to determine a patient's potential ability to use a prosthetic limb. Predictive scoring systems such as the Amputee Mobility Predictor may also aid the MDT in determining potential limb usage.[117] In a few cases, the amputee is too unwell in the early post-operative period but later may recover sufficiently to benefit from prosthetic rehabilitation. Therefore appropriate follow-up assessment should be arranged for this group of 'late bloomers'.

Amputees are unlikely to successfully ambulate with a prosthetic limb if they are extremely frail, have severe dementia, severe cardio-respiratory disease, gross fixed flexion contractures or severe arthritis. In these cases, amputee rehabilitation should focus on transfers and mobilising with a wheelchair. In borderline cases, the application of an early walking aid can be a useful trial to assess the suitability of a patient for potential prosthetic use before committing costs to the manufacture of an actual prosthetic limb.[118] Various borderline criteria (such as the BACPAR borderline criteria for transfemoral amputees) can also be used to assess suitability.[119]

In addition to assessing the patient, it is also important to assess the home environment of the patient and consider adaptations to facilitate mobility and activities of daily living. Driving advice and adaptations (including referral to the Regional Driving Assessment Centre), hobbies and employment should also be addressed as an integral part of the rehabilitation process.

EARLY WALKING AIDS

There are two main types of early walking aids used in the United Kingdom (Figs. 6.11 and 6.12). The most common is the pneumatic post-amputation mobility aid (PPAM Aid). The PPAM Aid can be used for transtibial, through-knee and TFAs and is useful in controlling post-amputation residuum oedema. Although the Femurette can also be used with through-knee amputations, it is an excellent early walking aid for transfemoral amputees as it mimics an active transfemoral prosthetic limb in terms of an ischial tuberosity-bearing socket configuration and knee joint as well as having a foot.[120] Early walking aids are also excellent morale boosters and are also used as assessment tools to estimate an amputee's potential for ambulating. Early walking aids facilitate residual limb desensitisation, assist in reduction of residuum oedema, promote wound healing, and allow re-training of postural reflexes, balance and gait. These aids should be considered 1 week

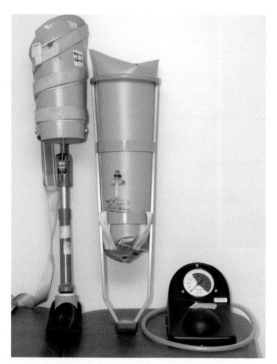

Figure 6.11   Early walking aids: Femurette (left) and pneumatic post-amputation mobility (PPAM) Aid (middle). A foot pump to inflate the PPAM Aid is shown on the right.

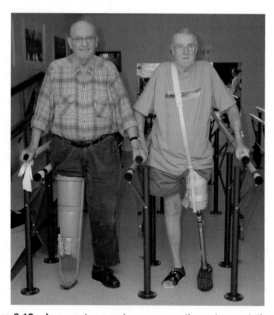

Figure 6.12   An amputee wearing a pneumatic post-amputation mobility (PPAM) Aid (left) and an amputee wearing a Femurette (right).

after amputation, under the judicious supervision of experienced therapists. However, in some cases where wound healing is poor or delayed, the introduction of early walking aids also needs to be delayed. In addition to being used as a trial to assess suitability for an actual prosthesis in borderlines cases, early walking aids can also be a temporary prosthesis for ambulatory training whilst the patient is waiting for his or her actual prosthetic limb to be designed, manufactured and fitted.

PRIMARY PROSTHETIC REHABILITATION

All amputees who receive a prosthetic limb should undergo prosthetic rehabilitation to achieve the best outcome. The role of the prosthetist in the fitting of a comfortable and functional prosthesis cannot be overemphasised. Prosthetic rehabilitation should aim to establish an energy-efficient gait based on normal physiological walking patterns. The physiotherapist should teach efficient control of the prosthesis through postural control, weight transfer, use of proprioception, and specific muscle strengthening and stretching exercises to prevent and correct gait deviations. Prosthetic rehabilitation will work towards the patient's own realistic goals and should include functional activities relevant to his or her lifestyle. All encouragement should be given to enable the patient to resume hobbies, sports, social activities, driving and return to work (where possible).

✔ Amputation rehabilitation guidelines for physiotherapy and occupational therapy have been published by the British Association of Chartered Physiotherapists in Amputee Rehabilitation (BACPAR)[121] and the UK College of Occupational Therapists.[122]

SPORTS ACTIVITIES FOR AMPUTEES

Amputation should not prevent an individual from actively participating in sports. This includes active and exertional sports such as running, cycling, swimming and soccer, but also less active/exertional sports that may be more appropriate for the older, vascular amputee, such as darts, billiards, bowling, fishing and golf.

Most sports will not require specially adapted prostheses and can be played alongside the able-bodied. Specialised adapted componentry are available for amputees who may want to run or swim. Beach/water activity limbs do not assist the user to swim but allow an amputee to access into and around the water for activities such as windsurfing, sailing and kayaking. Previous and current fitness, concurrent disabilities/co-morbidities and personal determination are all important factors in the individual returning to or engaging in a new sport. Amputees may seek sports advice from clinicians at their amputee rehabilitation centre, from peers, from groups such as the British Amputee and Les Autres Sports Association (BALASA), Limbless Association Sports Directory and the English Federation of Disability Sports. A systematic review was conducted in 2011 by Bragaru et al., which analysed 47 studies exploring the effects of sports participation by amputees. The authors found that sports participation gave general beneficial effects for the amputee in terms of cardiopulmonary conditioning, muscle training of the residual and other limbs, improved mobility and agility, physical functioning, psychological and social well-being and reducing obesity.[123]

PROSTHETIC DESIGN

The lower extremity prosthetic limbs used in the United Kingdom are mainly of an endoskeletal modular construction (Fig. 6.13). Compared to an exoskeletal prosthesis that

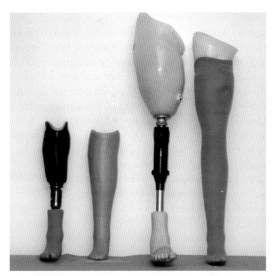

Figure 6.13 Modular endoskeletal prosthetic limbs for transfemoral and transtibial amputation, with and without cosmetic covers.

has a rigid outer shell, the endoskeletal design has a tubular structure that links each of the modular components.[124] This design allows for more rapid production, socket change, adjustments and repairs compared with the relatively older exoskeletal prostheses. For new amputees, the timeframe for a new limb, from measurement to delivery usually takes 1 week. The standard prosthesis usually incorporates thermoplastic materials like polypropylene or laminated plastics as socket materials and carbon fibre or lightweight alloy for the fabrication of the weight-bearing components. Traditionally, vascular amputees are measured for their first prosthesis at about 6 weeks post-amputation, although earlier fitting can take place subject to wound-healing status and the general condition of the residual limb. The residuum does *not* have to completely heal before limb fitting can take place. Where possible, earlier fitting using a preparatory prosthesis (sometimes as early as 1–2 weeks post-amputation) is beneficial for the patient in terms of reduced residuum oedema and muscle atrophy, improving patient confidence and facilitating early ambulation, reduced contractures and length of hospital stay.[125,126]

✔️ Early fitting and ambulation using a preparatory prosthesis (from 1–2 weeks post-amputation) should be considered where wound and patient conditions permit.[125,126]

There is ongoing controversy regarding the most optimal method of shape capture and casting of the residuum to accurately measure, manufacture and apply a well-fitting and comfortable socket. Traditionally, shape capture of the residuum was performed by hand casting and manual shaping using Plaster of Paris. In some rehabilitation centres, hand casting has been replaced by Computer-Aided Design (CAD) casting technology using MRI or Spiral X-ray Computed Topography, which is thought to be more accurate. However, more recent studies have cast doubt on this claim. In 2019 a systematic review of 22 studies comparing hand casting to CAD casting found no significant correlation between method of casting and the quality of the shape capture, socket fit and comfort as well as clinical efficiency. Although hand casting was more dependent on the individual

prosthetist's skill and had a steeper initial learning curve, in the hands of a well-trained and proficient prosthetist, hand casting yielded similar outcomes when compared to CAD.[127]

PROSTHESIS PRESCRIPTION AND RECENT DEVELOPMENTS

Transfemoral vascular amputees who are young and/or fit and active may have good musculature of the residual limb and adequate agility, general conditioning and manual dexterity to benefit from prostheses with suction socket fitting and sophisticated 'free knee' mechanisms like four-bar pneumatic or hydraulic swing phase controls. Fit and active transfemoral amputees who use their prosthesis daily may find conventional (passive) prosthetic limbs do not provide them with the desired stability especially when performing more exertional activities such as ambulating on an incline or on uneven terrain, which can lead to recurrent falls and stumbles. Therefore microprocessor-controlled knee (MPK) joints that provide enhanced control during the swing and stance phase of gait, may be suitable for these patients. In England, there are strict patient criteria for prescribing microprocessor knees on the National Health Service (NHS), including K3 activity level, able to ambulate 45 metres (50 yards) or more on flat ground, active commitment to the rehabilitation programme, sufficient cognitive ability, cardiovascular condition and muscle strength to activate the knee unit; a history of unstable gait, frequent falls or stumbles with a conventional transfemoral prosthesis and the requirement to use the MPK as a day-to-day prosthetic limb.[128]

In the United Kingdom, the majority of vascular transfemoral patients are middle-aged or elderly, and less active. If they are a potential limb user and accepted for a prosthetic rehabilitation programme, they are provided with non-suction prostheses with some form of waist-belt suspension and a 'locked' knee (bends only to sit down).

For knee disarticulation, Gritti–Stokes or long transfemoral amputees, prosthetic options are limited and many of these patients are non-limb users. Although prosthetic fitting at these levels is cosmetically and functionally challenging, the application of polycentric knee joints such as four-bar linkage knee mechanisms has eased some of the challenges by providing innate stability through a lower centre of rotation (Fig. 6.14). Since the polycentric knee unit folds back on itself at 90-degree flexion, it can also provide enhanced cosmesis for the patient when sitting.

✔️ For fit and active transfemoral amputees, microprocessor-controlled knee prosthetic limbs should be considered.[128]

OSSEO-INTEGRATED PROSTHETIC LIMBS

Osseo-integration (OI), also known as direct skeletal fixation, is a newer way of fitting the prosthesis to the residual limb. Used primarily in transfemoral amputees, an intra-medullary nail-like stem is inserted retrogradely into the medullary canal of the long bone within the residuum (i.e., the femur). The intra-medullary stem protrudes through the skin and has a distal metal abutment of which the prosthetic limb is attached to (Fig. 6.15). OI is usually performed in two surgical stages. The first stage involves excision of bony prominences

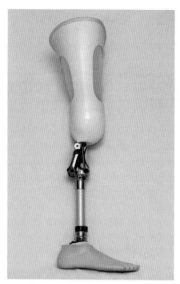

Figure 6.14   A knee disarticulation prosthesis with a four-bar linkage polycentric knee joint.

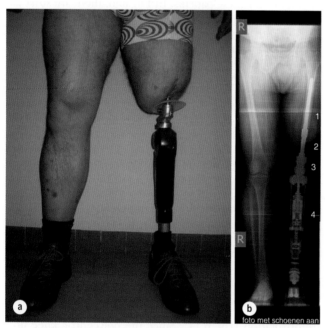

Figure 6.15   (a) Frontal view and (b) anteroposterior x-rays of an osseo-integrated transfemoral prosthetic limb. (From van de Meent H, Hopmanet MT, al. Walking ability and quality of life in subjects with transfemoral amputation: a comparison of osseointegration with socket prostheses. Arch Phys Med Rehabil. 2013;94(11):2174–8. Copyright 2013 by Elsevier Ltd. Reproduced with permission.)

of the distal femur, reaming of the medullary canal and insertion of the intra-medullary stem as well as refashioning of the residuum (including excision of excess skin, soft tissue and neuromas). If the femur is very short (i.e., <16 cm), cross screws or cross pins could be inserted through the stem transversely across the femur to secure fixation.[129] The wound is closed and post-operatively, the patient continues with physiotherapy exercises and progressive weight-bearing. The second stage involves surgically fixating a transcutaneous abutment adapter to the intra-medullary stem. This abutment adapter protrudes through the skin and is then attached to a torque control safety device, which in turn attaches to the interface of an external prosthetic limb.[130]

Previous studies, which secured the intra-medullary stem using screws, have recommended waiting up to 6 months between the two stages to allow for abundant bony ingrowth to the intra-medullary stem to enhance stability.[131,132] However, by using a 'press-fit' intra-medullary stem to achieve immediate stability, it is possible to undertake the second stage within 6 weeks after the first stage with promising results including earlier mobilisation and significant reductions of recovery time. Following the second stage, amputees in this study were able to use their prosthetic limb to ambulate without walking aids in about 4.5 months, instead of the usual 9 to 12 months with previous screw-fit stems.[130,132,133] Some teams have adopted a single-stage approach in which all the aforementioned procedures are carried out in one operative sitting, which can further shorten the recovery time by an additional 6 weeks.[134]

These initial studies, which focussed on younger patients with traumatic or combat injury amputation have been promising. OI can potentially avoid the problems associated with a traditional socket interface, such as skin issues, discomfort and pain, sweating, poor fitting and reduced control of the prosthetic limb leading to a lower QoL and prosthesis usage, and eventual cessation of limb use.[135] However, complications have been reported such as peri-prosthetic fractures, implant loosening and breakage, abutment failure and infection.[133]

Four systematic reviews have been conducted during the period 2017 to 2020 exploring the outcomes of OI. Each systematic review comprised between nine to 21 studies of OI primarily in younger traumatic amputees, with the total number of patients ranging from 211 to 809 in each review. The reviews all concluded that there were significant improvements in functional outcomes such as ambulation, mobility, prosthetic comfort and usage (both walking and sitting), general health and QoL and patient satisfaction.[133,135–137] However, three of the four systematic reviews also found that the most common complication encountered by patients was infection especially through the stoma site.[133,136,137]

This finding is corroborated in a longitudinal study of 18 patients that underwent OI prosthetic fitting for traumatic amputation during the period 1995 and 2018 in the United Kingdom with a median follow-up period of 12 years. The authors found that all but one patient (94%) had infection-related problems. Of these infected cases, five patients (28%) had their implants surgically removed either because of the infection itself or problems associated with infection such as loosening. The remaining 13 infected cases (including two deep peri-implant infections) were treated successfully with oral antibiotics.[138]

At the time of writing, there has only been one published study (pilot study in 2017 and follow-up study in 2021), exploring the use of OI in vascular amputees. The authors carried out a longitudinal case series of six vascular transtibial amputees, aged between 36 and 84 years. Five patients were originally followed up for initially 1 year post-single stage OI surgery, in the pilot study. These five, along with an additional patient, were subsequently followed up for 3-5 years in the follow-up study. One patient was reported to have diabetes mellitus. At 3-5 years follow up, four patients were able to ambulate un-aided using the OI prosthesis, and three of these patients were pain-free. However two patients had soft tissue infection requiring oral antibiotics. One patient had recurrent deep infection requiring removal of transtibial OI implant and a more proximal transfemoral amputation. This patient died two days post-revision surgery.[139,140]

With older vascular amputees, major concerns of OI include risk of infection (soft tissue infection and osteomyelitis) and loosening of the intra-medullary stem, which may require revision surgery. Therefore the NHS in England currently does *not* routinely recommend OI as a treatment option, especially for vascular amputees.[141] Further research into OI and vascular amputations is needed, especially studies with larger sample sizes, longer follow-up periods and including patients with concomitant diabetes mellitus.

✅ Osseointegration prosthesis is currently not recommended for vascular amputees.[141]

SOCKET SYSTEMS AND RESIDUUM SWEATING

For transtibial amputees, there are a variety of socket systems available to achieve optimal fit, suspension and comfort over the residuum. Innovations such as a pelite liner (a soft foam that is heat- and pressure-resistant) and supra-condylar suspension and silicone or gel suspension systems using pin or valve locking mechanisms have improved suspension as well as reduced friction and shear forces at the residuum–socket interface[142–144] (Fig. 6.16). This type of prosthesis uses a silicone or gel sleeve directly onto the residuum, which is then locked into the prosthetic socket or uses a suction valve for suspension, thus allowing for shorter residua to be fitted compared with the traditional patellar tendon-bearing prosthesis.

Sweating is a common problem of wearing a prosthetic limb, especially with silicone type liners.[145] Hyperhidrosis of the residuum can irritate the skin leading to rashes, blisters and skin breakdown, which in turn can cause pain and infection. Excessive sweat can also collect in the residuum-socket interface leading to impaired fit and loss of suction, which in turn can lead to reduced stamina in the prosthesis, falls and eventual cessation of prosthetic use.[146] To try to address this, prosthesis manufacturing companies have devised sweat management liners to allow the sweat to evaporate, however, their long-term effectiveness is currently inconclusive and further research, especially with longer usage periods (>6 months), is needed in this field.[147]

In the dermatological literature, topical aluminium chloride is often regarded as the first-line treatment for hyperhidrosis. Although effective amongst the general population, there are no studies exploring its specific use in amputees.[148] One cohort study reported the effectiveness of topical methamine has as an anti-perspirant in amputees.[149] Therefore further research is needed on topical treatments for hyperhidrosis in amputees.

Botulinum toxin injections can also be used for hyperhidrosis in amputees. Used alongside the starch-iodine test to focal identify areas of excessive sweating in the residual limb, targeted botulinum injections have been reported as effective in reducing hyperhidrosis.[148,150,151]

AMPUTEE REHABILITATION IN THE OBESE PATIENT

Obesity is increasing in prevalence in both higher income and lesser income countries. In 2018 28% of adults in the United Kingdom were classified as obese (i.e., body mass index [BMI] ≥30 kg/m^2). The amputated limb comprises approximately 11% of total body weight in TFA, 4.4% in knee disarticulation and 3.7% in TTA.[152] Therefore following amputation, the weight of the amputated limb needs to be taken into

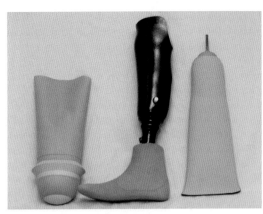

Figure 6.16 Left: An ICEROSS liner with a distal locking pin, which is applied by rolling onto the residuum; Middle: A transtibial prosthetic limb on which the residuum with the liner is to be inserted and locked in; Right: A Seal-in silicone liner that provides suspension by suction without the necessity of a locking pin.

consideration when calculation correct BMI and diagnosing obesity. Health risks associated with being overweight include diabetes mellitus, coronary heart disease, stroke and osteoarthritis. In addition, following limb loss and associated reduce mobility, amputees are also at risk of further weight gain. In 2015, Littman et al. conducted a retrospective study of 759 men who underwent lower extremity amputation and found that at 2 years post-amputation, there was an 8–9% weight gain amongst transfemoral and transtibial amputees.[153]

Obesity might also adversely affect a patient's prosthetic rehabilitation. Prosthetic limb wearing in the obese amputee has been reported to be associated with increased musculoskeletal pain, osteoarthritis, falls and other injuries, impaired mobility and functional capacity, reduced prosthesis fit and function as well as mechanical breakdown of componentry, which in turn can lead to prosthetic abandonment and a diminished QoL.[153,154] However, the extent of this association has been questioned and obesity alone should be a determining factor of whether an amputee is suitable for limb fitting.[155] Further research into the effects of obesity on prosthetic rehabilitation is needed.

✅ Although associated with adverse outcomes in prosthetic rehabilitation, obesity alone should not be the deciding factor when determining a patient's suitability for a prosthetic limb.[155]

LONG-TERM SEQUELAE OF AMPUTEES

OSTEOARTHRITIS

Traditionally, lower-extremity amputation caused by trauma has been associated with a long-term increased risk of developing osteoarthritis in the hip and knee joints the intact leg, compared to non-amputees. This was thought to be caused by increased weight bearing on the intact leg when ambulating following an amputation.[156] A retrospective cohort study of 75 male World War II amputee veterans 5 decades on, found a significantly higher incidence of hip osteoarthritis in the amputated leg (61%) compared to the intact leg

(23%). The authors hypothesised that vascular disruption during the initial traumatic amputation and subsequently altered gait and load distribution may be a plausible explanation to this finding.[157]

However, an association between osteoarthritis and vascular amputation has *not* been found. Welke et al. in 2019 conducted a retrospective database analysis of 1569 transfemoral amputees and matched (non-amputee) controls and found conversely a reduced prevalence of osteoarthritis in the mainly diabetic vascular amputee group compared to the control group, suggesting other factors such as physical lifestyle, manual labour employment and strenuous activities may also play a role in the development of osteoarthritis rather than amputation per se.[158] Further research is needed on the risk of developing osteoarthritis in vascular amputees.

BACK PAIN

Oosterhoff et al. conducted a systematic review in 2020 of 51 studies comprising a total of 10 201 lower extremity amputees. The authors found that back pain was present in over half those patients with no correlation between the level of amputation and the risk of back pain.[159] The exact aetiology of back pain post-amputation is not certain, however, contributory biomechanical factors include unequal limb length, altered gait pattern and associated changes in spinal kinematics, weight gain/obesity, muscle atrophy and weaknesses as well as referred pain from both the hip and knee of the amputated and intact legs.[159,160]

Following lower extremity amputation, the development of chronic back pain is associated with reductions in limb usage and mobility, difficulties with sitting, sleeping and travelling, and an overall reduction in QoL.[161] Like in the general non-amputee population, the treatment of chronic back pain in amputees is also challenging and complex with proposed treatment options such as NSAIDs, physiotherapy and lumbar strengthening exercise. However, in a systematic review comprising of 17 studies of back pain and lower extremity amputation, the authors found no substantial evidence in terms of the effectiveness of any particular treatment for back pain in amputees.[161] Further research is needed exploring the treatment of back pain in the amputee population.

RISK OF SUBSEQUENT CONTRALATERAL LIMB AMPUTATION

In patients who have had an initial lower extremity amputation because of peripheral vascular disease, the contralateral limb is at greater risk of future amputation.[162] A retrospective study of 391 patients who underwent major lower extremity amputation caused by dysvascularity found that within the first 5 years post-initial amputation, 63 of these patients (i.e., 16%) had a subsequent amputation of the contralateral limb.[163] A similar study carried out in the same year on 575 major lower extremity amputees found that 11.5% underwent subsequent contralateral amputation.[23]

Both studies also found that following initial amputation, the presence of end-stage renal disease, chronic renal insufficiency, atherosclerosis, diabetic neuropathy and revision surgery of the initial ipsilateral amputation to a more proximal level were associated with a higher risk of subsequent contralateral amputation. To reduce rates of subsequent contralateral amputation, a multidisciplinary and multi-specialty approach is needed to manage the aforementioned risk factors.

MORTALITY

There is significant mortality of patients following a major lower extremity amputation for peripheral vascular disease. A retrospective case note review of 201 vascular patients who underwent major lower extremity amputation found that at 5 years post-amputation, the survival rates for transtibial and TFAs were 30% and 60%, whilst the 10-year survival rates were 27% and 57%, respectively.[164] For vascular amputees who also have diabetes mellitus, the survival rates are even poorer, with rates of 64% at 1-year post-unilateral TTA.[165] Inderbitzi et al. in 2003 conducted a 12-year longitudinal study of 66 bilateral lower extremity amputees and found that patient survival at 2-years post-contralateral amputation was 62% and at 5 years 31%. The main causes of death amongst vascular amputees are coronary artery disease (37%), cerebral vascular events (15%) and pneumonia (10%).[166]

SUMMARY

Amputation is only the end of the beginning of a vascular patient's journey. It is imperative to have a coordinated interdisciplinary approach between vascular surgeons and the rehabilitation team to facilitate appropriate prosthetic fitting, reduce post-amputation complications and improve patient outcomes and QoL.

Key points

- In England, over 90% of all amputations carried out are caused by PAD, and an increasing proportion have diabetes.
- Selection of the ideal level of amputation depends on healing potential, rehabilitation potential and prosthetic considerations and the decision should be made in a multidisciplinary setting with the amputee rehabilitation team.
- Transtibial amputees have a much higher potential to achieve prosthetic mobilisation compared with those undergoing TFA.
- For patients who are unlikely to achieve prosthetic walking, a through-knee amputation is preferable to amputation at the transfemoral level.
- A comprehensive and holistic assessment of amputees or prospective amputees, followed by multidisciplinary rehabilitation, is likely to provide the optimal outcome.
- Amputation surgery should be considered as a constructive procedure to create the best possible residuum for limb fitting and should therefore be performed by experienced surgeons.
- A multimodal approach is needed to manage post-amputation pain and early involvement of the specialist pain management team is recommended.
- Appropriate use of early walking aids during the early post-amputation period is an essential part of assessment and preparation for prosthetic rehabilitation.
- Modern prostheses are modular and are custom-made to fit the individual requirements of the patient.
- The type of prosthesis and its components will be determined by the amputee's realistic goals, progress in rehabilitation and ability to benefit.
- Increasingly, more sophisticated components (such as microprocessor knees) are becoming available, although they tend to be applicable only for the more active amputee.
- OI prosthetic limbs is currently not recommended for vascular amputees.
- Associated long-term co-morbidities post-amputation include weight gain/obesity, osteoarthritis, back pain, risk of subsequent contralateral amputation and reduced life expectancy.

References available at http://ebooks.health.elsevier.com/

KEY REFERENCES

[44] Fortington LV, Dijkstra PU, Bosmans JC, Post WJ, Geertzen JHB. Change in health-related quality of life in the first 18 months after lower limb amputation: a prospective, longitudinal study. J Rehabil Med 2013;45(6):587–94

A longitudinal study of 82 patients exploring quality of life (QoL) following lower extremity amputation. Using the RAND-36 questionnaire, transtibial amputees reported better QoL scores compared to transfemoral amputees within the 18 months following an amputation. This was caused by a better walking ability leading to greater social participation amongst transtibial amputees.

[45] Davies B, Datta D. Mobility outcome following unilateral lower limb amputation. Prosthet Orthot Int 2003;27(3):186–90

An observational study of 281 unilateral lower extremity amputees found that amongst older (>50 years old) amputees at 1-year follow-up, approximately 50% and 60% of transtibial amputees were ambulating independently in the community or at home, respectively. Whereas for transfemoral amputees, the respective figures were 25% and 50%.

[71] Johnson WC, Wathins MT, Hamilton J, Baldwin D. Transcutaneous partial oxygen pressure changes following skew flap and Burgess-type below-knee amputations. Arch Surg 1997;132(3):261–3

A prospective cohort study of 20 transtibial amputees (10 Burgess flaps vs. 10 Skew flaps) and residuum transcutaneous partial oxygen pressure. The authors found that Burgess flaps had the greatest and most persistent reduction in oxygenation pressure (10 mmHg) at 20 days post-amputation.

[72] Jain SK. Skew flap technique in trans-tibial amputation. Prosthet Orthot Int 2005;29(3):283–90

A 15-year longitudinal study of 92 transtibial amputations performed using the Skew flap technique. The author found that 81.5% of these patients had 'good' to 'excellent' results at 5–15 years follow-up and the Skew flap produced a 'smooth, well-padded' residuum without 'dog-ears'.

7 Revision vascular surgery

Jan David Süss | Michael Gawenda

INTRODUCTION

Revision of vascular reconstructions and interventions is frequently required beyond the first 6 weeks because of progressive atherosclerosis, *graft occlusion, aneurysm formation* or *infection.* Up to 40% of femorodistal bypass surgery grafts require re-intervention within 5 years.[1] The same is true for endovascular intervention where it has been shown that up to 30% of the patients need a re-intervention within 5 years after endovascular aortic aneurysm reconstruction (EVAR).[2–7] Revision surgery requires experience and judgment; it is technically more difficult because of fibrosis and the loss of easily definable tissue planes, which necessitates careful sharp dissection to gain arterial control. The anatomy might be altered by previous operations or interventions and operating times, blood loss, infection rates and operative risk are therefore increased.

GRAFT OCCLUSION

Graft thrombosis usually presents acutely but is occasionally foreshown by increasing ischaemic symptoms, ranging from mild claudication to critical ischaemia. Nevertheless, asymptomatic graft occlusion can also occur. Occasionally, simultaneous distal embolisation causes digital ischaemia (blue toe syndrome or gangrene). Graft thrombosis with loss of runoff caused by distal embolisation is associated with a high risk of limb loss. Whereas graft thrombosis in the first 6 weeks is generally caused by technical error or poor run-off, most late occlusions result from intimal hyperplasia within the bypass or progressive inflow or run-off disease (see Chapter 4). Graft stenoses are usually asymptomatic and occur in 20–30% of infra-inguinal vein grafts, mostly in the first year.[8,9] Stenoses of greater than 70% (velocity >3 m/s or velocity ratio >3.0) compromise flow and often occlude if left untreated.[10]

FACTORS INFLUENCING GRAFT OCCLUSION

LOCAL FACTORS

These are essentially for the quality of the inflow, the run-off and the conduit itself (see Chapter 4).

Patency is better for supra-inguinal than infra-inguinal grafts and graft occlusion is more frequent in femorotibial than in femoropopliteal bypasses.[11]

Infra-inguinal bypass patency of autologous vein is better than Dacron, polytetrafluoroethylene (PTFE) or human umbilical vein.[12] Dacron and PTFE used in femoropopliteal bypass grafting did not differ in mid-term graft patency at 5 years.[13] The 1-year-results of a Scandinavian multicentre randomised trial revealed that a Heparin-bonded PTFE (Hb-PTFE) graft significantly reduced the overall risk of primary graft failure by 37%. Risk reduction was 50% in femoropopliteal bypass cases and in cases with critical ischaemia.[14] But at the 5-year results there was no difference in primary graft patency between Hb-PTFE and standard PTFE grafts. Patients receiving Hb-PTFE grafts for critical limb ischaemia were more likely to have a patent graft at 5 years than those with standard PTFE grafts.[15]

The results of reversed and in situ vein grafts are equivalent.[16,17] In a meta-analysis on the long-term primary and secondary patency and foot preservation following popliteal-to-distal bypass grafts, there was a superiority trend favouring reversed vein grafts.[18] (SCALPEL)

Arm veins are similar to long saphenous vein provided that angioscopically detected defects are corrected.[19] Preoperative ultrasound mapping seems to be crucial to use the best autogenous conduit available.[20] A recent published retrospective study of infra-inguinal bypasses for critical limb ischaemia (CLI) using arm vein conduit or prosthetic grafts revealed that arm vein conduits, even when spliced, are superior to prosthetic grafts in terms of mid-term assisted primary patency, secondary patency, and leg salvage in infrapopliteal bypasses for CLI.[21]

A recent published Cochrane Review disclosed a clear primary patency benefit for autologous vein when compared to synthetic materials for above knee bypasses. In the long term (5 years), Dacron confers a small primary patency benefit over PTFE for above knee bypass. PTFE with a vein cuff improved primary patency when compared to PTFE alone for below knee bypasses.[22] (SCALPEL)

The risk for ischemic complications and the need for emergency limb revascularisation are greater with occlusion of prosthetic grafts compared to venous grafts. This is because the thrombus in the prosthetic graft extends into the outflow artery. Vein cuffs at the distal anastomosis reduce the risk of outflow impairment after thrombosis of PTFE grafts (Fig. 7.1).[23]

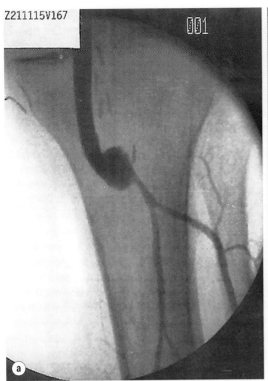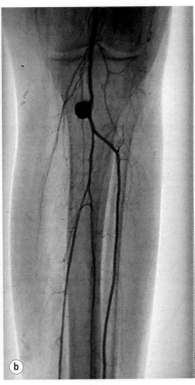

Figure 7.1 **(a)** Femoropopliteal bypass with venous cuff (Miller cuff) at the distal anastomosis. Perioperative angiography. **(b)** Preservation of outflow vessels after thrombosis at 3 years.

The Dutch BOA Study found no difference between venous and prosthetic graft material in the risk of amputation after infra-inguinal bypass occlusion.[24] (SCALPEL)

The quality and number of run-off vessels appear to potentially identify patients at high risk for a poor initial outcome by predicting patency in infra-inguinal bypass reconstructions.[25,26] Bypasses for gangrene occlude more frequently than for ulceration, rest pain or claudication.[27] This is probably related to the poorer run-off associated with worsening ischaemia.

GENERAL FACTORS

Continued smoking after lower limb bypass surgery results at least in a threefold increased risk of graft failure.[28] Diabetes and renal failure compromise patient survival but not graft patency.[28–30] (PEN NIB)

Raised fibrinogen, hyperlipidaemia, thrombophilias (e.g., protein C, protein S or antithrombin III deficiency, antiphospholipid antibodies), and increased platelet aggregation favour graft thrombosis,[31] whereas factor V Leiden mutation is debatable.[32,33]

Black race and female sex are risk factors for adverse outcomes after vein bypass surgery for limb salvage, with graft failure and limb loss being more common events in Black patients, and Black women being a particularly high-risk group.[34] (PEN NIB)

Even White women have more graft occlusions and recurrent stenoses and hormone replacement therapy potentiates this.[35,36]

PREVENTION OF GRAFT THROMBOSIS

Antiplatelet therapy with aspirin had a slight beneficial effect on the patency of peripheral bypass grafts but seemed to have an inferior effect on venous graft patency compared with artificial grafts.[37] The Dutch BOA trial revealed that aspirin is more effective for infra-inguinal prosthetic grafts, whereas warfarin is better for vein grafts.[38]

In the CASPAR trial, the combination of clopidogrel plus aspirin did not improve limb or systemic outcomes in the overall population of peripheral artery disease patients requiring below-knee bypass grafting. A subgroup analysis suggested that clopidogrel plus aspirin awards benefit in patients receiving prosthetic grafts without significantly increasing major bleeding risk.[39] (SCALPEL)

Surveillance for supra-inguinal bypass grafts does not seem to be cost effective. Occlusion is far more frequent after infra-inguinal bypass grafting and since most of the occlusions occur within 2 years after the implantation, patients should be carefully followed during this time period. This includes medical history, clinical examination and Doppler pressure measurements. Additional duplex scanning seems to not be effective after prosthetic bypass.

Some published reports tend to argue in favour of duplex surveillance on the basis of patency alone.[40] In a randomised trial with 596 patients, intensive surveillance with duplex scanning did not show any additional benefit in terms of limb salvage rates for patients undergoing femoropopliteal or femorocrural vein bypass graft operations.[41] (SCALPEL)

MANAGEMENT OF GRAFT STENOSIS (THE FAILING GRAFT)

Although there is some discussion about asymptomatic stenosis, it is clear that symptomatic graft stenosis should be treated by either angioplasty or surgical revision. Open surgical revision of femorodistal vein grafts provided an increased freedom from further re-interventions or major amputation; however, early success rates for endovascular procedures were similar, particularly for non-occluded grafts. And percutaneous transluminal angioplasty (PTA) of infra-inguinal vein grafts is safe and effective in the treatment of failing grafts. Graft angioplasties do not lose effectiveness when repeated and have shown cumulative benefit in prolonging graft survival.[42] With time, endovascular revisions required an increasing number of re-interventions and manifested higher rates of failure.[43] Surgical revision is probably more durable long term, but an endovascular approach is actually preferred because of the acceptable short-term patency and a low rate of complications, particularly for late graft stenosis (>3 months), short (<2 cm) and single stenoses.[43–45]

Short graft stenosis, whether mid-graft or anastomotic commonly responds well to angioplasty with high inflation pressures (up to 2020 kPa) (Fig. 7.2). Cutting balloons have been advocated, but seem to offer only small benefit at the expense of an elevated complication rate.[46–48] Stents (preferably self-expandable bare nitinol) should be used only selectively.[49]

A currently published randomised clinical study demonstrated that implantation of a polymer-free, paclitaxel-coated nitinol drug-eluting stent (DES) in patients with moderate-length lesions of the superficial femoral artery (SFA) and proximal popliteal artery was safe and associated with a superior 12-month patency compared with both PTA and provisional bare metal stent (BMS) placement. The proportion of treated re-stenosis in both cohorts was only 5.5 resp. 5.9%.[50] Two-year and the 5-year outcomes with the paclitaxel-eluting stent support its sustained safety and effectiveness in patients with femoropopliteal artery disease, including the long-term superiority of the DES to PTA and to provisional BMS placement.[51,52] (SCALPEL)

Longer graft stenoses are best treated by open surgery and may be bypassed using the contralateral long saphenous or superficial femoral vein.[19] Tibial or distal popliteal anastomotic stenoses resistant to angioplasty are best treated by a jump graft to a fresh run-off vessel to avoid the scar tissue or adherent tibial veins (Fig. 7.3).

MANAGEMENT OF THE FAILED GRAFT

If graft occlusion causes non-disabling claudication, a conservative approach might be preferred. Acute subcritical

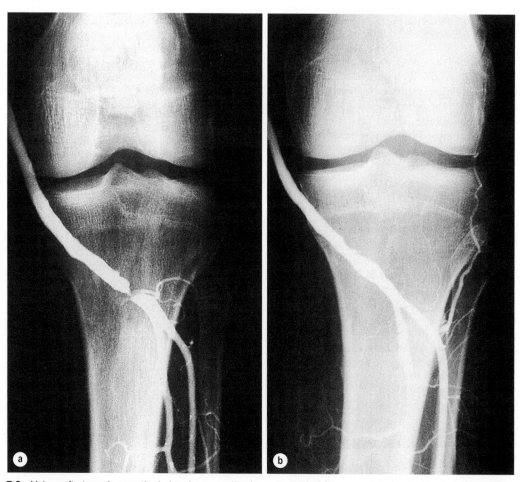

Figure 7.2   Vein graft stenosis near the below-knee popliteal anastomosis **(a)** successfully treated by balloon angioplasty **(b)**.

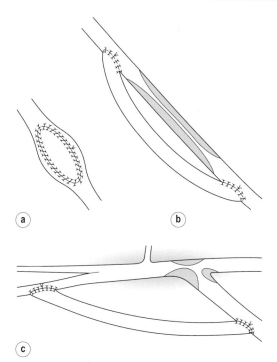

Figure 7.3 **(a)** Vein patch angioplasty, **(b)** bypass of long vein graft stenosis and **(c)** jump graft around stenosed distal anastomosis of a femoropopliteal bypass graft to the popliteal artery.

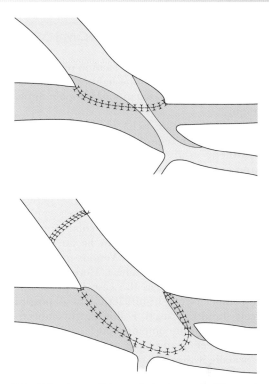

Figure 7.4 Extension graft to one limb of an aorto-bifemoral graft to treat a stenosis at the profunda femoris origin. In this case, the superficial femoral artery is occluded.

ischaemia allows time for thrombolysis or elective surgery, but an anaesthetic paralysed limb demands emergency revascularisation within a few hours (see Chapter 8).

ROLE OF THROMBOLYSIS

✔️ Local catheter-directed thrombolysis might be a valuable tool for a viable limb within 14 days of prosthetic graft occlusion provided that the patient has undergone surgery within 3 months.[53] (PEN NIB)

Although not applicable for supra-inguinal grafts, thrombolysis is still frequently used for femorodistal graft occlusion. The advantages are that redo surgery may be avoided and the graft will be cleared unmasking the underlying cause of thrombosis, which can often be treated endovascularly during the same session. The outflow vessels might also be cleared more effectively than with open surgery. Percutaneous mechanical thrombectomy or the use of high bolus therapy can reduce the duration of the procedure.[54–56] If thrombolysis is unsuccessful or reveals a problem that is not amenable to endovascular treatment, then open surgery can be performed with a clear knowledge of the cause of the problem and the state of the run-off. Although thrombolysis has a high initial success rate, it is also characterised by contraindications, haemorrhagic complications, poor long-term patency and persistent ischaemia.[57,58] This explains the reduced popularity of thrombolysis, and why the pragmatic solution to reserve thrombolysis for patients with associated extensive thrombosis of the outflow vessels is often applied.[59]

SUPRA-INGUINAL GRAFT THROMBOSIS

A unilateral limb thrombosis of an aorto-bifemoral graft can be thrombectomised through the groin even months after the occlusion. Thrombectomy is performed with Fogarty embolectomy catheters, an adherent clot catheter or a ring stripper. During these manoeuvres, the contralateral groin is compressed to avoid contralateral embolisation. The underlying cause is most frequently a stenosis at the distal anastomosis, which should be repaired by extension of the graft mostly into the profunda femoris artery (Fig. 7.4). Graft thrombectomy by a femoral approach is usually not possible in case of bilateral graft occlusion, as the problem is more likely to be in the proximal region (inflow problem). Here the graft should be replaced in situ instead or by an extra-anatomical bypass (axillo-bifemoral bypass).

The underlying cause of the occlusion in case of axillofemoral grafting is most frequently an anastomotic stenosis or stenosis of the inflow vessel.[60] Thrombectomy can then be performed from the groin, but most often a help incision along the graft is needed. The underlying cause needs to be taken care of. The inflow vessels (subclavian artery for axillofemoral graft) are checked pre- or peri-operatively and inflow stenosis is treated if necessary. A new graft in clean tissues offers the best solution in case of long-standing thrombosis or when thrombectomy is insufficient. For an occluded femorofemoral graft, the same principles applies and one often encounters bilateral stenoses, so that both groins need repair.

INFRA-INGUINAL GRAFT THROMBOSIS

In case of chronic occlusion, the decision regarding revascularisation should be taken in the light of the clinical examination and results of investigations (Doppler, duplex scan, angiography).

In patients with acute ischaemia, an immediate decision should be taken regarding thrombolysis or open surgery. Prosthetic grafts can usually be thrombectomised by a groin approach if the occlusion is less than 1 week old. Anastomotic stenosis must be corrected, and inflow and outflow vessels need to be checked by peri-operative angiography. If necessary, outflow vessels can be selectively approached by an infra-genicular approach, and intra-operative thrombolysis might be an adjunct in selected cases (see Chapter 8).[61] Venous grafts are usually more difficult to thrombectomise. Here it might be wise to place a new graft, as is the case in prosthetic grafts where thrombectomy is insufficient. If at all possible, a venous graft should be used. Following thrombectomy for acute ischaemia, four-compartment fasciotomy should be considered to relieve pressure and improve distal perfusion, especially if there is any calf swelling or tenderness pre-operatively.[62,63]

GRAFT INFECTION

Graft infection is relatively uncommon (1–5%) but has a high amputation and mortality risk.[64] In a recent multicentre audit of 55 graft infections, 31% died, 33% underwent amputation and only 45% left the hospital alive without amputation.[65] Treatment has therefore to focus on patient's survival, eradication of infection and revascularisation by a method, which is durable and does not become infected itself.

CAUSES

Graft infection is thought to occur most commonly by inoculation of bacteria from the patient's skin at the time of surgery (e.g., skin commensals) or by direct spread in the peri-operative period, often secondary to wound breakdown.[66] Surgical site infection after open surgery for lower extremity revascularisation is a serious complication that is associated with a more than twofold-increased risk of early graft loss and reoperation.[67]

Patients with gangrene, in elderly obese, and those undergoing reoperation during the same hospital admission have a higher risk. Pre-operative shaving, open surgical drainage for more than 3 days, operations lasting over 4 hours, emergency surgery, redo-surgery, female gender, diabetes, steroids, renal failure, recent angiography and wound haematoma are all risk factors.[67,68] Blood-borne bacteria from intravenous lines or systemic infections may also cause graft inoculation and sepsis.

Venous grafts are more resistant to infection than prostheses, but direct bacterial erosion can occur, especially when exposed in an open wound.

PREVENTION

Patients should be admitted as near to surgery as possible and isolated from patients with known infections, especially methicillin-resistant *Staphylococcus aureus* (MRSA). Many hospitals are adopting a policy of screening elective surgical patients for MRSA colonisation before admission and eradicating any infection before proceeding with the surgery.

Strict aseptic technique and laminar air-flow theatres minimise infection rates. Iodine-impregnated adhesive drapes help isolate the operative field.

Prophylactic antibiotics (cephalosporin or co-amoxiclav) reduce wound and graft infection. There is no evidence for using more than three doses (one intra-operative and two post-operative). Some surgeons add a single dose of gentamicin as this is active against many strains of MRSA. Vancomycin should be used if the patient is MRSA positive. Evidence for new generation antibiotics is still lacking.

Moreover, in a recently published randomised controlled trial, a silver-eluting alginate dressing placed over incisions after leg arterial surgery showed no effect on the incidence of wound complications.[69]

✔✔ Prophylactic systemic antibiotics reduced the risk of wound infection and early graft infection. Antibiotic prophylaxis for more than 24 hours appears to be of no added benefit. There was no evidence that prophylactic rifampicin bonding to Dacron grafts reduced graft infection at either 1 month or 2 years.[70] The same is true for the more recent silver-coated grafts.[71,72] There was no evidence of a beneficial or detrimental effect on rates of wound infection with suction groin-wound drainage[70] or of any benefit from a pre-operative bathing or shower regimen with antiseptic agents over unmedicated bathing.[73] (SCALPEL)

There is also little evidence regarding the need for prophylactic antibiotics before other surgical or dental procedures in the presence of prosthetic grafts.

PRESENTATION

Wound infections after vascular surgery are classified according to the depth of tissue involvement: type 1 involves the skin only, type 2, the subcutaneous tissue and type 3, the graft itself.[74] Prosthetic graft infection can present at any time from days to years after surgery with pyrexia, systemic sepsis, local abscesses and sinuses, graft exposure, thrombosis or anastomotic haemorrhage. On rare occasions, septic emboli can be the first sign (Fig. 7.5). Septic erosion of exposed vein grafts can occur at any point.

Infra-renal aortic grafts can erode the third or fourth part of the duodenum causing an aortoduodenal fistula, which may present with one or two sentinel gastrointestinal bleeds before the inevitable catastrophic haemorrhage. Occasionally, an aortic graft can also erode any other part of the bowel, including the appendix, and also the ureter. Such aortoenteric erosion will lead to localised peritonitis with retroperitoneal or groin abscesses (Fig. 7.6a and b) and ultimately catastrophic bleeding. The mortality rate of aortoenteric complications is high (>50%) with recurrent infection or aortic stump blowout in over 25%.[75]

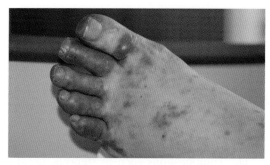

Figure 7.5 Septic emboli at the foot as the presenting sign of aortofemoral graft infection.

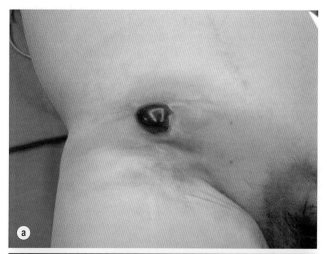

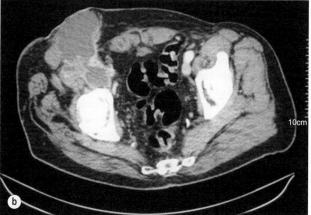

Figure 7.6 Aortoenteric fistula leading to retroperitoneal and groin abscesses **(a)** aspect of the groin **(b)** computed tomography scan.

BACTERIOLOGY

Most graft infections are caused by skin organisms.[76] *Staphylococcus epidermidis* is the least virulent, producing a biofilm or an infected seroma after months or years. It is difficult to culture, requiring homogenisation of explanted graft material to dislodge adherent bacteria. *S. aureus* is more virulent and usually presents earlier. MRSA infections have a particularly high morbidity and mortality, and the incidence unfortunately is increasing. Apart from staphylococcus, there is a wide variety of organisms that can cause graft infection. Gram-negative species include *Escherichia coli* and *Pseudomonas aeruginosa*, the latter being recognised by a

high tendency of anastomotic disruption and bleeding. It may be difficult or even impossible to culture the causative organism, particularly after prolonged periods of antibiotic therapy.

DIAGNOSIS

In most cases, there is a perigraft collection or sinus. Aspiration of frank pus or turbid fluid from around the graft and the subsequent culture of a causative organism are diagnostic. Computed tomography (CT), magnetic resonance imaging (MRI) or ultrasound usually demonstrates perigraft fluid and inflammation but can underestimate the extent of infection, especially if a sinus is present, and for the extent a sinography may be useful. For wholly intra-abdominal prostheses, there may be few signs, therefore diagnosis of aortic graft infection is often difficult, requiring a high index of suspicion and aggressive investigation. Leukocyte count, erythrocyte sedimentation rate and C-reactive protein are often raised. Persistence of perigraft fluid or perigraft soft-tissue attenuation beyond 3 months or perigraft gas (Fig. 7.7) beyond 4 to 7 weeks should be presumed to be infection and perigraft fluid should be aspirated using an image-guided technique and characterised for pathogens.[77] One in four anastomotic aneurysms result from graft infection, but this is not always evident from CT. Where doubt exists, indium-labelled leukocyte or positron emission tomography (PET) scanning is occasionally helpful. In aorto-enteric fistula (AEF), the graft may be seen eroding the duodenum at endoscopy (Fig. 7.8). Definitive confirmation of an infection is sometimes only made at the operation by the presence of pus around the graft and the absence of tissue incorporation (Fig. 7.9).

MANAGEMENT

GENERAL PRINCIPLES

Once infection is confirmed, semi-urgent treatment is required to pre-empt catastrophic haemorrhage, graft thrombosis or systemic sepsis. An infected prosthesis acts as a foreign body, rendering bacteria inaccessible to antibiotics. Conservative measures (including prolonged antibiotic therapy, drainage and irrigation of abscesses, muscle flaps) may be helpful and can buy time, but they are rarely curative.

The mainstay of vascular graft infection management is: first, excision of the graft as this as a foreign body may potentiate the infection; second, wide and complete debridement of devitalised and infected tissue to provide a clean wound in which healing can occur; third, establishment of vascular flow to the distal bed; fourth, the intensive and prolonged treatment with antibiotics, to reduce the risk for sepsis and secondary graft infection.[78]

Complete graft excision might be mandatory. Partial graft resection commonly requires later replacement.[79] Although contrary to conventional concepts, partial or complete graft preservation combined with aggressive drainage and groin wound debridement is an acceptable option for treatment of infection involving an entire aortic graft in selected patients with prohibitive risks for total graft excision.[80,81]

Simple graft excision without revascularisation can heal infection but usually results in major amputation, even in patients operated on initially for claudication.

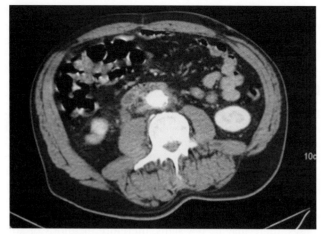

Figure 7.7   Perigraft gas bubbles in between duodenum and aortic graft.

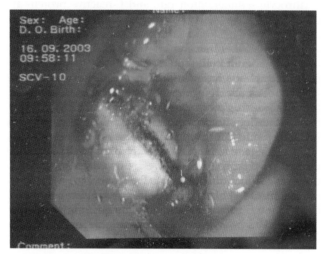

Figure 7.8   Aortic graft, eroding the duodenum as seen during endoscopy.

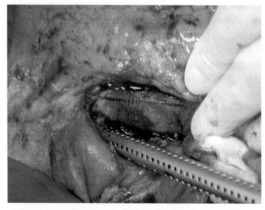

Figure 7.9   Situs intraoperatively with absence of tissue incorporation of the graft and discoloration by duodenal secretion.

Revascularisation is traditionally performed by extra-anatomical bypass (axillofemoral graft for infra-renal aortic graft infection, obturator bypass for infection at the groin, lateral bypass for infection of a femoropopliteal graft).[64]

✔ There is growing evidence that in situ reconstruction produces equal or better results than graft excision and extra-anatomical bypass, with regard to reinfection rate and particularly late patency and amputation rates.[82,83] (PEN NIB)

✔ An autologous conduit is preferable for in situ reconstruction.[84] (PEN NIB)

Arterial allografts are an alternative but they might dispose to late complications such as stenosis, occlusion or aneurysmal degeneration.[82,85] There are a few encouraging reports on the use of rifampicin-bonded grafts or silver-impregnated grafts, but they should be reserved for patients with low-grade infections (e.g., *S. epidermidis*).[86,87]

The duration of post-operative antibiotic therapy is still at discussion. Most authors will accept a period of 2 to 6 weeks depending on the causative organism.[88]

CASE DEFINITION AND GENERAL PRINCIPLES OF AORTIC GRAFT AND ENDOGRAFT INFECTION

Lacking a universally accepted case definition of aortic graft infection, the Management of Aortic Graft Infection Collaboration (MAGIC) provides criteria for diagnosing aortic graft infection (AGI).[89] Infection rates vary from 0.5–4% in the current literature.[90–93]

The main principles of therapy are eradication of the infected field and reconstitution of perfusion. Despite of a wide spectrum of surgical therapy options in combination with antimicrobial therapy, mortality remains extremely high (18–30%).[94–98] Diagnosis is challenging and often an odyssey for the patient. If AGI is suspected, the MAGIC criteria are a useful tool. MAGIC defines AGI as a combination of major and minor criteria with respect to clinical, surgical, radiological and laboratory findings (Table 7.1). These criteria based on expert consensus and systematic literature review.

The European Society of Vascular Surgery (ESVS) guideline from 2020 recommends the MAGIC criteria in case of a suspected vascular graft/endograft infection (Class of recommendation I, Level of evidence C).[99] Once graft infection is diagnosed, classification into early (<4 months) or late (>4 months) onset can be done. Early onset is associated with virulent pathogens (e.g., *S. aureus*) and more fulminant clinical presentation. However, late onset tends to have a chronic course with mild symptoms because of the less virulent pathogens (e.g., skin flora).

MAGIC criteria are very useful in diagnosing graft infections. But in clinical practice, a stepwise approach based on evidence are the recommendation of the ESVS guideline. Therefore a computed tomography angiography (CTA) scan is first-line diagnostic modality (Class I, Level B). When the CTA findings are questionable additional imaging with 18F-fluorodexyglucose-PET-CT is recommended (Class I, Level C). Above all, enforcement of microbiological proof of infection is necessary (Class I, Level C).

General therapeutic principles are antimicrobial and surgical therapy.

Antibiotics are the basic therapy to control infection and prevent sepsis. Broad spectrum or resistogram compatible

Table 7.1   MAGIC criteria (major and minor criteria with respect to clinical, surgical, radiological and laboratory findings)

Criterion	Clinical/surgical	Radiology	Laboratory
MAJOR			
	Pus (confirmed by microscopy) around graft or in aneurysm sac at surgery	Perigraft fluid on CT scan ≥3 months after graft insertion	Organisms recovered from an explanted graft
	Open wound with exposed graft or communicating sinus	Perigraft gas on CT scan ≥7 weeks after insertion	Organisms recovered from an intra-operative specimen
	Fistula development, e.g., aortoenteric or aortobronchial	Increase in perigraft gas volume demonstrated on serial imaging	Organisms recovered from a percutaneous, radiologically guided aspirate of perigraft fluid
	Graft insertion in an infected site, e.g., fistula, mycotic aneurysm, or infected pseudo-aneurysm		
MINOR			
	Localised clinical features of graft infection, e.g., erythema, warmth, swelling, purulent discharge, pain	Other, e.g., suspicious perigraft gas/fluid soft tissue inflammation; aneurysm expansion; pseudo-aneurysm formation: focal bowel wall thickening; discitis/osteomyelitis; suspicious metabolic activity on FDG-PET/CT; radiolabelled leukocyte uptake	Blood culture(s) positive and no apparent source except graft infection
	Fever ≥38°C with graft infection as most likely cause		Abnormally elevated inflammatory markers with graft infection as most likely cause, e.g., erythrocyte sedimentation rate, C-reactive protein, white cell count

CT, Computed tomography; *FDG-PET*, fluorodeoxyglucose positron emission tomography; *MAGIC*, Management of Aortic Graft Infection Collaboration.

antibiotics should be considered. Especially coverage of graft material with a biofilm and antifungal agents have to be of a certain concern. Duration of antimicrobial treatment differs in the literature without evidence-based recommendations. A minimum of 2 weeks up to lifelong therapy in respect to specific conditions are shown in the literature.[100] ESVS guideline recommends antimicrobial therapy in every patient with an infected graft/endograft (Class I, Level B).

Traditional surgical management consists of radical eradication of the infected field and in situ or extra-anatomical reconstruction. Anastomosis should be covered by biological materials (such as omentum, muscle etc.).

INFRA-RENAL AORTIC GRAFT INFECTION

General symptoms are not specific, and patients often suffer from typical infectious disease symptoms. In case of aortointestinal fistula, bleeding is the most common symptom (71.7%).[101]

Traditional management of aortic graft infection has contained of extra-anatomical bypass, specifically axillo-bifemoral or axillo-bipopliteal bypass, with complete removal of the infected aortic graft. A general important surgical step consists of securing the aortic clamping zone after laparotomy. Extra-anatomical reconstructions can be done as a stage procedure. Both reconstruction techniques are characterised by low patency and high amputation rates.[102] Certain risk of extra-anatomical reconstruction is stump rupture. Predictive factors are short stumps and incomplete debridement.

During the last 2 decades, methods have included debridement of infected tissue, with in situ replacement using cryopreserved allograft, autogenous vein or rifampicin-bonded prostheses (Fig. 7.10).

Similar to the thoracic aorta, extra-anatomical and in situ reconstruction methods serve to restore lower limb perfusion. Contrasting to the thoracic aorta meta-analyses are existing comparing in situ and extra-anatomical reconstruction (Table 7.2).[103] The meta-analysis found the in situ technique superior to extra-anatomical procedures in terms of rates of reinfection, amputation, early mortality and graft occlusion.

Several graft materials are available to perform in situ reconstruction (Fig. 7.11).

Another meta-analysis compared such graft materials with the following conclusions.[83] Prosthetic grafts can be rifampicin bonded or silver coated. Both show high reinfection rates but low amputation rates. About the silver grafts, high patency rates were reported.[104,105]

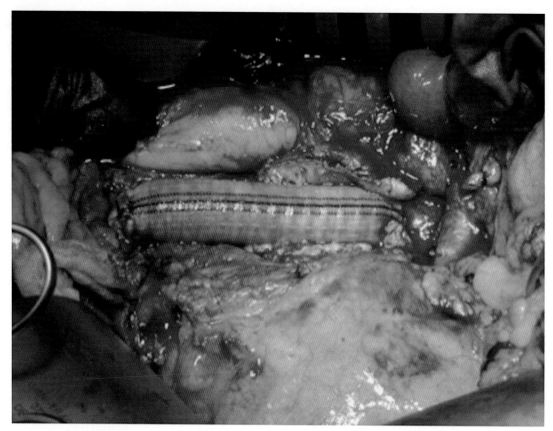

Figure 7.10 In-situ reconstruction with rifampicin-bonded polyester prosthesis.

Table 7.2 Meta-analysis of in situ and extra-anatomical reconstruction in infra-renal aorta

	Extra-anatomical (n=22)	In Situ (n=35)
Amputation	13%	8%
Reinfection	18%	10%
Early mortality	24%	17%
Graft occlusion	24%	13%

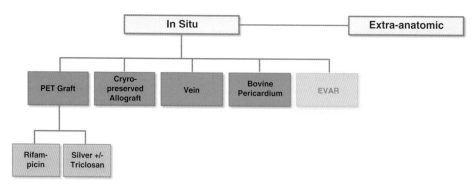

Figure 7.11 Graft materials for in situ reconstruction of the infra-renal aorta. *EVAR*, Endovascular aortic aneurysm reconstruction; *PET*, positron emission tomography.

✔✔ Autogenous vein use had the lowest rate of reinfection, followed by cryopreserved allograft. Later mortality was lowest for autogenous vein and cryopreserved allograft reconstruction. When all outcomes were considered, in situ options for aortic graft infection have shown considerable promise. (SCALPEL)

Other off-the-shelf products are xenografts like as bovine pericardium. Rates of freedom from reinfection appear to be very high in some studies.[106] Valid data are limited by small study populations and short follow-ups.

Autologous veins (femoral and popliteal veins) can be used to create Neoaortoiliac-System.[107] Venous morbidity caused by harvesting trauma and the potential necessity of fasciotomy are drawbacks. Low reinfection and graft thrombosis rates favour this method.[108]

The basic steps in this operation are:

1. Harvesting of the superficial femoral vein

   The patency of the femoral veins is checked pre-operatively by duplex scanning. The superficial femoral vein itself is approached by an incision anteromedially on the thigh, commonly used for harvesting of the greater saphenous vein. After incision of the fascia, the vein is identified just next to the SFA. The bifurcation with the profunda femoris vein is situated in the groin a couple of centimetres below the arterial bifurcation. When working from medially, this means that the venous bifurcation can be approached without entering the original and mostly infected groin incision. Distally, the adductor canal is opened and the dissection is continued to the level of the mid-popliteal artery. The vein is transected at the level of the knee joint and then freed upwards with ligation of the different side branches (Fig. 7.12). At the level of the adductor canal, there are usually dense adhesions with the artery and multiple fragile side branches. Proximally, the excision should be extended to the level of the venous bifurcation and the profunda femoris vein is carefully preserved since it receives important collateral circulation from the popliteal vein.

   Excision of one superficial femoral vein will usually be sufficient for aorto-bi-iliac reconstruction. In the event of an aorto-bifemoral reconstruction, the veins need to be harvested from both lower limbs. After excision, the veins are preserved in cold (4°C) solution and the wounds are closed.

2. Excision of the infected graft

   The preferred approach is median xyphopubic laparotomy. The retroperitoneal approach might be an alternative in selected cases, but the disadvantage is that it hampers a complete debridement and coverage of the new reconstruction with healthy tissue (omentoplasty). In addition, it renders the approach to the femoral vessels and reconstruction in this area more difficult. The infra-renal aorta is approached in the traditional way, but in case of dense adhesions, the right retrocolic approach can be a good option. It is frequently necessary to obtain aortic control at the supra-renal or supra-coeliac level. Once the aorta has been freed, the distal anastomoses at the iliac or femoral level are exposed. The aorta is clamped after systemic heparinisation, and the infected graft is excised completely. The periaortic tissues and any other sites of infection are generously debrided to achieve a healthy bed for the new graft. Existing retroperitoneal tunnels are irrigated and mechanically debrided by pulling open gauze sponges through them. Finally, the aorta itself and the femoral vessels are debrided to achieve a clean anastomotic site.

3. In situ reconstruction with the deep vein (Fig. 7.13)

   The veins can be used in reversed or non-reversed position, this after fracture of the valves with a valvulotome. The proximal aortic anastomosis is simply sutured with one vein end-to-end to the aorta. Taken into account the diameter discrepancy between the aorta and the veins, it is frequently necessary to downsize the aortic cuff somehow with two or three separate through and through stitches. The second vein graft is anastomosed afterwards to the first one some 5 centimetres below this proximal anastomosis. When replacing an infected

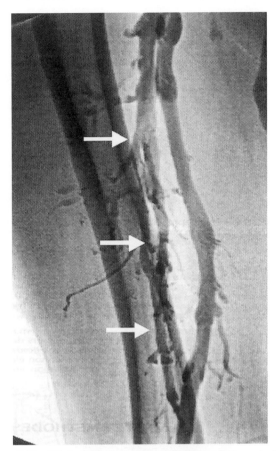

Figure 7.12 Phlebography showing the femoral vein. Important collaterals by the profunda femoris vein (*white arrows*) protect from venous hypertension after harvest.

aorto-bifemoral bypass, the vein grafts are brought to the groin through the old tunnels and anastomosed to the femoral vessels in the usual way. Afterwards, the vein grafts are covered both in the abdomen and at the femoral level with viable tissues leaving no residual cavities. Omentoplasty is generally used at the proximal anastomosis and muscle flaps are provided in the groin in case of extensive infection.

It is agreed that in situ reconstruction with the superficial femoral veins represents a technically demanding and time-consuming operation. The operation has also been criticised because of the risk of venous hypertension in the lower limbs and an increased need for fasciotomy as mentioned earlier.[109] Four point five percent of the patients required a fasciotomy within 30 days of the operation.[110]

As an alternative to the great vessel in situ reconstruction with the superficial femoral veins allogenic vessel transplants might be used (Fig. 7.14). Cryopreserved allografts are highlighted by low infection rates, but availability is limited, and degradation problems (aneurysm, dilatation, rupture) occur.[111,112]

Depending upon availability, one might use a fresh homograft or a cryopreserved one. We have almost exclusively used the cryopreserved ones from the German Transplant Donor Organisation.

As we rarely have got any aortic bifurcations, the thoracic aorta is more often provided. In such a case, we conduct a

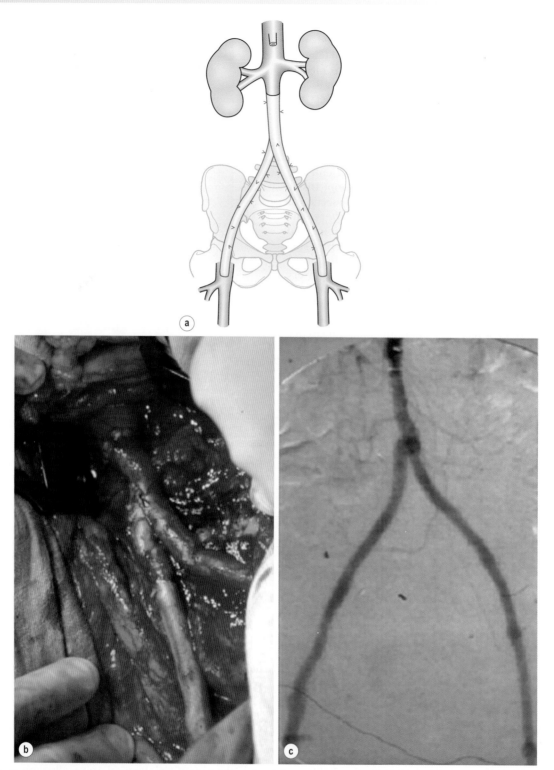

Figure 7.13   The reversed Y technique for in situ reconstruction of an infected aorto-bifemoral graft. **(a)** Schematic drawing, **(b)** Perioperative view, **(c)** Post-operative angiography.

new bifurcation just (see Fig. 7.14a) like when the first polyester grafts were produced and also the first stent grafts sizing is then normally reverse, so that the homograft is larger than the aorta, but by using purse string technique, the anastomosis is well fitting. It is wise to check for bleeding along the suture line before the graft is being tunnelled. Furthermore,

the length is more appropriate when the allograft is stressed with arterial pressure. If the section from the renal arteries to the femoral junction is to be replaced, it might not always suffice lengthwise with an allograft and then it is possible to extend with saphenous vein segments or a part of an artery that has been thrombendarterectomised (see Fig. 7.14b).

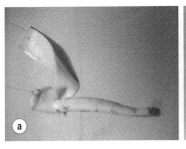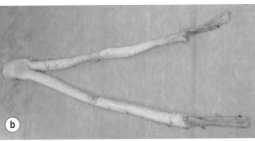

Figure 7.14 Cryopreserved allograft from thoracic aorta, **(a)** suturing a new bifurcation, **(b)** peripheral extension with thrombendarterectomised superficial femoral arteries

Lowering the rate after of reinfection after in situ reconstruction adjunctive therapy with coverage, the graft by pedicled omental flap, muscle, fascia or retroperitoneal tissue is recommended.

The role of endovascular reconstruction in graft infection, and particularly infra-renal aortic graft infection, seems limited.

Endovascular repair is often successful in the short-term achieving favourable immediate outcome. In the presence of systemic infection, however, EVAR alone as an ultimate solution is often followed by repeat infection and bleeding.[113] A staged combination of EVAR treatment for acute bleeding and aggressive infection treatment with systemic and local antibiotics, surgical abscess revision and fistula tract closure might be an option in fragile patients. For patients fit for open repair, EVAR can be used as a bridging procedure to definitive repair particularly in the setting of systemic infection.[114]

Endograft infection occurs in less than 1% of endovascular grafts implanted[90,91,115–117] (Fig. 7.15). Approximately one-third of patients present with evidence of an AEF (although less than half of these present with gastrointestinal haemorrhage), one third present with non-specific signs of low grade sepsis (malaise, weight loss) and the remainder with evidence of severe systemic sepsis.[90] Mortality was 18% overall, 36.4% after conservative treatment and 14% after surgical treatment. Mortality was 16% after surgical treatment with extra-anatomical bypass versus 5.8% for surgical treatment with in situ reconstruction.[91,117,118]

In conclusion, ESVS guideline recommends excision of all graft material and infected tissue for definitive treatment (Class I, Level B). In situ reconstruction with autologous vein is the preferred method (Class IIa, Level C). Using allografts lifelong control by image examination caused by the risk of degeneration is recommended (Class I, level C).

Relevant complications after abdominal aortic surgery as a worsening prognostic factor are fistulas. Graft enteric fistulas are associated with bowel injury, prior graft infection or suture line pseudo-aneurysm. During open repair, entering the fistula should be avoided.[119] Contrasting findings are existing about the method for aortic reconstruction. On the one hand, a systematic review favours extra-anatomical repair in a staged procedure concerning the lowest mortality.[120] Only PET grafts were used. Reinfection rate between extra-anatomical and in situ procedure showed no difference. On the other hand, a multivariable analysis reported in situ reconstruction as an independent factor for survival.[121]

If partial or total graft excision is mandatory remains unclear. There are several trials reporting no difference between both techniques. Length of follow-up was the only factor influencing the reinfection rate.[122]

Small bowel defects can be treated by direct suture, while extensive defects require resection and anastomosis.

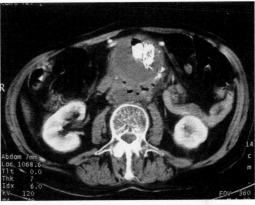

Figure 7.15 Computed tomography scan demonstrating gas bubbles inside the aneurysm sac following endovascular aortic aneurysm reconstruction with concomitant retro-aortic abscess formation.

Omental inlay is recommended to protect the vascular graft and reduce the risk of reinfection.

Aorto-ureteral fistulas are mostly related to open vascular grafts, especially after aorto-iliac reconstructions. Endovascular treatment is restricted to the emergency case with bleeding as mentioned earlier. The ESVS guideline recommends, as always, open surgery with graft explantation and fistula resection. Extra-anatomical reconstruction with femorofemoral crossover bypass and iliac artery ligation should be considered. Data are missing about in situ reconstructions concerning the choice of graft material, morbidity and mortality rates.[123]

GRAFT ANEURYSMS

TRUE ANEURYSMS

Following repair of a true aneurysm, the adjacent artery may also become aneurysmal. Aneurysms were frequent within some early PTFE grafts, but manufacturing improvements have almost eliminated this. Biological grafts such as the human umbilical vein graft frequently became aneurysmal before the addition of a Dacron wrap.[124] Xenografts such as bovine mesenteric vein and cryopreserved venous or arterial allografts are particularly subject to aneurysmal degeneration.[82,85] Dacron undergoes late degradation and dilatation, which becomes clinically significant in 2–3% of the cases. After 5–10 years, disruption can occur at points of stress (e.g., under the inguinal ligament) causing false aneurysms,[125] which may present with haemorrhage or thrombosis. Distraction during shoulder abduction may cause spontaneous rupture or axillary anastomotic disruption of PTFE axillofemoral grafts.[126]

Vein graft aneurysms are rare but more frequent in bypasses for popliteal aneurysms than for occlusive disease.[127] Information on the natural history of untreated graft aneurysms is lacking but repair is generally recommended and is essential to prevent rupture, thrombosis, or embolism. Treatment is either with a covered endovascular stent or by graft replacement.

FALSE ANEURYSMS

False aneurysms are essentially pulsating haematomas, which may occur at the arterial puncture site after angiography (or intervention), following intra-arterial injection by intravenous drug users, after trauma (usually penetrating), because of primary arterial infection (e.g., salmonella and HIV) and at disrupted arterial anastomoses. Puncture-site aneurysms often thrombose spontaneously.

✔✔ Although limited, the present evidence appears to support the use of thrombin injection as an effective treatment for femoral pseudo-aneurysm. A pragmatic approach may be to use compression (blind or ultrasound-guided) as first-line treatment, reserving thrombin injection for those in whom the compression procedure fails.[128] (SCALPEL)

Ultrasound-guided compression occludes over 80% and most others will thrombose following thrombin injection.[129] Direct surgical repair or a covered stent are rarely necessary. The management of infected (mycotic) aneurysms is dealt with in Chapter 13.

The incidence of anastomotic aneurysms is increasing, primarily because of the increased frequency of prosthetic vascular reconstructions involving groin anastomosis. The overall incidence following vascular anastomoses is about 2%, but this increases to 3–8% when the anastomosis involves the femoral artery. Although they are most common after prosthetic bypass, anastomotic aneurysms occasionally occur after vein bypass, semi-closed endarterectomy and open endarterectomy with a vein patch. Anastomotic aneurysms can occur anywhere, but they frequently develop near to a joint. About 80% occur at the groin, presumably because of movement-related strains.[130]

Aortic anastomotic aneurysms are not easily discovered by clinical examination, but when followed by CT, the incidence may be as high as 4%.[131] Some feel this justifies the need for life long follow-up after aortic reconstruction,[132] but many patients who develop an aneurysm above a previous aortic graft never come to revision because they are too old or the repair is too complex (involving the renal/visceral arteries).

Anastomotic aneurysms at the femoral level are best handled by open surgery and graft interposition,[132] although here are anecdotal reports of endovascular reconstruction.[133] The treatment of choice for iliac anastomotic aneurysms is now stent graft placement by the groin (Fig. 7.16). The procedure can be done under local anaesthesia and mortality and morbidity is minimal. Late complications include endoleak and occlusion in a minority of the cases.[134,135] Pre-operative embolisation of the internal iliac artery is frequently required, which may lead to gluteal claudication[136] and other pelvic complications (see Chapter 13).

Graft interposition for aortic anastomotic aneurysms is done by laparotomy or preferentially retroperitoneal approach. It is however, associated with a higher surgical risk than a primary vascular operation: perioperative mortality in the elective setting ranges from 0–17% and is definitely higher than 50% in case of rupture.[137,138]

✔ Endovascular reconstruction is actually preferred if the patient has a suitable morphology (Fig. 7.17).[139–144] A comparative study confirmed reduced blood loss, procedural time and a shorter hospital stay in the endovascular group. The operative mortality was 19% in the surgical group versus 10% in the endovascular series.[145] A recently published study demonstrated that endovascular repair of para-anastomotic aortic and iliac aneurysms after initial prosthetic aortic surgery is safe and durable in patients with an appropriate anatomy. The long-term follow-up showed fewer complications occurred after procedures with bifurcated stent grafts compared with procedures with tube grafts, aorto-uniiliac, or iliac extension stent grafts.[146] Although a tubular stent graft from a technical point of view can handle most aneurysms, there are indications that a bifurcated graft might be more effective at midterm follow-up.[147] (PEN NIB)

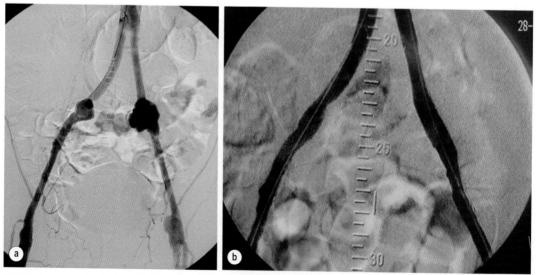

Figure 7.16   Pre-operative angiography with bilateral para-anastomotic iliac artery false aneurysm **(a)** pre-operative angiography **(b)** angiography after placement of tubular endoprostheses.

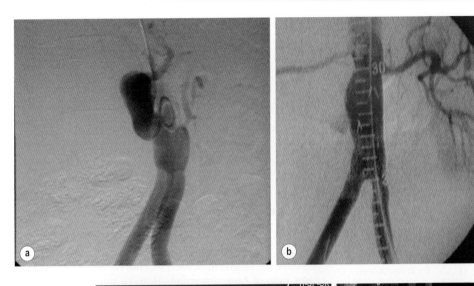

Figure 7.17 Pre-operative angiography with para-anastomotic false aneurysm in aortal localisation after interval of 4 years **(a)** and **(b)** angiography after placement of tubular endoprosthesis.

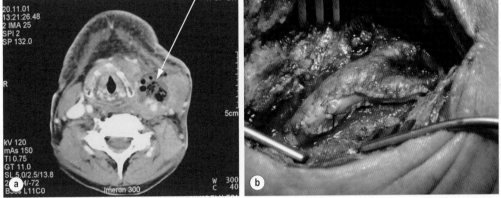

Figure 7.18 Computed tomography scan of infection following carotid endarterectomy with patch **(a)** and **(b)** situs intraoperatively with vein patch.

CAROTID ARTERY

INFECTION

Revision of the carotid artery surgery is either required post-operatively during the first 48–72 hours because of acute bleeding or thrombosis leading to hemispheric symptoms. These complications are extensively dealt with in Chapter 10 and will not be focused on here. During follow-up, the risk for patch infection is in the range of <1%[148,149] and the highest when foreign material has been used (Fig. 7.18). The patient normally presents with a swelling or a sinus with a positive bacterial isolate. Although carotid endarterectomy (CEA) is often performed under local anaesthesia, in cases of infection, general anaesthesia is preferred because of the risk for spreading the infection through the cannula, but also because the preparation is more tedious and is more extensive. Frequently, the scar tissue is so dense that one may not be able to have the external carotid artery dissected free but a balloon is necessary to prevent back bleeding. To gain full access to the healthy part of the internal carotid artery, it might be wise to use the Pruitt-Inahara shunt to stop the back bleeding from the internal carotid artery (ICA) thus one has secured the perfusion of the brain and does not come into time problems. Secondly one gains almost a cm of the carotid to use for the patch closing. We normally shift from polyester to a saphenous vein patch from the groin. Although there is no evidence based on randomised trials, it is suggested in the literature that the vein patch from the ankle should be less suitable.[150]

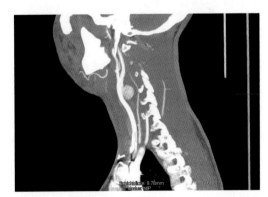

Figure 7.19 Carotid artery aneurysm after carotid endarterectomy.

Stents or stent grafts do not seem to play any definite role in the treatment of carotid artery infection but may play a bridging role to temporary stop a bleeding.

ANEURYSM FORMATION

The carotid artery aneurysm after CEA that is most frequently encountered, is on the basis of a 'low grade' infection or pseudo-aneurysm (Fig. 7.19).

Due to the turbulent flow, it is recommended that these aneurysms are operated upon when they have reached a 2-cm size or if they have been producing symptoms. The surgical exposure technique does not differ from the one using

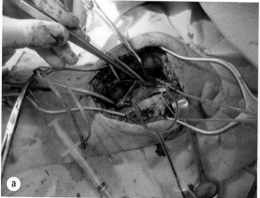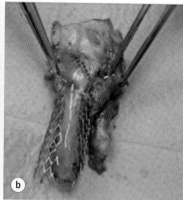

Figure 7.20 Carotid endarterectomy after carotid artery stent. **(a)** Situs intraoperatively, **(b)** specimen following thrombendarterectomy.

standard CEA but it might be necessary to resect the artery and use an interposition graft instead. There is no evidence for the use of carotid artery stenting (CAS) to treat aneurysm formation after CEA but may be possible with covered stents if surgery for some reason should not be possible.

REVISION AFTER CAROTID ARTERY STENTING

The risk for complications might be higher when doing CEA after CAS and if longer segments are being stented. Operative treatment should therefore mainly be reserved for patients that are neurologically symptomatic. The surgical exposure is the standard one like described in Chapter 10. The dissection of the common and carotid artery, though, might be extra cumbersome as there is often an inflammation around the artery where the stent is. Should the stent penetrate the arterial wall, then it is often necessary to insert an interposition graft instead of doing a thrombendarterectomy (Fig. 7.20).

REVISION SURGERY AFTER ENDOVASCULAR AORTIC ANEURYSM RECONSTRUCTION

EVAR is associated with a significant risk of late complications, which may occur at a rate of 5–10% per annum. Endoleaks are the most frequent complication and are described in more detail in Chapter 13. Most complications can be treated by endovascular re-intervention, if required.[151] Surgical techniques such as laparoscopic clipping of the side branches and remodelling of the aneurysm have not gained much enthusiasm (see Fig. 7.12).[152,153] Open surgery, on the other hand, is well accepted for graft limb thrombosis, for example, graft thrombectomy or femorofemoral crossover grafting.[151] But also open surgery is necessary for treating endoleaks. In the following, some technical details are described. Type I a and III endoleaks are associated with a high risk of rupture. Common approach for endograft explantation to treat relevant endoleaks is the transperitoneal by performing a mid-line incision. Extraperitoneal approaches are less used. Aortic cross clamping zones are infra-renal, supra-renal or supra-celiac. In cases of emergency, proximal occlusion can be gained by aortic occlusion balloons. Supra-coeliac clamping is most necessary in supra-renal active fixation of the endograft. With endografts with infra-renal fixation, there is often temporary supra-renal clamping required.

Supra-renal endograft fixation is associated with aortic wall injury. Avoiding such severe complications partial explantation of the endograft is advisable if there is no proximal endoleak.[154]

A recently published review revealed that the rate of early conversion ranged from 0.8–5.9%; the latest studies carried lower rates of early conversion. Mortality rates of early conversion varied between 0–28.5%, with an average mortality of 12.4%. The rates of late conversion ranged from 0.4–22% with a total average 1.9%; the mortality rate was 10%[155] (PEN NIB).

Although the operation is more challenging, the procedure is essentially performed according to the guidelines of primary aneurysm surgery. Dissection of the proximal infra-renal aortic neck might be more difficult because of periaortic inflammation caused by the stent graft. Supra-renal and preferably supra-coeliac clamping is frequently required, particularly in stent grafts with supra-renal fixation. Endografts with infra-renal fixation are easily removed once the aneurysm sac has been opened and the aorta is clamped below the renal arteries. In grafts with supra-renal fixation, particularly in those with hooks and barbs, it might be wise to leave the supra-renal portion in place and to amputate the infra-renal portion of the endoprosthesis by cutting the metal frame of the supra-renal attachment system.[156] The supra-renal fixation system is then incorporated into the proximal anastomosis, which is performed under supra-coeliac aortic clamping. By preference, the graft should be removed completely. In the usual case of a bifurcation graft, this means that the iliac arteries have to be dissected and that the external and internal iliac arteries have to be clamped selectively to perform a reconstruction to the iliac bifurcation.

Although it is understood that conversion is associated with increased risk of mortality and morbidity, different teams have reported a 0% mortality rate for elective late conversion. Mortality rates for early conversion range from 7–25%, going up to 40% in case of rupture.[157–159]

REVISION SURGERY AFTER INFECTED ENDOVASCULAR AORTIC ANEURYSM RECONSTRUCTION

EVAR as a primary treatment modality for abdominal aortic aneurysm is associated with short series of endograft infection, a rare complication with an incidence between 0.4–3%[116–118,160,161] but with a post-operative mortality as high as 40%, comparable to infection of open aortic grafts.[94,95,162] Whereas prevention of infection is essential, explantation is the only technique that can potentially result in cure of an aortic stent graft infection.[162] Preservation of the stent graft followed by appropriate antibiotic therapy and percutaneous drainage or surgical debridement has been described as an alternative treatment in selected high-risk patients who are unfit for extensive open repair.[94,115] A recently published extensive electronic health database search documented an overall mortality of 45% at 11.4 months. Patients with AEF have the worst outcome and there was evidence for lower mortality in patients who undergo an additional procedure, such as drainage, surgical debridement, sac irrigation, and/or omentoplasty. The authors concluded that surgical debridement or CT-guided percutaneous drainage followed by appropriate antibiotic therapy should be reserved for physically capable patients who are, however, poor candidates for major aortic reconstructive surgery.[163]

REVISION AFTER THORACIC ENDOVASCULAR AORTIC ANEURYSM RECONSTRUCTION

Although most of the complications after thoracic EVAR (TEVAR) are confined to endoleaks or migration of the stent graft, which may be dealt endovascularly (see Chapter 14), there are some situations that are more complicated and these are aortobronchial fistula, aortoesophageal fistula, and stent-graft infection.

AORTOBRONCHIAL FISTULA

Aortobronchial fistula after TEVAR is rare. Statistically, robust date are not available, but according to a national survey of 1113 TEVARs, the risk seems to be <2% when combined with aortoesophageal fistula.[164] A currently published analysis of an international multicentre registry (European Registry of Endovascular Aortic Repair Complications, EuREC) between 2001 and 2012 with a total caseload of 4680 TEVAR procedures (14 centres) revealed a prevalence of either central airway (aortobronchial) or pulmonary parenchymal (aortopulmonary) fistulation in the entire cohort after TEVAR in the study period was 0.56% (central airway 58%, peripheral parenchymal 42%). The incidence was 0.40/1000 interventions/year (range:

0.08–2.36).[165] Airway fistulas should be treated by open surgery according to the EuREC registry with a better survival with 63% after 2 years.[165] Operative techniques are primary repair of the defect, bronchial resection, lung resection (wedge resection) or pulmonary resection.

The symptoms before the haemoptysis are, if at all, vague. The typical patient will have some episodes of minor bleeding before the major one and the diagnosis is therefore often delayed.

Although a bronchoscopy might theoretically show the graft, sometimes the fistula is more peripheral in the lung tissue.

A new stent graft might serve as bridge solution to get the patient into a stable position, but the more radical solution with open surgery and replacement by a standard graft or an allograft is most likely a more long-lasting solution. In case of a new prosthetic graft, long-time therapy with antibiotics is needed. We prefer to use an allograft instead if timely possible (Fig. 7.21).

AORTOESOPHAGEAL FISTULA

The stent graft and its hooks or bare stent may penetrate the oesophagus because of mechanical reasons, but an

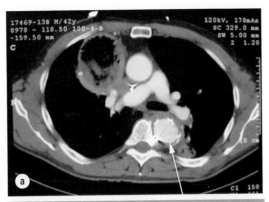
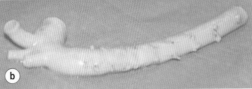
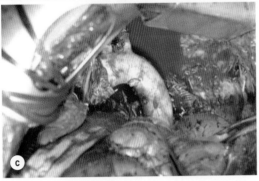

Figure 7.21 Infection following thoracic endovascular aortic aneurysm reconstruction in case of traumatic transection 4 years before. **(a)** Computed tomography scan, **(b)** cryopreserved thoracic allograft, **(c)** thoracic aortic reconstruction with allograft.

aortoesophageal fistula might also appear even in patients where the stent graft is not in contact with the oesophagus. Aortoesophageal arterial branches might be occluded by the stent graft, thereby leading to an ischaemic necrosis. TEVAR could serve as a bridge to surgery for emergency cases of AEF only, with definitive open surgical correction of the fistula undertaken as soon as possible.[166] In accordance with the ESVS guideline, this approach gains a recommendation (Class II, Level B).

Oesophageal fistulas can treated limited or radical. Limited treatment is the local closure of the oesophageal lesion with the risks of anastomotic leakage and mediastinitis. Radical fistula treatment consists of partial or total resection of the oesophagus and reconstruction with gastric or colonic pull up.

INFECTION

Stent graft infection occurs in 0.2–3% of endovascular grafts implanted.[80,90]

Because of the association of fistula creation (oesophagus, bronchial, pulmonary) first symptoms are often haematemesis or haemoptysis.

The infected stent graft is a challenge where the definite treatment is normally containing explantation of the

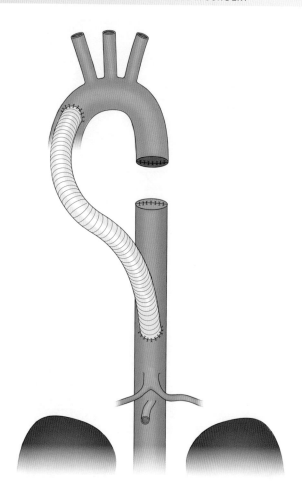

Figure 7.22   Ventral aorta, typical routed retrosternal.

stent graft. Although the antibiotic therapy over a long time might be an alternative for 'no surgery candidates', it might withhold the infection but rarely extinct it. As for several of the thoracic entities, there is no robust data but more case reports of on one or some cases.[91]

Surgical treatment options consist of in situ and extra-anatomical reconstructions as mentioned in infra-renal cases. Wide spectrum of graft material (similar to the abdominal aorta) can be used for in situ reconstruction as mentioned later. Adjunctive therapy for biological coverage of the vascular graft to decrease reinfection is recommended with intercostal, pericardial or omental flap.[167]

Surgical technique in an extra-anatomical scenario is the restoration of perfusion by an axillo-bifemoral or bilateral axillofemoral bypass in combination with aortic ligation. The most common extra-anatomical approach is the so-called *ventral aorta* (Fig. 7.22). This approach is limited by acute bleeding, involvement of the aortic arch. Aortic stump management is a central step during the operation. The stump is oversewn in a double-layer and covered (as mentioned earlier) to decrease the risk of stump rupture.

ESVS guidelines recommend total graft explantation (Class I, Level B) and coverage with autologous tissue in case of in situ reconstructions (Class I, Level C). Cryopreserved allografts may be considered the first-choice material (Class II b, Level C). Advantages of allografts are higher resistance to infection. Disadvantages are degeneration, rupture and

bleeding (especially in infections caused by *Pseudomonas aeruginosa* and *Candida* spp.).

Key points

- Late graft occlusion is caused by intimal hyperplasia or progression of atherosclerosis of the inflow or outflow.
- Graft stenoses occur in 20–30% of infra-inguinal vein grafts. Symptomatic stenoses require treatment. Angioplasty offers excellent early results. In the long-term, open surgery is probably better.
- Thrombolysis of occluded infra-inguinal grafts may be attempted in patients aged under 80 years with critical ischaemia, provided that limb viability is not severely threatened, that the patient has not undergone surgery within 3 months and that the occlusion is less than 14 days old.
- Graft infection results from a breakdown of sterility at surgery, by extension from a superficial wound infection or from bloodborne bacteria.
- Prosthetic graft infections cause perigraft abscesses, sinuses and anastomotic haemorrhage, including AEF and erosion. Vein grafts may be eroded by infection, particularly in open wounds.
- *Staphylococcus epidermidis* is the most frequent cause of low-grade infection. *Staphylococcus aureus* and gram-negative infections tend to present early and are more virulent. The incidence of MRSA infection is increasing.
- Any fluid around a graft after 3 months or gas beyond 4 to 7 weeks on CT or ultrasound suggests infection. Aspiration or perigraft fluid pus can usually secure the diagnosis.
- Conservative measures, such as prolonged antibiotic therapy, drainage and irrigation, or covering exposed grafts with muscle or omental flaps are rarely curative. The same goes on for partial graft excision.
- Simple graft excision without revascularisation usually causes severe ischaemia leading to amputation or death.
- Extra-anatomical revascularisation has been the 'gold standard' in the past. In situ revascularisation with autologous vein (e.g., femoral vein) has better patency and recurrent infection is rare. Arterial allografts are an alternative. In situ reconstruction with silver-bonded or rifampicin-bonded Dacron grafts is still semi-experimental.
- Endoprostheses can buy time in case of bleeding aortoduodenal fistula, but recurrence of infection is high.
- True aneurysms can occur within prosthetic or vein grafts or adjacent to previous aneurysms.
- False aneurysms may result from anastomotic distraction or infection. Treatment of femoral false aneurysms is surgical. Endovascular treatment offers an excellent alternative in case of non-infected iliac or aortic false aneurysms.
- Surgical conversion is rarely needed after endovascular treatment of abdominal aortic aneurysms. If necessary, surgery can be performed with excellent results.

 References available at http://ebooks.health.elsevier.com/

KEY REFERENCES

[3] de Bruin JL, Karthikesalingam A, Holt PJ, et al. Predicting reinterventions after open and endovascular aneurysm repair using the St George's Vascular Institute score. J Vasc Surg 2016;63. 1428–33.e1.

[4] Giles KA, Landon BE, Cotterill P, O'Malley AJ, Pomposelli FB, Schermerhorn ML. Thirty-day mortality and late survival with reinterventions and readmissions after open and endovascular aortic aneurysm repair in Medicare beneficiaries. J Vasc Surg 2011;53. 6–12,3.e1.

[5] Karthikesalingam A, Holt PJ, Hinchliffe RJ, Nordon IM, Loftus IM, Thompson MM. Risk of reintervention after endovascular aortic aneurysm repair. Br J Surg 2010;97:657–63.

Management of acute lower limb ischaemia

8

Rachael O. Forsythe | Robert J. Hinchliffe

INTRODUCTION

✓✓ The revised (2007) TASC Inter-Society Consensus defines acute leg ischaemia as any sudden decrease in limb perfusion causing a potential threat to limb viability.[1]

Symptoms of acute limb ischaemia (ALI) are usually present for less than 2 weeks. However, some overlap with chronic limb-threatening ischaemia (CLTI) is inevitable and increasingly common. The severity of ischaemia is best defined according to the modified Rutherford criteria (Table 8.1),[2,3] using the following categories:

- I Viable
- IIa Marginally threatened (salvageable if promptly treated)
- IIb Immediately threatened (salvageable if promptly revascularised)
- III Irreversible

The true incidence of ALI is unknown. Clinical presentation is variable, treatment is not standardised and often the incidence of ALI is reported together with that of CLTI in epidemiological studies. The Oxford Vascular Study found that the incidence of ALI was 10 per 100 000 per year between 2002 and 2012.[4]

The COhorte des Patients ARTeriopathes (COPART; a prospective multicentre registry of patients from three academic hospitals in Southwest France) found that ALI was responsible for 9% of hospitalisations compared to CLTI (91%) amongst patients hospitalised for lower limb peripheral artery disease (PAD).[5]

There is evidence that outcomes are improved when patients are managed by a vascular service providing 24-hour cover.[6] ALI is associated with a high cost to the community because of the significant risk of amputation (10–30% at 30 days) and prolonged hospitalisation.

AETIOLOGY

ALI is the result of occlusion of a native artery or vascular/endovascular prosthesis. Most commonly, embolism or in situ thrombosis can cause native arterial occlusion (Box 8.1).

EMBOLISM

Until about 30 years ago, embolic disease was the underlying cause of most cases of ALI. Emboli large enough to occlude major vessels usually arise in the heart. Rheumatic mitral valve disease was the most common cause, with large emboli forming in a dilated left atrium.

Atrial fibrillation caused by ischaemic heart disease is now the cardiac origin in 80% of embolic cases; mural thrombus following acute myocardial infarction causes most of the remainder.[7] Less commonly, embolisation originates from mural thrombi of the aorta, aortic or popliteal aneurysms and iliac arteries. Large emboli typically lodge at an arterial bifurcation, particularly in the common femoral or popliteal arteries (Fig. 8.1). Patients with cardiac embolism may also have co-existing PAD as a result of the underlying process of atherosclerosis. This increases the difficulty in establishing the cause of the ischaemia and in planning revascularisation. In 20% of patients with ALI, a source for the embolus cannot be found.

ATHEROEMBOLISM

Less common sources of emboli include proximal aneurysms or atherosclerotic plaques, usually located in the thoracic or abdominal aorta, or arising from popliteal artery aneurysm. Whereas cardiac embolism usually consists entirely of platelet-rich thrombus, embolism from proximal arteries can include atherosclerotic plaques or cholesterol-rich emboli. This has a much worse prognosis than cardiac embolism because embolectomy is less effective – small particles of atheroembolism can pass to very distal vessels in the foot. This digital embolism can result in the 'acute blue toe syndrome'. In this condition, the embolic source should be identified and treated if possible. Often, this is a proximal arterial plaque that has ruptured, and the emboli are a mixture of platelet-rich thrombus and cholesterol (Fig. 8.2).

Embolisation of cholesterol-rich atheroma can occur spontaneously, but also follows intra-arterial manipulation following endovascular intervention, or occasionally surgery (causing 'trash foot'). This can be disastrous, since both large and small arteries may be occluded, and it may not be possible to revascularise with either surgery or thrombolysis. This may result in limb or end-organ damage and is sometimes fatal (Fig. 8.3).

Table 8.1   Suggested clinical categories of acute limb ischaemia

Category	Prognosis	Capillary return	Motor deficit	Sensory loss	Doppler signals	
					Arterial	Venous
I Viable	Not immediately threatened	Intact	None	None	Audible	Audible
IIa Marginally threatened	Salvageable if promptly treated	Intact/slow	None	None or minimal (toes)	Inaudible*	Audible
IIb Immediately threatened	Salvageable if promptly revascularised	Slow/absent	Mild/moderate	More than toes	Inaudible	Audible
III Irreversible	Unsalvageable; major tissue loss and permanent nerve damage inevitable	Absent staining	Profound, paralysis (rigor*)	Profound, anaesthetic	Inaudible	Inaudible
	Requires primary amputation					

Reproduced from Rutherford RB, Flanigan DP, Gupta SK, et al, with modifications (*) according to European Society for Vascular Surgery (ESVS) 2020 Practice Guidelines on the Management of Acute Limb Ischaemia.[3] In the original 1997 classification by Rutherford et al,[2] aterial Doppler sounds are never present in Stage IIA, and rigor is always present in Stage III, however, the writing committee of the guidelines opine that exceptions to these rules exist.

Box 8.1   Aetiology of acute lower limb ischaemia

Thrombosis

- Atherosclerosis
- Popliteal aneurysm
- Bypass graft occlusion
- Endovascular stent or stent graft occlusion
- Iatrogenic (localised arterial dissection post endovascular intervention, for example, arterial closure device failure)
- Thrombotic conditions

Embolism

- Atrial fibrillation
- Mural thrombosis
- Vegetations
- Proximal aneurysms
- Atherosclerotic plaque

Rare causes

- Vasculitis
- Dissection
- Trauma (including iatrogenic)
- External compression
- Popliteal entrapment
- Cystic adventitial disease
- Iliac endofibrosis
- Paradoxical embolism
- Tumour embolism
- Foreign body embolism, e.g., intravenous drug use
- Acute compartment syndrome
- Low cardiac output states, e.g., hypotension, shock, sepsis

THROMBOSIS

In-situ thrombosis in a native artery is now the most frequent cause of ALI, commonly in patients with a high atherosclerotic burden. It may be the result of rupture of an atherosclerotic plaque or critical flow arrest at the site of an atherosclerotic stenosis. The advancing age of the population and the commensurate increase in atherosclerosis have increased the proportion of ALI caused by thrombosis. Acute native vessel arterial occlusion may also be caused by surgery (e.g., knee replacement disrupting the geniculate collateral vessels formed around a popliteal occlusion), heart failure, thrombotic tendency (polycythaemia, dehydration, malignancy, etc.) or trauma.

Acute thrombosis of a popliteal aneurysm poses the highest risk to the leg. Typically, this occurs in elderly men in association with aneurysms elsewhere (50% have an aortic aneurysm) or generalised arterial ectasia. As they enlarge, popliteal artery aneurysms can fill with lamellar thrombus, which may cause either acute thrombosis or distal embolisation that occludes the tibial vessels. The latter will place the leg in extreme jeopardy, with up to 30% risk of limb loss. It is much more common for a popliteal artery aneurysm to cause distal embolisation than to rupture.

OTHER CAUSES

The increasing use of both open and endovascular techniques to revascularise ischaemic limbs means that surgeons often have to deal with acute thrombosis of bypass grafts and arteries that have previously undergone endovascular treatment. Grafts occlude for a variety of reasons. Within 1 month of insertion, graft occlusion is usually the result of technical problems at the time of surgery or poor distal run-off. Graft occlusion within 1 year of placement is often caused by myointimal hyperplasia at an anastomosis or the development of stenoses within a vein graft. Occlusion after 1 year is usually caused by progression of distal atherosclerosis. Prosthetic grafts have

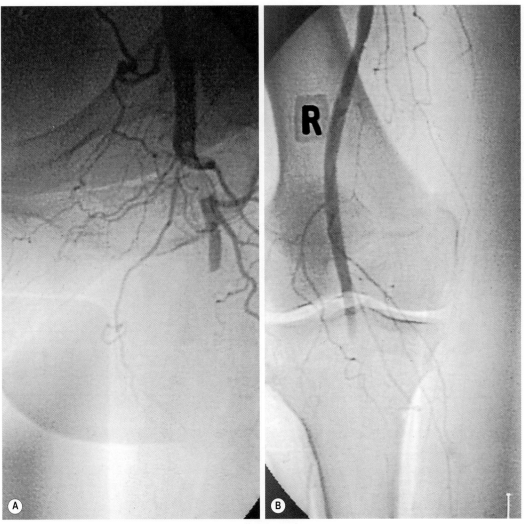

Figure 8.1   Arteriogram demonstrating an embolus lodged in the bifurcation of the common femoral artery (a) with further emboli occluding the distal profunda and popliteal artery (b).

a higher occlusion rate than autogenous vein grafts (see Chapter 7).

Iliac limb occlusions are observed after aorto-bifemoral bypass surgery if limbs become kinked or have poor outflow. Endovascular stent grafts used to repair abdominal aortic aneurysms (endovascular aneurysm repair [EVAR]) have similar modes of failure. Occlusion is more common when the iliac limb of the stent graft is extended into the external iliac artery. Occlusion may occur any time after implantation in up to 5% of patients.[8]

A special group of iatrogenic occlusion of external iliac and femoral vessels is related to the maldeployment or failure of arterial closure devices. These achieve closure of arteries after endovascular intervention using percutaneously delivered sutures or plugs. Inadvertently, they can cause arrest of flow through direct closure or stenosis of the artery, or by dissection of the vessel. Presentation is usually in the early post-intervention period but may be delayed.

Spontaneous native arterial thrombosis occasionally occurs without an underlying flow-limiting stenosis and these patients should be investigated for an intrinsic clotting abnormality/thrombophilia, for example, antiphospholipid syndrome, activated protein C deficiency or malignancy.

Occasionally, acute arterial occlusion may be caused by arterial dissection, trauma, extrinsic compression or illicit drug use (cocaine and 'crack' cocaine). In a young patient with acute popliteal artery occlusion, either popliteal entrapment or cystic adventitial disease should be considered (see Chapter 2 on chronic limb ischaemia).

RECENT CHANGES

A number of factors may have changed the presentation of ALI. The incidence of co-existing PAD is increasing, meaning that revascularisation can be more challenging in the acute setting. Medical therapy has improved and many patients are now treated with cardioprotective drugs such as antiplatelet therapy and statins if they have risk factors for cardiovascular disease. Antiplatelet therapy probably reduces the risk of deterioration and the need for limb revascularisation in those patients with established PAD.[9] Recent evidence suggests that low-dose (2.5 mg) rivaroxaban twice a day, in combination with low-dose (100 mg) aspirin may

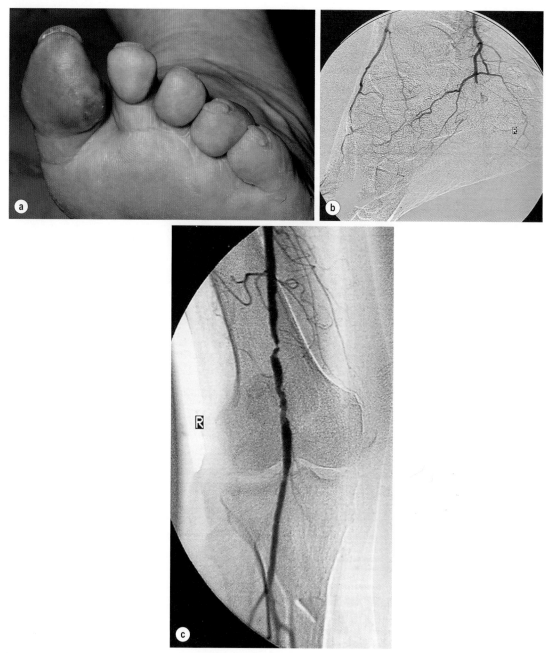

Figure 8.2   (a) 'Blue toe syndrome' caused by digital and pedal arterial atheroembolism (b) from a proximal atherosclerotic stenosis (c). Note the acute cut-off of the posterior tibial artery. Ultrasonography excluded a popliteal aneurysm, and the lesion was treated by balloon angioplasty.

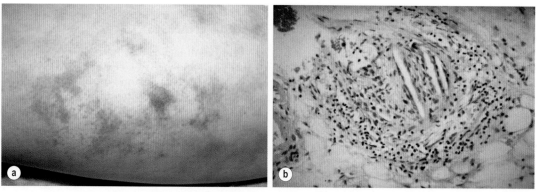

Figure 8.3   Livedo reticularis (a) caused by cholesterol embolism (b).

significantly reduce the risk of ALI when compared to aspirin alone.[10] Similarly, patients with atrial fibrillation are often established on anticoagulation to reduce their risk of embolic complications. However, despite adequate anticoagulation, some patients do still present with ALI.

A randomised double-blind placebo-controlled trial evaluating Vorapaxar used ALI as one of the endpoints. The investigators demonstrated that, in selected patients with symptomatic PAD without atrial fibrillation, Vorapaxar reduced the incidence of ALI regardless of the cause. With further research, this protease-activated receptor 1 antagonist could be used to reduce the risk of ALI in patients with known PAD, however it has not yet been widely adopted.[11]

CLINICAL FEATURES

The severity of ischaemia at presentation is the most important factor affecting outcome of the leg.[12,13] Complete occlusion of a proximal artery in the absence of preformed collateral vessels (as in cardiac embolism) results in the classical clinical presentation of pain, paralysis, paraesthesia, pallor, pulselessness and a perishingly cold leg (poikilothermia). In reality, all six of these signs are rarely encountered. The pain is severe and frequently resistant to analgesia. Calf pain and tenderness with a tense muscle compartment indicates severe muscle ischaemia or necrosis and often irreversible ischaemia. Sensorimotor deficit including muscle paralysis and paraesthesia is indicative of muscle and nerve ischaemia with the potential for salvage only if treated promptly. Initially, the leg is white with empty veins but after 6–12 hours vasodilatation occurs, probably caused by hypoxia of the smooth muscle. The capillaries then fill with stagnant deoxygenated blood, resulting in a mottled appearance that blanches on digital pressure (Fig. 8.4). If flow is not restored rapidly, the arteries distal to the occlusion fill with propagated thrombus and the capillaries rupture, resulting in a fixed blue staining

of the skin that is a sign of irreversible ischaemia. These features are typical of an acute arterial occlusion in the absence of existing collaterals and suggest an embolic cause.

When arterial occlusion occurs as part of a chronic process where collaterals have developed (in patients with pre-existing PAD), typically the leg is less severely ischaemic. Patients with peripheral atherosclerosis deteriorate in a stepwise fashion as thrombosis supervenes on an existing arterial plaque. Patients often report a sudden change in symptoms, which progress over a few days: the foot often has a dusky hue with slow capillary return. Previous claudication or absent pulses in the contralateral foot help make a clinical diagnosis of in situ thrombosis. Palpation of a mass in either popliteal fossa suggests thrombosis of a popliteal aneurysm. Young patients (<50 years), those with an atypical history (e.g., severe back pain associated with aortic dissection) or recent endovascular intervention raise the possibility of non-atherosclerotic/embolic ALI.

INITIAL MANAGEMENT

Patients presenting with ALI are often in poor general health, which contributes to the observed high mortality rate from associated cardiovascular disease. For some frail elderly patients, ALI may be a terminal event. Decisions about care must take into account the patient's pre-morbid frailty, fitness, comorbidities, as well as the projected quality of life associated with intervention. Most importantly, careful discussions with the patient (and relatives, particularly if the patient has cognitive impairment) is essential and should be documented clearly in the case notes. All patients with ALI should be urgently assessed by a vascular specialist in a vascular centre that offers the full range of open and endovascular interventions, ideally in a hybrid setting or operating theatre with a C arm.[3]

Dehydration, cardiac failure, hypoxia and pain should all be managed in the standard way. Intravenous unfractionated

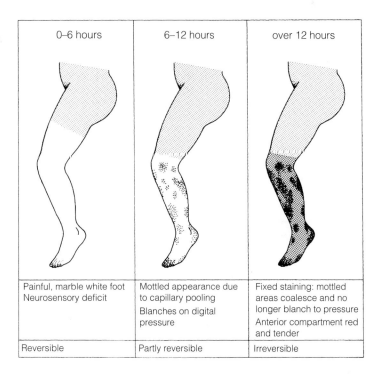

0–6 hours	6–12 hours	over 12 hours
Painful, marble white foot Neurosensory deficit	Mottled appearance due to capillary pooling Blanches on digital pressure	Fixed staining: mottled areas coalesce and no longer blanch to pressure Anterior compartment red and tender
Reversible	Partly reversible	Irreversible

Figure 8.4 Clinical outcome after acute leg ischaemia.

heparin (5000 IU or 70–100 IU/kg) should be given immediately, followed by systemic heparinisation titrated to a target activated partial thromboplastin time, APTT). The aim of heparinisation is to restrict propagation of thrombus and provide an anti-inflammatory effect, whilst allowing the intrinsic fibrinolytic pathway to break down the thrombus. Whilst there is evidence that heparinisation improves the prognosis, there are no data to suggest that unfractionated heparin is superior to other methods of anticoagulation. In reality, many patients do not achieve a stable target APTT[14] and in many units low-molecular-weight heparins have replaced unfractionated heparin because of their more reliable effect on anticoagulation. Anticoagulation should be delayed if urgent revascularisation is planned and the patient is likely to need epidural anaesthesia. The short half-life of unfractionated heparin is helpful in this situation. There is no role for systemic thrombolysis in the management of ALI.[3]

Venous blood should be taken for full blood count, urea, electrolytes, glucose and coagulation screen. There are no good data to support the use of biochemical markers of ischaemia, however, many units use creatine kinase (CK), which is a marker of skeletal muscle damage as a result of rhabdomyolisis and ischaemia. Whilst not validated for routine use, an elevated CK has been associated with a significantly increased risk of major amputation (56.2% vs. 4.6% if normal CK),[15] however, no biomarker should be used to decide whether to offer revascularisation or primary amputation.

An electrocardiogram (ECG) and chest radiograph may be of value in diagnosing and managing cardiac arrhythmias and heart failure. If a primary thrombotic tendency is suspected, investigation of this should be delayed as some of the diagnostic tests are inaccurate in the presence of fresh thrombus.

RADIOLOGICAL INVESTIGATIONS

Diagnostic imaging is recommended to guide treatment, unless it poses a significant delay to treatment, or if the need for primary amputation is obvious. The recent European Society for Vascular and Endovascular Surgery (ESVS) guidelines on acute limb ischaemia recommend computed tomography angiography (CTA) in the first instance.[3] Duplex ultrasound or contrast-enhanced magnetic resonance angiography (MRA) are alternatives, depending on availability. In practice, MRA is rarely used in the acute setting because of its long acquisition time and often limited immediate availability. Concerns about the use of contrast-enhanced imaging in the context of acute renal failure may be considered a relative problem when facing this life- and limb-threatening condition. Anatomical coverage of a standard lower limb CTA should extend from the renal arteries to the feet, with a second acquisition for the crural arteries if required.

REVASCULARISATION

The clinical assessment of the severity of limb ischaemia will help to decide the most appropriate form of therapy (Fig. 8.5).

IRREVERSIBLE (RUTHERFORD CATEGORY III) LEG ISCHAEMIA

A small number of patients will present in a moribund state or with irreversible leg ischaemia (muscle paralysis, tense swollen fascial compartments, fixed skin staining) and terminal care should be considered. For the irreversibly ischaemic leg, revascularisation is, by definition, inappropriate and may be dangerous, owing to the risk of ischaemia-reperfusion injury and subsequent systemic inflammatory response syndrome. This includes the patient who develops ALI while being treated for another condition, usually as an inpatient on an elderly care ward. Prognosis is particularly dismal in this group.[16] Surviving patients should be resuscitated and stabilised before considering primary amputation.

IMMEDIATELY THREATENED (RUTHERFORD CATEGORY IIB ISCHAEMIA)

The acute white leg with sensorimotor deficit requires urgent intervention to prevent limb loss. Although the differentiation between thrombosis and embolus can be difficult, it is in this group of patients that embolism is more likely. An acute white leg with no prior history of claudication, normal contralateral pulses and a probable embolic source, such as atrial fibrillation, would indicate that embolisation is the most likely cause. Urgent revascularisation is indicated in these patients, after resuscitation. Traditionally, patients with Rutherford IIb ischaemia have been managed preferentially with an open approach given the requirement for swift restoration of blood flow, however, this dogma has been challenged recently with improvements in the ability to restore flow rapidly using a variety of advanced endovascular tehcniques.[3] Operative approaches may include surgical thromboembolectomy, bypass, percutaneous catheter-directed thrombolysis (CDT), mechanical thrombectomy, thrombus aspiration (with or without CDT) and hybrid procedures such as thromboendarterectomy.

MARGINALLY THREATENED (RUTHERFORD CATEGORY IIA ISCHAEMIA)

The majority of patients presenting with ALI have acute onset of rest pain but no paralysis, with mild or no sensory loss. The cause is often acute thrombosis of either an atherosclerotic artery or a bypass graft.

There are a number of options for intervention depending on the likely aetiology, available expertise and disease burden. Surgical thromboembolectomy alone may be insufficient to revascularise an artery occluded by thrombus with co-existing atherosclerotic plaque; endarterectomy or arterial bypass may also be required. Nationwide registries suggest that surgical revascularisation is used three to five times more frequently than thrombolysis in everyday clinical practice for patients with ALI.[17] Alternatively, thromboembolectomy may be combined with simultaneous endovascular treatment of inflow or outflow disease, which is increasingly possible given the widespread use of hybrid theatres. It is recommended that the use of over-the-wire embolectomy catheters under fluoroscopic guidance should be considered for surgical thromboembolectomy, in preference to standard embolectomy to improve outcomes.

Primary or adjunctive CDT has the capacity to open small as well as large arteries. Intra-operative local thrombolysis may also be considered in patients with residual thrombus after surgical revascularisation and may be particularly valuable in the tibial arteries.

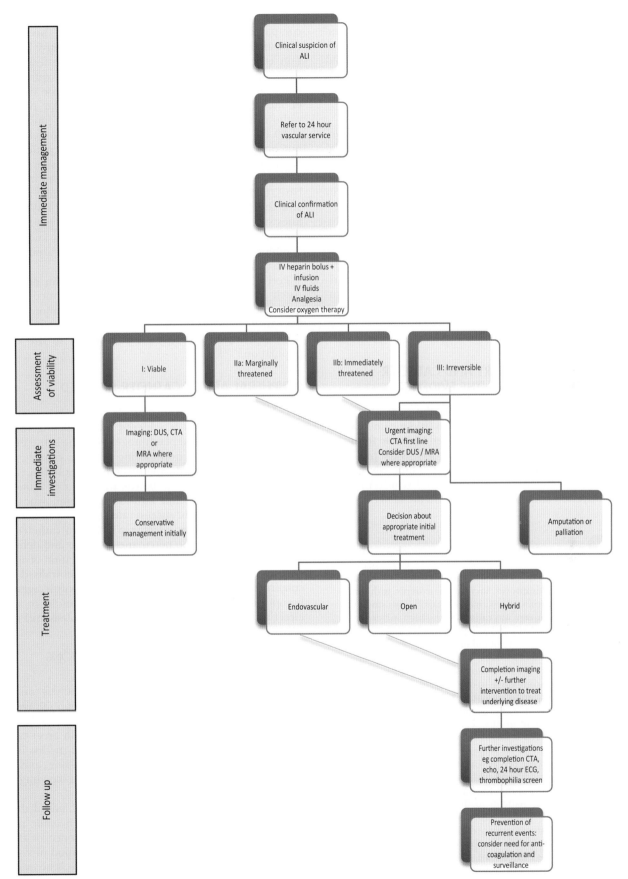

Figure 8.5 Clinical approach to the management of the acutely ischaemic leg. *ALI*, Acute limb ischaemia; *CTA*, computed tomography angiography; *DUS*, diagnostic ultrasound; *ECG*, electrocardiogram; *IV*, intravenous; *MRA*, magnetic resonance angiography.

Completion angiography is recommended in all patients to assess the success of revascularisation as well as the run-off.[3] Residual thrombus following attempted revascularisation is common and, if detected, further treatment should be carried out at the time to optimise the clinical result.

VIABLE (RUTHERFORD CATEGORY I ISCHAEMIA)

Some patients are admitted to hospital with acute thrombosis of a diseased peripheral artery (usually the superficial femoral artery) resulting in claudication without ischaemic rest pain. Revascularisation might appear an attractive option to treat claudication, but the risks are as high as in patients with immediately limb-threatening ischaemia,[18] with unacceptable risks of embolisation following endovascular management. Initial anticoagulation followed by expectant management, depending on the progression of symptoms, reduces the risk to both life and limb.[16] Some patients' symptoms improve and never require revascularisation. In others (especially those with short-distance claudication), it may be more appropriate to consider interval revascularisation 6–12 weeks after the acute event, when the thrombus has organised and embolic risk is reduced.

CHOICE BETWEEN SURGERY AND CATHETER-DIRECTED THROMBOLYSIS: THE EVIDENCE

There remains some controversy over the roles of surgery and CDT for ALI. A Cochrane Review in 2018 included >1200 patients from five randomised controlled trials and found no evidence in favour of open surgery or CDT as the preferred initial treatment strategy in ALI in terms of limb salvage, amputation or death at 30 days, 6 months or 1 year.[19] A further systematic review and meta-analysis found the same.[20]

Between 1994 and 1996, three randomised studies compared the effectiveness of thrombolysis with operative intervention.[21–26] The New York study was the first to show that thrombolysis improves survival in patients with limb-threatening ischaemia of less than 14 days.[21] This study was small and the advantage was caused by the high incidence of cardiorespiratory deaths following emergency surgery. The STILE study was much larger and included patients with ischaemia for longer than 14 days.[22] This study has been much criticised because of the failure to insert a catheter successfully for peripheral thrombolysis in one-third of cases. The study introduced the concept of amputation-free survival but failed to show any significant improvement in this primary endpoint between the treatment groups. In the subgroup of patients with ischaemia for fewer than 14 days, thrombolysis reduced the rate of amputation. Subsequent analysis of patients from this study up to 1 year revealed that thrombolysis was a better initial treatment for graft occlusions, whereas surgery was more effective and durable for native vessel occlusions.[23,24] However, few of the patients in the STILE study had critical ischaemia. The TOPAS trial was designed, using lessons learned from the aforementioned studies, to try to settle this debate. In the first phase, an optimal dose of thrombolytic therapy was selected (urokinase 4000 IU/h)[25] and in phase II, this was compared with urgent surgery in 544 patients.[26] Amputation-free survival was similar in both groups at 6 months and 1 year (72% and 65% for urokinase vs. 75% and 70% for surgery, respectively), though thrombolysis reduced the need for open surgical procedures.

Since these trials, a number of retrospective studies have compared the effectiveness of contemporary thrombolysis with surgery. Taha et al. concluded that operative intervention as an initial treatment had improved technical success in Rutherford II ischaemia, especially when caused by a failed stent or bypass.[27] This was at the expense of a higher mortality rate compared with endovascular treatment without any added advantage in patency or limb salvage at 30 days and 1 year. A systematic review showed similar outcomes between open surgery and CDT in patients with Rutherford IIb ischaemia.[28] Overall, the decision between surgery and thrombolysis should be made on an individual basis, taking into account the class of ischaemia, aetiology and the patient's comorbidities. The recent ESVS guidelines suggest that CDT can be considered in patients with Rutherford IIb ischaemia if initiated promptly and may be combined with adjuncts such as percutaneous aspiration or mechanical thrombectomy.[3]

Peri- and post-operative use of prostacyclin analogues (such as iloprost) may be considered as adjunctive therapy in patients undergoing open revascularisation, as they have been shown to reduce the rate of peri-operative mortality and major limb events, particularly in the elderly population.[29–31]

PERIPHERAL ARTERY CATHETER-DIRECTED THROMBOLYSIS

Thrombus dissolution is achieved by stimulating the conversion of fibrin-bound plasminogen into the active enzyme plasmin. Plasmin is a non-specific protease capable of degrading fibrin and producing thrombus dissolution.

In contrast to the thrombolytic treatment of acute myocardial infarction, systemic infusion of thrombolytic agents for ALI results in a poor success rate and unacceptable complications. However, by selectively placing a catheter within the thrombus via the percutaneous route and delivering the thrombolytic agent locally, the concentration of agent is maximised, and plasmin is less likely to be neutralised by circulating antiplasmins. The dose of thrombolytic agent can be optimised to the minimum level that results in a local effect without producing systemic thrombolysis and the attendant complications.

CONTRAINDICATIONS AND CONSIDERATIONS (BOX 8.2)

The risk of complications from thrombolysis must be weighed against the potential benefits of limb salvage. The elderly (>80 years) are at particularly high risk of bleeding complications and CDT should be used with great caution in this age group. Overall, whilst technical success is high at >80%, the risk of serious bleeding is 13–30%, and there is a small but significant risk of intracranial bleeding (0.4–2.3%), which is almost always fatal.[32,33]

Dacron grafts may take 3 months to seal, and if they do not become fully incorporated, they may become porous if thrombolytic therapy is used. The presence of cardiac thrombus theoretically increases the likelihood of systemic embolisation during thrombolysis, but there is no evidence that patient selection based on echocardiography affects management or outcome. Patients with end-stage renal disease fare significantly worse with CDT when considering amputation risk, primary, primary assisted and secondary

Box 8.2 Contraindications to thrombolysis for acute limb ischaemia[80]

Absolute:

1. Established cerebrovascular event (including transient isch-aemic attack) within the last 2 months
2. Active bleeding diathesis
3. Recent gastrointestinal bleeding (<10 d)
4. Neurosurgery (intracranial, spinal) within the last 3 months
5. Intracranial trauma within the last 3 months

Relatively major:

1. Cardiopulmonary resuscitation within the last 10 days
2. Major non-vascular surgery or trauma within the last 10 days
3. Uncontrolled hypertension: >180 mmHg systolic or >110 mmHg diastolic
4. Puncture of non-compressible vessel
5. Intracranial tumour
6. Recent eye surgery

Relatively minor:

1. Hepatic failure, particularly those with coagulopathy
2. Bacterial endocarditis
3. Pregnancy
4. Diabetic haemorrhagic retinopathy

Working Party on Thrombolysis in the Management of Limb Isch-emia. Thrombolysis in the management of lower limb peripheral arterial occlusion—a consensus document. J Vasc Interv Radiol. 2003 Sep;14(9 Pt 2):S337-49. https://doi.org/10.1016/s1051-0443(07)61244-5. PMID: 14514841.

patency rates, suggesting that patients with chronic kidney disease stage 5 are poor candidates for thrombolysis.[34]

TECHNIQUE

All patients should have adequate analgesia and a cannula inserted for venous access, analgesia and hydration. Patients should be managed in a unit where nursing and medical staff are experienced in thrombolysis and clear protocols exist to manage complications. A critical care environment is desirable for close monitoring during thrombolysis. The extent of occlusive disease needs to be defined by arteriography or duplex imaging before intervention.

Arterial puncture should be performed under ultrasound guidance and puncture attempts should be kept to a minimum to reduce the risk of puncture-site bleeding during treatment.

The initial diagnostic approach is tailored to the distribution of disease. For example, if there is an iliac artery occlusion, a contralateral femoral puncture will provide access for iliac thrombolysis using a crossover technique (Fig. 8.6).

As long as adequate inflow can be confirmed on pre-operative imaging, an antegrade puncture is appropriate to treat occlusions distal to the femoral bifurcation in order that adjuvant procedures such as angioplasty or thrombus aspiration can be performed from the ipsilateral side (see Fig. 8.6).

An occluded arterial bypass graft is optimally accessed from the native artery proximal to the graft so that any stenoses can be treated via the same puncture site. However, this is not always possible for technical reasons and direct puncture of the most proximal accessible part of the graft results in a high success rate from thrombolysis.

Once access has been achieved, a guidewire should be passed through the occlusion; indeed, the ability to do this (the guidewire traversal test) implies the presence of soft thrombus and is a good predictor of success. The catheter used to deliver the lytic agent is then placed within, or just proximal to the thrombus. A multiple side-hole catheter may be used to deliver the lysis over a longer segment of thrombus and to provide a degree of mechanical disruption.

Several techniques are described for delivering thrombolysis. The low-dose infusion method involves delivering the thrombolytic drug through the catheter over several hours. This may be combined with an initial high-dose bolus.

✓✓ High-dose techniques accelerate the rate of thrombus dissolution[35] by administering a number of high-dose boluses sequentially or by using the 'pulse spray' technique.[24] The latter involves high-pressure injection of tiny pulses of lytic agent through a catheter with multiple side-holes, and thus it combines enzymatic thrombolysis with mechanical disruption. The high-dose techniques accelerate thrombolysis and allow patients to be treated within the normal working hours of a radiology department.

Several randomised trials comparing low-dose and accelerated methods of thrombolysis have found that limb salvage rate and complication rates appear similar, though accelerated methods are quicker.[35–38]

Streptokinase and urokinase were the agents initially used for peripheral thrombolysis. Urokinase was used in the STILE and TOPAS trials discussed earlier; however, it is no longer available in North America. Tissue plasminogen activator (t-PA) is the most common lytic agent used in current practice. A number of recombinant t-PAs have subsequently been developed using molecular cloning and bioengineering techniques with the aim of lengthening the duration of bioavailability and avoiding the need for continuous infusion.

✓✓ There are very few high-quality trials to determine which drug is most effective, but most agree that t-PA and urokinase are superior to streptokinase.[39] Recombinant t-PAs have been found to be as effective and safe as urokinase[40] and are the agent of choice in the UK.

The STILE trial suggested that urokinase and t-PA had equivalent activity,[22] and this was confirmed in unpublished manufacturers' data.

Heparin is often administered systemically before and after thrombolysis to counteract the associated prothrombotic tendency. An alternative is concurrent administration of low-dose heparin (200 units/h) via the proximal arterial sheath to maintain patency while delivering the thrombolytic agent via an end-hole catheter. Because of data suggesting an increased risk of haemorrhagic complications without the benefit of improved outcomes, continuous systemic heparinisation during thrombolysis is no longer recommended.[3]

Heparin should be given routinely for 48 hours after completion of thrombolysis. Consideration will then be needed to determine whether individual patients need lifelong anticoagulation with warfarin. No data exist to guide appropriate therapy. In some patients, thrombolysis may be

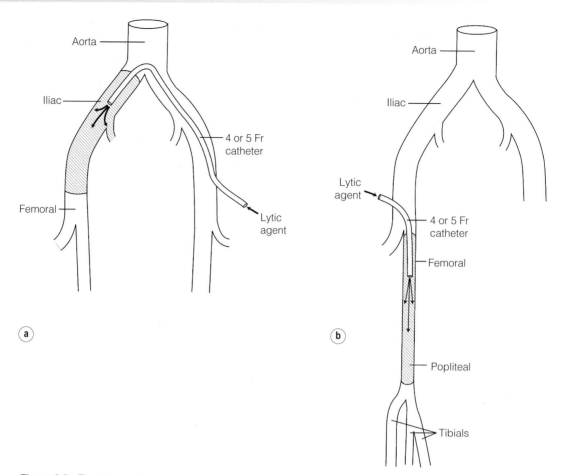

Figure 8.6   Technique of percutaneous thrombolysis: contralateral (a) and ipsilateral (b) transfemoral approaches.

considered a diagnostic process aimed at exposing any underlying flow-limiting lesion (Fig. 8.7). This should be found in the majority of patients using duplex ultrasonography of the suspect arterial segment and can often be managed by endovascular means. Where the disease appears too extensive, surgical reconstruction may be required.

PERCUTANEOUS THROMBECTOMY DEVICES

Percutaneous mechanical thrombectomy (PMT) devices have been developed to hasten thrombus removal and either replace the need for thrombolytic therapy or reduce the dose required.[41] The devices may be classified according to their mode of action. The most basic technique involves simply aspirating the thrombus by applying suction to a wide-bore catheter (e.g., Pat-Rat aspiration catheter ™, Angiomed Bard, Karlsruhe, Germany). Some devices simply macerate thrombus into particles so small that they are removed by natural fibrinolysis (e.g., Amplatz Thrombectomy™ Device, Microvena, White Bear Lake, MN, USA).

Mechanical Rotational Catheter systems (e.g., Rotarex™, Straub Medical, Wangs, Switzerland) use the principle of the 'Archimedes screw' to break up the clot and aspirate it. Other mechanisms include a clot aspiration system based on the Bernoulii or Venturi principle to remove fragments of thrombus and prevent distal embolisation (e.g., Angiojet™, Possis Medical Inc., Minneapolis, MN, USA).

Ultrasound catheters use ultrasound energy to lyse thrombus (e.g., the Acolysis™ catheter, Angiosonics, Morrisville, NC, USA). Thrombolysis is often required as a supplement to mechanical thrombectomy; in the Trellis Thrombectomy System™ (Covidien, Mansfield, MA, USA), the occluded segment of the artery is isolated by proximal and distal balloons. An oscillating wire fragments the thrombus while a thrombolytic infusion helps to dissolve it before the liquefied material is aspirated from the isolated segment. Only a few case reports have been published evaluating the performance of the Trellis system; however, these have reported promising results.

The most comprehensive data for percutaneous mechanical thrombectomy are for the Rotarex™ device. Recent studies report a greater than 90% technical success rate of primary reopening of infra-aortic vessels using either the Rotarex™ or Angiojet™ devices.[42] The amputation rate using the Angiojet™ device is between 4% and 11%. By contrast, the amputation-free survival rate at 12 months for the Rotarex™ catheter is 95–100%.[42] The results available for these devices need to be interpreted with caution as they are predominantly from small retrospective studies with heterogeneous groups.

Aspiration techniques tend to work best in acute (<14 days) thrombus. Technical success of thromboaspiration is reported in 70–97% of cases, but it has predominantly been used in Rutherford class I ischaemia. The 30-day mortality rate was 4.6% in a study examining a single centre's experience over 5 years, which is in line with previous studies.[43] The most common reason for incomplete thrombus removal is a mismatch between catheter size and artery diameter and this is more frequent above the knee when compared to the infra-popliteal arteries.

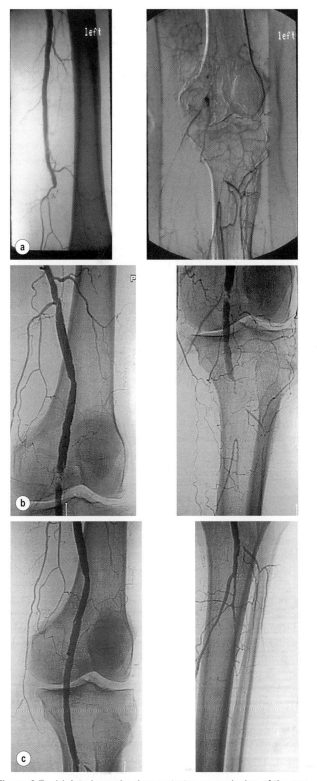

Figure 8.7 (a) Arteriography demonstrates an occlusion of the popliteal artery extending into the tibial vessels. (b) Thrombolysis reveals a popliteal stenosis but persistent occlusion of the tibial trifurcation. (c) The stenosis was treated by balloon angioplasty and the thrombus aspirated from the tibial vessels using an aspiration catheter.

These endovascular devices are significantly more expensive than CDT alone, however, the recent ESVS guidelines suggest that aspiration and mechanical thrombectomy may

be considered in patients with ALI. Multicentre prospective studies would provide more robust data for the efficacy and safety of pharmacomechanical thrombolysis in treating acute limb ischaemia.

COMPLICATIONS OF CATHETER-DIRECTED THROMBOLYSIS

There are significant risks associated with percutaneous thrombolytic therapy, most of which can be attributed to severe comorbidity of the patients and their advanced systemic atherosclerosis. Myocardial infarction and stroke are the commonest causes of death. The rate of reported adverse outcomes is variable, depending on the condition of the patients treated; the mortality after thrombolysis has been reported as 2–8%.[44]

The National Audit of Thrombolysis for Acute Limb Ischaemia (NATALI) database, which includes over 1100 episodes of thrombolysis (mostly for limb-threatening ischaemia), records a 12.4% mortality rate at 30 days.[45] Other large series report intermediate results.[46,47]

Minor haemorrhage

Minor haemorrhage is common (in approximately 40% of infusions) and usually occurs at the groin puncture site. It can be managed by direct compression or by exchanging the catheter system for a larger catheter or sheath. The decision about whether to continue CDT in the presence of minor haemorrhage is based on the balance of benefits and risks and can be challenging for a less experienced clinician.

Major haemorrhage

Major haemorrhage occurs in approximately 9% of patients, usually at a groin puncture site but occasionally in the retroperitoneum or within the abdomen. If major haemorrhage occurs during thrombolysis, aprotinin is an effective plasmin inhibitor and the administration of whole blood, fresh-frozen plasma and, in particular, fibrinogen concentrate will replenish the clotting factors. Stroke is seen in approximately 3% of patients (2.3% in the British Thrombolysis Study Group [TSG] database); this must be interpreted in the context of other risk factors for stroke in this population. Most occur after thrombolysis, during therapeutic anticoagulation. About half are thrombotic rather than haemorrhagic. If a stroke occurs, cerebral haemorrhage should be excluded by urgent CT. If haemorrhage is not the cause, then a clinical decision needs to be made whether to persist with thrombolysis to salvage the affected limb, with possible additional benefits to the intracerebral circulation.

There is some evidence that the monitoring of fibrinogen (which is depleted during thrombolysis) may help predict bleeding risk.[48] However, the data are conflicting and regular monitoring of fibrinogen is no longer recommended.[3]

Distal embolisation

Distal embolisation affects around 4% of patients and may occur either whilst crossing a lesion with a wire or catheter or during the infusion. It may be necessary to stop the infusion and consider an alternative surgical approach, however, in many cases it can be managed by aspiration thrombectomy or by increasing the infusion dose to help lyse the new embolus and allow treatment to continue. Reperfusion injury has been reported in 2% and pericatheter thrombosis in 1%.

Failure to rescue

It is important to remember that CDT takes time to work. Ischaemia may progress in the interim, mandating an alternative approach. However, in the early stages of CDT, the limb may initially look worse because of distal embolisation, which may subsequently resolve and improve with continued treatment. Experience is key when managing these patients, and the decision on whether and when to change tactics can be difficult. It is imperative that regular clinical review of the limb is undertaken and the treatment strategy adjusted if there is obvious clinical deterioration, or an absence of improvement after 6–12 hours of treatment.

OUTCOMES OF CATHETER-DIRECTED THROMBOLYSIS

Diffin and Kandarpa[49] report successful thrombolysis in 70% of treatments, with limb salvage in 93%, although many patients in the collected review did not have limb-threatening ischaemia. The TSG database records complete lysis in 45.5% and clinically useful lysis in a further 27.9% of infusions, leading to a limb salvage rate of 75.2%; 12.4% of patients required an amputation and 12.4% died.[45] Thrombolysis was similarly effective in bypass grafts and native vessels. The outcome seems dependent on the nature of the lesion treated and the clinical state of the patient. Patients with subcritical ischaemia appear less likely to need amputation than patients with critical ischaemia including a neurosensory deficit. In addition, the following are more likely to predict failure of thrombolysis: inability to traverse the occlusion with a guidewire or place a catheter within the thrombus, diabetes, multilevel disease, vein graft occlusion, advancing age and female sex.[46] In the long term, approximately 75% of successfully opened native vessels remain patent at 1 year and 55% at 2 years.[47,50] When an identifiable lesion is found after graft thrombolysis, the 2-year patency is approximately 85%. Long-term patency is less good where no underlying lesion is found in native vessels or grafts. In addition, successfully treated iliac occlusions and emboli have a better long-term outlook.[51,52]

The results of thrombolysis for vein graft occlusion have proved disappointing.[53] It is assumed that ischaemia of the vein graft reduces the chances of success. In contrast, the results of prosthetic graft thrombolysis are better. Where an underlying lesion is responsible for occlusion of a prosthetic graft, patency rates at 1 year are encouraging (86% vs 37%).[54]

Scoring systems may be used to try to identify patients unlikely to survive after thrombolysis.[55] Detailed analysis of available data and large databases may help identify patients at greater risk of a poor outcome. A detailed statistical analysis of the TSG database has shown that the following factors were associated with reduced amputation-free survival: increasing patient age, increasing severity of ischaemia (Rutherford Classification and presence of a sensorimotor deficit), shorter duration of ischaemia and diabetes.[45] Being on warfarin at the time of the occlusion improved the chance of amputation-free survival. The risk of death after thrombolysis was highest in patients with an embolic occlusion, in women, older patients and those with ischaemic heart disease. Amputation risk was highest in younger men, patients with a sensorimotor deficit, graft and thrombotic occlusions.

SURGICAL MANAGEMENT OF ACUTE LIMB ISCHAEMIA

With the increasing age of the population, underlying atherosclerosis often complicates ischaemia even if the cause is primarily embolic. Consequently, complex secondary procedures may well be necessary if initial surgical embolectomy fails (Fig. 8.8). It is therefore advisable that an experienced vascular surgeon performs or supervises the operation. Local anaesthesia may be considered in slim frail patients where success from a straightforward femoral embolectomy is considered likely. An anaesthetist should always be present to monitor the ECG and oxygen saturations, administer sedation or analgesia and convert to general anaesthesia if required, particularly given the risks of physiological demise caused by ischaemia reperfusion injury after reperfusion.

BALLOON CATHETER EMBOLECTOMY

Balloon catheter embolectomy should ideally be performed over-the-wire in a hybrid theatre.[3] Both groins and the entire leg should be prepared to permit surgical access and arteriography. The foot should be placed in a sterile transparent bag for easy inspection. The common femoral artery bifurcation is exposed via a groin incision and the vessels controlled with Silastic slings. Clamps should be avoided initially because they fragment thrombus that may otherwise be removed intact. A transverse arteriotomy is made in the common femoral artery proximal to the bifurcation, avoiding any obvious plaque (Fig. 8.9). A transverse arteriotomy is easier to close without narrowing and it can be converted to a diamond shape for proximal anastomosis if a bypass is required. Any thrombus at the bifurcation can be removed by gentle suction or forceps and momentary release of the sling or clamp. Some surgeons send the embolic material for histological and microbiological assessment, although there is little evidence to support this in routine practice.

If pulsatile inflow is not present, then a 4-Fr or 5-Fr balloon catheter is passed proximally up into the aorta, inflated and withdrawn carefully. Pressure should be applied to the contralateral femoral artery during this procedure to prevent contralateral embolisation, or a protection balloon can be inflated in the contralateral iliac artery. If adequate inflow cannot be achieved, then an alternative method of restoring inflow must be considered, such as a femorofemoral crossover, an axillofemoral bypass, or consideration of hybrid endovascular treatment. A saddle embolus can usually be retrieved by bilateral femoral embolectomy.

Next, a 3-Fr or 4-Fr balloon catheter is passed as far distally as possible down both the profunda and superficial femoral arteries. Force should not be used if resistance is met as dissection or perforation may result. The balloon is inflated only as the catheter is withdrawn and the amount of inflation adjusted to avoid excessive intimal friction. Tactile feedback when withdrawing the catheter can reveal the site of an underlying stenotic lesion. The procedure is repeated until no more thromboembolic material can be retrieved. Conventional embolectomy is performed blind, and the surgeon has no control over the direction of the catheter past the popliteal trifurcation. Use of

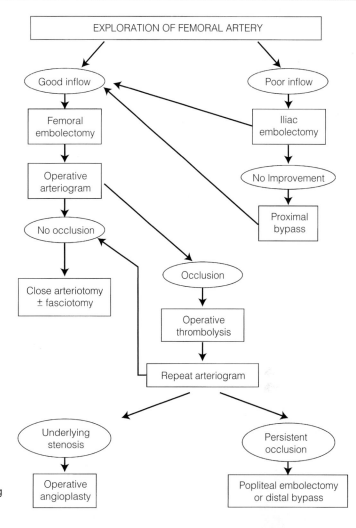

Figure 8.8 Possible treatment pathway required when exploring the femoral artery.

an over-the-wire embolectomy catheter is recommended, as it permits selective catheterisation of the tibial arteries under fluoroscopic control, which is preferable to performing an additional popliteal trifurcation exposure (Fig. 8.10).

COMPLETION ANGIOGRAPHY

✅ A completion arteriogram should always be performed because persistent thrombus may be present even if the catheter passes to the foot;[56] back bleeding is of no prognostic value as it may arise from established proximal collaterals. Hybrid operating theatres have excellent fluoroscopic facilities capable of high quality arteriography. Routine angiography results in a higher rate of extension of the procedure for a residual lesion and a lower re-occlusion rate at 24 months.[57]

The procedure involves flushing the distal arteries with heparin saline and if no thrombus is present on the arteriogram, the arteriotomy is repaired with 5/0 prolene. On removing the clamps, the foot should become pink with palpable pulses.

FAILED EMBOLECTOMY

If the arteriogram shows persistent occlusion, then 15 mg t-PA in 100 mL heparin saline can be infused via an umbilical catheter over 30 minutes and the arteriogram repeated (Fig. 8.11). This often results in complete lysis and reduces

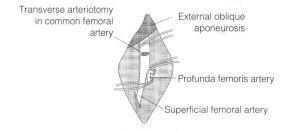

Figure 8.9 Exploration of the femoral artery using Silastic slings to control the vessels and a transverse arteriotomy proximal to the common femoral bifurcation.

the need for popliteal exploration.[58] The technique may also be used to lyse residual thrombus in the tibial arteries during bypass of a popliteal aneurysm.[59] If an underlying stenosis of the superficial femoral artery is revealed, then on-table angioplasty may be attempted. Persistent distal occlusion requires exploration of the below-knee popliteal artery and either popliteal embolectomy or distal vein bypass. The origins of the anterior tibial artery and tibioperoneal trunk should be controlled with slings and selective embolectomy performed via a longitudinal arteriotomy. The popliteal arteriotomy requires repair with a vein patch to prevent stenosis. Great saphenous vein is the conduit of choice if surgical bypass is required.

FURTHER MANAGEMENT

ISCHAEMIA REPERFUSION INJURY AND COMPARTMENT SYNDROME

Revascularisation of an ischaemic leg results in a sudden return of venous blood with anaerobic metabolites, low pH and a high potassium concentration. Ischaemia reperfusion injury may lead to arrhythmia, hypotension and pulmonary oedema, with the potential for systemic inflammatory response syndrome, multiorgan failure and death. Renal function may be impaired by myoglobinuria, which is improved by maintaining a good diuresis.

Even if revascularisation is performed under local anaesthetic, it is important to have an anaesthetist present to address the physiological issues associated with reperfusion, which may mandate post-operative management in the critical care unit. The importance of a specialist vascular anaesthetist is recognised in 'The Provision of Services for Patients with Vascular Disease 2015' executive statement[60] and the recent ESVS guidelines.[3]

✅ Revascularisation of ischaemic muscle can result in considerable swelling within the fascial compartments of the leg. This swelling leads to increased compartment pressures causing venous compression, worsening oedema and, if not treated promptly, permanent neurological insult. Patients with prolonged ischaemia or ischaemia from an embolic source are at highest risk of compartment syndrome,[61] which most commonly affects the anterior compartment resulting in deep peroneal nerve damage and subsequent foot drop if not treated expediently.

There is no role for routine prophylactic fasciotomies for all patients, however, in patients with prolonged or profound ischaemia or where the compartments are tense, it is wise to perform a fasciotomy at the time of the initial revascularisation procedure. Diagnosis of post-operative compartment syndrome is a clinical one; measurement of compartment pressures may be unreliable, however, a compartment pressure of >30 mmHg or <40 mmHg below the mean arterial pressure or diastolic blood pressure is suggestive of compartment syndrome. All four muscle compartments should be decompressed via full-length skin and fascial incisions from knee to ankle.[62] The anterior fasciotomy should be made about two fingerbreadths lateral to the anterior border of the tibia, which avoids the peroneal nerve. The posterior fasciotomy incision is made in a line about two fingerbreadths posterior to the medial condyle of the femur and the medial malleolus, which avoids the great saphenous vein. The soleal attachments to the tibia must be taken down to ensure the muscles of the deep posterior compartment are released. The skin defect can be closed later with sutures or a split-skin graft.

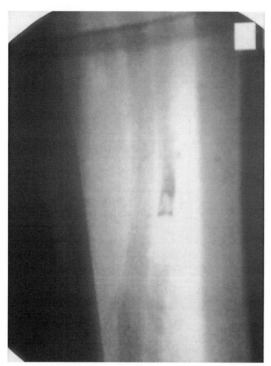

Figure 8.10 Angiographically controlled balloon catheter embolectomy. The balloon occluding the lumen and the thrombus above it can be seen as negative images against the contrast-filled artery.

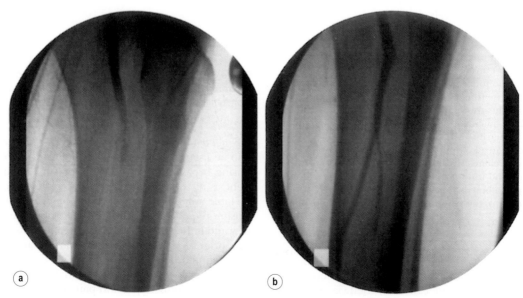

Figure 8.11 Completion angiogram after embolectomy showing persistent occlusion of the popliteal trifurcation (a) and complete lysis after intra-operative thrombolysis (b).

ANTICOAGULATION TO PREVENT FURTHER EVENTS

One of the most important aims of managing patients with ALI is the prevention of further events. In the case of arterial embolisation, the source of the embolus must be identified and treated. It is well established that patients with ALI caused by atrial fibrillation or intra-cardiac thrombus should be managed with lifelong anticoagulation; warfarin has typically been the therapy of choice, however, recent data suggest that direct oral anticoagulants are at least as effective as warfarin in reducing the risk of further events, and are associated with fewer bleeding complications.[63,64]

The evidence for lifelong anticoagulation in patients with ALI of embolic origin without atrial fibrillation or intra-cardiac thrombus is less well established, but this should be considered.[3] There are no data to support the routine use of anticoagulation in patients with ALI to prevent recurrent native arterial thrombosis, however, antiplatelet and statin therapy should be used to reduce overall cardiovascular events. For patients with thrombosis of a prosthetic graft, anticoagulation should be considered, according to registry data. In the Cardiovascular Outcomes for People Using Anticoagulation Strategies (COMPASS) trial, a small subgroup of patients with ALI receiving low-dose rivaroxaban and aspirin experienced a marked reduction in mortality and amputation rates.[10] It is important to note, however, that this was not the primary endpoint of the main trial and more studies are therefore required to investigate the use of long-term anticoagulation in patients with ALI caused by thrombosis.

FURTHER INVESTIGATION OF UNDERLYING CAUSES

In patients with embolic ALI, the source of embolus needs to be verified. Echocardiogram should always be undertaken during the index admission to investigate for a cardiac source. Acute myocardial infarction should be ruled out at the time of presentation, bearing in mind that a silent cardiac event may be initially undetected. If no obvious intra-cardiac source of thrombus is found, a 'completion' CTA of the rest of the aorta should be obtained, to look for aortic mural thrombus. A 24-hour ECG may also be considered if intermittent arrhythmia is suspected.

In patients presenting with likely thrombotic ALI, this may be caused by hypercoagulable states as a result of thrombophilia or cancer, particularly in younger patients. Incidental malignancy may be detected on the CTA, however, dedicated imaging should be obtained if cancer is suspected. Liaison with the haematology team for subsequent thrombophilia testing is necessary in patients with a suspected hypercoagulable disorder.

SPECIAL CONSIDERATIONS

POPLITEAL ARTERY ANEURYSM THROMBOSIS

ALI caused by popliteal aneurysm thrombosis remains a difficult clinical problem and is almost always treated with surgical vein bypass. The bulk of thrombus within the aneurysm restricts the use of thrombolysis within the popliteal artery itself because of the high risk of massive distal embolisation, the slow clearance and large amount of residual thrombus often persisting after re-canalisation. Pre-operative or peri-operative local thrombolysis should be considered in popliteal aneurysm thrombosis, but its only role is to reopen occluded tibial vessels in preparation for distal bypass. This is achieved by placing a catheter beyond the popliteal artery aneurysm into a tibial vessel and lysing until it becomes patent. Surgical revascularisation may be performed with on-table angiography and local thrombolysis to clear the run-off for bypass. Stent grafts are not recommended as first-line treatment for acute popliteal aneurysm thrombosis[3] because of the high risk of distal embolisation and worsening ischaemia. Regular post-operative duplex surveillance is recommended, in addition to screening of the contralateral popliteal artery, the iliac arteries, femoral arteries and abdominal aorta, ideally every 3 years.[3]

ACUTE AORTIC OCCLUSION CAUSING BILATERAL LOWER LIMB ISCHAEMIA

Acute aortic occlusion is a relatively rare but immediately life-threatening condition. Most commonly, it is caused by in situ thrombosis of a native atherosclerotic or aneurysmal aorta or common iliac arteries. Alternatively, it may be a result of a saddle embolus of cardiac origin following myocardial infarction or resulting from occlusion of a previous vascular graft or stent graft. Occasionally, it may occur in situations of low cardiac output, in patients with hypercoagulable disorders or as a result of false lumen compression because of acute aortic dissection.

The ischaemia-reperfusion injury associated with acute aortic occlusion is massive and is more of a threat to life than limb. Accordingly, outcomes of revascularisation are poor, with one Swedish study reporting a 30-days amputation rate of 9% and mortality of 20%.[65,66] When appropriate and depending on the aetiology and patient's condition, revascularisation options include thromboembolectomy, CDT, extra-anatomical bypass or aortic reconstruction in the form of either aorto-bifemoral or aorto-iliac bypass.

STENT GRAFT THROMBOSIS

Thrombosis of a stent graft following EVAR may cause unilateral or bilateral acute limb ischaemia, depending on whether the main body and/or the iliac limbs are affected. The risk of graft-related complications is three to four times higher following EVAR when compared to open repair.[67] Limb kinking and occlusion affects up to 8% of patients following EVAR (half of which will present with ALI), however, newer generation stent grafts may be more kink-resistant than early devices. One-third of patients with limb occlusion present within the first 30 days. Risk factors for limb occlusion include iliac artery angulation, tortuosity, presence of calcification, oversizing of the iliac limb stent graft >15% and when the distal landing zone is in the external rather than common iliac artery. Intervention options include CDT, graft thrombectomy with adjunctive stent relining or extra-anatomical bypass.[68] Urgent prophylactic treatment should be undertaken if limb kinking is detected on EVAR surveillance.

ACUTE LIMB ISCHAEMIA IN NEONATES, INFANTS AND YOUNG CHILDREN

ALI in childhood is rare and the principles of treatment are quite different from those of adults, particularly in very young children. In neonates and infants, iatrogenic injury is the commonest cause of ALI, usually as a consequence of catheterisation of the umbilical or femoral arteries.[69] Older children most commonly experience ALI as a result of trauma; the brachial artery is particularly vulnerable to disruption following a supra-condylar humerus fracture, which is the commonest cause of acute upper limb ischaemia in childhood. Unlike in adults with blunt trauma causing brachial artery disruption (see Chapter 9), the management of a child with a pink pulseless hand following supra-condylar fracture reduction should be conservative in the first instance.[3]

The diagnosis of ALI in infants and young children may be challenging, because of their inability to verbalise, as well as the propensity for rapid collateralisation in early life and the relative tolerance of neonatal muscle to hypoxia. The most common clinical presentation is cyanosis, with associated delayed capillary refill and absent Doppler signals. The normal ankle–brachial index of an infant <1 year old is 0.88.

There is little evidence to guide the management of ALI in neonates, infants and young children. However, consensus from expert opinion and small case series is that the mainstay of management in most cases should be conservative treatment with systemic heparinisation – either unfractionated or low-molecular-weight heparin.[3] Whilst this exposes the patient to a 3% risk of bleeding complications,[70] it is often sufficient to allow the development of collaterals and the restoration of adequate limb perfusion and function whilst sparing the need for operative intervention. Certainly, children under the age of 2 years should be managed with systemic heparinisation if at all possible; surgical revascularisation is difficult in this group of patients and confers no advantage in terms of outcomes.[69] It is estimated that around 15% of children with ALI managed conservatively will experience claudication or limb length discrepancy later in life.[70]

If heparinisation fails, then adjunctive systemic or CDT may be considered, or operative intervention. Contraindications to lysis in children include major surgery/haemorrhage within 7 days, invasive procedure within 3 days, seizure within 48 hours, prematurity less than 32 weeks, active bleeding and platelets <50. Re-imaging after 4–6 hours of lysis is important to assess progress.

Where revascularisation is necessary, the preferred conduit is debatable. Autologous great saphenous vein, which has good long-term patency, may be associated with future aneurysmal change. The internal iliac artery is an alternative choice and may 'grow with the child' if interrupted sutures are used for the anastomosis.[71] To allow for future growth, an end-to-side anastomosis may be preferable, using an oversized graft and a spatulated anastomosis.

In a child with previous ALI managed conservatively, consideration should be given to delayed revascularisation if the patient presents with disabling claudication or a limb length discrepancy of >2 cm, which has implications for hip stability and posture. In the elective setting, a temporary arteriovenous fistula can be created to arterialise the conduit before bypass. Any intervention should be deferred as late as possible, ideally until at least the teenage years.

A recent systematic review reports, an overall limb salvage rate of 88% for all management strategies.[72] An algorithm describing the management of ALI in children <3 years old can be found in Fig. 8.12.[73]

OVERALL PROGNOSIS IN ACUTE LIMB ISCHAEMIA

There has been little change in overall outcome from ALI because the improvements in radiological and surgical techniques have been balanced by the increasing prevalence of underlying atherosclerotic disease in ever older patients. Ten percent of patients presenting with ALI will have an unsalvageable lower limb. A Swedish population study demonstrated that between 1965 and 1983, there was an increasing incidence of ALI, without any improvement in amputation rates or survival,[74] although outcome after treatment in a university hospital was better than in a district hospital.[75] A prospective survey by the Vascular Surgical Society of Great Britain and Ireland that included 539 episodes in 474 patients recorded a limb salvage rate of 70% and an overall mortality rate of 22%.[76] An analysis of the Medicare population in the USA recorded an in-hospital mortality rate of 9% and an amputation rate of 11% at 1 year.[77] Patients with embolism have a higher mortality rate because of their underlying cardiac disease. In contrast, those with thrombosis are at increased risk of amputation.

Patients with a high mortality rate after embolectomy are characterised by:[78]

- poor cardiac function;
- associated peripheral artery disease;
- short duration of symptoms;
- the need for amputation.

The amputation risk appears higher in patients with a longer duration of ischaemia and poor pre-operative and post-operative cardiac function.[79] Patients with concomitant malignancy represent a very high-risk population and most studies have found that these patients have a very poor prognosis, however, active revascularisation should be considered in selected patients, as the immediate post-operative outcomes may be comparable to those without malignancy.[3]

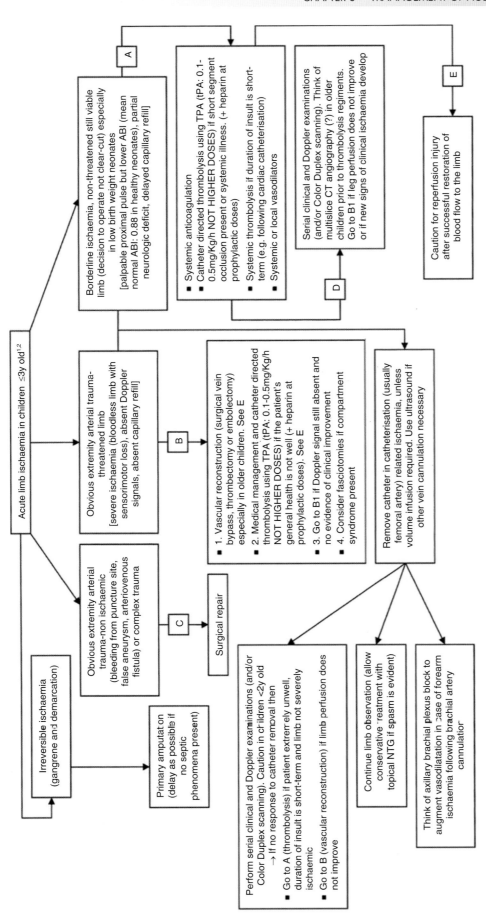

Figure 8.12 Proposed management algorithm for acute limb ischaemia in children <3 years old.[77]

ABI: ankle brachial index
TPA: tissue plasminogen activator
NTG: nitroglycerine

CONCLUSIONS

Although there have been huge changes in the therapeutic options for patients with ALI, there remains debate over the optimal management. Clinical trials in this area are difficult to organise and are often flawed by the great variation in the condition of the patients and their lower limb vasculature. However, further stratification of existing data could help define which occlusions are most suitable for thrombolysis, surgery or a hybrid approach. According to recent guidelines, CDT may be considered as an initial or adjunctive treatment in many cases of ALI and patients should be managed in a specialised vascular centre that can offer this option. The management of ALI in adults is quite different from young children, who should be managed conservatively with systemic heparinisation if at all possible.

Key points

- Patients with ALI have high morbidity and mortality rates.
- Optimal management is based on the severity of the ischaemia at presentation.
- Randomised trials have failed to show superiority of thrombolysis or surgery as primary management for all cases.
- The best results are achieved when management is agreed jointly by a team consisting of vascular surgeon and interventional radiologist using available expertise and local guidelines.
- Further research is required to identify which patients with salvageable legs at presentation may be better managed by primary amputation rather than futile attempts at revascularisation.
- For some patients, ALI heralds end of life and palliative care should be instituted.
- Infants and young children with ALI should be managed conservatively with systemic heparinisation if at all possible; operative revascularisation is technically challenging and often confers no additional clinical benefit. Catheter-directed or systemic thrombolysis may be required if systemic heparinisation fails.

 References available at http://ebooks.health.elsevier.com/

KEY REFERENCES

[3] Björck M, Earnshaw JJ, Acosta S, et al. Editor's Choice - European Society for Vascular Surgery (ESVS) 2020 C.practice guidelines on the management of acute limb ischaemia. Eur J Vasc Endovasc Surg 2020;59(2):173–218. https://doi.org/10.1016/j.ejvs.2019.09.006. Epub 2019 Dec 31. PMID: 31899099.
Updated guidelines on the management of patients with acute limb ischaemia from a working group of international experts. This guideline includes the management of acute limb ischaemia in children.
[19] Darwood R, Berridge DC, Kessel DO, Robertson I, Forster R. Surgery versus thrombolysis for initial management of acute limb ischaemia. Cochrane Database Syst Rev 2018;8(8):CD002784. https://doi.org/10.1002/14651858.CD002784.pub3. PMID: 30095170. PMCID: 6513660.

This Cochrane Review in 2018 included >1200 patients from five RCTs and found no evidence in favour of open surgery or CDT as the preferred initial treatment strategy in ALI in terms of limb salvage, amputation or death at 30 days, 6 months or 1 year.
[21] Ouriel K, Shortell CK, DeWeese JA, et al. A comparison of thrombolytic therapy with operative revascularisation in the initial treatment of acute peripheral arterial ischaemia. J Vasc Surg 1994;19:1021–30. PMID: 8201703.
This randomised controlled trial involved 114 patients who were randomised to thrombolytic therapy or operative management. It concluded that thrombolysis provided a safe alternative treatment for patients with acute limb ischaemia.
[22] The STILE Investigators. Results.of a prospective randomized trial evaluating surgery versus thrombolysis for ischaemia of the lower extremity. Ann Surg 1994;220:1–68. PMID: 8092895.
This multicentre study compared open revascularisation with catheter-directed thrombolysis (either urokinase or recombinant tissue plasminogen activator) for non-embolic leg ischaemia.
[23] Comerota AJ, Weaver FA, Hosking JD, et al. R.of a prospective randomized trial of surgery versus thrombolysis for occluded lower extremity bypass grafts. Am J Surg 1996;172:105–12. PMID: 8795509.
This randomised controlled trial of 134 patients compared surgery with catheter-directed thrombolysis for occluded lower limb bypass grafts. It showed that those with chronic ischaemia (>14 days) had better outcomes with surgery. In acute limb ischaemia successful thrombolysis improved limb salvage.
[24] Weaver FA, Comerota AJ, Youngblood M, et al. S.revascularisation versus thrombolysis for nonembolic lower extremity native artery occlusions: results of a prospective randomized trial. J Vasc Surg 1996;24:513–23. PMID: 8911400.
This randomised controlled trial involved 237 patients who were randomised to surgery or catheter-directed thrombolysis. It showed that at 1 year the incidence of recurrent ischaemia and major amputation was higher in the thrombolysis group.
[26] Ouriel K, Veith FJ, Sasahara AA, for the TOPAS investigators. A comparison of recombinant urokinase with vascular surgery as initial treatment for acute arterial occlusion of the legs. N Engl J Med 1998;338:1105–11. PMID: 9545358.
This multicentre randomised controlled trial compared surgery and thrombolysis in the treatment of acute limb ischaemia; 272 patients were randomised to surgery and 272 patients to thrombolysis. It found that thrombolysis with urokinase reduced the need for open surgery with no significant increase in the risk of amputation or death.
[33] Braithwaite BD, Buckenham TM, Galland RB, et al. On behalf of the T.S.G.P.randomized trial of high-dose bolus versus low-dose tissue plasminogen activator infusion in the management of acute limb ischaemia. Br J Surg 1997;84:646–50. PMID: 9171752.
This randomised trial involved 100 patients treated with either a high-dose bolus or conventional low-dose tissue plasminogen activator thrombolysis to treat acute lower limb ischaemia. It found that the high-dose bolus regime significantly accelerated thrombolysis without compromising outcome.
[38] Plate G, Jansson L, Forssell C, et al. T.for acute lower limb ischaemia – a prospective, randomised multicenter study comparing two strategies. Eur J Vasc Endovasc Surg 2006;31:651–60. PMID: 16427339.
This prospective randomised study involved 121 patients who were randomised to receive pulse spray or standard low-dose thrombolysis. It found that there was no obvious advantage with pulse spray thrombolysis.
[39] Berridge DC, Gregson RHS, Hopkinson BR, et al. R.trial of intra-arterial recombinant tissue plasminogen activator, intravenous recombinant tissue plasminogen activator and intra-arterial streptokinase in peripheral thrombolysis. Br J Surg 1991;78:988–95. PMID: 1913123.
This randomised trial involved 60 patients and compared three different thrombolysis agents. It found that intra-arterial recombinant tissue plasminogen activator is a more effective, safer thrombolysis agent than intra-arterial streptokinase.
[80] Working Party on Thrombolysis in the Management of Limb Ischemia. Thrombolysis.in the management of lower limb peripheral arterial occlusion—a consensus document. J Vasc Interv Radiol 2003;14(9 P.2):S337–49. https://doi.org/10.1016/s1051-0443(07)61244-5. PMID: 14514841.

Vascular trauma 9

Jacobus van Marle | Dirk A. le Roux

INTRODUCTION

Fewer than 10% of patients with polytrauma have associated vascular injuries, but these injuries can cause significant morbidity and mortality.[1] In most European countries, the majority of vascular trauma is caused by blunt (traffic accidents) and iatrogenic injuries.[2] In South Africa, injuries are mostly penetrating and have also changed from predominantly stab wounds to injuries caused by firearms.[3]

A clear understanding of the pathophysiology of vascular trauma and a logical approach to the management of those injuries are essential for a favourable outcome.

MECHANISM OF INJURY

Vascular injuries are classified according to the mechanism of the injury.

BLUNT TRAUMA

Direct trauma to the artery accounts for the majority of blunt vascular injuries. Indirect trauma is usually the result of shearing and distraction forces following dislocation of major joints, displaced long-bone fractures and acceleration/deceleration injuries as seen with high-speed motor vehicle accidents and falls from a height. Blunt trauma causes contusion of the arterial wall with disruption of the intima. This intimal tear may cause immediate obstruction because of an intimal flap or may predispose to thrombosis and delayed occlusion (Fig. 9.1a–d). As the vessel is stretched further, progressive layers of the media are disrupted until the continuity of the vessel is maintained only by the elastic adventitia or there is complete disruption.

PENETRATING TRAUMA

Penetrating trauma may result in partial or complete transection of a vessel. Bleeding is often brisk and distal flow may be interrupted. Stab and low-velocity missile injuries cause localised damage confined to the injury tract. High-velocity missiles cause total tissue destruction around the missile tract, surrounded by an area of doubtful tissue viability, causing extensive associated soft-tissue trauma. The shock wave of a high-velocity missile can also cause intimal injury.[4] The vessel may be macroscopically intact with minimal bruising, but on opening the vessel, there is an intimal tear with superimposed thrombosis. Shotgun injuries cause extensive local tissue destruction with often multiple sites of perforation (Fig. 9.2). Bomb blasts cause complex injuries because of the combination of extensive local tissue trauma, high-velocity fragments and thermal injury.

Iatrogenic injuries are becoming increasingly important and account for more than 40% of vascular trauma in many European countries.[2]

SEQUELAE OF VASCULAR INJURIES

Vascular injuries have significant sequelae (Box 9.1, Figs. 9.3 and 9.4). A contused artery may be patent initially but thrombose later. Subsequent propagation of thrombus may cause progressive ischaemia by obstructing essential collaterals. Acute ischaemia leads to degeneration and necrosis of muscle cells and Wallerian degeneration in nerves. Findings from large-animal studies indicate that early restoration of flow within 3 hours is associated with near-complete recovery, whereas delayed revascularisation at 6 hours was associated with significant muscle necrosis and nerve degeneration.[5]

Concomitant fractures, dislocations, injuries to accompanying veins and nerves, soft-tissue trauma and contamination of the wound with foreign material serve to compound vascular injury. Other determinants of the final outcome are the level of vascular injury, the quality of the collateral circulation and pre-existing occlusive arterial disease.

CLINICAL ASSESSMENT

HISTORY

Information regarding the mechanism of the trauma, blood loss before hospital admission and underlying vascular disease should be obtained.

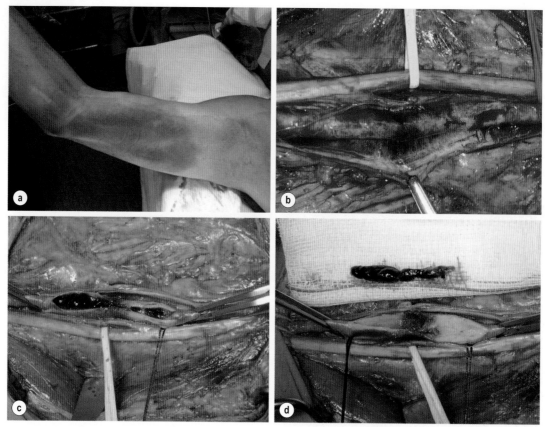

Figure 9.1   Blunt injury to the arm (a) causing contusion of the brachial artery, (b) predisposing to thrombosis, (c) because of underlying intimal damage (d).

EXAMINATION

Initial assessment should be carried out according to advanced trauma life support (ATLS) principles and life-threatening conditions managed. Vascular injury may present with any of the sequelae listed in Box 9.1. Clinical signs of vascular injuries can be divided into hard and soft signs.

Hard signs of vascular injury:
- Active pulsatile bleeding.
- Shock with ongoing bleeding.
- Absent distal pulses.
- Symptoms and signs of acute ischaemia.
- Expanding or pulsating haematoma.
- Bruits or thrill over the area of injury.

Soft signs of vascular injury:
- History of severe bleeding.
- Diminished distal pulse.
- Injury of anatomically related structures.
- Small non-expanding haematoma.
- Multiple fractures and extensive soft-tissue injury.
- Injury in anatomical area of major blood vessel.

Distal pulses may be difficult to evaluate in patients with extensive soft-tissue trauma, swelling and multiple wounds. A diminished or absent pulse is caused by arterial occlusion until proven otherwise and should not be attributed to vascular spasm, external compression or any other ill-defined factor.

Signs of acute arterial insufficiency (ischaemia) include pulse deficit (absent/diminished pulse), pain, pallor, paraesthesia and paralysis. Neurological deficit must be evaluated carefully to distinguish between ischaemic neuropathy and direct injury to the nerve.

DIAGNOSIS

✓✓ The value and accuracy of a thorough clinical examination in predicting significant vascular injury has been reported in various series.[6]

Arterial Doppler pressure measurement is a useful supplement to the clinical examination. An arterial pressure index (API) above 0.9 reliably excludes significant occult arterial injury.[7]

Special investigations should only be performed in patients who have been adequately resuscitated and who are haemodynamically stable. Haemodynamic instability, active bleeding and an expanding haematoma are indications for immediate surgery.

RESUSCITATION AND INITIAL MANAGEMENT

ATLS guidelines are followed, keeping in mind that the resuscitation of the unstable patient in urgent need of surgery may be best conducted in the operating room.

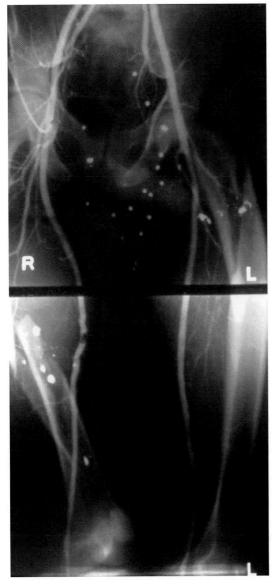

Figure 9.2 Arteriogram of the pelvis and thighs to demonstrate multiple arterial perforations together with extensive local trauma to bone and soft tissue caused by shotgun injury.

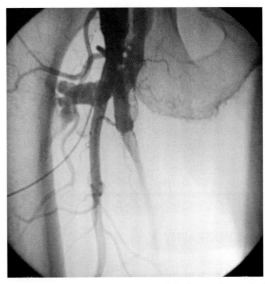

Figure 9.3 Arteriovenous fistula of the right femoral vessels following iatrogenic injury after diagnostic cardiac catheterisation.

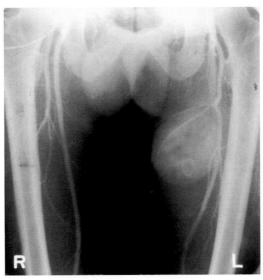

Figure 9.4 False aneurysm of the left thigh after gunshot wound.

Box 9.1 Sequelae of vascular injuries

Acute haemorrhage

- Overt external bleeding
- Contained bleeding (e.g., in muscle compartment)
- Concealed bleeding (e.g., pleural cavity)

Hypovolaemia, shock

- Haematoma with or without secondary infection
- Delayed bleeding and rebleeding
- Thrombosis: acute or delayed
- Ischaemia: acute or delayed
- Arteriovenous fistula (see Fig. 9.3)
- Pseudoaneurysm formation (see Fig. 9.4)

The amount, type and timing of fluid resuscitation is important. In uncontrolled haemorrhagic shock where bleeding has been temporarily stopped because of hypotension, vasoconstriction and thrombus formation, aggressive fluid resuscitation may lead to increased intravascular pressure, decreased blood viscosity and loss of the haemostatic plug, with resultant increased bleeding and mortality.[8] *Hypotensive resuscitation* (permissive hypotension) aims for a systolic blood pressure of between 70 and 90 mmHg to maintain cerebral and renal perfusion until operative control of bleeding has been achieved. *Haemostatic resuscitation* is indicated in patients with massive bleeding/blood loss. Immediate administration of plasma, platelets and red blood cells as part of the resuscitation protocol has resulted in improved survival.[9]

Temporary occlusion of the aorta with a percutaneously placed balloon has been used as an adjunct to resuscitation and haemorrhage control in abdominal and pelvic trauma (see section on abdominal trauma).

Active bleeding is an indication for urgent exploration, but can usually be temporarily controlled by direct pressure. Blind clamping of vessels in the depth of a wound is discouraged, because of the danger of injuring adjacent nerves and vessels. Tourniquets should be used in cases of massive bleeding that cannot be controlled with direct pressure.

Fractures must be stabilised during the period of resuscitation and diagnostic investigation to protect blood vessels and other soft tissue from further trauma. Preliminary reduction of a displaced fracture or dislocation may improve distal circulation.

SPECIAL INVESTIGATIONS

PLAIN RADIOGRAPHY

Plain radiographs are usually taken for associated skeletal injuries. A high index of suspicion for vascular trauma should exist with dislocations and displaced fractures (Fig. 9.5). Chest radiography is valuable in patients with chest trauma.

ANGIOGRAPHY

Computed tomographic angiography (CTA) is valuable in diagnosing blunt and penetrating vascular injuries in the neck, thorax, abdomen and extremities and should be the first-line investigation for all patients with suspected vascular trauma who do not require immediate surgical intervention.[10]

Digital subtraction angiography (DSA) may still be indicated for selected conditions in haemodynamically stable patients, and where endovascular management of the injury is considered. The use of magnetic resonance angiography (MRA) in trauma is limited because of time constraints and inaccessibility to the patient during the examination.

Surgical intervention should not be delayed for special investigations where vascular injury is evident, and the patient is unstable or the limb is at ischaemic risk. On-table arteriography can be performed in the operating room for vascular injuries where surgery cannot be delayed, and the additional information is considered valuable.

ULTRASOUND

Duplex Doppler examination is mostly used as a screening test in the absence of hard signs, in zone 2 neck injuries, in extremity vascular trauma and for follow-up evaluation in patients managed expectantly.

GENERAL PRINCIPLES OF MANAGEMENT OF VASCULAR INJURY

Procedures are performed under general anaesthesia in a suitably equipped theatre. Blood products should be available and arrangements for intra-operative autotransfusion should be made where further bleeding is expected. The value of prophylactic antibiotics in vascular surgery is established.

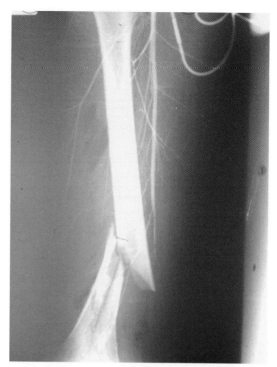

Figure 9.5 Displaced fracture of the femur with injury to the superficial femoral artery.

Adequate exposure is vital for obtaining proximal and distal control of injured vessels. This often requires inclusion of adjacent anatomical areas in the operative field, for example, preparing the neck in thoracic injuries (and vice versa) and the abdomen in groin injuries. An uninjured leg is prepared for possible vein harvesting should bypass be required. Vascular control must be achieved proximally and distally before directly approaching the area of injury. Bleeding may be temporarily arrested by digital compression or by endovascular means until clamps have been applied.

In blunt and high-velocity trauma, there is often extensive intimal damage, and careful debridement of the vessel is necessary until normal-appearing intima is found (Fig. 9.6). Antegrade and retrograde flow should be evaluated. Arteries are cleared of thrombus by careful passage of embolectomy catheters followed by irrigation with heparin-saline solution.

Simple laceration of the vessel wall is repaired by lateral suture, provided it does not lead to stenosis, when patch graft angioplasty is indicated. Where more than 50% of the circumference of a vessel wall is damaged, this area should be excised followed by end-to-end anastomosis. This requires mobilisation of the proximal and distal arterial stumps to achieve approximation without tension. Failing this, an interposition graft is indicated. Autologous vein is the preferred conduit for reconstruction. Where there is a mismatch in diameter between the vessel that needs to be repaired and the available autologous vein, either a panelled or spiral vein graft should be used. Prosthetic material may be used in the absence of available autologous vein or as part of a damage control strategy.[11]

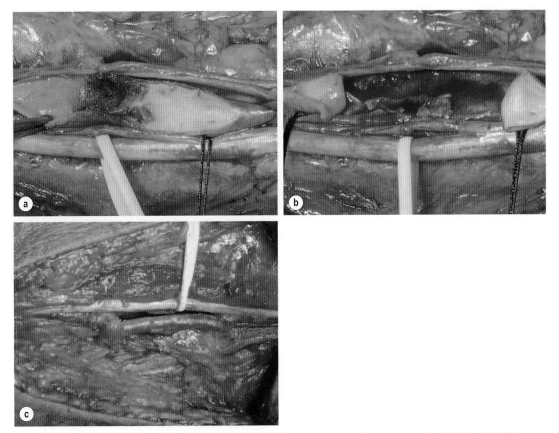

Figure 9.6   Blunt injury of the intima (a), resected (b) and replaced with a venous interposition graft (c).

✓✓ Where complex arterial repair will result in delay in revascularisation, intraluminal shunts should be used to maintain antegrade flow during repair, thereby reducing ischaemic time.[12]

Completion angiography should be performed to document a technically perfect repair and to assess the distal arterial tree. Associated injuries are addressed once vascular repair has been completed. Wound debridement should be performed with removal of all devitalised and contaminated tissue. Contaminated wounds are left open, but the vascular repair must be covered by soft tissue. Repeated wound inspections are performed, with delayed primary suture when the wound is clean.

VENOUS INJURIES

Venous injuries found during exploration for associated arterial injury should be repaired, if the repair itself can be done simply (e.g., lateral suture repair) and only if it will not significantly delay treatment of associated injuries or destabilise the patient's condition. Complex venous repair or bypass should only be attempted if the patient is haemodynamically stable. All veins, including the inferior vena cava (IVC), can be tied off in cases of haemodynamic instability.

ENDOVASCULAR MANAGEMENT OF VASCULAR TRAUMA

The application of endovascular techniques in the injured patient has many potential advantages. General anaesthesia is not required. Surgical trauma, with further blood loss, hypothermia, etc., as well as cross-clamping of major vessels, distal ischaemia and subsequent reperfusion injury, is avoided. The main advantage is the option of approaching complex arterial lesions in anatomically challenging locations from a remote site. A difficult exploration in an injured area is avoided, with less potential damage to surrounding structures, and preventing fresh bleeding.

Endovascular techniques are increasingly applied in vascular trauma, but still have certain limitations. These techniques are usually not applicable, mainly because of time constraints, in patients with active bleeding, in unstable patients or where there is end-organ ischaemia. Endovascular techniques are contraindicated where there are compression symptoms, infected wounds or where concomitant injuries require open exploration. Technical restrictions include inability to traverse the lesion by guidewire, where intraluminal thrombus prevents the safe passage of a guidewire because of the danger of distal embolisation or where luminal discrepancy exists between the proximal and distal involved segments.

Endovascular techniques are used to manage vascular trauma in three ways:

1. **To obtain haemostasis.** Damaged vessels are embolised using a variety of substances including haemostatic agents (gel foam), coils and balloons.

    ✓✓ Embolotherapy has become the standard treatment for managing significant bleeding following pelvic fractures[13] and also to control bleeding caused by penetrating and blunt trauma of the liver, kidneys and spleen.[14]

Embolotherapy is also the preferred option for treating vertebral artery lesions[15] and lesions of non-essential, inaccessible vessels in other regions.

2. **To obtain vascular control.** Temporary balloon occlusion of a damaged vessel at the time of diagnostic angiography can prevent exsanguinating bleeding until surgical control is achieved. It is especially valuable in relatively inaccessible regions and allows limiting the extent of the exposure to obtain surgical control.[16] This technique is valuable in injuries in zones 1 and 3 of the neck, the abdominal aorta, proximal subclavian and iliac arteries.

3. **For vascular repair.** Covered stent grafts are used for repairing vessels in anatomically challenging locations and to avoid major surgical exposures, for example, the thoracic aorta, thoracic outlet vessels, internal carotid and vertebral arteries (Fig. 9.7).[17-19] This will be discussed in more detail in the relevant sections. Covered stent grafts may also be used as a temporary measure to allow stabilisation of the patient until definitive open repair later.

In-stent stenosis, graft migration, stent breakage and endoleaks are well-known complications of stent graft repair. Durability is therefore of concern in the younger population, who are the main victims of trauma.

✓✓ Endovascular management of vascular trauma has gained wide acceptance and it is increasingly used in most vascular beds.[20]

CERVICAL VASCULAR INJURIES

CAROTID ARTERY INJURIES

The cervical vessels are involved in 25% of patients with neck trauma. Carotid artery injury constitutes 5–10% of all arterial injuries.[21] The mortality for carotid injuries ranges from 10–31%, with permanent neurological deficit ranging from 16–60%.[22]

MECHANISM

More than 90% of carotid injuries are caused by penetrating trauma. Blunt trauma is caused by a direct blow to the artery, hyperextension, hyper-rotation, or contusion by bone fragments associated with fractures of the mandible, temporal bone or cervical spine.

Penetrating injury may cause partial or complete transection of the vessel, pseudo-aneurysm or arteriovenous fistula (AVF; Fig. 9.8). Pseudo-aneurysm may have an acute or delayed onset, with progressive enlargement causing compression of the aerodigestive tract or brachial plexus. Blunt trauma may cause intimal flaps, intramural haematomas, dissection, complete disruption of the arterial wall with pseudo-aneurysms, AVFs and total occlusion (Fig. 9.9).

Neurological sequelae are caused by hypoperfusion (transected or thrombosed vessels) or embolisation from thrombus, pseudo-aneurysm or AVF.

CLINICAL SIGNS

Active external bleeding, rapidly expanding cervical haematoma, absent carotid pulse and a bruit or thrill are indicative of vascular injury. Signs that may indicate an associated vascular injury warranting further investigation include bleeding from wounds of the neck or the pharynx, a deficit of the superficial temporal artery pulse, ipsilateral Horner's sign, dysfunction of cranial nerves IX–XII, a widened mediastinum, fractures of the skull base and temporal bone, and fractures and dislocation of the cervical spine. Neurological deficit may be present but obscured because of concomitant head injury, shock or the use of alcohol or drugs. About 50% of patients with established blunt injury to the carotid and vertebral arteries could initially be asymptomatic, but 43–58% of these will eventually develop neurological signs after hospital admission.[23]

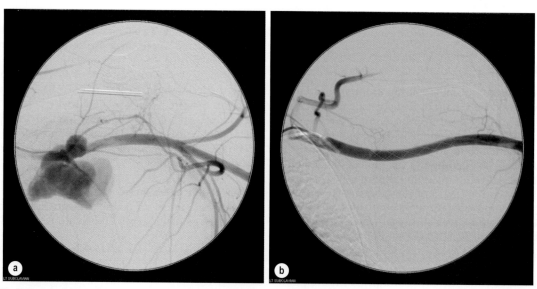

Figure 9.7   False aneurysm of left subclavian artery after infra-clavicular stab wound (a) repaired by means of a covered stent graft (b).

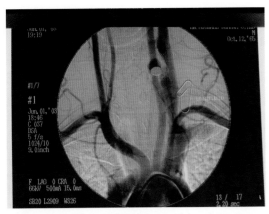

Figure 9.8 Arteriovenous fistula between the carotid artery and internal jugular vein caused by gunshot wound.

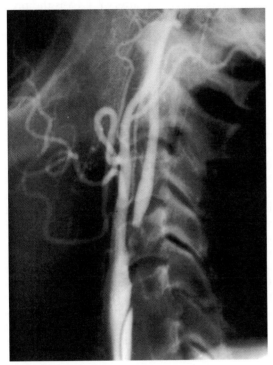

Figure 9.9 Dissection of the common carotid artery with blunt trauma to the neck following a motor vehicle accident.

DIAGNOSIS

Only patients who are haemodynamically stable and have a patent airway should undergo further appropriate investigations.

The neck has been divided into three anatomical zones to standardise diagnosis and management of cervical vascular injuries (Fig. 9.10).

Anteroposterior chest radiography can provide valuable information regarding associated haemothorax or pneumothorax, widening of the mediastinum, surgical emphysema of the neck with concomitant aerodigestive tract injuries.

CTA is accurate in detecting blunt and penetrating cervical vascular injuries and provides important information regarding associated bony and aerodigestive tract injuries.[24,25]

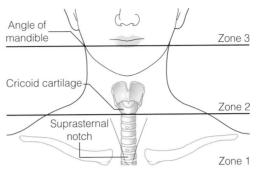

Figure 9.10 Zones of the neck.

Duplex Doppler examination is useful for investigating zone 2 vascular injuries and is now the preferred diagnostic modality in experienced hands.[26]

DSA is used in equivocal CTA findings and as part of the endovascular management.

Computed tomography (CT) of the brain should be used to investigate patients with associated head trauma, bone injuries of the spine and skull and neurological deficit. It is a good predictor of outcome: patients who have an infarct on initial CT on admission have a high mortality with poor chance of neurological recovery compared with those who have a normal CT on admission. MRA may be valuable in carotid artery and vertebral artery dissection.[27]

MANAGEMENT

Active external bleeding can be controlled in the emergency room by direct digital compression or a Foley catheter inflated in the wound tract to obtain balloon tamponade.[28]

Mandatory exploration of all penetrating neck injuries has been replaced by a selective approach.[29]

Active pulsatile haemorrhage, expanding cervical haematoma and airway compromise are indications for urgent surgical exploration. Some low-velocity penetrating injuries may be managed expectantly with careful observation, provided there is no active bleeding, and the distal circulation is normal.[30] These injuries include intimal defects, small pseudo-aneurysms (< 5 mm) and non-obstructive intimal flaps. The majority of penetrating carotid artery injuries, however, are best managed by primary arterial repair or endovascular stent grafting. Neurological deficit is only a contraindication to surgical repair in a deeply comatose patient with a dense neurological deficit, arterial occlusion and a huge infarct on cerebral CT.[31] All other patients with associated neurological deficit would benefit from arterial repair, with improved mortality and final neurological status.

Most blunt injuries of the carotid and vertebral arteries result in intimal disruption, with dissection and/or thrombosis, and the immediate goal of management is to restore cerebral perfusion and to prevent embolisation. Systemic anticoagulation is therefore the treatment of choice, because it limits the formation, propagation and/or embolisation of the thrombus. Intravenous heparin is administered in the acute phase, followed by oral anticoagulation for at least 3 months.[32]

OPERATIVE TECHNIQUE

Detailed description of operative technique falls outside the scope of this chapter and the reader is referred to the standard textbooks on operative surgery.[33] The general principles of management include the following:

- The patient should be in a supine position with a bolster between the scapulae and with the neck extended and the head rotated to the contralateral side. The patient must be draped to allow access from the base of the skull to the xiphisternum.
- Zone 2 injuries are explored by the standard carotid incision overlying the anterior border of the sternocleidomastoid muscle.
- Zone 1 injuries may require a median sternotomy.
- Various techniques have been described to improve exposure of the distal internal carotid artery in zone 3 injuries, including subluxation of the mandible, mandibular osteotomy, excision of the styloid process, etc.
- Some authors recommend routine shunting to maintain antegrade flow.
- Where simple repair is not feasible, a bypass should be performed. Saphenous vein should preferably be used in the internal carotid artery whereas polytetrafluoroethylene (PTFE) is used to repair the common carotid artery.
- The external carotid artery can be safely ligated if the internal carotid artery is patent. Internal carotid artery ligation is only recommended when the distal vessel is thrombosed with no back bleeding following extraction of thrombus.
- Minor venous injuries can be managed by lateral suture repair, but complex venous repair is not indicated as there is a high occlusion rate and it increases the magnitude of the operative procedure. Ligation of the jugular vein can be performed without significant sequelae.[34]
- In the presence of associated injuries to the trachea and oesophagus, the vascular repair should be protected by soft-tissue interposition (sternocleidomastoid muscle).

VERTEBRAL ARTERY INJURIES

The occurrence of vertebral artery injury is low, with the reported incidence in penetrating neck trauma ranging from 1–7.4%. Gunshot wounds are the most common mechanism of injury.[35] Blunt injury of the vertebral artery is even less common and is caused by fractures of the lateral mass of the cervical vertebrae involving the foramen transversarium, vertebral fractures, ligamentous cervical spine injury, or severe and sudden rotation and/or hyperextension of the head. These injuries are seen with motor vehicle accidents, near-hanging injuries and after extreme chiropractic manipulation.[36]

The majority of patients with vertebral artery injuries have associated injuries of the cervical spine, spinal cord and other vascular structures in the neck or aerodigestive tract.[37]

Angiographic embolisation is the treatment of choice in the majority of patients with vertebral artery injuries.[15,38] Operative management is only indicated for severe active bleeding or when embolisation has failed. Haemodynamically stable patients with a thrombosed vertebral artery do not need any intervention.

A detailed description of surgical approaches to, and management of, vertebral artery injuries is given by Hatzitheofilou et al.[39]

SUBCLAVIAN AND AXILLARY VASCULAR INJURIES

All patients with periclavicular trauma should be evaluated for possible vascular injury. Most of these injuries are caused by penetrating trauma. The presence of a peripheral pulse does not reliably exclude significant proximal arterial injury. A difference in blood pressure of more than 20 mmHg between the upper limbs warrants further investigation. The brachial plexus is injured in about one-third of patients with subclavian or axillary artery injuries. A thorough neurological assessment should be performed.

Duplex ultrasound reliably assesses arterial and venous injuries but has certain limitations, for example, visualising the origin of the subclavian artery.[40] CTA is the preferred diagnostic modality in cervico-mediastinal injuries. DSA has a therapeutic role in embolisation of injured vessels and for stent graft repair.

Where surgical repair is required, the neck and chest should be included in the operative field. The patient is placed supine and the arm is draped free and abducted to 30 degrees. The head is turned to the other side. The standard incision starts at the sternoclavicular joint and extends over the medial half of the clavicle, curving over the deltopectoral groove. For proximal subclavian artery injuries, this incision can be combined with a median sternotomy, which gives excellent exposure of both proximal subclavian arteries.[33] The so-called 'trapdoor' incision (supra-clavicular incision, upper third median sternotomy and left anterior thoracotomy) is not recommended because of significant post-operative morbidity.

The axillary artery is exposed through an infra-clavicular incision between the clavicular and sternal parts of the pectoralis major muscle. Dividing the clavicle should be avoided whenever possible because of post-operative morbidity.

Promising results have been obtained with endovascular repair of pseudo-aneurysms and AVFs in selected patients (see Fig. 9.7 and Fig. 9.11). Most studies report a significant incidence of brachial plexus injury associated with surgical repair of subclavian artery injuries; this may be avoided with endovascular repair.

ENDOVASCULAR MANAGEMENT OF CERVICAL VASCULAR INJURIES

An important advantage of endovascular repair of cervico-mediastinal trauma is the avoidance of general anaesthesia and the ability to monitor neurological status during the procedure. Endovascular therapies are used in three ways in the management of cervical vascular trauma:

1. **Angiographic embolisation.** This is indicated for (a) injury to the vertebral artery in the osseus vertebral canal and (b) persistent bleeding from external carotid artery branches (face, oro- and nasopharynx).[15,41]
2. **Temporary balloon occlusion.** This is used as an adjunct to support standard open vascular repair in neck zone 1 and 3 injuries. An occlusion balloon is placed via the femoral artery to provide proximal endoluminal control of

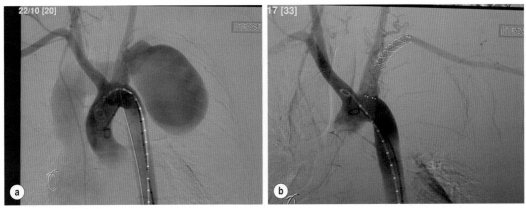

Figure 9.11 Arteriovenous fistula of the subclavian artery (a) repaired by stent graft (b).

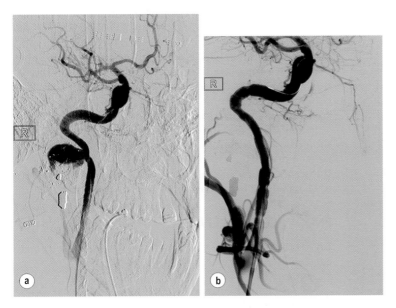

Figure 9.12 Stent graft repair of a pseudoaneurysm in the R-internal carotid artery, pre-stent (a) and post-stent (b).

the injured vessel, allowing surgical exposure in a more controlled fashion, and possibly avoiding sternotomy for proximal control.

3. **Covered stent grafts.** These are indicated for penetrating wounds, AVFs and pseudoaneurysms in (a) surgically inaccessible regions, and (b) in patients where extensive surgical exploration is to be avoided because of multiple traumas, local aggravating factors or high surgical risk resulting from medical comorbidities.

✔✔ Endovascular stent grafting should be considered in all patients with penetrating injuries of the brachiocephalic trunk, proximal common carotid, distal internal carotid and subclavian arteries[42–44] (Fig. 9.12).

THORACIC VASCULAR INJURIES

The majority of thoracic vascular injuries are caused by penetrating trauma, with a mortality rate as high as 90%.[45] Blunt aortic injury is considered as the second most common cause of death in trauma patients; 70–90% of patients sustaining these injuries will die before reaching a hospital and, if left untreated, 90% will die within 4 months.[46] The site of insertion of the ligamentum arteriosum, just distal to the origin of the left subclavian artery, is the typical point of injury. Deceleration or compression injury may also involve the brachiocephalic trunk, the pulmonary veins and the vena cava.

CLINICAL PRESENTATION AND INITIAL MANAGEMENT

Patients with penetrating thoracic vascular trauma are usually haemodynamically unstable, often with continuing haemorrhage into the pleural cavity or the mediastinum and should be taken for urgent thoracotomy. Patients with blunt thoracic trauma may initially be haemodynamically stable and the injury may not be immediately apparent because of the high incidence of concomitant trauma. The following clinical findings may be associated with underlying thoracic great vessel injury:

- shock/hypotension;
- difference in blood pressure or pulses between the two upper extremities;
- difference in blood pressure between upper and lower extremities (pseudo-coarctation syndrome);
- expanding haematoma at the thoracic outlet;

- left flail chest;
- infra-scapular murmur;
- palpable fracture of the sternum;
- palpable fracture of the thoracic spine;
- external evidence of major chest trauma;
- history indicating deceleration or compression injury to the chest.

DIAGNOSTIC STUDIES

The number and type of diagnostic studies performed will be determined by the patient's haemodynamic stability and general status, as well as the type of aortic lesion and concomitant injuries.

CHEST RADIOGRAPHY

A frontal chest radiograph is an important screening tool and should be obtained in all patients with penetrating and suspected blunt thoracic trauma. Radio-opaque markers are useful for identifying entrance and exit sites.

A widened mediastinum on chest radiography is associated with more than 90% of thoracic aortic injuries, with a 90% sensitivity and 95% negative predictive value.[47] Other radiographic findings associated with blunt injuries of the descending aorta include the following:

1. Mediastinal findings:
   a. widening of the mediastinum greater than 8 cm;
   b. obliteration of the aortic knob contour;
   c. depression of the left main stem bronchus greater than 140 degrees;
   d. loss of the paravertebral pleural line;
   e. lateral displacement of the trachea;
   f. deviation of a nasogastric tube;
   g. calcium layering of the aortic knob.
2. Fractures of sternum, first and second ribs and thoracic spine. Scapular and clavicular fractures in a polytrauma patient.
3. Other findings on (a) anteroposterior chest radiograph: apical pleural haematoma (apical cap), massive left haemothorax/effusion, ruptured diaphragm; (b) lateral chest radiograph: anterior displacement of trachea, loss of the aortopulmonary window.

Positive findings on chest radiography are indications for CTA.

ANGIOGRAPHY

✔ CTA is recommended as the primary diagnostic modality in patients with suspected blunt thoracic aortic injury.[48]

CTA is also preferred to conventional arteriography for penetrating trauma in haemodynamically stable patients with suspected injury to the innominate, carotid and subclavian arteries. CTA is less invasive, faster to obtain and more readily available than catheter angiography, and also provides important information regarding associated lesions. However, the relative inaccessibility to the patient during examination limits its use in unstable patients.

The proximity of a missile trajectory to the brachiocephalic vessels may in itself be an indication for CTA even without any physical findings of vascular injury. DSA is used as part of the endovascular management of the injured vessel.

OTHER IMAGING MODALITIES

Intravascular ultrasound is valuable for sizing and accurate placement of thoracic endografts during endovascular repair.[49]

TREATMENT

Indications for urgent surgery are haemodynamic instability, increasing haemorrhage from chest tubes and radiographic evidence of an expanding haematoma. An initial large volume of blood drained from a chest tube (>1500 mL) or ongoing haemorrhage of more than 200–300 mL/hour may indicate great vessel injury that requires thoracotomy.

The Vancouver classification of thoracic aortic injuries is useful in terms of staging the extent of injury and guiding intervention. Minimal aortic lesions, i.e. Vancouver grade I (intimal flap/intramural haematoma/thrombus <10 mm) or grade II (intimal flap/intramural haematoma/thrombus >10 mm) are managed non-operatively with close observation, whilst grade III lesions (pseudo-aneurysm, simple or complex but no extravasation) and grade IV lesions (active contrast extravasation) will require intervention.[50]

Patients selected for initial non-operative management should be closely monitored, with systolic blood pressure kept below 120 mmHg or mean arterial pressure below 80 mmHg. Intravenous beta-blockade, titrated to heart rate, was shown to be beneficial in patients with a blunt aortic injury.

ENDOVASCULAR REPAIR

Injuries to the arch outflow vessels can be successfully managed with endovascular stent grafting.[42–44]

✔✔ Endovascular stent grafting is currently the preferred method for treating traumatic rupture of the descending thoracic aorta. Mortality is significantly lower compared to open surgery (9% vs. 19%) with a decreased risk of spinal cord ischaemia, renal injury, graft and systemic infection (Fig. 9.13).[51]

Numerous recent studies have reported on the durability of thoracic stent grafts up to 10 years with low complication and re-intervention rates.[52]

SURGICAL REPAIR

Open surgery is reserved for unstable, hypotensive patients, for injuries of the ascending aorta and arch, and where endovascular treatment is not readily available. The basic surgical approaches are: median sternotomy, left anterolateral thoracotomy and left posterolateral thoracotomy. The reader is referred to the standard textbooks on thoracic surgery for a detailed description of these procedures.

ABDOMINAL VASCULAR INJURIES

Penetrating trauma accounts for 90–95% of abdominal vascular injuries (Fig. 9.14), with a high mortality because of the nature of these injuries as well as associated injuries to

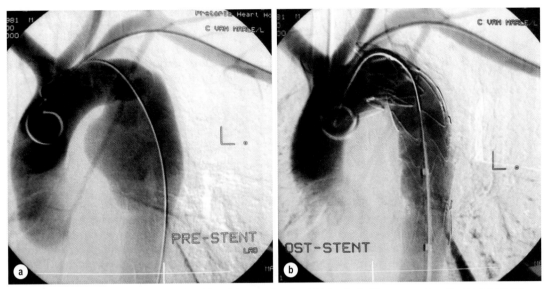

Figure 9.13   Thoracic aneurysm after blunt injury to the chest (a) treated with a covered aortic stent graft (b).

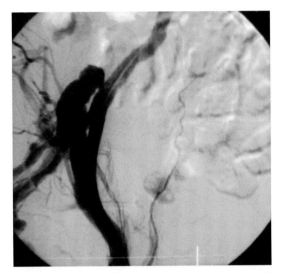

Figure 9.14   Arteriovenous fistula between the left common iliac artery and vein after a gunshot wound to the lower abdomen.

other intra-abdominal organs. It is important to consider intra-abdominal injury with all penetrating injuries from the fourth intercostal space anteriorly (level of T8 posterior) to the upper thighs.

RESUSCITATION

Resuscitative Endovascular Balloon Occlusion of the Aorta (REBOA) has recently been advocated to replace emergency room thoracotomy and aortic cross-clamping as a method to control haemorrhage below the diaphragm.[53–55] It involves placement of an endovascular balloon in the aorta to control haemorrhage and to augment afterload in traumatic arrest and haemorrhagic shock states. There seems to be less physiological disturbance and higher rates of technical success than aortic cross-clamping. A detailed description of the technique has been published in the Journal of Trauma.[56]

High quality evidence in support of this technique is, however, lacking. A recent systematic review of REBOA concluded that the evidence is weak, with no clear reduction of haemorrhage-associated mortality.[57] Guidelines for REBOA use and implementation have been published as a Joint Statement from the American College of Surgery Committee on Trauma and the American College of Emergency Physicians.[58]

The aorta is divided into three separate zones for the purposes of REBOA:

- Zone I of the aorta extends from the origin of the left subclavian artery to the coeliac artery, Zone II extends from the coeliac artery to the most caudal renal artery and Zone III extends distally from the most caudal renal artery to the aortic bifurcation.

REBOA is indicated in adult patients with traumatic life-threatening haemorrhage below the diaphragm. This includes patients with:
  - pulseless electrical activity arrest of less than 10 minutes secondary to exsanguination from sub-diaphragmatic haemorrhage and femoral vessels immediately identifiable on ultrasound (if not identifiable consider emergency thoracotomy),
  - severe hypovolaemic shock and a systolic blood pressure <70 mmHg,
  - an agonal state because of non-compressible exsanguinating haemorrhage, who are non/partial responders to rapid volume resuscitation and have had causes of obstructive shock, that is, cardiac tamponade and tension pneumothorax excluded, and suspected or diagnosed intra-abdominal haemorrhage because of blunt trauma or penetrating torso injuries (Zone I REBOA),
  - blunt trauma with suspected pelvic fracture and isolated pelvic haemorrhage (Zone III REBOA),
- Penetrating injury to the pelvic or groin area with uncontrolled haemorrhage from a junctional vascular injury (iliac or common femoral vessels) (Zone III REBOA).

DIAGNOSIS

The unstable patient with a possible abdominal vascular injury requires immediate surgery. The stable patient should be investigated according to the injuries. Plain abdominal radiography using radio-opaque markers (paperclips) placed on the entrance and exit wounds is of value in establishing the trajectory of missiles in penetrating injuries. DSA and CTA have little, if any, role in the diagnosis of abdominal vascular injury when the patient is unstable. CTA is the investigation of choice in stable patients with penetrating or blunt abdominal trauma.[10,59]

MANAGEMENT

Abdominal vascular injuries are usually associated with haemodynamic instability or concomitant bowel injuries requiring a laparotomy. The abdominal cavity should be entered rapidly as tamponade and haemodynamic stability may be lost with relaxation of the abdominal musculature at the induction of anaesthesia. A generous laparotomy incision is required from xiphisternum to supra-pubis. Four-quadrant packing of the abdomen is performed immediately and the proximal aorta is controlled at the diaphragmatic crus. Once the vascular injury is controlled, resuscitation with blood products is started. Bowel injuries are temporarily controlled until vascular repair is effected.

The retroperitoneum is divided into three anatomical zones for purposes of treatment. Central retroperitoneal haematomas (zone 1) are formally explored because of the high incidence of associated major vascular, pancreatic or duodenal injuries, and the high morbidity and mortality if these are overlooked. Flank/perinephric haematomas (zone 2) caused by penetrating injuries should routinely be explored, whilst haematomas caused by blunt trauma can be left alone if they are not expanding and the urogram on contrast-enhanced CT scan is normal. Zone 3 injuries, which are confined to or originate from the pelvis, are most often associated with pelvic fractures; exploration in these cases can be hazardous and is usually avoided. Retroperitoneal haematomas following penetrating injuries are usually explored to exclude major vascular injuries.

Different surgical exposures are used for specific injuries:

- Medial visceral rotation of the left-sided viscera (Mattox manoeuvre), i.e. spleen, tail of the pancreas, left colon and kidney allows access to the supra-coeliac aorta, coeliac axis with its branches to the left, superior mesenteric artery (SMA), inferior mesenteric artery, left renal artery and left iliac vessels.
- The Cattell–Braasch or extended Kocher manoeuvre (right-sided medial visceral rotation) allows access to infra-hepatic inferior vena cava, right renal vein, portal system and right iliac vessels.
- The infra-renal aorta and IVC are exposed by reflecting the transverse colon superiorly and the small intestine to the right and then dividing the mid-line retroperitoneum.
- The iliac arteries are exposed via separate incisions lateral to the caecum and sigmoid, respectively, avoiding injury to the ureters as they cross the common iliac arteries. The iliac veins may be accessible only after dividing the arteries that lie anterior to them.

AORTIC INJURY

Direct repair is used for simple lacerations; this should be done transversely to avoid narrowing. An interposition polyester or PTFE graft may be necessary where there is extensive destruction but should be avoided in a contaminated field.

✓✓ In the 'damage control' scenario, a temporary shunt using a sterile intercostal drain can be placed in the aorta. Definitive repair is performed once the patient is stable, and all physiological parameters are normal.[60]

In the absence of contamination, in situ graft replacement with either a PTFE or polyester (Dacron) graft soaked in rifampicin, can be used. In cases with contamination, the aorta is ligated and an extra-anatomical bypass (axillobifemoral bypass) is performed.[61] Autologous veins using the superficial femoral–popliteal veins have been used to replace infected aortic prosthesis, but this procedure is invasive, time-consuming and is associated with significant blood loss. It is therefore not indicated in the unstable patient.[62] Abdominal aortic dissection after blunt trauma ('seat-belt aorta') is relatively uncommon, but endovascular repair has been described in such cases.[63]

VISCERAL ARTERY INJURY

Injuries to the coeliac trunk and its branches are usually dealt with by primary ligation.[61] The SMA is divided into four zones.[64] Injuries to the first two zones (i.e., SMA trunk to the origin of the middle colic artery) should be repaired. Where primary repair is not possible because of extreme damage, bypass with saphenous vein or PTFE should be performed to maintain mid-gut viability. Injuries to the inferior mesenteric artery can usually be ligated.

RENAL ARTERY INJURY

Blunt injury, usually caused by acceleration/deceleration, results in intimal disruption with subsequent thrombosis of the vessels. These injuries should be repaired within 12 hours, since renal viability beyond this period is very slim. Proximal injuries are approached from the midline through the base of the mesentery, while distal injuries are approached laterally. Repair is performed by either primary repair or interposition grafting using saphenous vein.

Traumatic renal artery dissection can be managed endovascularly with either bare metal or covered stent grafts.[65]

INFERIOR VENA CAVA INJURY

The IVC consists of four parts: infra-renal, supra-renal, retrohepatic and intra-pericardial. The retrohepatic and intra-pericardial portions are usually affected by blunt trauma. Approximately 50% of patients die before reaching hospital and the in-hospital mortality ranges between 20–57%.[66]

Wounds in the infra-hepatic IVC can be temporarily controlled by means of digital pressure or intraluminal balloon catheters. When clamps are applied, one should be aware of the abundant lumbar collateral circulation. Repair is effected by means of lateral suture or, when there are large defects, even prosthetic material. The anterior laceration in a through-and-through lesion may need to be extended so that the posterior defect can be repaired first. In dire attempts to save an exsanguinating patient, this part of the IVC may be ligated. The retrohepatic IVC should be approached with extreme caution. If haemorrhage can be controlled with packing, this should be the method of treatment. Various strategies to repair these injuries have been described but the prognosis is still dismal, with a reported mortality of 70–90%.[67] The Shrock shunt, which is inserted through the right atrium, can be used to control these injuries temporarily. We use a modified technique by inserting an endotracheal tube through the infra-hepatic IVC and inflating the balloon in the right atrium. Total hepatic isolation (Heany manoeuvre) is associated with a high mortality, especially in an exsanguinated patient.

Emergency endovascular stent graft repair for traumatic injury of the IVC was described by Castelli et al.[68]

PELVIC VASCULAR INJURY

Haemorrhage is the primary cause of death in patients with pelvic fractures. The major sources of bleeding are branches of the internal iliac artery and vein, bone and soft tissues. These injuries are managed by embolising the relevant bleeding branches.[13] The common iliac, external iliac and common femoral arteries and corresponding veins are the source of catastrophic blood loss in about only 1% of pelvic fractures. Penetrating and blunt injuries to the common and external iliac arteries can be repaired by primary suturing or interposition grafting. In the case of severe contamination, ligation and femorofemoral bypass is an accepted technique.[61] The internal iliac artery may be ligated. Reports support a role for the endovascular management of iliac artery injuries.[69]

EXTREMITY VASCULAR TRAUMA

The incidence of peripheral vascular injury depends on the extent and type of trauma, ranging from 0.6–3.6% for isolated extremity fractures to 25–30% for all penetrating injuries of the extremities.[1] The risk of limb loss is greatest following blunt trauma and injuries from high-velocity missiles or close-range shotgun wounds.

DIAGNOSIS

Any extremity injury warrants a complete physical examination of the injured extremity and distal vessels. The absence of hard signs of vascular injury reliably excludes surgically significant arterial injury.[70]

✔✔ CTA has proven excellent sensitivity and specificity for diagnosing extremity vascular injury and can replace DSA as a diagnostic modality.[71]

The occurrence of delayed thrombosis stresses the importance of regular reassessment of the peripheral circulation for at least 24 hours after orthopaedic injury. There is a role for duplex Doppler studies in patients with soft signs of vascular injury or with proximity injuries.[72]

GENERAL PRINCIPLES OF MANAGEMENT

• Restoration of perfusion to an ischaemic extremity should be performed within 3–4 hours to optimise neuromuscular recovery of the injured limb.[5] Adjunctive therapies such as hypertonic saline resuscitation, temporary intravascular shunts, fasciotomy, limb cooling and ischaemic reconditioning may reduce the severity of ischaemic injury.[5,73]

• Restoration of perfusion to ischaemic muscle may cause an intense inflammatory response with serious local and systemic effects. This ischaemic reperfusion injury is mediated by reactive oxygen species and activated neutrophils, which cause cell membrane damage. Compliment activation (C3A, C5A) and cytokines (interleukin 1 & 6, thromboxane A2 and tissue necrosis factor), have been implicated in remote organ injury.[74,75] Measures should be taken to protect against the systemic effects of reperfusion injury and subsequent renal damage. A diuresis of at least 2–3 mL/kg per hour is maintained with the administration of adequate volumes of normal saline. This should be started during the operation and is continued post-operatively for as long as the serum myoglobin and creatine kinase remain elevated. Measures to treat hyperkalaemia and lactic acidosis may be required.

• Non-operative observation of asymptomatic non-occlusive arterial injuries is acceptable. These injuries can be defined as small pseudo-aneurysms, intimal flaps or irregularities, small AVFs and haemodynamically insignificant narrowing of the vessels. Should subsequent repair of these injuries be required, it can be done without significant increase in morbidity.[6]

• Extremity arterial trauma is usually addressed by conventional open surgical techniques. Endovascular treatment usually consists of embolisation of non-essential vessels after penetrating trauma.

• Simple arterial repairs do better than grafts. If complex repair is required, vein grafts appear to be the best choice.[76] PTFE is an acceptable conduit when no vein is available and may even be used in a contaminated field.[11] Effort should be made to cover the graft with soft tissue.

• Temporary shunting is valuable for maintaining antegrade flow to allow stabilisation of unstable fractures and/or dislocations before definitive arterial repair (Fig. 9.15).[12]

• Early four-compartment lower leg fasciotomy should be applied liberally. Indications for fasciotomy include: (i) ischaemic time greater than 4–6 hours; (ii) signs of acute ischaemia; (iii) extensive soft-tissue injuries; (iv) combined

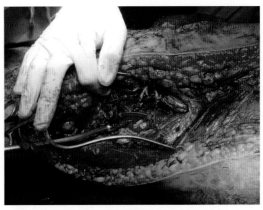

Figure 9.15 Temporary shunt in right superficial femoral artery, allowing distal perfusion while external fixator is applied to the femur.

arterial and venous injuries; (v) intra-compartmental bleeding; and (vi) increased compartmental pressure. Measurement of compartment pressures is an important adjunct and must be done in all compartments. Pressures should be interpreted in the context of each individual patient, because tissue perfusion is a balance between compartment pressure and blood pressure. Acceptable compartment pressures have been defined as absolute compartment pressures of less than 20 mmHg and at least 30 mmHg less than mean arterial pressure.[77]

- Completion angiogram should be performed after arterial repair to assess patency and technical perfection of the repair.
- Although amputation rates increase with longer ischaemia times, quantifying the relationship is difficult, because amputation rates also depend on other factors such as extent of soft-tissue damage, the capacity of collaterals, pre-existing arterial disease and the vessels injured.[78]
- In certain cases, primary amputation may be considered. Scoring systems such as the mangled extremity severity score (MESS) have been developed to help predict the outcome of limb salvage procedures.[79] A MESS score of 7 or more has a predicted amputation rate of 100%. Several MESS score calculators are available online. Given the significance of amputation, delaying the procedure even by a day or two is preferred as it allows careful examination of the limb and discussion with the patient and family.

VASCULAR INJURIES TO THE UPPER LIMB (FIG. 9.16)

BRACHIAL ARTERY INJURIES

The most common injuries to the brachial artery are associated with either a supra-condylar fracture or an elbow dislocation followed by penetrating vascular trauma.[80] Upper extremity vascular injuries are usually not life-threatening, but significant morbidity may occur. Return of function is often related to associated nerve injury. In the case of blunt injury, the fracture or dislocation should be reduced. If the distal pulse returns, the patient should be treated expectantly with regular, that is, 2-hourly, evaluation of the circulation. If the limb remains ischaemic or even if the hand is pink with no pulses, it is mandatory to explore and repair the arterial injury to avoid complications like an ischaemic contracture.[81] With penetrating trauma, the injury should be repaired by open surgical repair.

DISTAL ARTERIAL INJURIES TO THE UPPER LIMB

Most of the injuries to the forearm circulation are caused by a penetrating mechanism. When only one vessel in the forearm is injured, it may usually be ligated without any adverse effects. If both the radial and ulnar arteries are injured at least one should be repaired – preferably the ulnar artery as this vessel is in most cases the dominant supply to the hand. These injuries are often accompanied by injuries to the accompanying nerve and will require repair of the nerve.[80]

Venous injuries to the arm rarely require repair and even injuries to the brachial and axillary veins may be ligated because the collateral venous network is extensive.

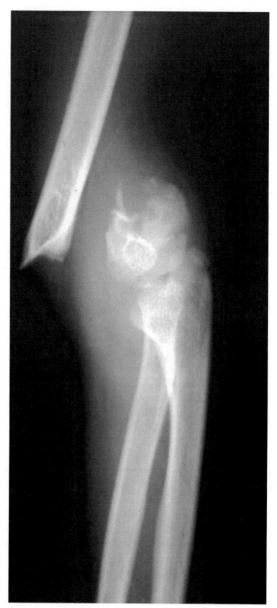

Figure 9.16 Fractures of the supra-condylar humerus are often associated with vascular injuries and should alert the physician to the possibility of a vascular injury.

VASCULAR INJURIES TO THE LOWER LIMB

These injuries are often associated with skeletal injuries, especially posterior dislocation of the knee, proximal tibial fractures and supra-condylar femur fractures. Immediate arterial repair should be performed when the skeletal injury is stable and not significantly displaced. When there is instability, severe displacement and where extreme orthopaedic manipulation is anticipated, a temporary shunt should be placed to restore blood flow while the orthopaedic repair is completed, after which definite arterial repair is performed. Patients may have significant bleeding from extremity vascular injuries and a tourniquet should be used if the bleeding cannot be controlled with direct pressure.[82]

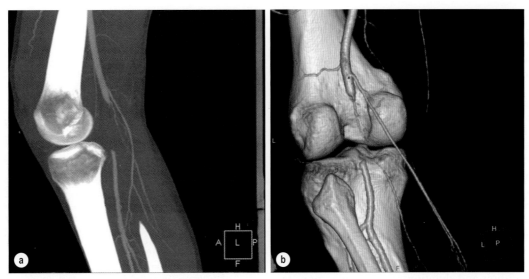

Figure 9.17   Popliteal artery injury after posterior dislocation of the left knee, angiogram (a), and three-dimensional reconstruction (b).

FEMORAL VASCULAR INJURIES

Bleeding from the femoral triangle can be difficult to control, particularly if both artery and vein are injured. The supra-inguinal region should be entered through a separate incision above the inguinal ligament to obtain proximal control of the vessels.

✓✓ Common femoral artery injuries should always be repaired as ligation has a 50% amputation rate.[78]

Effort should be made to also repair the common femoral vein.

Iatrogenic injuries (pseudo-aneurysms and AVF) secondary to attempted femoral access are fairly common. Primary treatment of small femoral pseudo-aneurysms consists of ultrasound-guided compression and thrombin injection while larger pseudo-aneurysms will require open surgical repair.[83,84]

POPLITEAL VASCULAR INJURY

The lower leg is almost totally dependent on the popliteal artery. Popliteal artery injury has an amputation rate of up to 16%.[78] The association between posterior knee dislocation and popliteal artery disruption is well known (Fig. 9.17). All patients with posterior knee dislocations should have a complete neurovascular examination of the affected limb. Most popliteal artery injuries present with hard signs of arterial injury. The absence of hard signs is usually sufficient to rule out injuries to the popliteal artery.[85]

✓✓ Selective angiography (CTA or DSA) following knee dislocation is safe as there is a strong correlation between results of serial physical examinations and the need for arteriography. Patients who are managed expectantly should be closely observed, with regular reassessment of the peripheral circulation.[86,87]

Injury to popliteal veins should be repaired to minimise post-operative swelling and compartment syndrome and to improve the patency of arterial repairs.

Compartment syndrome is a major risk factor for amputation following popliteal artery injury.[88] There is evidence that fasciotomy performed at the time of arterial repair, but before the development of compartment syndrome (prophylactic fasciotomy), may lower amputation rates, particularly in patients with long pre-operative delays, extensive injuries, injuries of the artery and vein, and venous injuries treated with ligation.[89]

Single tibial vessels may be ligated if there is documented collateral flow distally.

ARTERIOVENOUS FISTULA

Penetrating trauma and iatrogenic injury because of vascular access for catheter-based interventions, are the leading causes for acquired AVFs. The majority of AVFs occur in the lower limbs with 50% occurring in the groin. Clinical manifestations and complications depend on anatomical location, size, flow rate in, and duration of, the fistula. Presentation may be acutely after trauma or delayed for many years.

Shunting of blood from the high-pressure arterial system into the low venous-pressure system can have serious local and systemic effects.[90]

Local effects in the affected limb:
a. Venous hypertension with swelling, hyperpigmentation, skin induration, varicose veins, ulceration and bleeding.
b. Arterial insufficiency with claudication, trophic changes, and in the worst cases, ulceration and gangrene.
c. Increased flow leads to dilation of the supplying arteries and draining veins.

Systemic effects:
a. High output cardiac failure: in response to the decrease in total peripheral resistance, cardiac output is increased through increase in stroke volume and heart rate. To maintain blood pressure, blood volume can increase by 200 mL/m² up to 1000 mL/m² body surface.[91] These mechanisms lead to cardiac enlargement and high output cardiac failure.[92]

b. Renal failure: decrease in peripheral resistance causes stimulation of the renin-angiotensin aldosterone system, which results in vasoconstriction with decrease in renal blood flow and subsequent decrease in glomerular filtration rate.

The clinical diagnosis depends on the presence of a bruit or thrill over the affected area, local signs of chronic venous and arterial insufficiency. The Branham-Nicolaidoni sign is reflex bradycardia elicited by compression of the AVF causing an increase in the peripheral resistance (cardiac afterload).

Duplex ultrasound is the investigation of choice for evaluating patients with suspected AVF. CTA may be required for more precise anatomic information and planning of treatment.

While some small AVFs may occlude spontaneously, most will require intervention. It is recommended that post-traumatic AVFs be repaired as soon as possible.[93] Depending on the size, location and duration of the fistula, management may consist of ultrasound guided compression, open surgery or endovascular management.

Key points

- A high index of suspicion should be maintained regarding possible vascular injuries in the trauma patient.
- A thorough clinical examination is accurate in predicting significant vascular injury.
- Special investigations should only be performed in adequately resuscitated and haemodynamically stable patients.
- Haemodynamic instability, active bleeding and an expanding haematoma are indications for immediate surgery.
- The absence of hard signs of arterial injury justifies an expectant non-operative approach with careful observation.
- Restoration of arterial blood supply should be achieved as soon as possible; temporary intra-arterial shunts are valuable in this regard.
- Adequate surgical exposure is vital for proper management of vascular injuries.
- Fasciotomy should be applied liberally in lower-extremity vascular trauma.
- Endovascular treatment is useful in managing arterial lesions in anatomically challenging locations and is currently indicated for injuries of the descending thoracic aorta, proximal aortic arch branches, distal internal carotid and vertebral arteries, and common iliac arteries.

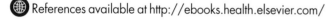 References available at http://ebooks.health.elsevier.com/

KEY REFERENCES

[6] Dennis JW, Frykberg ER, Veldenz HC, et al. Validation of non-operative management of occult vascular injuries and accuracy of physical examination alone in penetrating extremity trauma: 5–10 year follow up. J Trauma 1998;44:243–53. PMID: 9498494.
A prospective study with 10-year follow-up proving the accuracy of clinical assessment and conservative management of occult vascular trauma.

[7] Johansen K, Lynch K. Non-invasive vascular tests reliably exclude occult arterial trauma in injured extremities. J Trauma 1991;31:515–22. PMID: 2020038.
In this prospective study, it was shown that an API of more than 0.9 has a negative predictive value of 99% for excluding significant arterial trauma. Reserving arteriography for limbs with an API of less than 0.9 is safe, accurate and cost-effective.

[8] Bickell WH, Wall MJ, Pepe PE, et al. Immediate vs delayed fluid resuscitation for hypotensive patients with penetrating torso injuries. N Engl J Med 1994;331:1105–9. PMID: 7935634.
In a randomised controlled trial of patients with penetrating torso injuries, reduced mortality and complications were seen when fluid resuscitation was delayed until haemorrhage was controlled.

[9] Johansson PI, Stensballe J, Oliveri R, et al. How I treat patients with massive haemorrhage. Blood 2014;124:3052–8. PMID: 25293771.
Comprehensive literature review on haemostatic resuscitation with recommendations regarding the monitoring of haemostasis and targeted administration of blood products.

[10] Patterson BO, Holt PJ, Cleanthis M, et al. On behalf of the London vascular injuries Working Group. Imaging vascular trauma. Br J Surg 2012;99:494–505. PMID: 22190106.
A systematic review of the literature on the radiological diagnosis of vascular trauma. CTA was found to have acceptable sensitivity and specificity for diagnosing blunt and penetrating vascular injuries and is recommended as the primary investigation for vascular trauma.

[12] Inaba K, Aksoy H, Seamon MJ, et al. Multicentre evaluation of temporary intravascular shunt use in vascular trauma. J Trauma 2016;80:359–64. PMID: 26713968.
This multicentre report represents the largest civilian experience of temporary intravascular shunts used for damage control, staged procedures and for referral caused by insufficient surgeon skill. Description of the indication, technique and outcome in a range of vascular injuries.

[13] Velmahos GC, Toutouzas KG, Sarkisyan G, et al. A prospective study on the safety and efficacy of angiographic embolisation for pelvic and visceral injuries. J Trauma 2002;53:303–8. PMID: 12169938.
One hundred consecutive patients were evaluated by angiography for bleeding from major pelvic fractures (n=65) or solid visceral organ injuries (n=35). Angiographic embolisation was found to be highly effective in controlling bleeding in patients with selected injuries of the pelvis and abdominal visceral organs.

[14] Stratil PG, Burdick TR. Visceral trauma: principles of management and role of embolo therapy. Semin Intervent Radiol 2008;25:271–80. PMID: 21326517.
This article reviews the general management of visceral injuries with special reference to embolising lesions of the liver, kidneys and spleen.

[20] Glaser JD, Kalapatapu VR. Endovascular therapy of vascular trauma – current options and review of the literature. Vasc Endovascular Surg 2019;53(6):477–87. https://doi.org/10.1177/1538574419844073.
This article is an extensive review of the existing literature regarding the endovascular management of vascular trauma.

[29] Feliciano DV. Penetrating cervical trauma. World J Surg 2015;39:1363–72. PMID: 25561188.
Detailed discussion on the management of patients with penetrating cervical trauma.

[42] Du Toit DF, Odendaal W, Lampbrechts A, et al. Surgical and endovascular management of penetrating innominate artery injuries. Eur J Vasc Endovasc Surg 2008;36:56–62. PMID: 18356085.
The authors discuss the diagnosis and management of patients with penetrating innominate artery injuries with special reference to surgical and endovascular technique.

[43] Du Toit DF, Coolen D, Lampbrechts A, et al. The endovascular management of penetrating carotid artery injuries: long-term follow up. Eur J Vasc Endovasc Surg 2009;38:267–70. PMID: 19570690.
This article discusses the indications and technique of carotid artery stenting and reports on the long-term follow-up.

[44] Du Toit DF, Lampbrechts A, Stark H, et al. Long-term results of stentgraft treatment of subclavian artery injuries: management of choice for stable patients? J Vasc Surg 2008;47:739–43. PMID: 18242938.
The authors report their extensive experience with endovascular management of subclavian artery injuries discussing their technique, with immediate results and long-term follow-up (mean 49 months, range 5–104 months).

[48] Fox N, Schwartz D, Salazar JH, et al. Evaluation and management of blunt traumatic aortic injury: a practice management guideline from the Eastern Association for the Surgery of Trauma. J Trauma Acute Care Surg 2015;78:136–46. PMID: 25539215.
These guidelines represent a comprehensive overview of the literature

regarding the evaluation and management of blunt thoracic aortic injury (BTAI). Three important and evidence-based recommendations regarding BTAI are made: (1) CTA is strongly recommended for the identification of clinically significant BTAI. (2) The use of endovascular repair is strongly recommended in patients with BTAI who do not have contraindications to endovascular repair. (3) The use of delayed repair in patients with BTAI is suggested with strict blood pressure control.

[51] Lee WA, Matsumura MD, Mitchell RS, et al. Endovascular repair of traumatic thoracic aortic injury: clinical practice guidelines for the Society for Vascular Surgery. J Vasc Surg 2011;53:187–92. PMID: 20974523.

A systematic review and meta-analysis of the literature including 7768 patients from 139 studies. The mortality was significantly lower in patients who underwent endovascular repair compared with open repair (9% vs. 19%). Endovascular repair also had decreased risk of spinal cord ischaemia, renal impairment, graft and systemic infections.

[60] Aucar JA, Hirshberg A. Damage control for vascular injuries. Surg Clin North Am 1997;77:853–62. PMID: 9291986.

A good review of the different techniques in vascular damage control.

[71] Jens S, Kerstens MK, Legemate DA, et al. Diagnostic performance of computed tomography angiography in peripheral arterial injuries due to trauma: a systematic review and meta-analysis. Eur J Vasc Endovasc Surg 2013;46:329–37. PMID: 23726770.

A systematic review and meta-analysis of literature comparing CTA with surgery, DSA or follow-up in extremity vascular trauma. Excellent sensitivity and specificity was found with CTA and it is recommended that CTA replaces DSA as diagnostic modality.

[78]. Hafez HM, Woolgar J, Robbs JV. Lower extremity arterial injury: results of 550 cases and review of risk factors associated with limb loss. J Vasc Surg 2001;33:1212–9. PMID: 11389420.

The authors review their experience with 641 lower limb arterial injuries in 550 patients with reference to diagnosis, management, results and risk factors for amputation.

[86] Stannard JP, Shiels TM, Lopez-Ben RR, et al. Vascular injuries in knee dislocations: the role of physical examination in determining the need for arteriography. J Bone Joint Surg 2004;86:910–4. PMID: 15118031.

In a prospective study of 138 consecutive patients with acute multiligamentous knee injury, a strong correlation was found between the results of physical examination and the need for arteriography. It was concluded that selective arteriography, based on serial physical examination, is a safe and prudent policy following knee dislocation.

[87] Holtis JD, Daley BJ. 10-year review of knee dislocations: is arteriography always necessary? J Trauma 2005;59:672–6. PMID: 16361911.

In this retrospective review of patients with knee dislocation, the result of routine arteriography was compared to that of physical examination. It was concluded that routine arteriography was unnecessary in patients with a normal physical examination after reduction of the knee.

10 Extracranial cerebrovascular disease

A. Ross Naylor | Jos C. van den Berg

INTRODUCTION

Stroke is the third commonest cause of death and is a major cause of neurological disability. It is defined as an acute loss of focal cerebral function with symptoms exceeding 24 hours (or leading to death), with no apparent cause other than a vascular origin. A transient ischaemic attack (TIA) has the same definition but lasts <24 hours. In the UK, the annual incidence of stroke is 2:1 000 and 150 000 patients will suffer their first stroke each year.[1] Although mortality has diminished by about 20%, attributed to improved survival rather than a declining incidence, overall stroke incidence could increase by 30% by 2033 because of the ageing population.[1] About 36 000 patients suffer a TIA each year, giving an annual UK incidence of 0.5:1 000.[2]

RISK FACTORS

About 80% of strokes are ischaemic and 20% are haemorrhagic (intracerebral/subarachnoid). Approximately 80% of ischaemic strokes affect the carotid territory. Risk factors include increasing age, smoking, hypertension, ischaemic heart disease, cardioembolic source, previous TIA, diabetes, peripheral artery disease (PAD), high plasma fibrinogen and hypercholesterolaemia.

AETIOLOGY

The Trial of ORG 10172 in Acute Stroke Treatment (TOAST) classification of TIA/ischaemic stroke includes five categories: (1) large artery atherosclerosis with ≥50% stenosis of an extracranial or intracranial artery; (2) cardioembolic; (3) small vessel occlusion (e.g., caused by lipohyalinosis, microatheroma); (4) stroke of other determined aetiology (e.g., arteritis, dissection) and (5) stroke of undetermined aetiology (e.g., two potential causes, no cause identified, or incomplete investigations).[3]

LARGE-ARTERY ATHEROSCLEROSIS

Commonest cause is thromboembolism from a stenosis at the origin of the internal carotid artery (ICA) (Fig. 10.1). Haemodynamic failure accounts for <2% of strokes. Stenoses develop at the ICA origin because of a region of low shear stress, flow stasis and flow separation that predisposes towards atherosclerotic plaque formation. If the plaque undergoes acute disruption (rupture, ulceration, haemorrhage), the core of sub-endothelial collagen is exposed, triggering thrombus formation and secondary embolism.

SMALL-VESSEL OCCLUSION

Occlusion of penetrating end-arterioles causes lacunar infarcts. The occlusive process follows fibrinoid necrosis (hypertensive encephalopathy), lipohyalinosis, micro-atheroma (chronic hypertension) or microcalcinosis (diabetes). The commonest sites for lacunar infarction include the basal ganglia, thalamus and internal capsule.

CARDIOEMBOLIC

Sources include ventricular mural thrombus (post-myocardial infarction [MI], cardiomyopathy), left atrial thrombus (atrial fibrillation) and valvular lesions (vegetations, prostheses, calcified annulus, endocarditis).

STROKE OF OTHER DETERMINED ORIGIN

HAEMATOLOGICAL DISORDERS

Myeloma, sickle-cell disease, polycythaemia, the oral contraceptive pill and related prothrombotic disorders predispose towards stroke.

NON-ATHEROMATOUS CAROTID DISEASES

Fibromuscular dysplasia

Fibromuscular dysplasia (FMD) is a rare disorder of unknown aetiology affecting the renal (60–75%) and carotid arteries (25–30%) in young to middle-aged women. The commonest presentation is hypertension. FMD is classified as: (i) intimal fibroplasia, (ii) medial dysplasia (medial fibroplasia, perimedial fibroplasia, medial hyperplasia) and (iii) adventitial (peri-arterial) fibroplasia. The commonest is medial fibroplasia (75–80% of cases), characterised by alternating stenotic webs and dilatation/aneurysm formation (Fig. 10.2). In up to 60%, FMD is bilateral. Patients with carotid FMD may be asymptomatic or symptomatic (TIA/stroke, dissection, false aneurysm). Management is conservative in asymptomatic individuals, but surveillance is recommended. Once symptomatic, patients should be treated as for symptomatic atherosclerotic disease. Options include resection and interposition bypass, open graduated internal dilatation or (more commonly) percutaneous angioplasty.

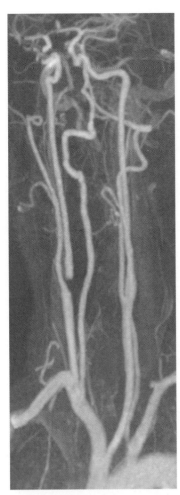

Figure 10.1 Contrast-enhanced magnetic resonance angiography in the right anterior oblique orientation providing overview anatomical imaging, i.e. from the arch origin to the circle of Willis. There is an extremely tight stenosis (>95%) at the right carotid bulb/proximal internal carotid artery.

CAROTID WEBS

A carotid web (thought to be an intimal variant of FMD) can occasionally be found in the carotid bulb and creates a pocket for local thrombus accumulation and secondary brain embolisation (Fig. 10.3a–d). A systematic review identified 37 studies involving 158 patients (median age 46 years; 68% female; 76% symptomatic). In the symptomatic cohort, 56% of those who were initially treated medically suffered a recurrent stroke at a median of 12-months after symptom onset.[4] Treatment requires a high degree of suspicion and most symptomatic cases are now treated surgically by resection of the web plus patching or segmental resection and anastomosis.

ARTERITIS

Takayasu's arteritis (TA) is a transmural, granulomatous inflammatory condition, ultimately causing occlusion through fibrosis. TA predominantly affects younger females (female:male ratio 7:1) and presentation may be a relatively innocuous illness comprising malaise, fever and arthralgia/myalgia. In the acute phase, there is a granulomatous vasculitis

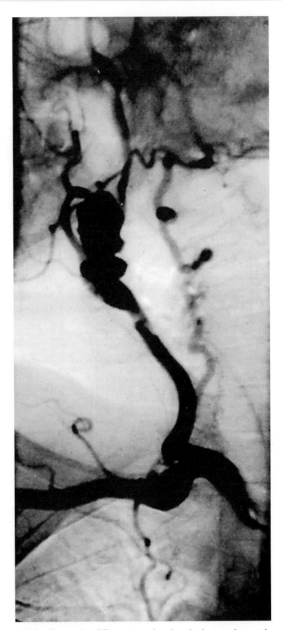

Figure 10.2 Example of fibromuscular dysplasia causing early aneurysm formation in the carotid artery.

with medial disruption, followed by transmural fibrosis. Occasionally, focal aneurysms form after disruption of the internal elastic lamina and media. Neurological symptoms follow vessel occlusion or via renovascular hypertension. Type I TA (arch branches) and Type IIa (ascending aorta, aortic arch, arch branches) present with cerebral vascular/ocular symptoms or asymptomatic stenoses. Type III TA (arch vessels plus abdominal aorta and its branches) accounts for 65% of cases and is associated with stroke, renovascular hypertension and mesenteric ischaemia.

The mainstay of treatment is immunosuppression (steroid/cyclophosphamide/methotrexate). Surgery should be avoided in the acute phase where possible. Neither endarterectomy nor angioplasty/stenting is really an option with involvement of the carotid vessels because of the long segments of fibrotic disease. If surgery becomes necessary, bypass is the preferred option, and the inflow should be taken

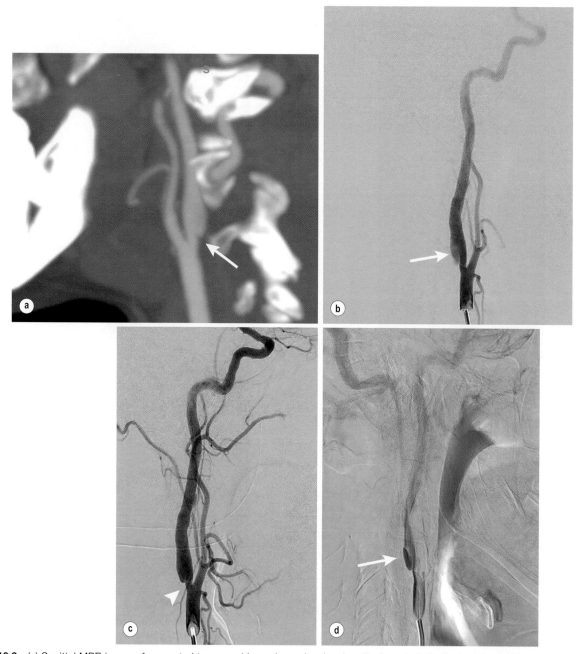

Figure 10.3 (a) Sagittal MPR image of computed tomographic angiography showing diaphragmatic lesion in the proximal segment of the left internal carotid artery (ICA) (*arrow*), indicative of the presence of a carotid web. (b) Angiographic image of selective digital subtraction angiography (DSA) of left common carotid artery (CCA) in early phase demonstrating slow filling of the space behind the carotid web (*arrow*). (c) Selective DSA showing only 'diaphragmatic' lesion at the level of the carotid bulb (*arrowhead*), indicating the carotid web. (d) Selective DSA late phase showing stagnation of contrast in the 'pouch' created by the carotid web (*arrow*).

from the ascending aorta (as opposed to the subclavian artery) as the latter may be involved in the disease process.

Giant-cell arteritis (GCA) is the most common vasculitis in adults and primarily affects older females (female:male ratio 4:1). There are three recognised subtypes (systemic inflammatory syndrome; cranial arteritis and large vessel arteritis). The intracranial vessels are unaffected. The commonest presentation is malaise, headache and myalgic pain. Jaw claudication occurs in 50%, while 50% will develop pain over the temporal artery. Stroke is rare, the commonest presentation being transient/permanent blindness. Ocular symptoms (blindness, corneal ulcers/cataracts) can occur

up to 6 months after initial presentation. Treatment is corticosteroid therapy.

CAROTID ANEURYSM

Carotid aneurysms are rare (<2% of peripheral aneurysms, 0.2% of all carotid interventions). The accepted definition is a diameter >150% of the common carotid artery (CCA) or twice the diameter of the distal ICA. The aetiology is unknown but may be 'atherosclerotic' or follow trauma/infection. Presentations include pulsatile swelling (with/without pain), Horner's syndrome, thrombosis, dissection, rupture or embolisation (TIA/stroke). Treatment involves exclusion and primary re-anastomosis or interposition bypass. Endovascular exclusion is the preferred option in patients with distal ICA aneurysms.

CAROTID DISSECTION

Acute carotid dissection causes 2% of strokes, increasing to 20% in young adults. One-fifth of trauma patients with an unexplained neurological deficit will have a dissection and 25% will be bilateral. Dissection can be spontaneous (FMD), iatrogenic (angioplasty/stenting), be part of a type A dissection or follow blunt trauma (forced hyperextension or forced rotation with compression of the ICA between the mastoid process and the transverse process of C2). Type I carotid dissections involve irregularity, but no significant stenosis (Fig. 10.4a); type II involves a 70–99% stenosis and/or >50% dilatation, while type III dissections present with a characteristic 'flame'-shaped occlusion about 2–3 cm distal to the bifurcation (Fig. 10.4b). The latter is caused by compression of the true lumen by thrombus in the false channel.

The commonest presentation is ipsilateral head/neck pain (70%), but 50–75% of patients will present with TIA/stroke (usually embolic), pulsatile tinnitus, syncope, ocular signs or cranial nerve palsies (III, IV, VI, VII, IX, X, XII). Cranial nerve signs probably follow mechanical compression from mural haematoma or stretching. Up to 60% with spontaneous dissection will have ocular signs (oculosympathetic paresis, amaurosis fugax, aggravated by sitting/standing), hemianopia, ischaemic optic neuropathy and painful Horner's syndrome). The latter follows segmental

ischaemia of the post-ganglionic fibres distal to the superior cervical ganglion and may persist in 50%.

✓ Recognition of ocular symptoms in patients with suspected dissection is important as up to 25% may suffer a stroke within 7 days.

Patients suspected of having an acute dissection should undergo Duplex ultrasound (DUS) and computed tomographic angiography (CTA)/magnetic resonance angiography(MRA) (to include axial T2 fat-saturated images). This typically shows the dissection to start 2–3 cm beyond the origin of the ICA (see Fig. 10.4b). The distal limit is variable (occasionally the petrous segment) with varying combinations of stenosis, dilatation, intimal flaps and occlusion in the intervening segment. The majority of dissections are managed conservatively. The aim is to reduce the risk of thrombosis and embolism.

✓ Most acute carotid dissections are treated with anticoagulation (heparin then warfarin), but systematic reviews suggest that there is no evidence that this is preferable/safer to antiplatelet therapy.[5]

Surgery (or endovascular intervention) is mainly reserved for complex symptomatic trauma cases (usually type II) but may be indicated in patients with recurrent cerebral events despite medical therapy. Overall, dissection carries a 20% mortality and a 30% rate of disability. About 10–40% of dissection patients will develop a false aneurysm, usually in the distal ICA. A systematic review of 166 non-operated

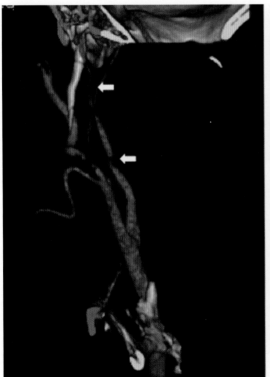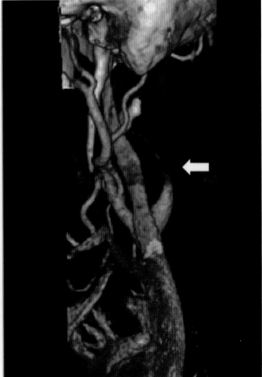

Figure 10.4 Three-dimensional computed tomographic angiography (CTA) reconstruction showing bilateral carotid dissections in the same patient. Left panel shows asymptomatic, spontaneous internal carotid artery (ICA) dissection (type 1 lesion) with entry and exit tears (*small arrows*), causing no significant stenosis. Right panel: symptomatic 'flame'-shaped type 3 dissection with sub-occlusion of the ICA, 2–3 cm beyond the bifurcation.

distal ICA false aneurysms revealed that in 95% of cases, the false aneurysm either stayed the same size or regressed, while <3% became symptomatic.[6]

✅ Most distal false aneurysms following carotid dissection do not increase in size or cause symptoms. The majority should therefore be managed conservatively. Interventions are only warranted if the aneurysm increases in size or causes symptoms.

CAROTID BODY TUMOUR

The carotid body is located within the adventitia of the posterior aspect of the carotid bifurcation and is responsible for monitoring blood gases/pH. A carotid body tumour (CBT) is derived from cells originating from the neural crest ectoderm (chemoreceptor cells). It is typically located in the space between the ICA and external carotid arteries (ECA) and consists of nests of neoplastic epithelioid chief cells. As it enlarges, the bifurcation splays (Fig. 10.5a). In a recent systematic review (104 studies, 4 588 CBTs), mean age at diagnosis was 47 years (1M:2F), 10% were bilateral and 4% were malignant.[7] A palpable neck mass was the presenting symptom in 75% (86% asymptomatic), with cranial nerve palsies and dysphagia being the next commonest presenting symptoms. Stroke/TIA is rarely a clinical presentation (0.4%).[7]

Diagnosis requires awareness, supplemented by DUS, MRA/CTA. Treatment involves excision, although a conservative approach may be preferable in elderly patients with small asymptomatic tumours. Pre-operative embolisation or insertion of a covered stent into the proximal ECA may reduce intra-operative bleeding, but this is probably only necessary with large CBTs. Patients with bilateral CBTs or a family history of CBTs should be referred for testing for mutations of the succinyl dehydrogenase gene as they may

be associated with worse disease-free survival after resection in patients with carotid body paragangliomas and may therefore benefit from resection at an earlier stage.[8] Differential diagnoses include glomus vagale/glomus jugulare tumours. A glomus vagale tumour arises from chemoreceptor cells within the vagus nerve and can be differentiated from a CBT because the bifurcation is not splayed. Instead, the tumour causes deviation of the ICA above the bifurcation (Fig. 10.5b). It is important to consider a glomus vagale tumour pre-operatively as resection leads to swallowing problems (injury to vagal motor fibres) and hoarseness (recurrent laryngeal nerve) and the patient has to be warned about this. CBT resection is associated with a 4% stroke rate and a 20% incidence of cranial nerve injury (CNI; half permanent). Surgical risks increase as the tumour enlarges and increasingly encircles the bifurcation, ICA and ECA.[7]

PRESENTATION OF CAROTID DISEASE

ASYMPTOMATIC CEREBROVASCULAR DISEASE

Using DUS, the incidence of moderate (>50%) and severe (>70%) asymptomatic carotid stenosis (ACS) in 23 706 people (mean age 61 years, 46% male) recruited from four population-based studies was 2.0% and 0.5%, respectively.[9] The prevalence of >70% ACS increases with age. In males aged 50–59 years it is 0.7%, increasing to 2.1% at age 70–79 years. The respective prevalences for females are 0.5% and 1%.[9]

SYMPTOMATIC CEREBROVASCULAR DISEASE

CAROTID TERRITORY
'Classical' carotid territory symptoms include: (1) hemimotor/sensory signs, (2) transient monocular blindness (TMB)

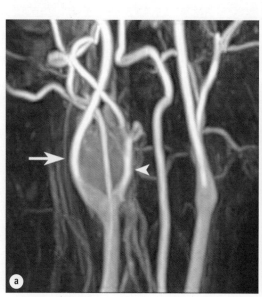
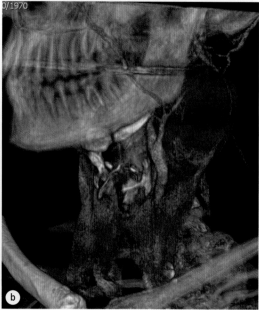

Figure 10.5   (a) Maximum intensity projection reconstruction of magnetic resonance angiography (MRA) of a highly vascular right carotid body tumour causing splaying of the bifurcation (right internal carotid, *arrow*; right external carotid artery, *arrowhead*). (b) Three-dimensional computed tomography angiogram of a probable glomus vagale tumour. Note that the tumour does not splay the bifurcation, but it pushes between the external and internal carotid arteries from a posterior location higher up in the neck.

Box 10.1 'Classical' carotid and vertebrobasilar features

Carotid territory

Hemimotor/hemisensory signs
Monocular visual loss (amaurosis fugax)
Higher cortical dysfunction (dysphasia, visuospatial neglect etc.)

Vertebrobasilar

Bilateral blindness
Problems with gait and stance
Hemi- or bilateral motor/sensory signs
Dysarthria
Homonymous hemianopia
Diplopia, vertigo and nystagmus (provided it is not the only symptom)

and (3) higher cortical dysfunction (Box 10.1). TMB usually develops over a few seconds and clears within a few minutes. Failure to resolve within 24 hours is analogous to a stroke.

✔ A history of TMB in the absence of a source of embolisation should prompt urgent referral to an ophthalmologist to exclude anterior ischaemic optic neuropathy (microvascular disease of the posterior ciliary arteries), which causes acute ischaemia of the optic nerve head.

Differential diagnoses for carotid territory events include epilepsy, tumour, giant aneurysm, hypoglycaemia and migraine (i.e. stroke mimics). Where TIAs are precipitated by a heavy meal, hot bath, exercise or where there is a 'limb shaking' TIA, a haemodynamically critical ICA stenosis should be suspected.

Conventional teaching advises that the risk of stroke after a TIA/minor stroke is 1–2% at 7 days and 2–4% at 30 days. This, in conjunction with a historical reluctance to perform carotid surgery within the early time period after onset of symptoms (concerns about increased procedural risks), has led to little urgency regarding referral, investigation and management. However, there is now compelling evidence that the incidence of recurrent stroke after the index TIA in patients with 50–99% ICA stenoses ranges from 5–8% at 48 hours, 4–17% at 72 hours, 8–22% at 7 days and 11–25% at 14 days.[10] Interestingly, pooled data from patients randomised to 'best medical therapy' (BMT) in the European Carotid Surgery Trial (ECST), North American Symptomatic Carotid Endarterectomy Trial (NASCET) and the Veterans Affairs trials observed only a 21% risk of ipsilateral stroke at 5 years in patients randomised to BMT.[11] This would suggest that most patients who were destined to suffer an early recurrent stroke after their TIA were rarely randomised quickly enough within these trials. The decision to refer a recently symptomatic patient should never be influenced by the presence/absence of a carotid bruit.

VERTEBROBASILAR

Vertebrobasilar (VB) symptoms (see Box 10.1) include bilateral blindness, problems with gait/stance, hemilateral/bilateral motor or sensory impairment (10% will have hemisensory/motor signs), dysarthria, homonymous hemianopia,

nystagmus, dizziness, diplopia and vertigo (provided the latter three are not isolated).

✔ VB TIAs carry early stroke risks comparable to carotid territory events, especially if they have an ipsilateral 50–99% stenosis (20–30% stroke risk within 90 days).[12] Patients reporting VB symptoms need to be treated more urgently in future.

NON-HEMISPHERIC

The term 'non-hemispheric' is applied to patients with isolated syncope (blackout, drop attack), presyncope (faintness), isolated dizziness, isolated double vision (diplopia) and isolated vertigo.

✔ 'Non-hemispheric' symptoms should never be considered to be carotid or VB in origin unless other 'classical' symptoms are present. It is very important to exclude a cardiac or inner ear pathology.

INVESTIGATION OF PATIENTS

✔✔ The Intercollegiate Stroke Working Party recommends that any patient with a suspected acute TIA should be assessed and imaged <24 hours by a specialist physician in a single-visit neurovascular clinic or an acute stroke unit.[13]
The Intercollegiate Stroke Working Party recommends that any patient with a suspected TIA that occurred more than 7-days prior should be assessed and imaged within 7 days by a specialist physician in a single-visit neurovascular clinic.[13] Every centre should know which carotid stenosis measurement method is being used in their unit (i.e. ECST or NASCET).[13]

There are three methods for measuring stenosis severity, each using the luminal diameter at the point of maximum stenosis as the numerator (Fig. 10.6). In ECST, the denominator was the estimated artery diameter at the same point, usually the carotid bulb. In NASCET, the denominator was the diameter of a disease-free point in the ICA above the stenosis where the walls of the vessel were parallel. These two methods produce different values for the 'same' stenosis. Stenoses measured using the ECST method generate 'higher' grades of stenosis than those using the NASCET method. In practice, a 50% NASCET stenosis is broadly equivalent to a 70% ECST, while a 70% NASCET stenosis broadly equates to an 85% ECST stenosis. Neither trial used the CCA method, in which the denominator is the diameter of CCA proximal to the bifurcation. While the CCA method may be the most reproducible, most guidelines of practice now recommend using the NASCET measurement method.

DUPLEX ULTRASOUND

Stenosis severity is usually evaluated using DUS, which combines B-mode (real-time) imaging with waveform analysis using pulsed-wave Doppler. Advantages include: (i) low cost, (ii) accessibility within 'single-visit' clinics and (iii) being non-invasive. There are recognised limitations, however, mostly relating to operator expertise. With highly experienced sonographers, DUS can identify up to 95% of lesions responsible for carotid territory symptoms and there is no evidence that operating on the basis of DUS (alone) compromises patient safety.[14] A joint working group of the Vascular Society of Great Britain and Ireland and the Society of Vascular Technologists[15] published consensus criteria for diagnosing the severity of carotid disease based on the NASCET measurement method (Table 10.1).

In some UK centres, carotid endarterectomy (CEA) procedures are planned on the basis of DUS alone. However, DUS can only insonate the cervical portion of the extracranial ICA and is relatively unreliable at excluding disease elsewhere and cannot be used for planning carotid artery stenting (CAS). Any suspicion of additional lesions (damped proximal CCA waveform, unable to image above the stenosis) requires alternative imaging (MRA/CTA). Because the benefit conferred by CEA in patients with 50–69% stenoses falls significantly with delays to surgery (see later), it has been recommended that if 4 weeks or more have elapsed after the index event, corroborative

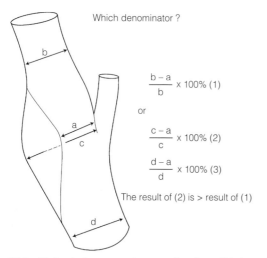

Figure 10.6 Methods for measuring severity of carotid stenosis by the European Carotid Surgery Trial (ECST) method (equation 2), North American Symptomatic Carotid Endarterectomy Trial (NASCET) method (equation 1) and common carotid method (equation 3), where 'a' is the residual luminal diameter, 'b' is the diameter of internal carotid artery above stenosis, 'c' is the diameter of the carotid bulb at the point of measuring 'a', while 'd' is the diameter of the distal CCA below the stenosis.

imaging with either contrast-enhanced MRA (CEMRA) or multidetector CTA (MDCTA) should be undertaken to confirm stenosis severity. If, however, DUS was performed within 4-weeks of the index event, a Health Technology Assessment (HTA) felt it reasonable to proceed to CEA on the basis of DUS alone, as the number of strokes prevented through rapidly performed surgery exceeded the potential risk to patients with <50% stenoses undergoing inappropriate surgery.[16]

The Gray–Weale classification[17] categorises plaques according to whether they are echolucent (type 1), predominantly echolucent (type 2), predominantly echogenic (type 3) or echogenic (type 4). Unfortunately, correlation with histology and clinical risk is variable. The Grey Scale Median (GSM) is a computerised measurement of plaque echogenicity that was developed to differentiate echogenic carotid plaques (that have a fibro-calcified content that is thought to be associated with a stable plaque) and echolucent plaques (with a thin fibrous cap and a higher lipid or haemorrhagic content that are supposedly unstable). The presence of a low GSM is associated with a higher incidence of neurological events after CAS.[18] Several studies have indicated that plaque echogenicity on high-resolution B-mode ultrasound is related to the histological components of carotid plaques, and low echogenicity (or echolucency) is associated with the development of neurological events, especially in asymptomatic patients.[19]

CATHETER ANGIOGRAPHY

Digital subtraction angiography (DSA) was previously the gold standard in carotid imaging. It is, however, associated with a small risk of peri-operative stroke. Minor adverse reactions include groin haematoma, unstable angina, need for blood transfusion, leg ischaemia and iliac artery dissection. The main advantages of angiography are its high resolution and ability to demonstrate flow dynamics within the diseased artery and of the collateral circulation (circle of Willis and ECA). In the era of high-quality non-invasive imaging, no centre would currently advocate any role for routine DSA, because of the risk of angiographic stroke and arterial access site complications.

Table 10.1   Diagnostic velocity criteria for NASCET based carotid stenosis measurement

% stenosis NASCET	PSV ICA cm/sec	PSV$_{ICA}$/PSV$_{CCA}$ ratio	St Mary's ratio PSV$_{ICA}$/EDV$_{CCA}$
<50%	<125	<2	<8
50-69%	≥125	2.0-4	8-10
60-69%			11-13
70-79%	≥230	≥4	14-21
80-89%			22-29
>90% but not near occlusion	≥400	≥5	≥30
Near-occlusion	High, low – string flow	Variable	Variable
Occlusion	No flow	Not applicable	Not applicable

CCA, Common carotid artery; *EDV,* end diastolic velocity; *ICA,* internal carotid artery; *NASCET,* North American Symptomatic Carotid Endarterectomy Trial; *PSV,* peak systolic velocity.
Reproduced with permission from Oates C, Naylor AR, Hartshorne T, Charles SM, Humphries K, Aslam M, et al. Reporting carotid ultrasound investigations in the United Kingdom Eur J Vasc Endovasc Surg 2009;37:251-261.

Table 10.2 Meta-analysis of the accuracy of non-invasive imaging for carotid stenosis subgroups and imaging modalities

	Sensitivity		Specificity	
	50%-69% ICA stenosis	70%-99% ICA stenosis	50%-69% ICA stenosis	70%-99% ICA stenosis
DUS	0.36 (0.25-0.49)	0.89 (0.85-0.92)	0.91 (0.87-0.94)	0.84 (0.77-0.89)
TOF-MRA	0.37 (0.26-0.49)	0.88 (0.82-0.92)	0.91 (0.78-0.97)	0.84 (0.76-0.97)
CE-MRA	0.77 (0.59-0.89)	0.94 (0.88-0.97)	0.97 (0.93-0.99)	0.93 (0.89-0.96)
CTA	0.67 (0.30-0.90)	0.77 (0.68-0.84)	0.79 (0.63-0.89)	0.95 (0.91-0.97)

CE-MRA, Contrast-enhanced MRA; *CTA*, computed tomographic angiography; *DUS*, duplex ultrasound; *MRA*, magnetic resonance angiography.
Adapted from Wardlaw et al.[16] "Accurate, practical and cost-effective assessment of carotid stenosis in the UK". Health Technology Assessment 2006;Vol 10:No. 30. Department of Health Crown copyright material is reproduced with the permission of the Controller of the HMSO and Queen's Printers for Scotland. Document available at: http://www.hta.ac.uk/fullmono/mon1030.pdf

In the Asymptomatic Carotid Atherosclerosis Study (ACAS), selective catheter angiography incurred a stroke/death risk of 1.5% (>50% of the overall surgical risk).[20] It is no longer part of the routine work-up of a recently symptomatic patient.

MAGNETIC RESONANCE ANGIOGRAPHY

CEMRA uses the paramagnetic agent gadolinium and (compared to non-enhanced TOF-MRA), images are obtained more rapidly. CEMRA incurs fewer flow-related artefacts and provides a much greater field of view that enables high-resolution imaging from the aortic arch up to the circle of Willis (see Fig. 10.1), whilst retaining the ability to evaluate flow directionality. CEMRA is, however, limited by availability, accessibility, and (occasionally) patient incompatibility (e.g., pacemaker) or claustrophobia. Whilst MRA is non-invasive and avoids ionising radiation, gadolinium has recently been identified as a cause of nephrogenic systemic fibrosis (NSF).

Plaque bleeding or the presence of a lipid-rich necrotic core may lead to an increase in symptoms and therefore it can be anticipated that crossing these lesions may lead to a higher burden of cerebral emboli detected using transcranial Doppler (TCD).[21]

NSF is a systemic scleroderma like condition, which affects 3–5% of patients with pre-existing renal impairment exposed to gadolinium-based compounds. Five percent of affected individuals exhibit a rapidly progressive course.

COMPUTED TOMOGRAPHIC ANGIOGRAPHY

MDCTA permits rapid acquisition of large amounts of cross-sectional data that can be reformatted into any plane and produce three-dimensional reconstructions. The advantages of CTA include: (i) being minimally invasive, (ii) overview anatomical imaging with short scan times, while thinner 'slices' mean less artifact, (iii) CTA is more accessible than MRA and (iv) CTA is generally well tolerated. Disadvantages include: (i) requirement for iodinated contrast, (ii) radiation burden, (iii) inability to impart dynamic information, for example, 'trickle flow' is not reliably identified and (iv) heavy calcification makes it more difficult to reliably estimate stenosis severity. CTA yields optimal accuracy in the detection of carotid artery stenoses when careful analysis of all axial slices is performed.[22,23] The problem of severely calcified lesions can be overcome by newer CT technology (dual energy [DE] or dual source CT) and can yield similar accuracy in measuring stenosis severity as CEMRA (with DSA as the gold standard).[24] Maximum intensity projection images obtained with DE-CTA tend to overestimate stenosis severity because of a partial exclusion of the lumen as a consequence of the plaque subtraction algorithm, emphasising the importance of evaluating all axial slices.

COMPARISON OF METHODS

An HTA performed a meta-analysis of the accuracy of non-invasive imaging for all carotid stenosis subgroups and imaging modalities (Table 10.2).[16] CEMRA had the highest sensitivity (94%; 95% CI, 0.88–0.97), specificity and least heterogeneity. A more recent systematic review that evaluated pre-operative DUS and CTA demonstrated comparable sensitivities and specificities for both methods when measuring >70% stenoses. Accordingly, DUS may be used as the sole imaging modality to diagnose a >70% stenosis, provided criteria are audited,[24] but many centres now prefer to corroborate DUS with CTA or CEMRA.

MANAGEMENT OF CEREBROVASCULAR DISEASE

'BEST MEDICAL THERAPY'

All patients benefit from optimisation of risk factors, antiplatelet/statin therapy and exclusion of important comorbidities. Everyone should undergo an electrocardiogram to exclude occult cardiac pathology. Baseline blood tests will exclude diabetes, arteritis, polycythaemia, anaemia, thrombocytosis, sickle-cell disease and hyperlipidaemia.

Angina therapy should be optimised in patients with carotid disease as the principal cause of late death is cardiac. Systematic reviews suggest that reducing diastolic blood pressure (BP) by 5 mmHg lowers the relative risk (RR) of stroke by 35%, while the RR of MI falls by 25%.[25] However, evidence suggests that only 60% of patients with known hypertension will receive treatment before suffering their first stroke and only half will have a documented diastolic BP <90 mmHg.[26] The 2018 European Society for Cardiology/European Society for Hypertension now recommends a target BP <130 mmHg / <80 mmHg in non-diabetic patients under 65 years of age, and <140 mmHg/ <80 mmHg in non-diabetic patients ≥65 years old.[27]

✔✔ The Heart Protection Study showed that patients randomised to statin therapy had a 25% relative risk reduction (RRR) in: (i) any major coronary event, (ii) any stroke and (iii) the need for revascularisation at 5 years. This benefit was irrespective of age, gender or presenting cholesterol level.[28]

Evidence suggests that a target total cholesterol level might be <3.5 mmol/L[27] with a low-density lipoprotein (LDL)-C <1.8 mmol/L,[28,29] or at least a 50% reduction in LDL-C versus baseline.[30] It is also reasonable to add ezetimibe in patients with symptomatic carotid stenosis who do not achieve their lipid targets whilst on maximum doses or maximum tolerated doses of statins.[29,30] In a meta-analysis involving six studies (n=7 503), patients taking statins before CEA had significantly lower peri-operative mortality versus statin-naïve patients (odds ratio [OR], 0.26; 95% CI, 0.1–0.61).[31] In another meta-analysis (11 studies, n=4 088), patients taking statins before CAS had significantly lower peri-procedural mortality (OR, 0.30; 95% CI, 0.10–0.96) and significantly lower procedural stroke risks (OR, 0.39; 95% CI, 0.27–0.58) versus statin-naïve patients.[32]

No randomised controlled trial (RCT) has evaluated the role of antiplatelet agents in asymptomatic patients. However, most guidelines recommend low-dose aspirin to minimise the risk of late cardiovascular events.[33] Since the last edition, there has been a change in advice regarding antiplatelet therapy in recently symptomatic patients, which previously recommended monotherapy with either clopidogrel or aspirin.

✔✔ Meta-analyses of three RCTs have shown that starting aspirin + clopidogrel dual antiplatelet therapy (DAPT) as soon as possible after minor ischaemic stroke/TIA is associated with significant reductions in early non-fatal recurrent ischaemic and haemorrhagic stroke, moderate/severe functional disability and poor quality of life.[34]

DAPT only needs to be continued for 10–21 days after onset of symptoms, as the highest risk period for recurrent stroke was the first 10 days and the patient faced increased bleeding risks if DAPT continued for longer.[34] After 21 days, all recently symptomatic patients should revert to clopidogrel monotherapy, unless contraindicated. An algorithm for prescribing DAPT to patients undergoing urgent CEA in the peri-operative period is detailed in (Fig. 10.7).

The early risk of stroke after suffering a TIA is much higher than previously thought. This has led to a review of practice regarding the timing of surgery (see later), but also regarding the benefit of very early implementation of BMT. The EXPRESS study evaluated early stroke rates in two cohorts of TIA patients. In the first (2002–2004), patients were seen in a daily TIA clinic (appointment based, usual referral delays, etc.) with treatment recommendations faxed to the referring doctor. The patient then contacted their doctor to obtain their prescription, but an average of 19 days elapsed before medications were started. In the second cohort (2004–2007), there was a daily 'walk-in' service, but statin and antiplatelet therapy were started in the outpatient clinic.[35] The 90-day stroke risk fell from 10% in the first cohort to 2% in the second. The reduction in risk was independent of age and gender, with no increase in rates of haemorrhagic stroke.

✔✔ Rapid institution of 'BMT' significantly reduces the risk of early stroke and should be started in the TIA clinic.

MANAGEMENT OF CAROTID DISEASE

SYMPTOMATIC CAROTID ARTERY DISEASE

The Carotid Endarterectomy Trialists Collaboration (CETC) combined data from ECST, NASCET and the Veterans Affairs trials, having re-measured pre-randomisation angiograms using the NASCET measurement method. This database[11,36,37] now provides 5-year outcome data in >6000 patients (Table 10.3). Notwithstanding concerns regarding the 'historical' nature of the RCTs, the 5-year CETC data should now be quoted in preference to the constituent RCTs.

✔✔ CEA is not indicated in symptomatic patients with <50% NASCET stenoses. CEA confers modest (but significant) benefit in recently symptomatic (<6 months) with a 50–69% NASCET stenosis (ECST 70–85%). CEA confers maximum benefit in recently symptomatic (<6 months) with a 70–99% NASCET stenosis, excluding those with the 'string sign'.

✔ Surgeons must know and also quote their own operative risks, rather than justifying practice on the basis of the RCTs.

ECST/NASCET have published over 50 papers since 1991, most being secondary analyses that have increased knowledge about the role of CEA in patients with symptomatic cerebral vascular disease.[10] These should not be used to *exclude* patients from intervention, but rather to identify clinical and/or imaging predictors of increased risk of stroke on BMT (Box 10.2).

One of the most important issues facing CEA and CAS practitioners is the effect of 'delay to intervention'. Previously, there was no impetus for expediting carotid interventions, other than recommending that CEA be performed 'as soon as reasonably possible'. This approach has, however, been challenged because of increasing evidence that the most vulnerable patients are suffering recurrent strokes before they can undergo CEA. A

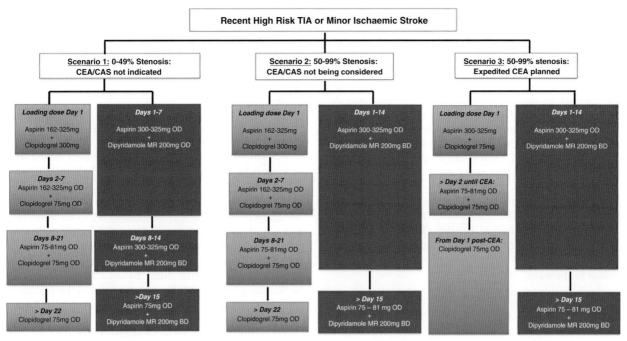

Figure 10.7   Algorithm detailing timing, dose and duration of peri-operative dual antiplatelet therapy in the early phase after onset of high-risk transient ischaemic attack (TIA) or minor ischaemic stroke in patients not on antiplatelet therapy*. *CAS*, Carotid artery stenting; *CEA*, carotid endarterectomy; *MR*, modified release; *od*, once daily; *bd*, twice daily. (* Reproduced with permission from: Naylor AR, McCabe DH. New data and the Covid-19 pandemic mandate a rethink of antiplatelet strategies in patients with ischaemic TIA or minor stroke because of atherosclerotic carotid artery disease. Eur J Vasc Endovasc Surg. 2020;59:861-865.)

Table 10.3   Carotid endarterectomy trialists ollaboration: 5-year risk of any stroke (including 30-day stroke/death) from a pooled individual patient meta-analysis from the VA, ECST and NASCET trials*

NASCET stenosis	n=	30d death/ stroke after CEA	5 year risk		ARR in stroke at 5 years	RRR in stroke at 5 years	NNT	Strokes prevented per 1000 CEAs at 5y
			CEA	BMT				
<30%	1746	no data	18.4%	15.7%	-2.7%	NB	NB	none at 5y
30-49%	1429	6.7%	22.8%	25.5%	+2.7%	10%	37	27 at 5y
50-69%	1549	8.4%	20.0%	27.8%	+7.8%	28%	13	78 at 5y
70-99%	1095	6.2%	17.1%	32.7%	+15.6%	48%	6	156 at 5y
near occln	262	5.4%	22.4%	22.3%	-0.1%	NB	NB	none at 5y

*Data derived from the CETC[11,36,37] with all pre-randomisation angiograms remeasured using NASCET method.
ARR, Absolute risk reduction; *BMT*, 'best medical therapy'; *CEA*, carotid endarterectomy; *NB*, no benefit conferred by CEA; *NNT*, number needed to treat; *RRR*, relative risk reduction.

recent review suggested that the incidence of recurrent stroke after the index TIA in patients with 50–99% ICA stenoses ranged from 5–8% at 48 hours, 4–17% at 72 hours, 8–22% at 7 days and 11–25% at 14 days.[38] Second, the CETC has published evidence that 'delays to surgery' significantly reduces the benefit conferred by CEA.[11,36,37] By implication, the same will apply to CAS. Table 10.4 presents a re-analysis of CETC data showing long-term stroke prevention conferred by CEA in male and female patients with NASCET 50–99% stenoses, stratified for delays from randomisation to surgery. In practice, the median delay from symptom onset to randomisation was about 7 days (P. Rothwell, personal communication). Note that the benefit conferred in males with 70–99% stenoses persisted with increasing delays,

but rapidly diminished in males with 50–69% stenoses. By contrast, the benefit conferred in females appeared to disappear after 4-weeks had elapsed, even in those with 70–99% stenoses.[11,36,37]

✔✔   Maximum benefit, regarding late stroke prevention, was observed when surgery was performed within 2 weeks.[11,36,37]

✔   Symptomatic women gain less benefit from CEA than men and maximum benefit was only conferred if CEA was performed as soon as possible. Excessive delays to treatment could mean that female patients face all the risks of intervention with little prospect of gaining any benefit.[11,36,37]

However, there have been concerns that expedited CEA may be associated with increased 30-day risks of death/stroke, which may negate any potential benefit from intervening early. In a review of 1046 symptomatic patients undergoing CEA in New York, the 30-day death/stroke rate was three times higher (5.1%) if CEA was performed within 4 weeks, as compared with 1.6% if surgery was deferred for >4 weeks.[39] Data like these have been used as a reason to delay interventions to achieve the 'lowest' procedural risks. However, three national registries have now published 30-day death/stroke rates after CEA stratified for delays to surgery (Table 10.5). Only one (SwedVasc[40])

observed a very high procedural risk (11.5%) when CEA was performed within 48-hours of symptom onset; the German and UK registries did not.[41,42] After 48-hours, all three national registries reported acceptably low procedural risks when CEA was performed in the first 7–14 days after symptom onset.[40–42]

✅ Evidence suggests that more strokes will be prevented in the long term through rapid intervention, even if the procedural risk is slightly increased. Future guidelines must consider whether it is reasonable to accept a slightly higher procedural risk if the operation is carried out early.

CAS is now an alternative to CEA (see later). The Carotid Stent Trialists Collaboration (CSTC) undertook a meta-analysis of outcomes from Endarterectomy Versus Angioplasty in Patients with Symptomatic Severe Carotid Stenosis (EVA-3S), Stent-Protected Angioplasty versus Carotid Endarterectomy (SPACE) and International Carotid Stenting Study (ICSS) stratified for delays from index symptom to intervention.[43] Patients undergoing CEA within the first 7-days after the index TIA/stroke had a 30-day death/stroke rate of 2.8%, compared with 9.4% in patients undergoing CAS during the same time period (hazard ratio [HR], 3.4; 95% CI, 1.01–11.8; P = 0.03) after adjusting for age, sex and type of qualifying event. Patients treated between 8 and 14 days had a peri-procedural death/stroke rate of 3.4% after CEA, versus 8.1% following CAS (HR, 2.42; 95% CI, 1.0–5.7; P = 0.04).[43] These data would therefore suggest that (for now) CEA is probably safer than CAS in the first 7–14 days after symptom onset, especially as a recent systematic review of procedural risks following CAS in symptomatic patients in large administrative datasets showed that 70% of registries reported death/stroke rates that exceeded the accepted 6% procedural risk.[44] Twenty percent of registries reported death/stroke rates in excess of 10% after CAS.[44]

Box 10.2 Which patients with symptomatic 50–99% stenoses are at higher risk of suffering a stroke on 'best medical therapy'?*

Clinical features

Male versus female gender
Increasing age (especially >75 years)
Hemispheric versus ocular symptoms
Cortical versus lacunar stroke
Recurrent symptoms for >6 months
Increasing medical comorbidity
Symptoms within 1 month

Imaging features

Irregular versus smooth plaques
Increasing stenosis but not near occlusion
Contralateral occlusion
Tandem intracranial disease

* Derived from Naylor AR, Sillesen H, Schroeder TV. Clinical and imaging features associated with an increased risk of early and late stroke in patients with symptomatic carotid disease. Eur J Vasc Endovasc Surg 2015;49:513–23.

Table 10.4 Absolute risk reduction conferred by CEA in the 5-year risk of ipsilateral carotid territory ischaemic stroke (including the peri-operative risk) in patients with a NASCET 50-69% and 70-99% stenosis, stratified for delay from index event to randomisation and gender (*)

	50 – 69% stenosis			70-99% stenosis		
(1) ALL PATIENTS	**ARR**	**NNT**	**CVA/1000**	**ARR**	**NNT**	**CVA/1000**
< 2 weeks	14.8%	7	148	23.0%	4	230
2-4 weeks	3.3%	30	33	15.9%	6	159
4-12 weeks	4.0%	25	40	7.9%	13	79
>12 weeks	-2.9%	NB	NB	7.4%	14	74
(2) MALES						
< 2 weeks	15.2%	7	152	23.3%	4	233
2-4 weeks	6.8%	15	68	23.8%	4	238
4-12 weeks	5.0%	20	50	18.3%	5	183
> 12 weeks	6.3%	16	63	20.4%	5	204
(3) FEMALES						
< 2 weeks	13.8%	7	138	41.7%	2	417
2-4 weeks	-5.7%	NB	NB	6.6%	15	66
4-12 weeks	-2.2%	NB	NB	-2.2%	NB	NB
> 12 weeks	-21.7%	NB	NB	-2.4%	NB	NB

*Data derived from the CETC[11,36,37] with all pre-randomisation angiograms remeasured using the NASCET method. CVA/1000: number of ipsilateral strokes prevented at five years by performing 1000 CEAs.
ARR, Absolute risk reduction; CEA, carotid endarterectomy; CETC, Carotid Endarterectomy Trialists Collaboration; NASCET, North American Symptomatic Carotid Endarterectomy Trial; NB, no benefit; NNT, number needed to treat.

Table 10.5 30-day death/stroke after CEA, stratified for delay from index symptom onset to undergoing CEA, in national audits of practice

National audit	0-2 days	3-7 days	8-14 days	≥15 days
Sweden[40]	17/148	29/804	27/677	52/967
n=2,596	(11.5%)	(3.6%)	(4.0%)	(5.4%)
UK[41]	29/780	128/5126	132/6292	254/11037
n=23,235	(3.7%)	(2.5%)	(2.1%)	(2.3%)
Germany[42]	157/5198	480/19117	427/16205	370/15759
n=56,279	(3.0%)	(2.5%)	(2.6%)	(2.3%)

CEA, carotid endarterectomy.

RANDOMISED TRIALS COMPARING CAROTID ENDARTERECTOMY WITH CAROTID ARTERY STENTING IN SYMPTOMATIC PATIENTS

Table 10.6 details 30-day procedural risks in a meta-analysis involving 5797 symptomatic patients randomised to CEA or CAS in 10 RCTs.[45] Compared with CEA, CAS was associated with significantly higher rates of stroke (OR, 1.73; 95% CI, 1.38–2.18); death/stroke (OR, 1.71; 95% CI, 1.38–2.11); death and disabling stroke (OR, 1.42; 95% CI, 1.00–2.02) and death/stroke/MI (OR, 1.61; 95% CI, 1.21–2.14). However, once the 30-day peri-operative period had elapsed, meta-analyses suggest that there was no significant difference in 5- and 9-year rates of ipsilateral stroke, suggesting that CAS was just as durable as CEA.[46]

✓✓ At present, CAS carries higher 30-day risks of stroke and death/stroke compared with CEA in recently symptomatic patients. However, once the peri-operative period has elapsed, 5- and 9-year rates of ipsilateral stroke are identical indicating that CAS is as durable as CEA.

Accordingly, the key issue as to whether CEA or CAS is preferable (safer) in recently symptomatic patients will be the predicted 30-day risks in individual patients. In a systematic review of secondary analyses from 20 RCTs comparing CEA with CAS, a number of pre-operative predictors were identified, which were associated with increased rates of 30-day death/stroke following CAS. These included: (i) age >70 years; (ii) performing CAS within 7–14 days of symptom onset, (iii) the presence of sequential plaques or remote lesions beyond the carotid bulb, (iv) plaque length >13 mm, (v) the use of open cell stents, (vi) the use of two or more stents during CAS and (vii) an Age-Related White Matter Change (ARWMC) score ≥7.[45]

RCTs have shown that CAS was associated with better health-related quality of life (HRQoL) during the early recovery period (compared with CEA), especially for physical limitations and pain *(P = 0.01)*. These differences were significant at 4-weeks, but by 1 year, there was no difference in any HRQoL measure. Perhaps most importantly, peri-procedural stroke was associated with poorer 1-year HRQoL scores across all domains, while peri-procedural MI and CNI were not.[47] In the CREST trial, peri-operative MI and stroke were both associated with increased mortality at 10-years.[48]

✓✓ After the perioperative period has elapsed, CAS appears to be as durable as CEA with similar rates of long-term ipsilateral stroke.[46]

The key to determining whether CEA or CAS is preferable (in individual patients) will be largely governed by factors that increase the 30-day risk of death/stroke.

Performing CAS in the first 7–14 days after symptom onset is associated with significantly higher rates of death/stroke, compared to CEA.[43]

CEA appears to be safer (than CAS) in recently symptomatic patients aged >70 years.[49]

CAS had similar procedural risks to CEA in patients aged <70 years.[49]

Peri-operative stroke and MI (clinical and/or biomarker) were both associated with poorer long-term survival.[48]

NEW ISCHAEMIC BRAIN LESIONS ON MAGNETIC RESONANCE IMAGING

ICSS undertook a sub-study where CEA and CAS patients underwent diffusion weighted imaging (DWI) MRI, 1–7 days before treatment, followed by a second scan 1–3 days after treatment and a third scan 27–33 days after treatment.[50] Sixty-two of 124 CAS patients (50%) and 18/107 CEA patients (17%) had at least one new ischaemic brain lesion (NIBL) on the first post-treatment scan (OR, 5.21; 95% CI, 2.78–9.79) *P* < 0.0001). When the scans were repeated at 1-month, there were persisting changes on fluid-attenuated inversion recovery MR sequences in 28/86 CAS patients (33%), compared with 6/75 CEA patients (8%) (OR, 5.93; 95% CI, 2.25–15.62), *P* = 0.0003).[50] In a meta-analysis (46 studies; 5018 patients); 68% of 1873 CEA patients and 56% of 3145 CAS patients were symptomatic. The weighted prevalence of NIBLs was 18.1% (95% CI, 14–22.7) after CEA versus 40.5% (95% CI, 35.4–45.7) after CAS.[51]

The clinical relevance of NIBLs remains uncertain. There is no evidence that NIBLs after CEA/CAS are associated with cognitive impairment in the various carotid RCTs.[45] However, the NeuroVISION study reported that 7% developed NIBLs following non-cardiac surgery, of whom 42% developed cognitive impairment within 1-year, versus 29% in patients without NIBLs (HR, 1.98; 95% CI, 1.22–3.2).[52] In ICSS, the 5-year incidence of recurrent stroke/TIA was 22.8% in CAS patients with NIBLs, versus

Table 10.6   Meta-analysis of peri-operative outcomes in 10 RCTs comparing CAS versus CEA in 5797 symptomatic patients*

	Death	Stroke	Death/ Stroke	Disabling Stroke	Death/ Disabling stroke	MI	Death/ Stroke/MI
	9 RCTs	9 RCTs	10 RCTs	6 RCTs	5 RCTs	6 RCTs	6 RCTs
	n=4257	n=5535	n=5754	n=4855	n=3534	n=3980	n=3719
CEA	1.4%	4.6%	5.08%	1.8%	3.2%	1.6%	5.1%
	(0.9-2.0)	(3.26-6.37)	(3.7-6.9)	(1.1-3.1)	(2.5-4.1)	(1.0-2.3)	(4.13-6.30)
CAS	1.9%	8.5%	9.3%	3.28%	5.21%	0.8%	8.4%
	(1.4-2.6)	(5.87-12.14)	(6.8-12.6)	(1.6-6.7)	(3.0-8.9)	(0.5-1.4)	(5.0-13.8)
OR (95%CI)	1.38	1.73 **	1.71**	1.35	1.42**	0.50	1.61 **
	(0.81-2.34)	(1.38-2.18)	(1.38-2.11)	(0.91-1.99)	(1.00-2.02)	(0.24-1.02)	(1.21-2.14)

*Data derived from Batchelder A, Saratzis A, Naylor AR. Overview of Primary and Secondary Analyses from 20 randomised controlled trials comparing carotid artery stenting with carotid endarterectomy. Eur J Vasc Endovasc Surg 2019;58:479-493.
**p<0.05.
CAS, Carotid artery stenting; *CEA*, carotid endarterectomy; *OR*, odds ratio; *95%CI*, 95% confidence intervals; *MI*, myocardial infarction.

8.8% in CAS patients with no new DWI-MRI lesions (HR, 2.85; 95% CI, 1.05–7.72], P = 0.04). ICSS concluded that NIBLs after CAS may be a marker for an increased risk of recurrent cerebrovascular events and that DWI +ve CAS (CEA) patients might benefit from more aggressive and prolonged DAPT.[53]

ASYMPTOMATIC CAROTID ARTERY DISEASE

Although five RCTs have compared CEA + BMT with BMT alone, only two (ACAS and the Asymptomatic Carotid Surgery Trial [ACST]) have influenced practice.[20,54,55] The 5- and 10-year outcomes from ACAS/ACST are summarised in Table 10.7.

Although ACAS and ACST reported a small but significant benefit favouring CEA (over BMT) at 5-years (ACAS/ACST) and 10-years (ACST), the findings are now somewhat historical and the risk of stroke on BMT may now be lower than when the trials were recruiting.

✓✓ The risk of stroke on modern medical therapy may be declining. A meta-analysis of 41 studies reported an ipsilateral stroke rate of 2.3:100 person years in studies completing recruitment before 2000, compared with 1:100 person years for those between 2000–2010 (P < 0.001).[56]

The decline in ipsilateral stroke risk was attributed to improvements in BMT and smoking cessation. In studies where >25% of participants took statins, ipsilateral stroke risk was 1.2/100 person years, compared with 2.3/100 person years where fewer participants took statins (P = 0.009).[56] Another systematic review reported that the temporal trend towards declining stroke rates in medically treated patients was consistent across all grades of stenosis (50–99%, 60–99% and 70–99%) and was also evident in ACAS and ACST, where annual rates of any and ipsilateral stroke declined by about 60% between 1995 and 2010.[57]

COMPARISON OF CAROTID ENDARTERECTOMY AND CAROTID ARTERY STENTING IN RANDOMISED TRIALS

Table 10.8 details 30-day procedural risks in a meta-analysis involving 3467 asymptomatic patients randomised to CEA or CAS in seven RCTs.[45]

✓✓ In asymptomatic patients, CAS was associated with significantly higher rates of 30-day stroke (OR, 1.73; 95% CI, 1.06–2.84) and 30-day death/stroke (OR, 1.64; 95% CI, 1.02–2.64).[45] However, once the peri-operative period had elapsed, late ipsilateral stroke after CAS was no different to CEA, indicating that CAS was durable.

Despite declining stroke rates on BMT, it is inevitable that a small cohort of asymptomatic patients will gain benefit from intervention. The 2023 European Society for Vascular Surgery (ESVS) guidelines recommend that otherwise fit patients (expected to survive 5-years) with a 60–99% ACS and one or more clinical/imaging criteria making them 'high-risk for stroke' on BMT should be considered for CEA (Class IIa/B) or CAS (class IIb/B).[33] The ESVS 'high risk for stroke' clinical/imaging criteria are detailed in Table 10.9.

CAROTID ENDARTERECTOMY/CAROTID ARTERY STENTING AND CORONARY BYPASS

Recently symptomatic patients who are unable to undergo CEA/CAS because of unstable cardiac disease should undergo staged or synchronous CEA + coronary bypass (CABG) as soon as possible. This is because the risk of stroke is highest in the early period after onset of symptoms. In reality, this applies to <5% of all cardiac surgery patients.[58] A recent meta-analysis suggested that CAS + CABG carried a much higher risk of peri-operative stroke (15%) compared with CEA + CABG in patients with a prior history of stroke/TIA.[59] The role of prophylactic CEA/CAS in CABG patients with ACS remains controversial. In the USA, about 96% of staged/synchronous interventions

Table 10.7   Perioperative and late outcomes following CEA and BMT in VACS, ACAS and ACST

RCT	30-day death/ stroke after CEA	Ipsilateral stroke plus perioperative death or stroke		any stroke plus perioperative death or stroke	
		CEA	BMT	CEA	BMT
ACAS[20]	2.3%	5.1% at 5y	11.0% at5y	17.8% at 5y	12.4% at a5y
ACST-1[54]	2.8%	Not available	Not available	6.4% at 5y	11.8% at 5y
ACST-1[55]	2.8%	Not available	Not available	13.4% at 10y	17.9% at 10y

ACAS, Asymptomatic Carotid Atherosclerosis Study; *ACST*, Asymptomatic Carotid Surgery Trial; *BMT*, 'best medical therapy'; *CEA*, carotid endarterectomy.

Table 10.8   30-day morbidity and mortality in 7 randomised trials comparing CEA and CAS in 3467 asymptomatic patients*

	Death	Stroke	Death/ Stroke	Disabling Stroke	Death/ Disabling stroke	MI	Death/ Stroke/MI
	7 RCTs n=2286	7 RCTs n=3467	7 RCTs n=3467	5 RCTs n=2918	Insufficient data	5 RCTs n=2948	5 RCTs n=2948
CEA	0.7% (0.3-1.8)	1.9% (1.3-2.9)	2.1% (1.5-3.1)	0.5% (0.2-1.2)	Insufficient data	1.8% (1.1-2.8)	3.1% (2.2-4.3)
CAS	0.7% (0.3-1.7)	3.0% (2.3-3.8)	3.1% (2.4-4.0)	0.5% (0.3-1.0)	Insufficient data	0.8% (0.5-1.4)	3.3% (2.5-4.2)
OR (95%CI)	1.02 (0.18-5.90)	1.73** (1.1-2.8)	1.64 ** (1.02-2.64)	1.57 (0.40-6.19)	Insufficient data	0.53 (0.24-1.16)	1.14 (0.72-1.81)

*Data derived from Batchelder A, Saratzis A, Naylor AR. Overview of Primary and Secondary Analyses from 20 randomised controlled trials comparing carotid artery stenting with carotid endarterectomy. Eur J Vasc Endovasc Surg 2019;58:479-493.
**p<0.05.
CAS, Carotid artery stenting; *CEA*, carotid endarterectomy; *OR*, odds ratio; *95%CI*, 95% confidence intervals; *MI*, myocardial infarction.

Table 10.9   Clinical/imaging criteria for being considered 'higher risk for stroke on medical therapy*

Clinical	Prior contralateral TIA/stroke
CT/MRI	Ipsilateral silent brain infarction
Ultrasound based	Stenosis progression >20%
	Spontaneous embolisation on TCD
	Impaired cerebral vascular reserve
	Large area plaques (>80mm^2)
	Echolucent plaques
	Large juxta-luminal black area (>8mm^2)
MRI based	Intra-plaque haemorrhage
	Large lipid rich necrotic core

*Criteria derived from: Naylor AR, Ricco JB, de Borst GJ, Debus S, de Haro J, Halliday A et al. Management of atherosclerotic carotid and vertebral artery disease: 2017 Clinical practice guidelines of the European Society for Vascular Surgery (ESVS). Eur J Vasc Endovasc Surg 2018;55:3-86.

are undertaken in patients with ACS, the majority with unilateral stenoses.[58] In a pooled series of 23 557 patients undergoing CABG without prophylactic CEA/CAS, 95% of 476 observed post-operative strokes could not be attributed to underlying patterns of carotid disease.[60–62] Accordingly, most of the evidence suggests no causal relationship between a significant (asymptomatic) unilateral stenosis and post-operative stroke in the majority of cardiac surgical patients. This would suggest that other aetiologies play a more important role, particularly aortic arch atheroembolism.

✔✔ In a meta-analysis of 190 449 patients undergoing CABG,[63] the risk of stroke was 1.7% (95% CI, 1.5–1.9).

✔✔ A meta-analysis observed that three 'carotid' factors were predictive of post-CABG stroke: (i) carotid bruit, (ii) a prior history of stroke/TIA and (iii) the presence of a severe carotid stenosis or occlusion.[63]

✔ In an updated meta-analysis (which excluded symptomatic patients, those with bilateral stenoses and patients with unilateral carotid occlusion), patients undergoing isolated CABG in the presence of a unilateral, asymptomatic stenosis, incurred a 2% risk of procedural stroke. It is unlikely that prophylactic CEA/CAS could confer significant benefit, although it would still be reasonable to consider prophylactic interventions in CABG patients with bilateral severe asymptomatic disease.[64]

Table 10.10 details 30-day outcomes from a series of meta-analyses[59,65–67] regarding outcomes after synchronous/ staged CEA or CAS in CABG patients. In practice, the majority will involve patients with asymptomatic unilateral carotid stenoses.

Table 10.10   Peri-operative morbidity and mortality following staged/synchronous carotid interventions in patients undergoing cardiac surgery*

Parameter	n=	Death % (95%CI)	Stroke % (95%CI)	MI % (95%CI)	Death/stroke % (95%CI)	Death/stroke/MI % (95%CI)
synchronous CEA + CABG with CEA done pre-bypass	5386	4.5% (3.9-5.2)	4.5% (3.7-5.3)	3.6% (2.8-4.4)	8.2% (7.1-9.23)	11.5% (10.1-13.1)
synchronous CEA + CABG with CEA done on bypass	844	4.7% (3.1-6.4)	3.8% (2.0-5.5)	2.9% (1.3-4.6)	8.1% (5.8-10.3)	9.5% (5.9-13.1)
synchronous CEA + OPCAB	324	1.5% (0.3-2.8)	n/a	n/a	2.2% (0.7-3.7)	3.6% (1.6-5.5)
staged CEA – then CABG	917	3.9% 1.1-6.7)	2.7% (1.6-3.9)	6.5% (3.2-9.7)	6.1% 2.9-9.3)	10.2% (7.4-13.1)
reverse staged CABG then CEA	302	2.0% (0.0-6.1)	6.3% (1.0-11.7)	0.9% (0.5-1.4)	7.3% (1.7-12.9)	5.0% (0.0-10.6)
staged CAS then CABG (this study)	2196	4.8% (3.3-6.8)	5.4% (4.5-6.5)	4.2% (3.2-5.6)	8.5% (7.3-9.7)	11.0% (9.4-12.9)
Same-day CAS + CABG (this study)	531	4.5% (2.9-7.0)	3.4% (2.0-5.9)	1.8% (0.9-3.7)	5.9% (4.0-8.5)	6.5% (4.6-9.3)

*Based on data derived from a series of themed meta-analyses.[59,65,66,67]
OPCAB, Off pump coronary artery bypass.

✔ Morbidity and mortality rates after staged/synchronous CEA + CABG were considerably higher than when CEA or CAS were performed on their own. In a cohort of predominantly asymptomatic patients with unilateral stenoses, the procedural risks probably exceed the risk of performing isolated CABG, suggesting that cardiac surgery patients with unilateral, asymptomatic carotid stenoses will gain little additional benefit by performing staged or synchronous CEA/CAS.

EMERGENCY CAROTID ENDARTERECTOMY

In the 1960s emergency CEA for acute stroke was associated with significant mortality and morbidity, because of haemorrhagic transformation of areas of ischaemic infarction. This led to the abandonment of this strategy and a recommendation that patients should wait 6 weeks before undergoing CEA to stabilise the area of infarction. This is clearly at odds with current recommendations to expedite CEA analyses.[33] A meta-analysis has, however, shown that procedural risks for early CEA in patients with minor stroke and full/partial recovery were similar to those in patients for whom surgery was deferred.[68]

Although several single-centre studies have demonstrated the feasibility of CAS in the early period after onset of symptoms,[69] a pooled analysis of data from the CSTC showed that the risk of CAS, compared to CEA, was greatest in patients treated within 7-days of symptom onset.[43] It was also noted that CAS patients suffering peri-procedural complications underwent stenting significantly earlier, compared with patients whose treatment was uneventful. CAS therefore does not seem to be the treatment of choice in emergency cases.

✔ Emergency re-exploration (i.e. immediate) should be reserved for patients who suffer an acute thrombotic occlusion of the carotid artery after either CEA or CAS. Urgent CEA (<24 hours) is recommended in patients with stroke-in-evolution, stuttering hemiplegia or crescendo TIAs. There is no evidence that patients with an extensive neurological deficit should be considered for an early carotid intervention.

VERTEBRAL ARTERY REVASCULARISATION

The VB territory is affected in 15–25% of ischaemic strokes. In the past, it was believed that the majority of VB strokes were haemodynamic. However, the New England Posterior Circulation Registry reported that 40% were embolic (cardiac [60%], artery to artery [40%]; 32% haemodynamic), while 28% had miscellaneous causes (trauma, dissection, aneurysm, arteritis).[70] Of those TIAs secondary to vertebral/basilar artery stenoses or occlusions; 62% were located within the extracranial vertebral artery (VA) (origin 39%; near VA origin 30%; V2/V3 segment 31%), 30% affected the intracranial VA, while 8% affected the basilar artery. In a meta-analysis of early and long-term outcome data in patients with VB stroke/TIA and an extracranial VA stenosis, 30-day death/stroke was 1% in stented patients but by 3 years, there was still no benefit observed for stenting over BMT (HR, 0.63; 95% CI, 0.27–1.47).[71] The ESVS guidelines currently recommend extracranial VA stenting in patients with recurrent symptoms despite BMT.[33]

Three VB related syndromes are worthy of mention. An occlusion/severe stenosis at the subclavian artery origin may cause reversed flow down the ipsilateral VA to perfuse the arm (subclavian steal). Arm exercise may precipitate forearm claudication or dizziness. Intervention is usually recommended in patients with symptomatic lesions, especially involving the dominant arm. Both surgery and endovascular interventions carry a small risk of procedural stroke. At present, the latter is generally the first-choice intervention. A similar syndrome (coronary steal) occurs in patients who have undergone CABG using the internal mammary artery (usually the left). Should a proximal subclavian stenosis be missed pre-operatively (or develop subsequently) angina can be precipitated by arm exercise. In this situation, the angina can be treated by carotid–subclavian bypass or angioplasty/stenting. There is no evidence that either strategy is preferable. Third, it is traditionally believed that rotational (positional) dizziness/vertigo follows osteophyte compression of the extracranial VA. Evidence suggests that this is almost always never the case, and an alternative aetiology should be sought.[33]

SURGICAL MANAGEMENT OF CAROTID DISEASE – CAROTID ENDARTERECTOMY

ANAESTHESIA

CEA under locoregional anaesthesia is the only reliable method for predicting who needs a shunt, but it will not prevent thromboembolism (the main cause of intra-operative stroke).

✓✓ In a meta-analysis of 31 studies (152 376 patients), there was no evidence that choice of anaesthesia (general or locoregional) influenced 30-day outcomes.[72]

TECHNIQUE

CEA is usually performed using loupe magnification with the extended head turned away from the side of the operation and placed on a rubber ring. An incision is made over the anterior border of the sternocleidomastoid muscle and dissection continued down to the carotid bifurcation after division of the common facial vein.

✓ A meta-analysis of four non-randomised trials and two RCTs (740 CEAs) found no evidence that retrojugular (versus antegrade) exposure was associated with reductions in peri-operative death (0.6% vs. 0.5%) or stroke (0.9% vs. 0.7%).[73]

✓✓ A meta-analysis of four RCTs found no evidence that carotid sinus nerve blockade reduced hypotension, hypertension or arrhythmias after CEA.[74]

The distal ICA is mobilised 1 cm beyond the upper limit of the plaque, facilitated by ligation and division of the sternomastoid vessels, which tether the hypoglossal nerve (with/without division of the digastric muscle). If surgeons are worried about the need to proceed higher in the neck, access can be facilitated (pre-operatively) by nasolaryngeal intubation or temporomandibular subluxation. The latter must be planned in advance as it cannot be performed once the operation has started. The main cranial nerves (hypoglossal, vagus) are identified. With high dissections, the glossopharyngeal nerve is at risk. Contrary to classical teaching, however, most post-operative swallowing problems do not follow glossopharyngeal nerve injury but are secondary to damage to the motor branches of the vagus, which cross the ICA anteriorly, just distal to the hypoglossal nerve.

✓✓ Any patient who has undergone a contralateral CEA, neck dissection or thyroidectomy must undergo a pre-operative check of recurrent laryngeal and hypoglossal nerve function. Bilateral injuries can be fatal.

Following systemic heparinisation, clamps are applied to the ICA, CCA and ECA. A longitudinal arteriotomy is made across the plaque and into the distal ICA. If a shunt is to be deployed, it is inserted now.

✓ A Cochrane review of six RCTs (1270 CEAs) concluded that no meaningful recommendations could be made regarding shunting strategies because of poor-quality data. The choice of whether to selectively, routinely or never shunt is, therefore left to the discretion of the surgeon.[75]

✓ If the surgeon is a 'selective shunter', the only way of knowing who needs a shunt is to perform CEA under locoregional anaesthesia.

The endarterectomy plane is developed using a Watson–Cheyne dissector and it is conventional to divide the plaque proximally and then mobilise it towards the distal ICA. The upper end usually feathers but can be tacked down. Loose intimal fragments are removed in a radial, as opposed to axial, direction. An alternative technique is 'eversion' endarterectomy. Here the ICA origin is transected and reimplanted after eversion of the atheromatous core.

✓ Systematic reviews suggest that eversion endarterectomy confers similar benefits to traditional endarterectomy provided the arteriotomy is closed with a patch. Patched CEA and eversion CEA are associated with better early and late outcomes than where the arteriotomy is routinely primarily closed.[76]

PERI-OPERATIVE MONITORING AND COMPLETION ASSESSMENT

The aim of monitoring is to prevent cerebral ischaemia before permanent neurological injury occurs. The simplest is a subjective assessment of ICA backflow or stump pressure, but this may bear little relation to intracranial perfusion in the presence of circle of Willis abnormalities. TCD is probably the most versatile of monitoring methods and uses a low-frequency (2 MHz) pulsed-wave ultrasound beam directed through the temporal bone. This permits insonation of the middle cerebral artery (MCA), which receives 80% of ICA inflow. The quality of the signal depends on the thickness of the cranium and an inaccessible window may be present in about 10% of patients.

A single monitoring modality, however, is no guarantee of protection. During CEA, TCD fulfils four roles: (i) diagnosing embolisation during carotid dissection (unstable plaque), (ii) ensuring mean MCA velocity remains >15 cm/s, (iii) ensuring the shunt is working (3% abut on a distal ICA coil or kink and malfunction) and (iv) diagnosing the very rare case of on-table thrombosis following flow restoration.[77] Neurological activity can be monitored using locoregional anaesthesia and this is the gold standard for determining who needs a shunt. However, it will not prevent thromboembolic complications. Neurological activity can be evaluated indirectly by electroencephalogram (EEG) or sensory-evoked potential (SEP) measurement. Once perfusion falls below 18 mL/100 g brain per minute there is loss of high-frequency activity on the EEG, whereas below 15 mL/100 g brain per minute, the EEG becomes isoelectric.[78] The advantage of intra-operative SEP measurement is that it reflects the function of the afferent pathway from a peripheral nerve (usually the median nerve) to the somatosensory cortex. Ischaemia causes a reduction in the amplitude of the primary cortical wave and prolongation of central conduction time.

✔ The surgeon should remember that just because an EEG trace may be flat, it does not mean that neurological injury is inevitable, as this only occurs once perfusion falls below 10 mL/100 g brain per minute.[78] Loss of EEG function is a warning that insertion of a shunt or elevation of systemic BP is warranted.

The role of completion assessment is to identify technical error (incomplete endarterectomy, intimal flaps, luminal thrombus, residual stenoses, wall irregularities). The most important is exclusion of luminal thrombus, which often originates from bleeding from transected vasa vasorum onto the endarterectomised vessel surface. Quality control techniques include TCD, completion angiography, DUS, CW-Doppler and angioscopy. TCD ensures optimal shunt function and is the only method capable of also diagnosing embolisation, on-table thrombosis and post-operative occlusion. Angiography (which must be biplanar) provides anatomical data but requires ionising radiation and can only be performed after restoration of flow (i.e. any thrombus could be swept distally). The latest colour DUS probes are smaller and more accessible because of the development of L-shaped probes, but usually require the presence of a technician in theatre. The principal advantage of angioscopy is that it is performed *before* restoration of flow. Its main role is to identify the 3–5% of patients with residual luminal thrombus and the 1% with large intimal flaps.[77]

OPERATIVE COMPLICATIONS

CRANIAL NERVE INJURIES

✔✔ CNI are an important source of morbidity, but very few are permanent or disabling.

In a meta-analysis of 7535 patients in 13 RCTs comparing CEA with CAS; CNI after CAS was 0.5% (95% CI, 0.3–0.9), versus 5.4% (95% CI, 4.7–6.2) after CEA (OR, 0.07; 95% CI, 0.04–0.1).[45] In another meta-analysis of 16 749 CEA patients, the incidence of CNI was 4.2% for the recurrent laryngeal nerve, 3.8% for the hypoglossal nerve, 1.6% for the mandibular branch of the facial nerve, 0.2% for the glossopharyngeal nerve and 0.2% for the spinal accessory nerve.[79]

WOUND COMPLICATIONS

In six RCTs (2988 CEA patients), 2.2% (95% CI, 1.2–3.9) developed a haematoma requiring re-exploration.[80] Risk factors included; female gender, anticoagulation, atrial fibrillation. A systematic review and meta-analysis of outcomes in 3817 CEA patients receiving protamine and 6070 CEA patients not receiving protamine, reported that protamine administration was associated with a significant reduction in the incidence of neck haematoma requiring re-exploration (OR, 0.42; 95% CI, 0.22–0.8; $P = 0.008$), with no evidence of an increase in peri-operative stroke (OR, 0.71; 95% CI, 0.49–1.03; $P = 0.07$).[80] Early vein patch rupture complicates <1% of CEAs, but is virtually abolished provided saphenous vein is harvested from the groin.

PERI-OPERATIVE STROKE

Peri-operative stroke is classed as intra-operative if the patient recovers from anaesthesia with a new deficit and post-operative if the event occurs some time thereafter. In historical series, intra-operative stroke predominated and were more likely to affect patients with a combination of cerebral infarction and partial/total haemodynamic compromise. This suggests that high-risk patients are more vulnerable to otherwise minor changes in perfusion or emboli, so that the margin for technical error is reduced or possibly non-existent.

Intra-operative stroke has been virtually abolished at the Leicester Vascular Institute (0.25% in 2900 cases), mainly attributed to removing residual luminal thrombus (identified by angioscopy) before flow restoration.[77] The source of residual luminal thrombus was found to be bleeding from transected vasa vasorum. The commonest causes of post-operative stroke are: (i) ICA thrombosis (especially in the first 6 post-operative hours), (ii) hyperperfusion syndrome (HS) and (iii) intracranial haemorrhage (ICH). Patients destined to suffer an early post-operative stroke because of thrombosis/embolism have platelets that are more sensitive to aggregation to adenosine diphosphate (ADP). This complication can be prevented by prescribing DAPT (aspirin and clopidogrel) pre-operatively.[77] ICH and HS complicate 1–2% of CEAs and are more common in patients with severe bilateral extracranial disease, in association with impaired cerebral vascular reserve, defective autoregulation and poor collateral flow patterns.

Most cases of ICH and HS are preceded by post-CEA hypertension and units should have clear guidance for the urgent management of this condition. In Leicester,[77] a systolic BP >170 mmHg in theatre recovery is treated by boluses of intravenous labetalol +/- infusion, with the second line agent being hydralazine. Back on the ward, treatment of patients with a systolic BP >170 mmHg (in the absence of headache, seizures or neurological deficit) depends on whether patients are already taking anti-hypertensive therapy. If not, the first-line oral agent is 10 mg nifedipine retard (never crush a capsule), with 5 mg bisoprolol added if required. If the patient is already on anti-hypertensive therapy, the ABCD system is helpful; *(A = angiotensin-converting enzyme[ACE] inhibitor, B = B-Blocker, C = Calcium Channel Blocker, D = Diuretic).* If the patient is taking A, add C (nifedipine LA 10 mg). If the patient is taking C, add A (ramipril 5 mg). If the patient is taking D, add A (ramipril 5 mg). If the patient is taking A+C, add in D (bendrofluazide 2.5 mg). If the patient is taking A+D, add in C (nifedipine LA 10 mg), while if the patient is taking A+C+D, add in B (bisoprolol 5 mg).[77] Any patient developing a systolic BP >160 mmHg in the presence of headache, seizure or neurological deficit should be considered a neurological emergency. The first-line treatment is control of seizures with intravenous lorazepam (and/or appropriate anti-epileptic drugs) followed by boluses of labetalol (+/- infusion) as per the protocol used in theatre recovery, with iv hydralazine as second line. Bolus treatment with iv labetalol must be started immediately and the patient transferred to high dependency care unit/intensive care unit for further monitoring and treatment.[77]

✔ Emergency medical units must recognise the importance of rapid BP treatment in the CEA patient who presents with seizures, usually 5–7 days after surgery. These patients have a high risk of ICH, and the mainstay of treatment is control of seizures and aggressive BP control.

The strategy for managing peri-operative stroke depends on: (i) timing (intra-operative/post-operative), (ii) whether it follows thrombosis, embolism or haemorrhage and (iii) the severity of the deficit. The more extensive the deficit, the more likely that the ICA/MCA has occluded. For those without access to TCD or DUS, the surgeon has to assume that any deficit following recovery from anaesthesia or in the first 24 hours is thromboembolic and the patient should be re-explored. Although re-exploration will not benefit patients with MCA branch embolism or haemodynamic stroke, this cannot be avoided. The management of MCA embolisation will be discussed in the section on CAS. For those with access to TCD, decision-making is easier. The immediate priority is to identify patients with ICA thrombosis, as they require immediate exploration. Provided flow is restored within 1 hour, good neurological recovery can be expected.

✔ TCD features of early carotid thrombosis include flow reversal in the ipsilateral anterior cerebral artery, enhanced flow in the ipsilateral posterior cerebral artery and, most importantly, flow velocities in the ipsilateral MCA that mimic those observed during carotid clamping.

✔ The administration of 75 mg clopidogrel the night before surgery (in addition to regular aspirin) was found to virtually abolish stroke because of early post-operative carotid thrombosis.[77]

LONG-TERM FOLLOW-UP AND RESTENOSIS

A number of centres perform serial DUS surveillance after CEA and CAS although a definite association between a recurrent asymptomatic stenosis and late ipsilateral stroke has never convincingly been demonstrated. A recent meta-analysis of DUS surveillance data in patients who were randomised within 11 RCTs found no evidence that an asymptomatic 70–99% restenosis after CAS was associated with a higher risk of late ipsilateral stroke (0.8% at mean 50 months follow-up), compared with 2.0% in CAS patients without a significant restenosis (OR, 0.87; 95% CI, 0.24–3.21).[81] By contrast, CEA patients with an untreated asymptomatic restenosis >70% incurred a 4.5% risk of late ipsilateral stroke at a mean of 37 months, compared with 1.5% in CEA patients with no evidence of a significant restenosis (OR, 4.38; 95% CI, 2.08–9.25).[81] However, once the peri-operative risk of redo CEA or CAS was factored in, very few CEA patients with asymptomatic restenoses >70% will gain benefit from reintervention.

✔ Patients who present with recurrent TIA/stroke after CEA and who have a 50–99% recurrent stenosis should be considered for treatment by CAS or redo CEA.

PATCH INFECTION

Patch infection complicates <1% of CEAs. If infection is suspected, the CCA must be controlled below the original incision. The prosthetic patch should be removed and replaced (where possible) with vein (bypass/patch). Infected prosthetic patches should not be treated by insertion of further prosthetic material, as there is a very high risk of reinfection.[82] Ligation should only be considered as a last resort (uncontrollable haemorrhage) and preferably if some form of monitoring (e.g., TCD, awake neurological testing at the original procedure) suggests that collateral flow is satisfactory.

✔ No abscess overlying a CEA wound should be incised before being seen by a vascular surgeon.

ENDOVASCULAR TREATMENT OF CAROTID DISEASE

ASSESSING SUITABILITY FOR CAROTID ARTERY STENTING

Careful case selection is mandatory, and most patients being considered for CAS require 'overview' anatomical imaging (arch to the circle of Willis) with CTA/MRA to allow evaluation of the anatomy of the access vessels, configuration of

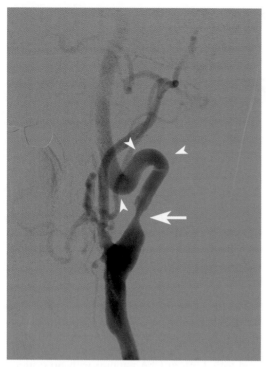

Figure 10.8 Digital subtraction angiogram of the left carotid bifurcation demonstrating a high-grade stenosis (*arrow*) and severe tortuosity of the distal left internal carotid artery (*arrowheads*) that may preclude the use of distal protection devices (filters and distal balloons).

the aortic arch, tortuosity and length of the CCA and ICA, and to exclude significant disease involving the ECA. Absolute contraindications include an occluded ICA (except in cases of acute stroke with a so-called tandem occlusion of ICA and ipsilateral MCA) or visible thrombus. Anatomical factors that increase the technical difficulty of CAS include those related to ICA access (low carotid bifurcation/short CCA, tortuous CCA, diseased CCA and disease or occlusion of the ECA), the configuration of the aortic arch (severe arch atheroma, severe arch origin disease, type III arch and bovine arch) and characteristics of the target vessel (pinhole stenosis, angulated ICA origin, angulated distal ICA and circumferential ICA calcification).[83] A difficult origin to the brachiocephalic artery/left CCA or severe CCA tortuosity are relative contraindications. Tortuosity of the ICA above the stenosis (Fig. 10.8) may prevent use of filter or distal occlusive protection systems. This sort of tortuosity can potentially be transformed into a kink or occlusion following stent deployment. The absence of (occlusive) disease of the ECA is essential to enable placement of a long guidewire into the ECA to perform an exchange of the diagnostic catheter for a long introduction sheath or guiding catheter. ECA patency is also a prerequisite for the use of proximal embolic protection devices that use an occlusive ECA balloon (see later).

DUAL ANTIPLATELET THERAPY

It is routine practice to prescribe DAPT before CAS; 75 mg of clopidogrel is commenced 1 week before intervention in addition to 75 mg aspirin daily. In recently symptomatic patients, 300–600 mg clopidogrel (depending on body weight) is given at least 15-hours pre-intervention. The

dual antiplatelet regime should continue for at least 28 days post-procedure.

✓✓ Randomised trials have confirmed the benefit of peri-operative DAPT before CAS.[84]

CAROTID ARTERY STENTING TECHNIQUE

The most commonly used access route is via the common femoral artery. Brachial, radial or direct carotid approaches are alternatives if there is a difficult arch ('type III' or 'bovine'). In a type III arch, the origin of the brachiocephalic is significantly lower than a horizontal line drawn across the highest point of the arch. In a 'bovine' arch, there is a conjoint origin to the brachiocephalic and left CCA.

During the procedure, anticoagulation (usually heparin) should be administered to reduce the risk of thrombus formation around intra-arterial sheaths, catheters and guidewires. The optimal dose of heparin ranges from 75 to 100 units/kg. In a standard patient, a single dose of 5000–7500 units will usually be sufficient throughout the entire CAS procedure, provided it does not take more than 45 minutes and (therefore) activated clotting time (ACT) measurement is not routinely necessary. The effect of heparin is generally allowed to subside in a physiological way, and protamine sulphate reversal is not usually recommended. Lesion access depends on anatomy, experience and choice of protection. Methods include: (i) exchange technique (ipsilateral ECA accessed with a selective catheter and hydrophilic guidewire with subsequent exchange for supportive exchange-length guidewire over which a long sheath is advanced); (ii) co-axial technique with advancement of a dedicated catheter and long 6-Fr sheath over a wire into the CCA, thus avoiding interaction with the bifurcation; and (iii) 'direct probing' with an 8-Fr guiding catheter that is positioned just beyond the ostium of the great vessel of interest (helpful in patients with a type III arch), and which is therefore slightly more vulnerable to catheter prolapse and loss of secure access during the procedure.

The stenosis is then either crossed with a distal cerebral protection device (CPD) or after deployment of a proximal CPD (see 'Cerebral protection devices'). Stent delivery systems are mostly 5-Fr or 6-Fr compatible. Occasionally, it is possible to cross the lesion with the delivery system without pre-dilatation, but plaque 'snow-ploughing' must be avoided. Severe stenoses (80–90%) require 3-mm pre-dilatation to permit safe passage of the stent-delivery system. Stent length should be chosen such that it will cover the carotid artery over at least 5 mm proximal and 5 mm beyond the stenosis. Extreme elongation or kinks situated close to the stenosis should also be taken into account when choosing stent length, to avoid arterial redundancy and a tendency to increase the amount of kinking. One must avoid placing the distal end of the stent into kinks and tortuosities of the ICA, because these kinks cannot be eliminated and tend to be displaced distally. Stent diameter should be oversized by at least 1 mm with respect to the reference vessel diameter. In the event that the stent needs to extend from the CCA into the ICA (i.e. covering the origin of the ECA), a tapered stent should be used. The stent is delivered across the stenosis using road mapping (when filter protection is used) or by reference to a 'control' image with bony anatomy once flow arrest/flow reversal has been established. Once deployed, the stent can be dilated to ensure good apposition against the arterial wall. It is important to avoid aggressive post-dilatation as emboli are generated during this phase of the procedure. Many practitioners are comfortable with leaving some degree of residual stenosis. This is on the understanding that most Nitinol stent systems will continue to expand after deployment and because the 'potato masher effect' should be avoided. Atropine (0.6–1.2 mg) or 200 µg glycopyrrolate (synthetic derivative with less cardioaccelerator effect) is delivered just before balloon dilatation and stent placement either via the sheath or intravenously to block the carotid sinus baroreceptors.

✔️ Atropine/glycopyrrolate will cause short-term unilateral mydriasis if administered via the arterial sheath. Staff looking after the patient upon return to the ward should be notified about this harmless finding.

Angiography is performed in at least two planes after completion of the procedure with attention directed towards excluding plaque prolapse into the lumen through stent interstices (or platelet/thrombus aggregates) (Fig. 10.9). This requires gentle re-ballooning or 'double scaffolding' (placement of a second stent inside the first). Plaque prolapse may be less likely to occur with dual-layer or micromesh stent systems that consist of a nitinol outer layer and a micromesh inner layer with very small cell size. A small RCT (104 patients with lipid-rich plaques) showed that the use of a dual layer stent resulted in a 13–29% reduction in micro-embolic signals during stent deployment.[85]

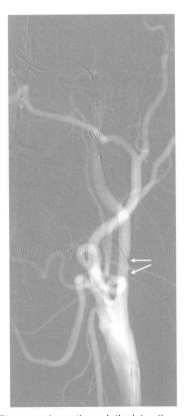

Figure 10.9 Plaque prolapse through the interstices of a closed-cell stent (Abbott XAct; *arrows*). This was treated by placing a second stent inside the first, i.e. 'double scaffolding'.

Spasm (usually well tolerated) is managed by careful cephalad movement of the filter, the administration of diluted nitroglycerine (100–200 µg) or (200 µg diluted in a 10-mL solution injected slowly as a 2–3 mL bolus) into the long sheath and timely completion of the procedure. A full filter (causing sluggish flow) requires aspiration with a 0.014-inch compatible rapid-exchange system. Proximal CPD devices avoid these issues, but a proportion of patients are intolerant, leading to yawning, lack of responsiveness, obtundation or seizure. This can be dealt with by either intermittent flow reversal or by stopping flow reversal and using a distal filter.

An evaluation of 627 protected CAS procedures has yielded important information regarding the timing of complications during (after) CAS.[86] At 30-days there were 10 major strokes (two fatal), 18 minor strokes (2.9%) and one cardiac death. Four major strokes occurred in phase 1 (catheterisation of the arch, target vessel and CCA) and six in phase 3 (stent deployment, pre- and post-dilatation). It was concluded that a large proportion of major strokes (4/10) during CAS occurred during catheterisation and that these could not have been prevented by the use of a protection device.

CEREBRAL PROTECTION DEVICES

No RCTs have determined whether CPDs reduce the risk of post-CAS stroke. A Cochrane Review on stenting for symptomatic carotid artery stenoses (based on outcomes from EVA-3S, SPACE and ICSS)[87] concluded that for the outcome of death or any stroke within 30-days after treatment, there was no evidence that the use of filter-type CPDs was beneficial. By contrast, a meta-analysis of 22 non-randomised studies (n = 11 655) reported significantly lower rates of peri-operative stroke/death favouring the use of CPDs (OR, 0.57; 95% CI, 0.43–0.76; $P < 0.01$).[88] Notwithstanding the conflicting data, most CAS practitioners currently use some form of cerebral protection during the procedure. A recent meta-analysis has shown no difference in outcome between proximal and distal CPDs.[89]

DISTAL BALLOON OCCLUSION

Although the rationale is simple, there are a number of disadvantages. Angulated lesions may be difficult to cross, the distal balloon can damage the ICA wall, 10% of patients are intolerant of ICA occlusion and the stenosis cannot be imaged whilst the ICA is occluded. These devices are not widely used anymore.

DISTAL FILTER DEVICES

These devices can be divided into mesh-like filters, or filters that make use of a porous membrane that can be eccentric or concentric. These devices are either premounted onto a wire that comes with the delivery system (wire-mounted filters) or are inserted over a previously positioned guidewire (bare-wire filters). The filter is placed in a way similar to the placement of a bare guidewire. Pre-dilatation before passage of the filter is typically not performed. Care should be taken to deploy the filter in a segment of the ICA that is straight, to allow for proper wall appositioning of the filter. Furthermore, the filter should be placed at a distance from the stenosis that allows the tip of the stent delivery system and distal part of the stent to cross the lesion. In cases of severe tortuosity (where the filter cannot be advanced), the use of an adjunctive wire ('buddy wire') will help to straighten out the ICA, thus facilitating passage of the protection device. The filter is retrieved following final stent dilatation. There is the potential for filter through-flow (controlled by pore size) and filter peri-flow. Self-limiting spasm of the ICA is relatively common (Fig. 10.10a–c).

FLOW REVERSAL/FLOW ARREST (ENDOVASCULAR CLAMPING)

The working principle of proximal CPDs is by either completely interrupting or reversing blood flow in the ICA. In this way, 'endovascular clamping' can be achieved, with cerebral perfusion relying on collateralisation via the circle of Willis. These devices cannot be used in all cases, because complete occlusion/flow reversal is not tolerated by up to 30% of patients.[90] Embolic particles can be aspirated, and the systems offer the advantage that the ICA stenosis is only crossed once the protection device is in place and thus all manipulation needed to cross the lesion is performed during protection. The currently available proximal CPD systems create occlusion of the ECA and ICA with separate balloons.

MoMa (Medtronic-Invatec) consists of an 8-Fr or 9-Fr sheath that provides an effective working channel of 5-Fr or 6-Fr, respectively, with two balloons that can be inflated independently (Fig. 10.11a–e). The distal balloon is located close to the sheath tip and is used to occlude the ECA. The proximal balloon is located on the body of the sheath and is inflated within the CCA. When inflated, both balloons prevent antegrade flow from the CCA and retrograde flow from the ECA, leading to complete flow cessation. The device is advanced into the ECA. The distal ECA balloon should be placed proximal to the origin of the superior thyroid artery to provide flow interruption/reversal. Once the device is in place, the stenting procedure can be performed. Following CAS, three 20-mL syringes of carotid blood are aspirated and checked for debris before deflating the distal and then the proximal balloons, thus re-establishing cerebral blood flow.

The ENROUTE system (otherwise known as *Transcarotid Artery Revascularisation* [TCAR]) involves flow reversal via a mini proximal CCA incision and does not require occlusion of the ipsilateral ECA to achieve flow reversal into the femoral vein. This is achieved by means of low-resistance, wide-bore dialysis tubing that completes the extracorporeal circuit. Direct access via the CCA cut-down avoids wire and sheath manipulation within the aortic arch.[91]

DOES STENT DESIGN INFLUENCE OUTCOME?

A systematic review of 32 studies (1363 procedures) found that closed-cell stents significantly reduced NIBLs on diffusion-weighted MRI, compared with open-cell stents.[92] In SPACE, the closed-cell WallStent was associated with significantly better outcomes than open cell Acculink or Precise stents,[93] while ICSS also observed better outcomes where CAS was performed using closed-cell designed stents.[94] A recent meta-analysis (two RCTs, 66 cohort studies; 46 728 procedures) reported that short-term and intermediate term clinical major adverse event (MAE) rates were similar for patients treated with open versus closed cell or hybrid stents.[95] The Acculink stent was associated with a higher risk of short-term MAEs, compared with the Wallstent (RR, 1.5; *P* = 0.03), as was the Precise stent versus Xact stent (RR, 1.55; *P* < 0.001). The use of open cell stents is associated with a 25% higher chance (RR, 1.25; *P* = 0.03) of developing post-operative NIBLs. The incidence of restenosis, stent fracture, or intra-procedural hemodynamic depression was similar between the various stent designs.[95]

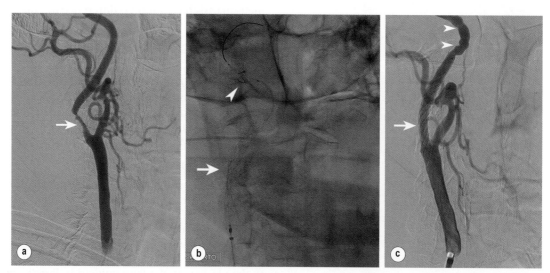

Figure 10.10   (a) Digital subtraction angiogram (DSA) image of high-grade symptomatic stenosis (*arrow*) of the right internal carotid artery (RICA). The straightforward anatomy allows use of a distal filter-type protection device. (b) Fluoroscopic image after placement of dual layer stent (*arrow*); filter device is still in place (*arrowhead*). (c) Completion DSA showing restoration of flow, with smooth stent surface (*arrow*). Note non-flow limiting spasm in the distal RICA at the level of the previous position of the embolic protection device (*arrowhead*). In this case, no treatment was necessary.

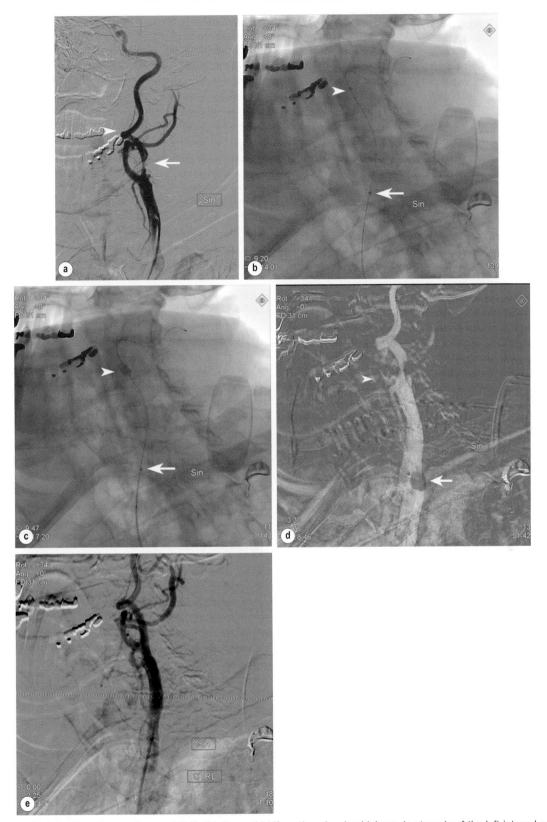

Figure 10.11   (a) Digital subtraction angiogram (DSA) of left carotid bifurcation showing high-grade stenosis of the left internal carotid artery (LICA) (*arrow*). Note tortuosity of the distal LICA (*arrowhead*), rendering the use of a distal cerebral protection device (CPD) unfavourable. (b) Fluoroscopic image with MoMa device inserted over a guidewire into the left external carotid artery (ECA). Markers for the distal ECA balloon (*arrowhead*) and proximal common carotid artery (*arrow*) are clearly visible. (c) Fluoroscopic image with distal ECA balloon inflated (*arrowhead*), proximal balloon marker indicated by *arrow*. (d) Roadmap image with both distal (*arrowhead*) and proximal (*arrow*) protection balloons inflated. The roadmap image is used for stent positioning. (e) Completion DSA after stent placement and removal of proximal CPD.

PERI-PROCEDURAL HAEMODYNAMIC PROBLEMS

HAEMODYNAMIC DEPRESSION

Haemodynamic instability is common during CAS and is probably baroreceptor mediated. Measures for preventing haemodynamic instability include adequate hydration and withholding antihypertensive medications on the morning of CAS. Early CAS literature suggested that without anticholinergic prophylaxis, the incidence of intra-procedural hypotension was 17–22%, while 28–71% developed bradycardia. Post-procedural hypotension is common (usually lasting about 24 hours) but is usually benign. Treatment is reserved for symptomatic patients or those in whom sustained hypotension may cause cardiovascular compromise (e.g., patients awaiting CABG or aortic valve replacement). Treatment in symptomatic or 'at-risk' patients includes antimuscarinic and/or selective alpha agonists. A recent study evaluated the use of vasopressors in the critical care unit (CCU) for the treatment of persistent post-CAS hypotension in 623 patients.[96] The authors concluded that in patients with a systolic BP ≤90 mmHg, especially those protracted cases where the BP was low for ≥24 hours, there was a significant increase in the risk of stroke/death/MI.[96] Furthermore, compared with the mixed alpha/beta-agonist dopamine, the more selective alpha-agonists (norepinephrine and phenylephrine) were associated with a shorter infusion time and reduced CCU lengths of stay and fewer major adverse events. Patients that develop clinically significant haemodynamic instability are more likely to experience periprocedural stroke, as compared to patients that are haemodynamically stable (8% vs. 1%, respectively). Patients that received prophylactic anticholinergic therapy did not show any increase in procedural stroke, even if they developed clinically significant haemodynamic instability. Haemodynamic depression after CEA occurs less frequently, and its management is the same as for post-CAS hypotension. Haemodynamic disturbances are an important cause of stroke during both CEA and CAS in ICSS. In CAS patients, it was the most frequent cause of stroke, and is probably related to carotid sinus manipulation and baroreceptor dysfunction related to stenting.[97]

HYPERPERFUSION AND INTRACRANIAL HAEMORRHAGE

No consensus criteria exist for diagnosing cerebral hyperperfusion syndrome (CHS), but clinical presentation includes headache (35%), +/- confusion, hemiparesis, seizures, decreased level of consciousness and nausea and vomiting. The average time between CEA/CAS and onset of symptoms is 12 hours.[98,99] Several mechanisms may be associated with CHS, including failure of autoregulation, baroreflex disturbances, and disturbances in the trigeminovascular reflex. Hyperperfusion (and ICH) are more frequently seen after CAS (pooled estimate 4.6% [range 0–25%]) than after CEA (range 0–3%), possibly because CAS is accompanied by intra-procedural hypotension, followed by a state of compensatory hypertension.

In a meta-analysis, the pooled frequency of ICH in patients diagnosed with CHS was 38%, incurring a 51% mortality rate.[100] Hypertension and ipsilateral high-grade stenoses are risk factors for ICH,[100] reinforcing the importance of careful BP control after carotid revascularisation. Prophylactic pharmacotherapy (short-acting beta-blockers) is considered in patients deemed high risk and may reduce the incidence of HS and ICH.[101]

✓ Intra-procedural haemodynamic instability is an important cause of stroke. Baseline systolic BP >180 mmHg in a patient without prior good control of BP is an independent risk factor for an increased incidence of intra- and peri-procedural hypotension/hypertension. If hypotension develops, the magnitude of BP drop correlates linearly with the severity of subsequent neurological insult. Permissive tolerance of an elevated systolic BP in patients with good BP control is supportive during CAS procedures with proximal protection. Withholding ACE inhibitors and calcium antagonists before the procedure generally allows a pressure that will withstand 'endovascular clamping'. A procedural systolic BP of ≥160 mmHg generally supports the use of proximal embolic protection.

MANAGEMENT OF POST-CAROTID ARTERY STENTING AND POST-CAROTID ENDARTERECTOMY EMBOLIC STROKE

The endovascular treatment of acute stroke has been demonstrated to provide significant clinical benefit over intravenous thrombolysis in five RCTs[102] and many of these endovascular techniques can now be applied to treating acute embolic stroke after CEA or CAS (especially embolisation of the MCA mainstem).[103,104]

DISTAL EMBOLISM

In cases of stroke secondary to macro-emboli, these can be removed mechanically or via thrombolysis.[103,104] Mechanical removal has a theoretical advantage over thrombolytic therapy because it carries a lower risk of bleeding (especially in cases where hyperperfusion is more likely to occur) and because the material that may be dislodged can be expected to be more organised and/or non-thrombotic.[103] Mechanical removal of embolic material from the intracranial branches of the ICA is possible using neuro-interventional retrieval systems. Proximal devices include aspiration catheters, while distal devices include spiral-shaped or basket-like devices. These are typically introduced through a guiding catheter or long introduction sheath and are advanced beyond the point of occlusion in an undeployed state (Fig. 10.12).

For aspiration thrombectomy (at the intracranial level), several microcatheters that originated from cardiac practice have been used in the past, but nowadays specific devices for intracranial use are available. Catheters fit for this purpose should have a large inner lumen, and because of the tortuous intracranial anatomy, they should be kink-resistant. The latter is typically provided by micro-braiding the catheter shaft. Sufficient aspiration power can be obtained by using a dedicated vacuum pump. If this system is not available,

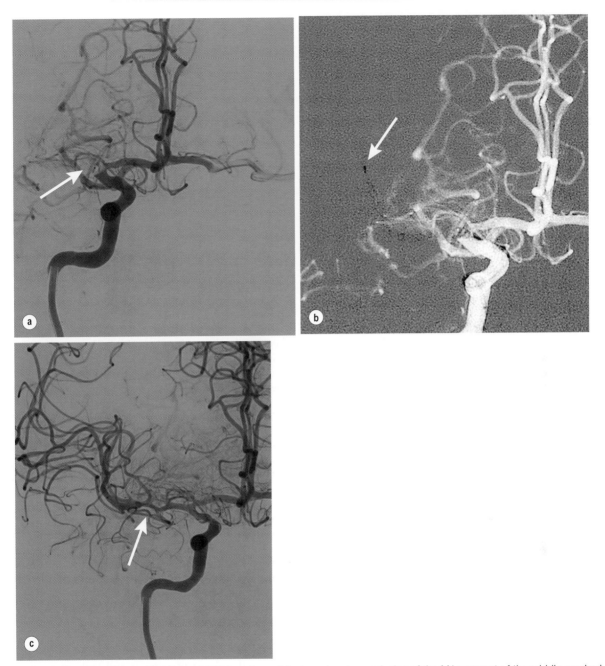

Figure 10.12   (a) Selective angiography of the right internal carotid artery showing occlusion of the M1 segment of the middle cerebral artery (*arrow*) after treatment of acute stent thrombosis with thrombo-aspiration (same patient as in Fig. 10.13). (b) Roadmap image of the right internal carotid artery with stent retriever (*arrow*) in place. (c) Digital subtraction angiogram (DSA) of control angiography demonstrating restoration of flow in the middle cerebral artery (*arrow*).

negative pressure can be obtained by using a 50-mL syringe for larger bore catheters (used in the CCA or the cervical portion of the ICA), but when using microcatheters: smaller syringes (<10 mL) can be used, although the vacuum is less efficient. The catheter should be advanced until it contacts the thrombus, and then negative pressure should be applied. One specific advantage of aspiration catheters is that they can be used in situations where there is limited space beyond the occlusion where distal retrieval devices cannot be used (e.g., distal MCA mainstem branches or bifurcations).

In the absence of dedicated retrieval devices, restoration of antegrade flow can be achieved by fragmenting the embolus using balloon angioplasty or guidewire manipulation.[102,103] Wire fragmentation should be performed using a flexible hydrophilic-tipped guidewire (0.008–0.010 inches). The wire tip should be formed into a J-shape to avoid vessel perforation. Penetration and fragmentation of the thrombus can be achieved by gently advancing and rotating the wire. Balloon angioplasty tends to be relatively ineffective, because of the spongy nature of the clot/embolus that tends to recoil. In cases of recoil, additional stent placement at the level of the (residual) embolus may be performed. To be able to reach the lesion, flexible stents and stent delivery systems should be used. A major disadvantage of the fragmentation technique (and to a lesser extent stenting) is the relatively high risk of distal embolisation.

Intra-arterial thrombolysis is an effective therapy for acute thrombotic occlusion of cerebral vessels.[103,104] The site of occlusion, type of thrombus and presence of leptomeningeal collateralisation influences the chance of recanalisation. Typically, occlusions of the proximal carotid terminus and M1 segment of the MCA respond poorly to intra-arterial thrombolysis, mainly because of the large clot burden, which requires a longer time to achieve complete thrombolysis. Although a thrombus in the MCA mainstem may be successfully treated, clinical success may be negatively influenced by non-recanalisation of smaller lenticulostriate branches. Thrombolytic agents include urokinase and recombinant tissue plasminogen activator (rTPA), and these are delivered through a super-selectively placed microcatheter. An infusion microcatheter (<3.0-Fr) with a single end-hole should be placed into the proximal third of the thrombus using a steerable micro guidewire. Using a so-called coaxial catheter technique, the microcatheter is advanced through a Y-connector, attached to a diagnostic catheter with a lumen of at least 0.038 in. The Y-connector also allows for continuous flushing of the microcatheter with heparinised saline. If intra-thrombus positioning of the microcatheter is not possible, the tip of the catheter needs to be placed as close to the proximal aspect of the embolic occlusion as possible for thrombolytic infusion. A superselective angiogram needs to be performed through the microcatheter to confirm correct positioning of the catheter. High-dose urokinase regimens are generally administered (500 000 IU urokinase with half being administered as a single bolus). Alternatively, continuous infusion (without a bolus) of up to 1 250 000 units of urokinase over 90 minutes can be performed. rTPA may be given as a 5-mg bolus, followed by slow-infusion (maximum dose 20 mg). It is important to perform serial angiograms (every 15 minutes) and to continue thrombolytic therapy until complete recanalisation has been achieved (to a maximum of 1 hour). If the proximal thrombus dissolves, the tip of the microcatheter needs to be advanced into the next portion of residual clot. Mechanical disruption of the clot can be performed in cases where no advancement of lytic activity is observed. As mentioned previously, intra-arterial thrombolysis increases the risk of haemorrhagic complications. Selective intra-arterial administration of 5 mg abciximab (ReoPro, Lilly Pharmaceuticals, Indianapolis, IN, USA) followed by a bolus of 5 mg abciximab intravenously has also been used for the treatment of neurological sequelae because of distal embolisation after carotid artery angioplasty and stent placement.

THROMBOSIS

Thrombosis occurring during the CAS procedure seems to be associated with the use of embolic protection devices (e.g., filters), but acute thrombosis of the stented target lesion has also been described. A large embolic load may block the filter completely, leading to proximal flow stasis. In addition, thrombus forming on the wire of the filter system has been described, despite maximum anticoagulation. Treatment consists of local administration of abciximab or aspiration of thrombus, followed by retrieval of the filter device using the guiding catheter or sheath already in place. Care should be taken not to close the filter system completely, as its embolic contents may be squeezed out and embolise distally.[103,104]

Acute stent thrombosis is a potentially fatal complication, with an incidence of 0.5–2% and seems to be related to the lack of (pre)treatment DAPT, although cases can occur whilst the patient is on DAPT because of antiplatelet resistance. Treatment consists of intra-arterial thrombolysis or administration of intra-arterial abciximab.[103,104] Intra-arterial thrombolysis involves administration of urokinase or rTPA as described earlier. A successful dosage regime of 0.25 mg/kg of abciximab intra-arterially, followed by a continuous intravenous infusion (9 μg/min for 12 hours) has been successfully used. Alternatively, intra-carotid injection of 5 mg rTPA, followed by systemic administration of 5 mg rTPA and intra-carotid administration of a half-dose bolus of abciximab (0.125 mg/kg) is an alternative. In cases where additional endovascular therapy with thromboaspiration (Fig. 10.13) or systemic pharmacological treatment does not resolve the occlusion in a timely fashion, conversion to surgery using either thrombendarterectomy with stent removal and patch closure or thrombectomy using aspiration after transverse arteriotomy of the ipsilateral CCA should be considered.

DISSECTION

Dissection is a rare complication during CAS. Dissection can be related to stent placement and balloon angioplasty (as in other vascular territories), as well as being caused by distal balloon CPDs. In cases where flow reduction is limited, a wait-and-see policy may be used. In cases of severe flow impairment, treatment consists of either inserting a second stent, or urgent surgical repair, which will involve removal of the stent and carotid bypass.[103,104]

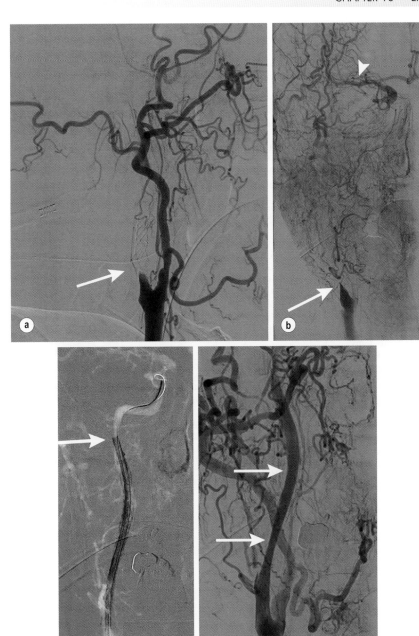

Figure 10.13 (a) Angiographic image of the right carotid bifurcation in a patient that presented with acute thrombotic occlusion (*arrow*) of a dual-layer stent (RoadSaver) in the right internal carotid artery (same patient as in Fig. 10.12). (b) Late phase angiographic image demonstrating preserved distal flow in the right middle cerebral artery (*arrowhead*), as well as the occlusion of the right internal carotid artery (*arrow*). (c) Roadmap image demonstrating position of thrombo-aspiration catheter in the right internal carotid artery, distally from the stent. (d) Control angiography after thrombo-aspiration demonstrating restoration of flow in the right internal carotid artery (*arrows*)

Key points

- 'Best medical therapy' and risk factor control is mandated in everyone.
- There is compelling evidence that recently symptomatic patients benefit from treatment (medical therapy, intervention) in the early time period after onset of symptoms.
- The beneficial role of CEA is supported by level 1 evidence in selected asymptomatic and symptomatic patients. In symptomatic patients, the benefit conferred by CEA is dependent on being performed early with a low operative risk and requires surgeons to quote their own operative risks rather than trial data.

- Randomised trials have shown that CAS is an alternative to CEA in selected patients. The decision as to which treatment strategy should be implemented in individual patients will depend on unit experience, recency of symptoms, patient age and overall cardiovascular risk.
- Interventions should not be delayed to achieve a lower procedural risk. The highest risk period for stroke is the first few days after onset of symptoms. CAS is not currently indicated in the very early time period after onset of symptoms.

References available at http://ebooks.health.elsevier.com/

KEY REFERENCES

[5] Menon R, Kerry S, Norris JW, Markus HS. Treatment of cervical artery dissection: a systematic review and meta-analysis. JNNP 2008;79:1122–7.

[11] Rothwell PM, Eliasziw M, Gutnikov SA. For the Carotid Endarterectomy Trialists Collaboration. Analysis of pooled data from the randomised controlled trials of endarterectomy for symptomatic carotid stenosis. Lancet 2003;361:107–16.

[16] Wardlaw JM, Chappell FM, Stevenson M, et al. Accurate, practical and cost-effective assessment of carotid stenosis in the UK. Health Technol Assess 2006;10. iii–iv, ix–x,1–182.

[20] Executive Committee for the Asymptomatic Carotid Atherosclerosis Study. Endarterectomy for asymptomatic carotid artery stenosis. JAMA 1995;273:1421–61.

[25] MacMahon S. Antihypertensive drug treatment: the potential, expected and observed effects on vascular disease. J Hypertens 1990;8(Suppl. l):S239–44.

[26] Kalra L, Perez I, Melbourn A. Stroke risk management: changes in mainstream practice. Stroke 1998;29:53–7.

[27] Williams B, Mancia G, Spiering W, Agabiti Rosei E, Azizi M, et al. 2018 ESC/ESH Guidelines for the management of arterial hypertension. Eur Heart J 2018;39:3021–104.

[28] Heart Protection Study Collaborative Group. MRC/BHF Heart Protection Study of cholesterol lowering with simvastatin in 20536 high-risk individuals: a randomised placebo controlled trial. Lancet 2002;360:7–22.

[30] Powers WJ, Rabinstein AA, Ackerson T, Adeoye OM, Bambakidis NC, Becker K, et al. Guidelines for the early management of patients with acute ischaemic stroke: 2019 update to the 2018 Guidelines for the early management of acute ischaemic stroke: a guideline for Healthcare Professionals from the American Heart Association/American Stroke Association. Stroke 2019;50:344–418.

[33] Naylor AR, Rantner B, Ancetti S, de Borst GJ, de Carlo M, Halliday AH et al. European Society for Vascular Surgery (ESVS): 2023 Clinical Practice Guidelines on the Management of Atherosclerotic Carotid and Vertebral Artery disease. Eur J Vasc Endovasc Surg 2023;65:7–11.

[34] Hao QH, Tampi M, O'Donnell M, Foroutan F, Siemieniuk RAC, Guyatt G. Clopidogrel plus aspirin versus aspirin alone for acute minor ischaemic stroke or high risk transient ischaemic attack: systematic review and meta-analysis. BMJ 2018;363:k5108.

[36] Rothwell PM, Eliasziw M, Gutnikov SA. For the Carotid Endarterectomy Trialists Collaboration. Endarterectomy for symptomatic carotid stenosis in relation to clinical subgroups and timing of surgery. Lancet 2004;363:915–24.

[37] Rothwell PM, Eliasziw M, Gutnikov SA. Sex difference in the effect of time from symptoms to surgery on benefit from carotid endarterectomy for transient ischaemic attack and minor stroke. Stroke 2004;35:2855–61.

[43] Rantner B, Goebel G, Bonati LH, Ringleb PA, Mas JL, Fraedrich G. The risk of carotid artery stenting compared with carotid endarterectomy is greatest in patients treated within 7 days of symptoms. J Vasc Surg 2013;57:619–26.

[45] Batchelder A, Saratzis A, Naylor AR. Overview of primary and secondary analyses from 20 randomised controlled trials comparing carotid artery stenting with carotid endarterectomy. Eur J Vasc Endovasc Surg 2019;58:479–93.

[56] Hadar N, Raman G, Moorthy D. Asymptomatic carotid artery stenosis treated with medical therapy alone: temporal trends and implications for risk assessment and the design of future studies. Cerebrovasc Dis 2014;38:163–73.

[63] Naylor AR, Mehta Z, Rothwell PM. Stroke during coronary artery bypass surgery: a critical review of the role of carotid artery disease. Eur J Vasc Endovasc Surg 2002;23:283–94.

[64] Naylor AR, Bown MJ. Stroke after cardiac surgery and its association with asymptomatic carotid disease: an updated systematic review and meta-analysis. Eur J Vasc Endovasc Surg 2011;41:607–24.

[65] Naylor AR, Cuffe R, Rothwell PM, Bell PRF. A Systematic review of outcomes following staged and synchronous carotid endarterectomy and coronary artery bypass. Eur J Vasc Endovasc Surg 2003;25:380–9.

[66] Naylor AR, Cuffe R, Rothwell PM, Bell PRF. A Systematic review of outcomes following synchronous carotid endarterectomy and coronary artery bypass Influence of patient and surgical variables. Eur J Vasc Endovasc Surg 2003;26:230–41.

[67] Fareed K, Rothwell PM, Mehta Z, Naylor AR. Synchronous carotid endarterectomy and off-pump coronary bypass: an updated systematic review of early outcomes. Eur J Vasc Endovasc Surg 2009;37:375–8.

[71] Markus HS, Harshfield EL, Compter A, Kuker W, Kappelle LJ, Clifton A, et al. Stenting for symptomatic vertebral artery stenosis: a preplanned pooled individual patient data analysis. Lancet Neurol 2019;18(7):666–73.

Vascular disorders of the upper limb

11

Jean-Baptiste Ricco | Romain Belmonte | Iris Lebuhotel | Thanh-Phong Le

INTRODUCTION

Arterial diseases of the upper limb are relatively rare in comparison with those involving the lower extremity. The good collateral supply around the shoulder and elbow explains why chronic occlusive disease is commonly asymptomatic, but acute occlusion caused by embolism can result in limb-threatening ischaemia. In addition, thoracic outlet syndrome, subclavian–axillary vein thrombosis and occupational vascular problems need to be considered. In this chapter, we do not review vasospastic disorders, connective tissue disease, vasculitis and Raynaud's disease, as these are covered in Chapter 12, nor vascular trauma, which is covered in Chapter 9. The main causes of upper limb vascular disease are summarised in Box 11.1.

CLINICAL EXAMINATION

Vascular assessment of the upper limb should include the thoracic outlet. Palpation and auscultation of the supraclavicular region may help to detect a cervical rib, a subclavian artery stenosis or aneurysm. The arm pulses should be examined with the arm placed in the neutral position and then in abduction and external rotation (surrender position) to detect arterial thoracic outlet compression. Pulse palpation is important and must include the axillary, brachial, radial and ulnar pulses. The nail folds should be examined for infarcts and splinter haemorrhages. The blood pressure should be measured in both arms, preferably using a hand-held Doppler. A difference of more than 15% is abnormal.

Examination in cases of hand ischaemia is not complete unless Allen's test is performed. The examiner compresses the radial and ulnar arteries at the wrist. The examiner then asks the subject to clench the fist to empty the hand of blood. The radial artery is then released, and the hand is observed for return of colour. The test is then repeated for the ulnar artery. The test is normal if refilling of the hand is complete within less than 10 seconds from either side. Any portion of the hand that does not blush is an indication of incomplete continuity of the palmar arch.

OCCLUSIVE DISEASE

Occlusive lesions of the brachiocephalic and subclavian arteries occur in relatively young patients with mean ages ranging from 50 to 60 years. These lesions are less frequent than those involving the carotid bifurcation.[1] Atherosclerosis is the predominant cause in Europe, with Buerger's disease and Takayasu's arteritis rarely seen. The symptoms of occlusive disease of the upper extremities include muscle fatigue and ischaemic rest pain. Digital necrosis or atheroembolisation is

---

Box 11.1 Causes of upper limb vascular diseases

Arterial obstruction

Large artery

Atherosclerosis
Radiotherapy
Thoracic outlet syndrome
Arteritis (giant cell, Takayasu's)

Small artery

Atherosclerosis
Connective tissue disease
Myeloproliferative disease
Buerger's disease
Vibrating tools

Arterial vasospasm

Large artery

Ergot-containing medications and other pharmacological causes

Small artery

Raynaud's disease
Vibrating tools

Embolism: proximal sources

Heart
Ulcerated arterial plaques (aortic arch, brachiocephalic and subclavian arteries)
Aneurysm (brachiocephalic, subclavian, axillary, brachial, ulnar arteries)
Thoracic outlet syndrome

Subclavian–axillary vein thrombosis

Primary: Paget–Schroeter syndrome (thoracic outlet syndrome)
Secondary: catheter, hypercoagulable states

Hypercoagulable states

Heparin antibodies
Deficiencies of antithrombin III, proteins C and S
Antiphospholipid syndrome
Malignancy
Cryoglobulinaemia
Aneurysms

Table 11.1   Direct reconstruction of the supra-aortic vessels: complications and late patency

Authors, year	No. patients	Mean follow-up (month) [range]	Complications (%)	Primary patency (%)
Takach et al., 2005[58]	113	61.2 ± 6 [3–264]	Death: 2.7 Stroke: 2.7 MI:* 1.8	10 years:* 94.4 ± ± 4
Berguer et al.,[4] 1998	100	51 ± 4.8 [1–184]	Stroke + death: 16 Morbidity: 27	5 years:† 94 ± 3
Uurto et al.,[7] 2002	76	158 [6–136]	Death: 2.6 Morbidity: 19.7	1 year: 95 5 years:‡ 91 15 years:‡ 89

*22 patients were followed at 10 years.
†34 patients followed at 5 years.
‡54 patients followed at 5 years and 25 at 15 years.
MI, myocardial infarction.

less common than in the lower extremities, accounting for no more than 5% of patients with limb ischaemia.[2]

BRACHIOCEPHALIC ARTERY

Stenotic lesions of the brachiocephalic artery are uncommon and may be asymptomatic in 13–22% of patients.[3,4] Symptomatic patients may present with ischaemia of the right upper extremity, carotid territory symptoms or vertebrobasilar symptoms.[5] The diagnosis is suspected by physical examination (i.e., right supra-clavicular/cervical bruit, absent right subclavian or axillary pulse) and confirmed by duplex scanning, conventional angiography, or computed tomographic angiography (CTA) or magnetic resonance angiography (MRA). Most patients (61–84%) with brachiocephalic artery occlusion have multiple lesions of the aortic arch vessels.[6] Symptomatic stenotic lesions of the brachiocephalic artery may be treated surgically or radiologically. Surgically, this can be approached by median sternotomy with direct bypass grafting from the aortic arch, or indirectly by extra-anatomical bypass such as subclavian–subclavian, contralateral carotid–carotid or subclavian–carotid bypass.

AORTO-BRACHIOCEPHALIC BYPASS

✓✓ Extra-anatomical bypasses have a lower morbidity and mortality but direct bypasses from the aortic arch are more durable. In total, the combined post-operative death and stroke rate for direct reconstruction of the supra-aortic trunks ranges from 2.6–16% (Table 11.1). The primary patency is about 90% with a 72% survival rate at 10 years.[7]

A median sternotomy is used with extension into the neck. The left brachiocephalic vein is identified (Fig. 11.1a). A partial occluding clamp is applied to the ascending aorta proximal to the brachiocephalic artery to avoid the risk of fracturing atheromatous plaque (Fig. 11.1b). An 8–10-mm prosthetic graft is anastomosed at this site with deep suture placement in the aortic wall (Fig. 11.1c). Once the anastomosis is completed, a clamp is applied across the graft and systemic heparin is given. The brachiocephalic artery is clamped, sectioned and the proximal stump oversewn. The patent distal artery is spatulated and the graft attached in an end-to-end fashion (Fig. 11.1d). Air is evacuated from the graft by back-bleeding the

subclavian artery, then flow is released into the arm and then into the carotid artery. The mortality of direct bypass ranges from 5.8–8% in Kieffer's and Berguer's series,[3,4] with a primary patency rate at 5 years of 94% in both series.

BRACHIOCEPHALIC ENDARTERECTOMY

The proximal location of the disease with extension into the aortic arch makes this technique hazardous. Attempts to remove an orifice lesion may initiate an aortic dissection or distal embolisation. For this reason, bypass or endovascular therapy are preferred for all brachiocephalic lesions where treatment is indicated, except perhaps for those located in the distal segment.

ENDOVASCULAR TREATMENT

Percutaneous transluminal angioplasty (PTA) and stenting of the brachiocephalic artery is being performed with increased frequency and is the preferred primary approach in many patients. The approach may be percutaneous from either the femoral or brachial artery or through an anterolateral cervical approach with clamping of the right common carotid artery to avoid atheroembolisation during angioplasty. Because of a relatively small number of cases, most papers concerning angioplasty of the brachiocephalic artery include results for the subclavian artery. Only four series report PTA of the brachiocephalic artery alone[8–11] (Table 11.2). The benefit of adjuvant stenting is not well established.[8,9,12] Open surgery gives better mid-term results, but angioplasty is much less invasive.

SUBCLAVIAN ARTERY

Symptomatic lesions of the subclavian artery are associated in 72% of cases with concomitant lesions of carotid and vertebral vessels.[1] The indications for intervention are those of vertebrobasilar insufficiency and marked upper extremity ischaemia. Atheroembolisation is quite common in this location.[13] If surgery is contemplated and the ipsilateral common carotid artery is healthy, carotid–subclavian bypass or carotid–subclavian transposition is the method of choice.

CAROTID–SUBCLAVIAN BYPASS

Access is achieved by a horizontal supra-clavicular incision with division of both heads of the sternomastoid muscle. Scalenus anterior and the phrenic nerves are exposed, and

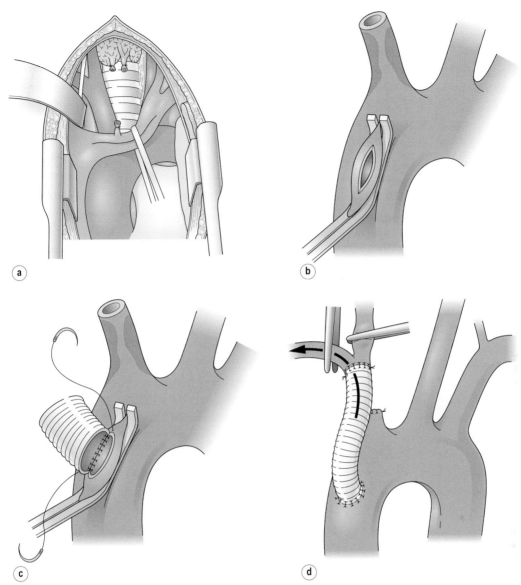

Figure 11.1 (a) The left brachiocephalic vein is retracted to expose the brachiocephalic artery. (b) A clamp is applied laterally to the ascending aorta. (c) A polyester graft is implanted on the ascending thoracic aorta proximal to the brachiocephalic artery. (d) Completed bypass. Flow is released into the arm and then into the common carotid artery.

then scalenus anterior is divided near its insertion into the first rib (Fig. 11.2a). On the left side, the thoracic duct is ligated to prevent unrecognised traction injury. The carotid sheath is opened, safeguarding the vagus nerve. After heparinisation, the common carotid artery is clamped as low as possible. A vein or polytetrafluoroethylene (PTFE) graft is then anastomosed to the lateral aspect of the common carotid artery in an end-to-side fashion (Fig. 11.2b). Use of a prosthetic graft seems to give better results than the vein graft in this location. The graft under arterial tension is then passed behind the jugular vein. Graft length should be cautiously estimated and the graft anastomosed end-to-side to the superior aspect of the distal subclavian artery. If the proximal subclavian lesion is ulcerated, it should be excluded by ligation. If the distal subclavian artery is too diseased for distal implantation, the graft should be passed behind the clavicle and implanted on the axillary artery exposed via a short infra-clavicular incision.

✔✔ Prosthetic carotid–subclavian bypass has an excellent patency. Post-operative mortality is less than 1%, with a primary patency of 95% at 10 years.[14,15]

CAROTID TRANSPOSITION

Re-implantation of the subclavian artery into the common carotid artery is an alternative that avoids graft material but requires a more extensive cervical dissection.[16] Dissection should avoid the recurrent laryngeal nerve, which is closely related to the posterior aspect of the subclavian artery. A curved clamp is applied across the subclavian artery, which is transected and the proximal stump oversewn. The site of anastomosis to the common carotid artery should be chosen to avoid kinking and angulation of the vertebral artery. The clamps on the common carotid artery should be rotated anteriorly to present the posterolateral surface for anastomosis with the subclavian

Table 11.2 Angioplasty of the brachiocephalic artery: post-operative complications and late patency

Authors, year	No. patients	Mean follow-up (month) [range]	Complications (%)	Primary patency (%)	Secondary patency (%)
Paukovits et al., 2010[8]	72	42.3 [2–103]	Total: 8.3 Death: none TIA: 2.6 Access site bleeding: 5.2	12 months: 100 24 months: 98 ± 1.6 96 months: 69.9 ± 8.5	12 months: 100 24 months: 100 96 months: 81.5 ± 7.7
Van Hattum et al., 2007[9]	30	n/a Median = 24 [4 weeks – 92]	Total: 10.0 Death: none TIA: 4.0	24 months: 79	n/a
Hüttl et al., 2002[10]	89	n/a [12–117]	Stroke: 5.6 Local: 3.0	6 months: 98 ± 25 months: 95 ± 3	96 months: 98 ± 2
Mordasini et al., 2011[11]	18	32.4 [4–110]	Neurological: 11.1	n/a	n/a
van de Weijer et al., 2015[12]	51	52 [2–163]	None	Restenosis-free survival 12 months: 94.1 24 months: 90.2	n/a
Zacharias et al., 2020[59]	33	51 [30–70]	Stroke: 3.0	Restenosis free survival 51 months:91.0	n/a

n/a, Not available; *TIA*, transient ischaemic attack.

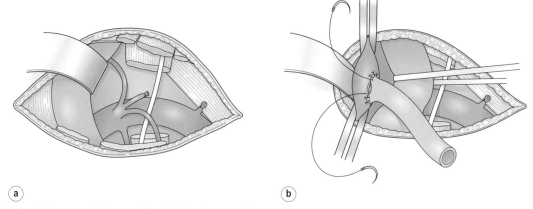

Figure 11.2 (a) Cervical approach for carotid-subclavian bypass. The sternomastoid muscle is divided and the subclavian artery is exposed by sectioning the scalenus anterior. (b) A PTFE graft is anastomosed to the lateral aspect of the left common carotid artery.

artery (Fig. 11.3). An ellipse is excised from the wall of the common carotid artery and the subclavian artery anastomosed in end-to-side fashion.

✓✓ Subclavian–carotid re-implantation is an excellent technique that seems to give better results than the subclavian–carotid bypass in the series of Cinà et al.[17] (Table 11.3). Post-operative mortality is less than 1%, with a long-term patency of 100% in the series of Sandmann et al.[18] and Kretschmer et al.[19]

CROSSOVER GRAFTS

Subclavian revascularisation may also be achieved by crossover subclavian–subclavian or axillo-axillary bypass. These grafts are relatively simple to construct, although their greater length and reversed angle of take-off may reduce durability. Furthermore, problems may arise if subsequent median sternotomy is needed for coronary bypass. The donor and recipient arteries are exposed by a short supraclavicular incision on either side (Fig. 11.4). A tunnel is created from one side of the neck to the other passing

behind the sternomastoid muscles and anterior to the carotid vessels. Crossover axillo-axillary bypass is easier to perform but the graft should pass subcutaneously over the sternum, with risks of compression or erosion. The post-operative death rate for crossover axillo-axillary bypass is 1.6% with a 5-year primary patency of 86.5% in the series of Mingoli et al.[20]

ENDOVASCULAR TREATMENT

PTA of subclavian artery stenoses is a relatively safe and often simple procedure to perform. Access is usually obtained from the femoral artery or from the brachial artery and the lesion dilated to 5–8 mm (Fig. 11.5). Because there is usually retrograde flow in the vertebral artery, stroke is rare. When there is no retrograde flow, an occlusion balloon may be placed in the vertebral artery from the arm while the stenosis is dilated. Simple stenoses are adequately dilated by balloon. Occlusions are more difficult to cross and less frequent in most endovascular series;[21–23] they often require catheterisation from the brachial artery with the use of balloon or self-expandable stents.

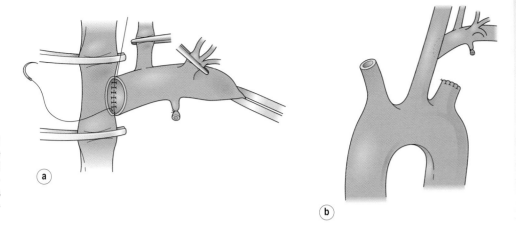

Figure 11.3 Carotid-subclavian transposition: (a) clamps on the common carotid artery are rotated anteriorly to present the postero-lateral surface for anastomosis with the subclavian artery; (b) end-to-side anastomosis completed.

Table 11.3 Carotid transposition: post-operative complications and late patency

Authors, year	No. patients	Mean follow-up (month) [range]	Complications (%)	Primary patency (%) at mean follow-up
Cinà et al., 2002[17]	27	25 ± 21	Morbidity: 11.1	100
Schardey et al., 1996[16]	108	70 [1–144]	Stroke: 1.8 Morbidity: 15	100*

*84 patients followed.

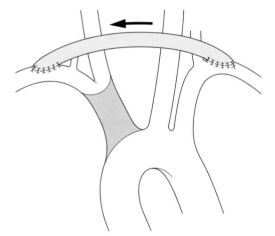

Figure 11.4 Brachiocephalic artery occlusion. Revascularisation by a cross-subclavian PTFE graft. Tunnelisation is done behind the sternomastoid muscles and anterior to the carotid vessels.

✓✓ PTA with or without stenting is an appropriate treatment for symptomatic patients with localised subclavian artery stenosis with a 2-year primary patency of 90% in most series[21–23] (Table 11.4), but a long-term patency inferior to that obtained with carotid–subclavian bypass or transposition.[24]

UPPER ARM ARTERIES

Patients with chronic atherosclerotic occlusion of the axillary or brachial arteries usually present with fatigue on using the arm. Some of these patients have radiation-induced occlusive disease. Severe ischaemia with rest pain or digital necrosis is uncommon because of collateral blood supply,

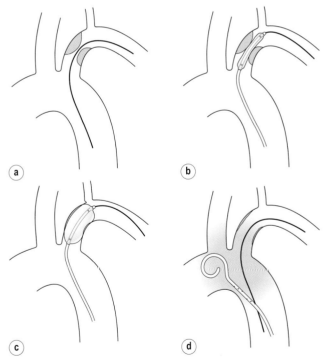

Figure 11.5 Retrograde approach from the brachial artery by percutaneous puncture, or better by cut-down if stenting is necessary: (a) the guidewire is placed through the subclavian stenosis; (b) balloon is advanced over the guidewire and balloon angioplasty performed; (c) arteriography completed by withdrawing the balloon with the same catheter; (d) more accurate arteriographic control can be achieved by using a second transfemoral pigtail catheter positioned in the aortic arch. (From Schneider PA. Endovascular skills; 2003. Reproduced by permission of Informa Healthcare.)

Table 11.4 Angioplasty of the subclavian artery: post-operative complications and late patency

Authors, year	No. patients	Mean follow-up (month) [range]	Complications (%)	Primary patency (%)
De Vries et al., 2005[21]	110	34 [3–120]	Stroke + death: 4.5 Local: 3.6	2 years:* 89 3 years:† 89
Berger et al., 2011[22]	72	82 [3–299]	Death: 19.6 Local: 4.9 Transient monoplegia: 1.5	10 years: 85.2
Soga et al, 2015[23]	553	39 [1–129]	Death: 0.7 Stroke: 1.8	1 year: 90.6 2 years: 83.4 5 years: 80.5
Özdemir-van Brunschot, 2016[24]	47	n/a	n/a	1 year: 72 5 years: 54

*64 patients followed at 2 years. †36 patients followed at 3 years.
n/a, Not available.

unless there have been repeated episodes of embolism because of proximal ulceration or aneurysmal degeneration. Direct reconstructive surgery is feasible since the occlusive lesions tend to be segmental with preserved distal patency. Axillobrachial occlusions can be managed with a bypass procedure if symptoms justify it. These sites can usually be approached with limited incisions and the bypass tunnelled subcutaneously between the two incisions (Fig. 11.6). In these cases, the autogenous saphenous vein is the preferred graft material. When unavailable, the basilic or cephalic vein may be considered. Upper limb bypass using the saphenous vein has a 5-year patency rate of 60–90%.[25] PTFE has a lower patency rate at this level and is generally avoided.

AXILLARY AND BRACHIAL ACCESS COMPLICATIONS

The brachial and axillary arteries have demonstrated adequacy as access vessels to perform lower extremity, visceral or complex endovascular procedures. In the Vascular Quality Initiative, brachial access was associated with an increased complication rate compared to femoral access (9.0% vs. 3.3%, P< 0.001), including haematomas (7.2% vs. 3.0%, P = 0.01) and occlusion.[26] Larger sheath sizes >5 Fr, percutaneous access and female sex were risk factors for such complications. The small diameter of the brachial artery makes it more prone to thrombosis and complications associated with percutaneous closure devices. It is also important to consider the risk of nerve injury with brachial and axillary access. The most common cause is compression from an axillary hematoma. Treatment involves urgent decompression of the fascial compartment and brachial artery repair.

LOWER ARM AND HAND ARTERIES

The causes of chronic occlusion in the forearm or hand vessels include atherosclerosis, Buerger's disease, immunological and connective tissue disorders (see Chapter 12) and occupational trauma. An arch-CTA scan to exclude proximal embolic disease, and selective arteriography are essential in evaluating these patients with distal disease. Most of these patients can be managed conservatively. Avoidance of

cold and abstinence of tobacco are essential. Vasodilator or sympatholytic agents may also be used. Patients with digital necrosis may require local debridement or amputation if gangrene is extensive. Some patients with radial, ulnar or palmar arch occlusion and critical ischaemia may be managed, if run-off is present, by vein graft bypass using microsurgical techniques. Cervico-dorsal sympathectomy by thoracoscopy may also be considered in patients with severe distal forearm ischaemia. However, the results of sympathectomy have often been disappointing, particularly in patients with diffuse arteritis. Radial artery access, increasingly used for coronary interventions, is associated with a 7.7% rate of occlusion at 24 hours, often without sequelae because of palmar arches and collaterality in the hand.[27]

ANEURYSMAL DISEASE

True aneurysms of the upper limb arteries are uncommon. The subclavian artery is the most frequent site, usually caused by thoracic outlet compression. These patients may present with distal ischaemia, embolisation or acute thrombosis. False aneurysms from trauma or infection often produce motor or sensory impairment because of brachial plexus compression. As described later, subclavian artery aneurysms are best managed by a combined supra-clavicular and infra-clavicular approach. Aneurysms of the brachiocephalic artery are rare. In the series of Kieffer et al.,[28] the perioperative death rate was 11%, with most deaths occurring in patients operated on in an emergency setting.

An aberrant right subclavian artery arising from the descending thoracic aorta is a common anomaly. Rarely, the artery compresses the oesophagus against the trachea, producing a condition described as dysphagia lusoria. Aneurysmal degeneration, known as *Kommerell's diverticulum*, may also occur. The largest experience has been reported by Kieffer et al.[29] Because of the possibility of rupture, resection of the aneurysmal artery with aortic prosthetic reconstruction via a thoracic approach is recommended. As this technique carries a relatively high post-operative mortality, hybrid procedures with aortic stent grafts are more commonly used with good reported outcomes.[30,31]

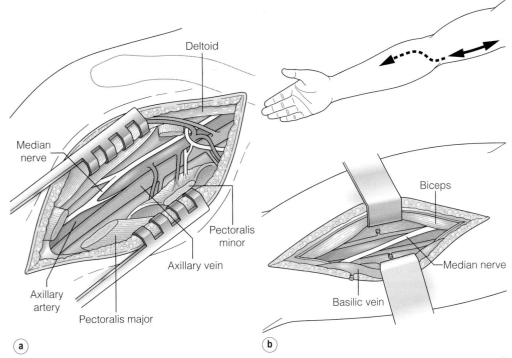

Figure 11.6 (a) Axillary artery approach. The pectoralis minor muscle is divided, and the neurovascular bundle is exposed. If access to the axillobrachial junction is needed, the pectoralis major tendon should also be resected. (b) Brachial artery approach. Incision along the medial border of the biceps. If necessary, the bicipital aponeurosis is divided to expose the brachial artery division.

UPPER ARM ARTERY ANEURYSMS

Axillary artery aneurysms are usually caused by blunt or penetrating trauma. Degenerative or congenital aneurysms are rare in this location. False aneurysms of the axillary artery occur with humeral fractures and anterior dislocation of the shoulder. These aneurysms can lead to neurological complications because of compression of the brachial plexus. Duplex scan and arteriography allow an accurate diagnosis. The axillary artery is exposed by a delto-pectoral incision with division of the pectoralis minor. The aneurysm is resected followed by interposition of a reversed saphenous vein graft. Stent grafts have been used for emergency control of upper limb aneurysms but their long-term integrity is often compromised by compression between the first rib and clavicle or by excessive arterial flexion.[32]

LOWER ARM AND HAND ARTERY ANEURYSMS

Radial artery aneurysms are usually caused by inadequate compression or infection following removal of an intra-arterial blood pressure cannula. If the Allen test shows good filling of the hand from the ulnar artery, then the radial artery can simply be ligated above and below the aneurysm. If not, reconstruction using a vein graft is required.

ULNAR ARTERY ANEURYSM OR HYPOTHENAR HAMMER SYNDROME

It is important to recognise an ulnar artery aneurysm because it may lead to digital necrosis. The condition known as *hypothenar hammer syndrome* develops in workers who suffer repetitive trauma to their hands, including carpenters and pipe fitters. Those who play sports such as volleyball or karate are also at risk. The pathophysiology is related to the vascular anatomy of the hand. The distal ulnar artery is vulnerable to external trauma between the distal margin of Guyon's canal and the palmar aponeurosis. Over this short distance, the artery lies anterior to the hook of the hamate bone and is covered only by the palmaris brevis muscle and the skin. Trauma of the ulnar artery at this level causes thrombosis or aneurysm formation and distal embolisation in the fourth and fifth fingers, with pain, coldness and cyanosis. The thumb is always spared because of its radial blood supply. Angiography with magnification is essential in these patients.

When the ulnar artery is chronically thrombosed, calcium channel blockers may be helpful. In all cases, patients should avoid further hand trauma.

✔✔ Surgical therapy includes microsurgical arterial reconstruction with or without adjunctive pre-operative thrombolytic therapy to restore patency to digital arteries. Resection of the aneurysm with the placement of an interposition vein graft is the treatment of choice. Satisfactory long-term results have been reported by Vayssairat et al. using this approach.[33]

UPPER LIMB EMBOLISM

Embolic arterial occlusion is the major cause of acute upper limb ischaemia; upper limb emboli represent 20–32% of major peripheral emboli.[34] A cardiac origin is found in 90% of cases and is related to arrhythmia, myocardial infarction, valvular disorder or ventricular aneurysm. Noncardiac sources include ulcerative atherosclerotic plaques or aneurysms in the arch or subclavian–axillary arteries and thoracic outlet compression. The brachial bifurcation is the most frequently involved site for an embolus to lodge. Clinical examination and a duplex scan can locate the level of the arterial occlusion. Pre-operative conventional angiography or CTA is indicated to exclude a proximal arterial embolic lesion if a cardiac source is not evident or if the subclavian pulse is either absent (because of dissection or occlusion) or unduly prominent (because of a subclavian aneurysm or underlying cervical rib). Immediate systemic heparinisation is essential to limit the propagation of thrombus and to prevent recurrent embolism.

Most emboli can be retrieved through a distal brachial transverse arteriotomy. This site has the advantage that both forearm arteries can be directly cannulated. An S-shaped incision is made under local anaesthesia in the antecubital fossa and the brachial artery division exposed by dividing the bicipital aponeurosis. A transverse arteriotomy is made proximal to the bifurcation. It is important to clear both forearm vessels with a 2-Fr Fogarty catheter (Fig. 11.7). Heparinised saline is then instilled distally, and after confirming proximal patency, the arteriotomy is closed with 6/0 Prolene interrupted sutures. Completion on-table angiography should be performed. If there is retained distal thrombus, the ulnar and radial artery can be opened at the wrist and a 2-Fr Fogarty catheter passed distally. Alternatively, intraoperative thrombolysis can be used (see Chapter 8). Emboli in the axillary or subclavian arteries may also be removed by the same approach, using trans-brachial retrograde catheterisation. However, sometimes a large proximal embolus cannot be removed via the brachial arteriotomy, in which case an axillary or subclavian embolectomy will be required. Percutaneous thrombo-aspiration with or without local thrombolysis via a femoral approach has also been used in this situation.

OTHER CAUSES OF ACUTE ISCHAEMIA

The pharmacological causes of upper extremity ischaemia are summarised in Box 11.2. Inadvertent arterial injection by drug abusers often results in intense vasospasm because of particulate microembolism. Intra-arterial infusion of prostacyclin analogues such as iloprost or other vasodilators may help. Forearm compartment syndrome is rare except in this situation and requires careful, complete forearm fasciotomies. Limb loss is common.

THORACIC OUTLET SYNDROME

Thoracic outlet syndrome describes a variety of symptoms caused by compression of the brachial plexus or subclavian vessels at the thoracic outlet. In more than 90% of all cases of thoracic outlet syndrome,[35] symptoms are neurological with pain and weakness resulting from C8 or T1 root compression. Arterial or venous symptoms resulting from compression are uncommon, accounting for 5% of cases in large published series, though some present with a mixed clinical picture.[36] Standards have been reported by the Society of Vascular Surgery.[37]

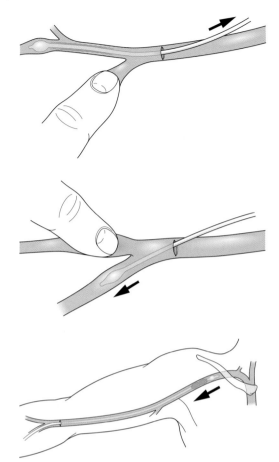

Figure 11.7 Brachial artery embolectomy. A transverse arteriotomy is performed. A Fogarty catheter is directed into the radial and ulnar arteries in turn, using alternate digital compression and/or Silastic slings. A subclavian–axillary embolectomy is carried out by retrograde catheterisation from the antecubital fossa.

Box 11.2 Upper extremity ischaemia caused by pharmacological agents

Ergot poisoning
Beta-blockers
Drug abuse, cocaine use
Dopamine overdose
Cytotoxic drugs

NEUROGENIC THORACIC OUTLET COMPRESSION SYNDROME

The neurovascular bundle may be compressed between the first rib and the clavicle because of a low-lying shoulder girdle or loss of muscle tone. Other anatomical factors include congenital fibromuscular bands crossing the thoracic outlet that tent up the brachial plexus, and abnormalities/hypertrophy of the scalene muscles. Bony lesions may also be the cause. These include cervical ribs, a broad first rib, and fracture or exostoses of the first rib or clavicle. The scalene triangle is the commonest site of nerve compression. It contains the brachial plexus and the subclavian artery. Neurogenic thoracic outlet compression syndrome (N-TOCS) probably represents a

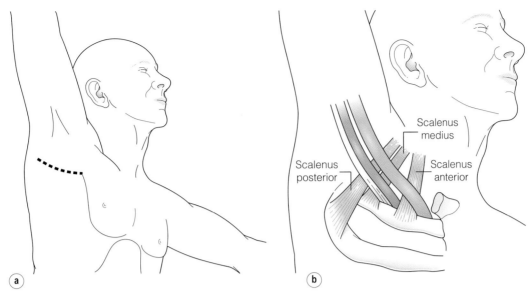

Figure 11.8 Transaxillary resection of the first rib: (a) operative position and skin incision; (b) the neurovascular bundle is pulled away from the first rib by traction on the arm.

repetitive stress injury as there are well-defined at-risk occupations (e.g., typists) and sports (e.g., swimming). Most patients with N-TOCS are in the 25- to 45-year age group and 70% of them are women. The symptoms are arm pain, paraesthesia and weakness, with involvement of all the nerves of the brachial plexus or with specific patterns related to the upper plexus (median nerve) or lower plexus (ulnar nerve).

DIAGNOSIS

Positive findings on clinical examination include supra-clavicular tenderness and paraesthesia in the ipsilateral upper extremity in response to pressure over the scalene muscles. Rotating the head and tilting the head away from the involved side often produces radiating pain in the upper arm. Abducting the arm to 90 degrees in external rotation and repeated slow finger clenching in this position often reproduces the symptoms (Roos' test). Diagnostic tests include a scalene muscle block, and a good response to this test correlates well with successful surgical decompression.[38] Neurophysiology testing is helpful in excluding other sites of nerve compression, for example, cervical root and carpal tunnel. Duplex scanning is a useful surrogate marker if it shows arterial compression in the stress position. Cervical spine films may detect cervical or abnormal first ribs but will not detect non-bony causes of compression. Magnetic resonance imaging is more useful for excluding cervical disc lesions than confirming N-TOCS.

TREATMENT

Therapy for N-TOCS should always begin with non-operative treatment, including postural exercises and physiotherapy. Patients should avoid heavy lifting and working with the arm above shoulder level. Conservative treatment should be continued for several months. Many patients will improve significantly and will not require surgery. Indications for surgery include failure of conservative therapy after several months and persistent disabling symptoms that interfere with work and activities of daily living. The goal of surgery is

to decompress the brachial plexus. A cervical rib can usually be removed via a supra-clavicular approach.

Transaxillary resection of first rib

The transaxillary approach described by Roos[39] is indicated for neurogenic complications of N-TOCS and can be summarised as follows. The patient is placed in the lateral position leaving the arm free. The assistant elevates the shoulder by applying upward traction on the upper arm. This manoeuvre opens the costoclavicular space and pulls the neurovascular bundle away from the first rib. A horizontal skin incision is made at the lower border of the axillary line over the third rib (Fig. 11.8). The intercostal nerve emerging from the second intercostal space should be preserved. The fascial roof of the axilla is opened to expose the anterior portion of the first rib. Scalenus anterior is separated from the artery and sectioned at its attachment to the first rib (Fig. 11.9). The tendon of the subclavius muscle is divided with care because of its close relation with the subclavian vein. The scalenus medius is then pushed off the rib. The intercostal muscles are similarly detached from the lower part of the rib. The rib is then sectioned at the chondrocostal junction and maintained by bone-holding forceps to distance it from the neurovascular bundle (Fig. 11.10). The T1 root is displaced medially. The rib is then divided and excised to within 1–2 cm of the vertebral transverse process using rongeurs. The stump must be smooth since sharp bony spicules may lacerate the plexus. Serum saline is then injected in the wound to ensure that the pleura is intact. The wound is closed in the usual way with suction drainage.

Complications of transaxillary rib resection include subclavian vein or artery injury, extra-pleural haematoma or brachial plexus injury caused by traction of the arm or damage to the T1 root retraction. Good illumination and visualisation are crucial to this approach and can help with both.

Other operative techniques for N-TOCS include a supra-clavicular approach. Axelrod et al.[40] reported the results of

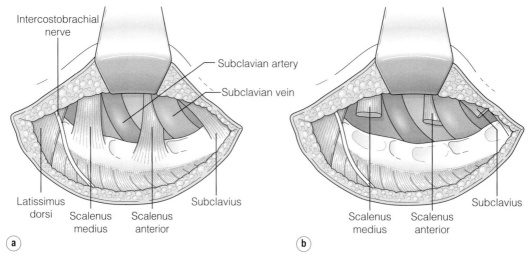

Figure 11.9 Transaxillary resection of the first rib: (a) exposure of the first rib, scalene muscles and subclavian–axillary vessels; (b) detachment of the scalenus anterior, medius and subclavius muscles from the first rib.

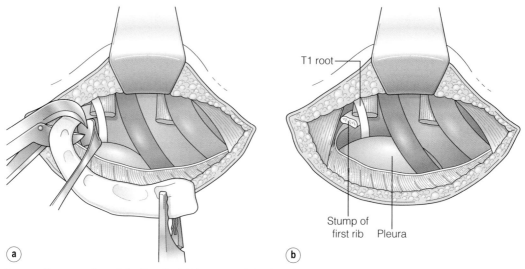

Figure 11.10 Transaxillary resection of the first rib. (a) Exposure of the first rib. The rib has been disarticulated at the chondrocostal junction. T1 root is protected by a retractor. (b) Extra-periosteal resection of the first rib is complete.

surgery in 170 patients operated for N-TOCS. No major operative complication occurred in those patients who underwent decompression via a supra-clavicular approach. Only 11% of patients experienced minor complications, most commonly, the need for chest tube placement because of pneumothorax. At short-term follow-up (10 months), most patients had improved pain levels (80%) and range of motion (82%). However, at long-term follow-up (47 months), residual symptoms were present in 65% of patients, and 35% took medication for pain. Nonetheless, 64% said they were satisfied with the result. Scali et al.[41] performed a long-term follow-up after first rib resection (average 8.7 years). An equivalent or better functional outcome was observed in 72.7% of the patients. Cordobes-Gual et al.[42] showed the importance of a precise questionnaire (DASH) to evaluate the functional recovery after N-TOCS surgery.

✔️ Controversy still exists concerning the surgical treatment of N-TOCS, and a randomised study of thoracic outlet surgery versus conservative treatment is lacking for this indication.

ARTERIAL THORACIC OUTLET COMPRESSION SYNDROME

Arterial complications are often associated with bony abnormalities, including a complete cervical rib or fracture callus of the first rib or clavicle. The initial arterial lesion is fibrotic thickening with intimal damage and post-stenotic dilatation, leading to aneurysmal degeneration with mural thrombus and the risk of embolisation. Most emboli are small and located in the hand vessels, with pallor, paraesthesia and coldness suggestive of Raynaud's syndrome. If unrecognised, severe digital ischaemia with gangrene may occur. Early recognition of this condition is essential, and a duplex scan should be performed in all patients with unilateral Raynaud's syndrome and asymptomatic patients with a cervical bruit. Loss or reduction of the radial pulse during Adson's manoeuvre (abduction and external rotation of the shoulder) is not very reliable as it is found in 9–53% of healthy volunteers.[35] The arteriographic changes may be obvious but sometimes minimal, with moderate dilatation beyond a bony abnormality at the thoracic outlet and radiological

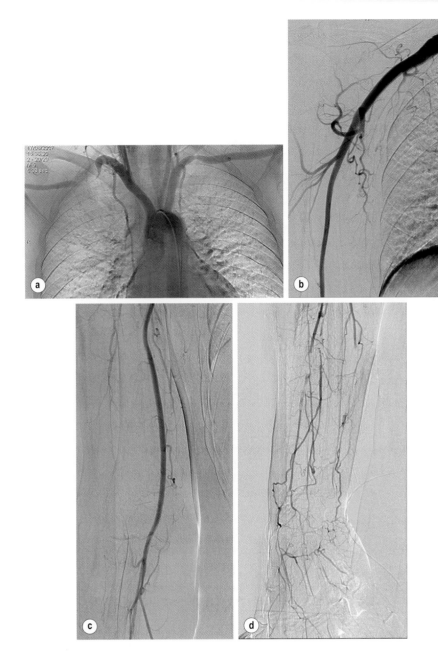

Figure 11.11   Angiography of a thoracic outlet compression syndrome with arterial compression. (a) Right subclavian artery compression when the arm is abducted to 90 degrees in external rotation. (b) Post-stenotic dilatation of the right subclavian artery. (c) Right brachial artery. (d) Distal arterial embolisation.

evidence of distal embolisation (Fig. 11.11). Subclavian stenosis is not always evident on anteroposterior view and oblique stress views are often necessary.

SURGICAL MANAGEMENT

Subclavian lesions associated with cervical ribs can usually be repaired via a supra-clavicular approach, after excision of the cervical rib or better by a combined supra-clavicular and infra-clavicular approach.

Combined supra-clavicular and infra-clavicular approach

The combined supra-clavicular and infra-clavicular approach offers a complete exposure. The infra-clavicular dissection is commenced first with an S-shaped incision. Pectoralis major is detached from the upper sternum and clavicle (Fig. 11.12). The subclavius is resected and the artery and the axillary vein are then freed behind the clavicle. Via a supra-clavicular

incision, the clavicular head of the sternomastoid and the external jugular vein are divided to expose the scalenus anterior and the phrenic nerve. The scalenus anterior is then sectioned near the first rib. The subclavian artery and vein are freed (Fig. 11.13). The intercostal muscles are detached from the first rib and the rib is disarticulated at the costochondral junction. The rib is then sectioned without attempting to reach the posterior segment. Access to the rib stump is achieved via the supra-clavicular exposure by reflecting the brachial plexus laterally and the artery medially. The scalenus medius is then detached from the first rib and, after protecting the T1 root, the rib is sectioned near the transverse process.

In patients with aneurysm or post-stenotic dilatation secondary to first rib or cervical rib, there is often sufficient length of artery to permit resection of the arterial lesion and direct anastomosis (Fig. 11.14). When arterial lesions are more extensive, graft replacement is required using reversed great saphenous vein or PTFE if no vein is available. Intra-operative angiography

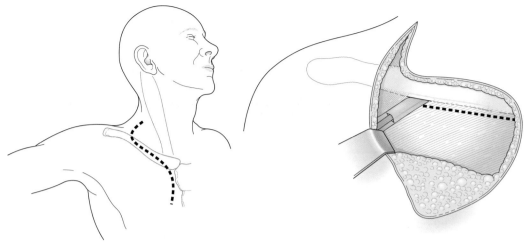

Figure 11.12   Combined supra-clavicular and infra-clavicular approach for first rib resection when extensive arterial or venous reconstruction is required. Skin incision and section of the pectoralis major from the clavicle.

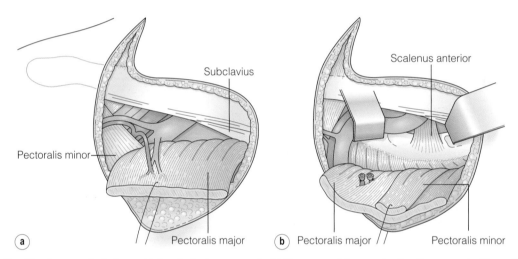

Figure 11.13   Combined supra-clavicular and infra-clavicular approach. (a) Exposure of the proximal axillary vessels. The axillary vessels are held aside with a retractor to show the first rib and insertion of the scalenus anterior. (b) The infra-clavicular dissection with detachment of the intercostal muscles from the first rib. The anterior portion of the rib will be removed, and the first rib stump will be shortened via the supra-clavicular exposure, not shown here.

is recommended in all cases. In patients with a recent distal embolic event, catheter embolectomy should be attempted. If embolectomy is impossible, a distal bypass using the great saphenous vein may be needed to revascularise one of the forearm arteries. Additional sympathectomy may also be considered where there is an extensive long-standing distal embolic occlusion. Difficulty in clearing the distal arterial bed accounts for the incomplete revascularisation observed in advanced cases with disabling ischaemic sequelae.

✔✔ Arterial reconstruction and first rib or cervical rib resection are indicated in all patients with arterial complications of thoracic outlet syndrome.

SUBCLAVIAN–AXILLARY VEIN THROMBOSIS

Spontaneous or effort-related venous thrombosis in a fit young patient is known as *Paget–Schroetter syndrome*, the first

cases being published separately by these two authors over a century ago. Hughes, who in 1949 collected 320 cases recognised the distinct entity and coined the eponym. As the indications for central venous access have increased, so has the incidence of catheter-related subclavian–axillary vein thrombosis (SVT).[43]

Acute deep venous thrombosis (DVT) of the upper limb has many causes, with treatment and prognosis depending on the specific cause. SVT can be divided into two groups, primary and secondary. Primary SVT (Paget–Schroetter syndrome) is caused by anatomical venous compression in the thoracic outlet during exercise and comprises about 25% of all cases. Secondary SVT is the result of multiple aetiological factors, although in most series, trauma caused by central venous catheters dominates this category (40% of all cases of SVT). SVT is responsible for 1–4% of all cases of DVT. Monreal et al.[44] reported a 15% incidence of pulmonary emboli in 30 consecutive patients with SVT who were investigated with ventilation–perfusion scanning.

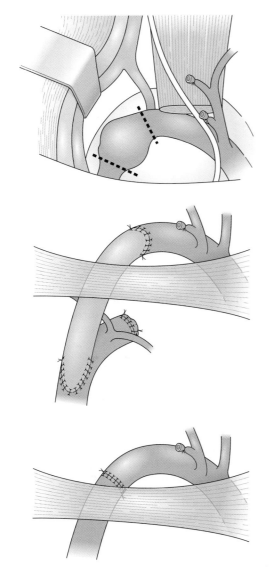

Figure 11.14 Combined supra-clavicular and infra-clavicular approach. Exposure of the subclavian and axillary vessels. Depending on the extent of arterial resection, end-to-end anastomosis or graft replacement is done.

PRIMARY SUBCLAVIAN–AXILLARY VEIN THROMBOSIS

In a review of the literature, Hurlbert and Rutherford[45] reported a male-to-female ratio of 2:1, with an average age of 30 years for patients with primary SVT that represents only 3.5% of all cases of TOCS. Venous thrombosis is seen three times more frequently in the right than the left upper limb, but bilateral venous compression also occurs frequently. Thrombosis is probably caused by repetitive trauma from compression. Virtually every patient with primary SVT has some degree of upper extremity swelling associated with pain that worsens with exertion. Some patients may have cyanosis of the arm. Unlike lower-extremity DVT, symptoms in the upper extremity are more related to venous obstruction than reflux. Venous outflow through the collateral vessels is limited, resulting in venous hypertension, swelling and occasionally venous claudication. Venous gangrene is an extremely rare complication of SVT.

DIAGNOSIS

Clinically, the arm may be swollen and cyanosed, with dilated shoulder girdle collateral veins. Duplex is the first-line investigation and has a sensitivity of 94% and a specificity of 96% compared with venography.[46] MRA has poor sensitivity for non-occlusive thrombi and short-segment occlusion. CTA has been used to diagnose upper-extremity DVT, but its specificity and sensitivity are undetermined. Venography is still considered as the reference in evaluating SVT (Fig. 11.15). The basilic vein is the preferred site for injection, with the arm abducted at 30 degrees. The catheter used for the venogram should be left in position as it can be used for subsequent thrombolysis and/or heparin infusion. The cephalic vein is not used because it joins directly with the subclavian vein and may miss an axillary vein thrombosis.

TREATMENT

For many years, treatment of SVT relied on rest and elevation of the upper limb with anticoagulant therapy. However, the morbidity associated with this conservative treatment is high. More recently, investigators have realised that many patients with SVT have compression at the thoracic outlet. Initially, in patients with primary SVT, subclavian vein patency was restored by open thrombectomy associated with first rib resection.[47] Although now supplanted by thrombolysis, open thrombectomy has proved effective and should be considered in patients with contraindications or failure of thrombolysis therapy. Catheter-directed techniques of thrombolysis allow for immediate venous evaluation and assess extrinsic compression with positional venography after thrombolysis.[48] However, Sheeran et al.[49] have shown that recanalisation of the vein by thrombolysis without decompression of the thoracic outlet has poor outcomes, with 55% of patients remaining symptomatic. Conversely, Machleder[50] reported the success of combined treatment, with 86% of 36 patients becoming asymptomatic. The appropriate time interval between thrombolysis and thoracic outlet decompression is still debated. Machleder waited 3 months, whereas Lee et al.[51] recommended immediate first rib resection within 4 days after thrombolysis. Waiting too long risks repeat thrombosis, whereas operating immediately risks bleeding because of the thrombolytic agent.

✔✔ Patients with thoracic outlet syndrome and SVT should have early treatment with thrombolysis followed by first rib resection.[52]

Specific problems may arise in some patients after thrombolysis. In a small group, no residual lesion or compression is seen on positional venography after thrombolysis. In these cases, anticoagulation therapy is recommended without thoracic outlet decompression. In other patients, intrinsic stenosis is seen on venography after thrombolysis (see Fig. 11.15). In these cases, operative vein bypass or patch angioplasty with first rib resection is needed and should be performed in the days after thrombolysis because the risk of repeat thrombosis appears to be quite high. In this setting, percutaneous balloon angioplasty with or without stenting has been suggested. The results of this technique without thoracic outlet decompression are poor, with a primary patency of 35% at 1 year.[53] Obviously, this technique does not obviate the need for surgery because thoracic outlet decompression is still needed. Even after thoracic outlet

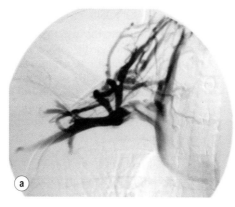 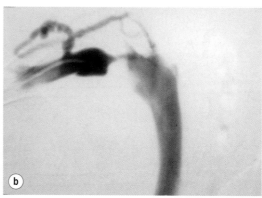

Figure 11.15 (a) Venogram via basilic vein demonstrating subclavian–axillary vein thrombosis with collaterals. (b) Thrombolysis revealed an underlying stenosis of the subclavian vein. This was treated by excision of the first rib and vein patch.

decompression, some venous stenoses are resistant to dilatation or present intrinsic elastic recoil. Various types of stents have been used to treat residual stenoses, but are associated with a worse prognosis than balloon angioplasty alone after vein decompression.[54]

✓✓ Stenting in primary SVT is not appropriate. As surgery is usually needed for thoracic outlet decompression, it seems logical to repair the subclavian vein with patch angioplasty or a short autogenous bypass at the same time.

In a significant number of patients, seen more than 10 days after the onset of primary upper-limb DVT, late thrombolysis fails. Most of these patients should be treated conservatively with anticoagulation unless the occlusion is short. In these cases, open thrombectomy with vein reconstruction and first rib resection can be considered with acceptable results.[55] The technique involves internal jugular vein transposition or cephalic vein bypass with a temporary arteriovenous fistula. Prosthetic bypass has shown inferior results in this location.

SECONDARY SUBCLAVIAN–AXILLARY VEIN THROMBOSIS

The main cause of secondary SVT is central venous catheterisation (CVC). Overall, one-third of patients with central-line catheters develop SVT, although only 15% of them are symptomatic. The aetiology of catheter-associated thrombosis is multifactorial but may be related to the fibrin sheath that forms around the catheter. The method of insertion, size, composition and duration of use of the catheter are also important. A reduced rate of thrombosis has been found with soft and more flexible catheters. Large catheters used for haemodialysis have a higher incidence of SVT. Another risk factor is the type of fluid infused through the catheter. Cancer chemotherapeutic agents are aggressive to vascular endothelium and may increase the risk of thrombosis. Furthermore, many patients with central-line catheters also have systemic risk factors for thrombosis, that is, malignancy, sepsis, congestive heart failure and prolonged bed rest.

Symptomatic patients have oedema and distended veins around the shoulder. Pulmonary embolism is not uncommon, with 16% of patients positive on ventilation–perfusion scan.[56] Therapy guidelines are based on observational reports as no controlled studies are available. In all cases, anticoagulation using intravenous heparin via the affected arm is indicated to prevent clot extension until the catheter is removed. Thrombolytic therapy has a role in reopening thrombosed catheters. Prevention of thrombus formation has been emphasised, and for high-risk patients, it may be advantageous to administer low-dose coumadin[57] or low-molecular-weight heparin to reduce the risk of catheter-associated thrombosis. A further discussion about CVC management can be found in Chapter 16.

Case 1 Paget-Schroetter syndrome

A 21-year-old woman presented to the hospital for left lower neck pain and swelling over her left upper arm after she attempted heavy weightlifting (Fig. 11.16). On admission, physical examination was positive for swelling and tenderness in the upper left arm. Venous ultrasound of the left upper extremity showed a large echogenic thrombus of the subclavian vein (Fig. 11. 17). Coagulation studies showed a normal protein S activity along with a negative factor V Leiden, anticardiolipin and prothrombin mutation. The patient was subsequently placed on a heparin infusion and was scheduled to undergo thrombolysis. Venography performed before procedure showed complete occlusion of the subclavian vein (Fig. 11.18). The patient underwent intravenous catheter thrombolysis with alteplase bolus continued with intravenous infusion for 24 hours without any complications. An interval venography, which was performed after 24 hours of the procedure demonstrated a persistent thrombus at the first rib within the triangle formed by the scalene anterior muscle posterior to the subclavian vein, the first rib beneath the vein and the clavicle above the vein. Balloon angioplasty with pressure of 10 atm was performed with improvement of the previous findings (Fig. 11.19). No embolism following balloon angioplasty has been observed. The patient was discharged on rivaroxaban and received thoracic first rib resection 3 weeks later. Six months after the surgical procedure, venous ultrasound showed a patent subclavian vein and rivaroxaban was interrupted.

Keys

- The presentation of severe pain in the upper extremities in young patients following strenuous exercise should raise a high index of suspicion for Paget-Schroetter syndrome and should be worked up as quickly as possible.
- Thrombolysis is most effective in patients treated within 2 weeks of onset of symptoms. Incomplete results following thrombolysis may lead to percutaneous angioplasty followed by surgical decompression with first rib resection, which is known to lower rates of recurrent thrombosis. Stenting should be avoided in this context.

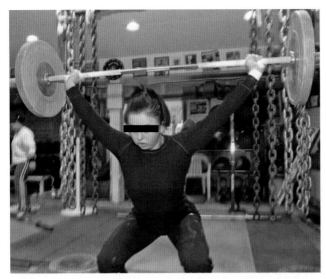

Figure 11.16 Case 1: Woman presented to the hospital for left lower neck pain and swelling over her left upper arm after she attempted heavy weightlifting.

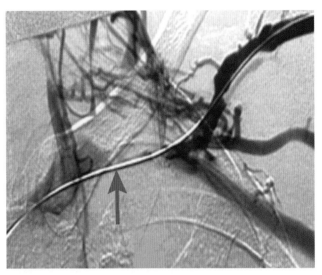

Figure 11.18 Case 1: Venography performed before procedure showed complete occlusion of the subclavian vein.

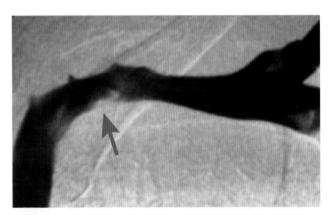

Figure 11.19 Case 1: No embolism following balloon angioplasty.

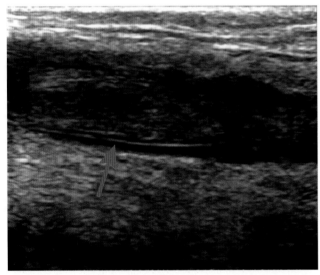

Figure 11.17 Case 1: Venous ultrasound of the left upper extremity showed a large echogenic thrombus of the subclavian vein.

Case 2 Radiation arteritis

Sixty-seven-year-old woman with a background of hypertension, smoking cessation, no diabetes, history of neoplasia of the left breast, with lumpectomy and radiotherapy 5 years previously presented with exertional pain in the right upper limb. Examination revealed a significant blood pressure drop on the symptomatic side, of 30 mmHg. Duplex echography demonstrated a tight and long stenosis of the right axillary artery confirmed by angiography (Fig. 11.20). Angioplasty and stenting of the right axillary artery by retrograde brachial puncture was performed, with a nitinol stent (5 mm x 80 mm, Lifestent, BARD®). One year later, she developed a recurrence of the exertional pain, with a restenosis confirmed by duplex ultrasound, probably by myointimal hyperplasia. Further balloon angioplasty (5 mm x 80 mm, Lutonix, BARD®) was performed and dual-antiplatelet agents prescribed for 1 year. There has been no further recurrence after 2 years(Fig. 11.21).

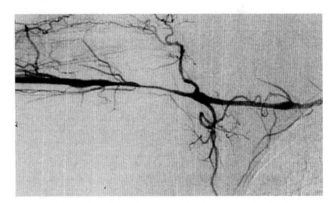

Figure 11.20 Case 2: Duplex echography demonstrated a tight and long stenosis of the right axillary artery confirmed by angiography.

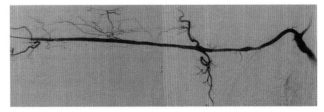

Figure 11.21 Case 2: Further balloon angioplasty was performed on the patient and dual-antiplatelet agents prescribed for 1 year. There has been no further recurrence after 2 years.

Key points

- Vascular diseases of the upper limb are rare in comparison to those involving the lower limbs, except for arterial embolism.
- Clinical examination, including the Allen test, is important.
- There are good mid-term results of endovascular treatment of supra-aortic trunk stenoses.
- The long-term results of carotid bypass or carotid transposition are excellent.
- It is important to consider arterial disease in the work environment, for example, hypothenar hammer syndrome.
- There is controversy concerning the diagnosis and treatment of N-TOCS.
- The combined supra-clavicular and infra-clavicular approach for first rib resection and arterial bypass is of value in the treatment of patients with arterial thoracic outlet compression syndrome.
- Early thrombolytic therapy followed by surgical thoracic outlet decompression is indicated in patients with primary SVT.

 References available at http://ebooks.health.elsevier.com/

KEY REFERENCES

[2] McCarthy WJ, Flinn WR, Yao JST, et al. Result of bypass grafting for upper limb ischemia. J Vasc Surg 1986;3(5):741–6. PMID: 2939264.

Between 1978 and 1984, the authors performed 33 bypass grafts to relieve hand and forearm ischaemia in 27 patients. A reversed saphenous vein graft was used in 22 cases and PTFE in the remaining 11 procedures. Follow-up of 31 grafts from 6 to 72 months (mean 35.5 months) revealed an overall patency rate of 73% at 2 years and 67% at 3 years. More proximal grafts fared better: the 2-year patency rate was 83% for grafts at or above the brachial artery but only 53% for bypass distal to the brachial bifurcation.

[3] Kieffer E, Sabatier J, Koskas F, et al. Atherosclerotic innominate artery occlusive disease: early and long-term results of surgical reconstruction. J Vasc Surg 1995;21(2):326–37. PMID: 7853604.

During a 20-year period (1974–93), the authors operated on 148 patients with brachiocephalic (innominate) artery atherosclerotic occlusive disease. Approach was through a median sternotomy in 135 (91%) patients. Endarterectomy was performed in 32 (22%) patients, whereas 116 (78%) patients underwent bypass. Eight (5.4%) patients died in the peri-operative period. There were five (3.4%) peri-operative strokes. Mean follow-up was 77 months. Survival was 51.9% at 10 years. The probability of freedom from ipsilateral stroke was 98.6% at 10 years. The primary patency rate was 98.4% at 10 years. In conclusion, surgical reconstruction of brachiocephalic artery atherosclerotic occlusive disease yields acceptable rates of peri-operative complications with excellent long-term patency and freedom from neurological events and reoperation.

[14] Vitti MJ, Thompson BW, Read RC, et al. Carotid-subclavian bypass: a twenty-two-year experience. J Vasc Surg 1994;20(3):411–8. PMID: 8084034.

A retrospective review of 124 patients who underwent carotid–subclavian bypass from 1968 to 1990 was done to assess primary patency and symptom resolution. Graft conduits were PTFE in 44 (35%) and Dacron in 80 (65%) cases; 30-day mortality was 0.8%, 30-day primary patency was 100%. Primary patency rate was 95% at 10 years. Survival rate was 59% at 10 years. Symptom-free survival rate was 87% at 10 years. Carotid–subclavian bypass appears to be a safe and durable procedure for relief of symptomatic occlusive disease of the subclavian artery.

[29] Kieffer E, Bahnini A, Koskas F. Aberrant subclavian artery: surgical treatment in thirty-three adult patients. J Vasc Surg 1994;19(1):100–11. PMID: 8301723.

The authors reviewed their experience with surgery for aberrant subclavian arteries (ASA). During a 16-year period they surgically treated 33 adult patients with ASA. Twenty-eight patients had a left-sided aortic arch with a right ASA, whereas five had a right-sided aortic arch with a left ASA. Eleven patients had dysphagia caused by oesophageal compression, five patients had ischaemic symptoms, 10 patients had aneurysms of the ASA and seven patients had an ASA arising from an aneurysmal thoracic aorta. In all cases, the distal subclavian artery was revascularised, most often by direct transposition into the ipsilateral common carotid artery. The cervical approach was combined with a median sternotomy or a left thoracotomy in 17 patients. Aortic cross-clamping was required in 12 patients to perform the transaortic closure of the origin of the ASA with patch angioplasty or prosthetic replacement of the descending thoracic aorta. Cardiopulmonary bypass was used in six patients. Four patients died after operation. Satisfactory clinical and anatomical results were obtained in the remaining 29 patients. Provision should be made for cardiopulmonary bypass in patients with aneurysm of ASA or associated aortic aneurysm.

[32] Sullivan TM, Bacharach JM, Perl J, et al. Endovascular management of unusual aneurysms of the axillary and subclavian arteries. J Endovasc Surg 1996;3(4):389–95. PMID: 8959496.

Aneurysms of the upper extremity arteries are uncommon and may be difficult to manage in emergency with standard surgical techniques. The authors report the exclusion of three axillary–subclavian aneurysms with covered stents. Palmaz stents were covered with either PTFE (two cases) or brachial vein and deployed to exclude pseudoaneurysms in one axillary and two left subclavian arteries. Endovascular exclusion of axillary and subclavian aneurysms with covered stents may offer a useful alternative to operative repair in patients with ruptured aneurysm or significant comorbidities.

[33] Vayssairat M, Debure C, Cormier J-M, et al. Hypothenar hammer syndrome: seventeen cases with long-term follow-up. J Vasc Surg 1987;5(6):838–42. PMID: 3586181.

The authors report 17 patients who had either ulnar thrombosis or ulnar aneurysm; most also had embolic occlusions of the digital arteries. Main pathological findings were thrombosis on the intima and fibrosis in the media. The authors adopted a surgical procedure consisting of resection with end-to-end reconstruction for patent aneurysms to avoid downstream emboli and more conservative treatment when the ulnar artery was thrombosed. No patient required digital amputation and all except one improved and were able to live and work normally.

[40] Axelrod DA, Proctor MC, Geisser ME, et al. Outcomes after surgery for thoracic outlet syndrome. J Vasc Surg 2001;33(6):1220–5. PMID: 11389421.

This study determined whether there is an association between psychological and socio-economic characteristics and long-term outcome of operative treatment for patients with sensory N-TOCS. Multivariate logistic regression models were developed as a means of identifying independent risk factors for post-operative disability. Operative decompression of the brachial plexus via a supra-clavicular approach was performed for upper-extremity pain and paraesthesia, with no mortality and minimal morbidity in 170 patients. After an average follow-up period of 47 months, 65% of patients reported improved symptoms and 64% of patients were satisfied with their operative outcome. However, 35% of patients remained on medication and 18% of patients were disabled. Pre-operative factors associated with persistent disability include major depression, being unmarried and having less than a high-school education. Operative decompression was beneficial for most patients. The impact of the pre-operative treatment of depression on the outcome of TOCS decompression should be studied prospectively.

[43] Rutherford R. Primary subclavian–axillary vein thrombosis: consensus and commentary. Cardiovasc Surg 1996;4(4):420–3. PMID: 8866074.

Fifteen multiple-choice questions concerning options in the management of primary subclavian–axillary vein thrombosis (SVT) were discussed by a panel of experts and then voted upon by 25 attending vascular surgeons with experience in SVT. The large majority favoured or agreed upon: (i) early clot removal for active healthy patients with a need/desire to use the involved limb in work or sport; (ii) catheter-directed thrombolysis as initial therapy; (iii) further therapy based on follow-up positional venography; (iv) surgical relief of demonstrated thoracic outlet compression after a brief period of anticoagulant therapy; (v) conservative therapy if post-lysis venogram showed either no extrinsic compression or a short residual occlusion; and (vi) intervention for residual intrinsic lesions with over 50% narrowing.

[44] Monreal M, Lafoz E, Ruiz J, et al. Upper-extremity deep venous thrombosis and pulmonary embolism. Chest 1991;99(2):280–3. PMID: 1989783.

The authors prospectively evaluated the prevalence of pulmonary embolism in 30 consecutive patients with proved DVT of the upper extremity. Ten patients had primary DVT and 20 patients had catheter-related DVT. Ventilation–perfusion lung scans were routinely performed at the time of hospital admission in all but one patient. Lung scan findings were normal in nine of 10 patients with primary DVT. In contrast, perfusion defects were considered highly suggestive of pulmonary embolism in four patients with catheter-related DVT. The authors conclude that pulmonary embolism is not a rare complication in upper-extremity DVT and that patients with catheter-related DVT seem to be at higher risk.

[50] Machleder HI. Evaluation of a new treatment strategy for Paget–Schroetter syndrome: spontaneous thrombosis of the axillary–subclavian vein. J Vasc Surg 1993;17(2):305–17. PMID: 8433426.

The authors conducted a study to determine an acceptable treatment approach to primary subclavian vein thrombosis. A retrospective review evaluated 11 patients in an 8-year period. All patients with occlusion received urokinase therapy and underwent surgical decompression within 5 days of thrombolytic therapy. Five percutaneous transluminal angioplasties were attempted before operative intervention. Eleven decompressions were performed. All patients received coumadin for 3–6 months after the operation. Urokinase therapy established wide venous patency in nine of 11 patients treated, with the remaining two requiring thrombectomy. One patient who underwent transluminal angioplasty before the operation had re-thrombosis, and the remaining four showed no improvement in venous stenosis after the intervention. Eight of nine extremities treated by first rib resection and one of two treated by scalenectomy were free of residual symptoms at follow-up. The authors conclude that pre-operative use of percutaneous balloon angioplasty is ineffective and should be avoided in this setting. Surgical intervention within days of thrombolysis enables patients to return to normal activity sooner.

[52] Urschel Jr HC, Razzuk MA. Paget–Schroetter syndrome: what is the best management? Ann Thorac Surg 2000;69(6):1663–8. PMID: 10892903.

The authors evaluated the results of 312 extremities in 294 patients with Paget–Schroetter syndrome to provide the basis for optimal management. Group I (35 extremities) was initially treated with anticoagulants only. Twenty-one developed recurrent symptoms after returning to work, requiring transaxillary resection of the first rib. Thrombectomy was necessary in eight. Group II (36 extremities) was treated with thrombolytic agents initially, with 20 requiring subsequent rib resection after returning to work. Thrombectomy was necessary in only four. Of the most recent 241 extremities (group III), excellent results accrued using thrombolysis plus prompt first rib resection for those evaluated during the first month after occlusion (199). The results were only fair for those seen later than 1 month (42). The authors conclude that early diagnosis (less than 1 month), expeditious thrombolytic therapy and prompt first rib resection are critical for the best results.

[57] Bern MM. Very low doses of warfarin can prevent thrombosis in central venous catheters. Ann Intern Med 1990;112(6):423–8. PMID: 2178534.

The goal of this study was to determine whether very low doses of warfarin are useful in thrombosis prophylaxis in patients with central venous catheters. Patients at risk for thrombosis associated with chronic indwelling central venous catheters were prospectively and randomly assigned to receive, or not to receive, 1 mg of warfarin beginning 3 days before catheter insertion and continuing for 90 days. Subclavian, innominate and superior vena cava venograms were done at onset of thrombosis symptoms or after 90 days in the study. A total of 121 patients entered the study and 82 patients completed the study. Of 42 patients completing the study while receiving warfarin, four had venogram-proven thrombosis. All four had symptoms from thrombosis. Of 40 patients completing the study while not receiving warfarin, 15 had venogram-proven thrombosis and 10 had symptoms from thrombosis (P <0.001). In conclusion, very low doses of warfarin can protect against thrombosis without inducing a haemorrhagic state. This approach may be applicable to other groups of patients.

12 Primary and secondary vasospastic disorders (Raynaud's phenomenon) and vasculitis

Patrick D.W. Kiely | Mark E. Lloyd

INTRODUCTION

A range of vasospastic and inflammatory disorders can present with ischaemia and thus come to the attention of the vascular clinician. These include primary and secondary Raynaud's phenomenon (RP), and conditions that cause vasculitis (the vasculitides). Diagnostic accuracy is important as management is directed by the underlying pathogenic process, be it vasospasm or inflammation. Diagnosis can be challenging, not least because presenting features of the vasculitides and some of the connective tissue diseases associated with secondary Raynaud's are non-specific, and features of atherosclerosis, vasculitis and vasospasm may overlap. The aim of this chapter is to provide the vascular clinician with a grounding of knowledge in these conditions so that the initial diagnosis can be made. It describes the clinical features, diagnostic tests, with particular emphasis on serology and imaging, and delineates treatment, highlighting guidelines where they exist.

RAYNAUD'S PHENOMENON

DEFINITION AND CLINICAL FEATURES

Vasospasm is the key feature of RP, illustrated in Fig. 12.1. Maurice Raynaud's original description was of episodic digital ischaemia induced by cold and emotion.[1–4] There is no single accepted clinical definition of RP. The classic 'French tricolour'

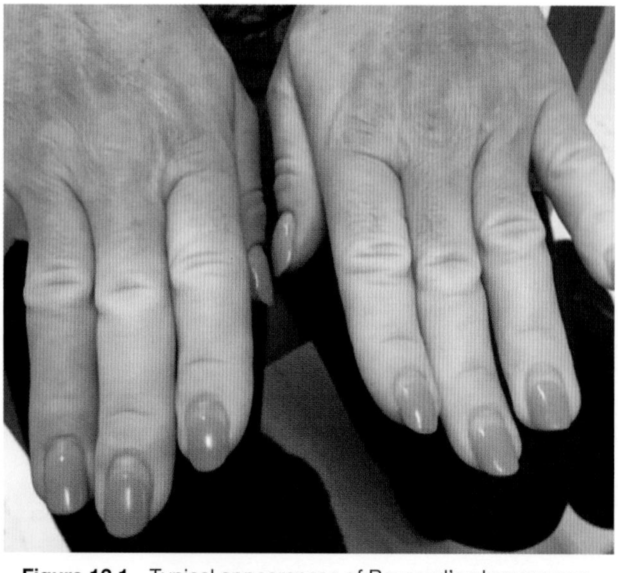

Figure 12.1 Typical appearances of Raynaud's phenomenon.

is pallor (vasospasm), then cyanosis (deoxygenation of static venous blood) and finally rubor (reactive hyperaemia). This full triphasic colour change is not essential for the diagnosis of RP, and a history of monophasic cold-induced blanching may be sufficient. The condition may be asymmetrical and may not involve the whole digit. Other stimuli can provoke attacks, such as stress, chemicals (including drugs and those in tobacco smoke[2]), and trauma. In addition to the digits, vasospasm may involve the nose, tongue, ear lobes and nipples.

There is inconsistent terminology around RP. The nomenclature recommended in recent European Society for Vascular Medicine (ESVM) guidelines suggests the terms *primary Raynaud's phenomenon (PRP)* where there is no underlying associated condition, and *secondary Raynaud's phenomenon (SRP)* where there is.[4] The terms *Raynaud's disease* and *Raynaud's syndrome* are best avoided.

✅ Use the term 'Raynaud's phenomenon'.

✅ Colour change may only be monophasic – have a low index of suspicion for diagnosis.

✅ **Primary** Raynaud's phenomenon (PRP) is not associated with any underlying condition.

✅ **Secondary** Raynaud's phenomenon (SRP) is associated with an underlying condition, most often rheumatological.

EPIDEMIOLOGY

A meta-analysis of observational studies suggests a prevalence of RP of approximately 5% in the UK[5] but may affect 20–30% of women in younger age groups.[4] Primary RP comprises 80–90% cases, is nine times more common in women and has a genetic contribution in 50% of cases.[4,6,7]

DISTINGUISHING BETWEEN PRIMARY RAYNAUD'S PHENOMENON AND SECONDARY RAYNAUD'S PHENOMENON

This can be difficult but is critical to management. Conditions associated with SRP are shown in Box 12.1 and features, which can be helpful to distinguish them in Table 12.1.

✅ Distinguishing PRP and SRP can be clinically difficult.

✅ Have a low threshold for further investigation and referral to rheumatology.

Box 12.1 Conditions associated with secondary Raynaud's phenomenon

Connective tissue diseases

Systemic sclerosis
Idiopathic inflammatory myositis, amyopathic disease, anti-synthetase syndrome
Systemic lupus erythematosus
Sjögren's syndrome
Mixed connective tissue diseases/overlap syndromes
Undifferentiated connective tissue diseases
Rheumatoid arthritis

Obstructive vascular

Atherosclerosis
Buerger's disease (thromboangiitis obliterans)
Microemboli
Thoracic outlet syndrome (especially cervical ribs)

Increased plasma viscosity

Cryoglobulinaemia, cryofibrinogenaemia
Paraprotein
Malignancy, paraneoplastic phenomenon

Drug/chemical exposure

Anti-migraine therapies: ergot alkaloids, e.g., methysergide
Non-selective beta-blockers, including eye drops
Bromocriptine
Clonidine
Cytotoxics, e.g., bleomycin, cisplatin
Ciclosporin
Drugs of misuse: amphetamines, cannabis, cocaine
Ephedrine, in ear, nose and throat preparations
Interferon α and β
Oestrogen replacement therapy without progesterone
Vinyl chloride monomers

Occupational

Vibration white finger disease
Frozen food industry

Other causes or associations

Reflex sympathetic dystrophy
Hypothyroidism
Phaeochromocytoma

PRP is generally a benign condition with few if any significant sequelae. Nevertheless, individuals with PRP still report impaired quality of life.[8]

SRP is more severe, has the potential to cause ischaemic damage to the digit (Fig. 12.2) and often requires pharmacological intervention. Recognition of SRP is important as it enables identification of an associated reversible cause (see Box 12.1), or connective tissue disorder (CTD) and the opportunity to optimise management of this at an early stage.

The age of onset is one useful feature, SRP generally occurring at a later age, for example, at a median of 36 years compared to 14 years in PRP.[9] Around 80% of patients over 60 years presenting with new digital ischaemia will have an associated condition.[10] Conversely RP occurring in very young children, whilst rare, is frequently caused by an underlying CTD. Thumb involvement suggests SRP.[3]

The CTDs are the most common group of disorders underlying SRP, with the prevalence of RP in each listed in Table 12.2. Of these, systemic sclerosis (SSc) is the most frequent association and linked with digit loss in up to 16% of patients.[11] A 'top to toe' screen to identify possible features of a CTD is recommended (Box 12.2). Nonetheless, SRP may be the only feature of an underlying CTD and precede other symptoms by years. One study reported that 12.6% of patients referred for assessment of RP progressed to SSc after a median follow-up of 4 years.[12] Another reported a 9% transition in patients presenting with RP alone and 30% from 'possible' secondary RP after a 12.4-year mean follow-up.[10]

 Systemic sclerosis (SSc) and systemic lupus erythematosus (SLE) are the commonest and most serious connective tissue disorders (CTDs) associated with SRP.

 RP may be the only presenting symptom.

EXAMINATION

Close examination of the hands may reveal signs of ischaemic damage, which excludes PRP, and features of CTDs associated with SRP. Ischaemia is indicated by digital pulp loss, skin cracks or breaks, ulcers and at worse, gangrene. Features of CTDs include subcutaneous calcification

Table 12.1 Features suggestive of primary and secondary Raynaud's phenomenon

	Primary Raynaud's	Secondary Raynaud's
Age at onset	Generally young	Can be older
Involvement of thumbs	Usually spared	Involved
Temperature trigger	Severe cold	Trivial temperature drop
	Long exposure	Short exposure
Recovery time on rewarming	Short; often <10 minutes	Long; may be >30 minutes
Ischaemic damage	Absent	Digital pain, pitting, ulcers, gangrene
	No pain between episodes	
ANA	Negative	Positive; >1 in 80
	Weak positive 1 in 80	Supplementary antibodies positive; ENA, SSc specific, myositis specific
Nailfold capillaroscopy	Normal	Abnormal
Peripheral pulses	Normal	Impaired/absent if obstructive cause
ESR, plasma viscosity	Normal	Raised if hyperviscosity causal

ANA, Antinuclear antibody; ENA, extractable nuclear antigens; ESR, erythrocyte sedimentation rate; SSc, systemic sclerosis.

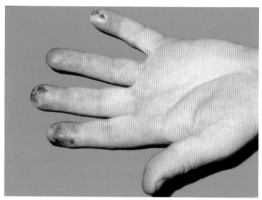

Figure 12.2 Digital ulceration in secondary Raynaud's phenomenon.

Table 12.2 Incidence of Raynaud's phenomenon in connective tissue disorders

Systemic sclerosis	95%
Mixed connective tissue disease	85%
Systemic lupus erythematosus	29–40%
Idiopathic inflammatory myositis	40%
Sjögren's syndrome	33%
Rheumatoid arthritis	10%

Box 12.2 'Top to toe' screen for connective tissue disorders (systemic lupus erythematosus, Sjögren's, myositis) in a patient with Raynaud's

- hair thinning, alopecia
- dry mouth or eyes
- oral ulcers
- rash, photosensitivity
- arthralgia
- difficulty swallowing, choking
- cough, breathlessness on exertion
- muscle pain or weakness
- fatigue

Table 12.3 Autoantibody associations with secondary Raynauds, and clinical phenotypes

Antibody	Disease	Specific association
Centromere	Limited SSc	
Topoisomerase I (Scl70)	Diffuse SSc	ILD, cardiac
RNA polymerase III	Diffuse SSc	Renal crisis
Double stranded DNA	SLE	Renal disease
RNP, Sm	SLE	PH
U1RNP	mixed CTD	
SSA (Ro), SSB (La)	Sjogren's syndrome, SLE	
Jo-1, PL-7, PL-12*	Anti-synthetase syndrome	ILD
Pm/Scl-75/100	Myositis, SSc	ILD
Ro-52	Sjogren's, myositis	ILD
MDA-5	Dermatomyositis	ILD
SAE	Dermatomyositis	Oesophageal disease
TIF1γ, NXP-2	Dermatomyositis	Malignancy
CCP	Rheumatoid arthritis	
ANCA, PR3, MPO	Small vessel vasculitis	ILD and renal disease

*8 antibodies are recognized in the anti-synthetase syndrome: Jo-1, PL-7, PL-12, EJ, Ha, KS, OJ, Zo.
ANCA, anti-neutrophil cytoplasm antibody; CTD, connective tissue disease; ILD, Interstitial lung disease; MPO, myeloperoxidase; PH, pulmonary hypertension; PR-3, proteinase 3; SSc, systemic sclerosis; SLE, systemic lupus erythematosus.

INVESTIGATIONS

Basic tests include full blood count, erythrocyte sedimentation rate (ESR) and C-reactive protein (CRP), urea and electrolytes, liver and thyroid function tests, antinuclear antibody (ANA) and urinalysis. In systemic lupus erythematosus (SLE), myeloma and other hyperviscosity syndromes, the ESR may be raised but CRP normal. This should prompt serum protein electrophoresis and serum free light chain testing. Imaging for obstructive causes including a cervical rib may be appropriate.

IMMUNOLOGICAL TESTS

Most patients with SSc or SLE will have a positive ANA. However, the test is positive in around 10% of healthy individuals, usually at low titre (1/80–1/160). If the ANA is positive, check extractable nuclear antigen (ENA) antibodies and anti-double stranded deoxyribonucleic acid antibodies and specific antibodies for SSc and myositis. Autoantibodies have clinical utility as they are associated with specific autoimmune diseases, patterns of disease and organ involvement, summarised in Table 12.3. As such, their detection enables prediction of likely clinical phenotypes, greatly enhancing patient care, with targeted screening and preemptive treatment before critical organ damage ensues.

SSc has the strongest association with RP. It is present in virtually all cases, sometimes preceding other clinical manifestations by several years. Limited SSc is associated with anti-centromere antibodies and specific clinical features and signs including telangiectasiae, calcinosis cutis, sclerodactyly and

(calcinosis cutis), ragged cuticles and visible nailfold capillaries. The latter are caused by abnormal giant capillary loops and haemorrhage from these, confirmed by capillaroscopy (see later section). The skin of the fingers should be examined for SSc where early features include puffiness followed by the classic waxy tightening of sclerodactyly, and ultimately progressive sclerodermatous change extending proximally up the arms and legs, involvement of the trunk, back and face with peri-oral puckering, tendon friction rubs and joint contractures. Roughening of the skin, on the radial aspect of the fingers and ulnar side of the thumb, called 'mechanic's hands' is seen almost exclusively in inflammatory myositis.

Peripheral pulses should be checked for strength and symmetry, blood pressure compared in both arms, and subclavian arteries checked for bruits. Thoracic outlet syndromes can be checked using dynamic tests such as Adson's.

oesophagitis (previously known as 'CREST'). Diffuse cutaneous SSc is a more aggressive disorder associated with internal organ involvement including renal and interstitial lung disease (ILD) and pulmonary hypertension. Antibodies to topoisomerase I (Scl70) are associated with ILD and cardiac involvement[13] and antibodies to ribonucleic acid (RNA) polymerase III with renal disease.[14,15] Early detection of ILD enables commencement of immunosuppressants such as cyclophosphamide and mycophenolate mofetil to prevent progression. Detection of anti-RNA polymerase III enables enhanced monitoring for renal crisis with blood pressure and estimated glomerular filtration rate (eGFR) assessment, avoidance of steroids, which increase the incidence, and early commencement of angiotensin-converting enzyme (ACE) inhibitors to significantly improve outcome from this rare but fatal complication.

Isolated patches of sclerodermatous skin, called *morphoea*, may also be associated with RP and the presence of autoantibodies or abnormal nailfold capillaries confers a high likelihood of a systemic disease.[16]

In patients with SLE, the presence of RP associates with anti-Sm and anti-RNP autoantibodies[17,18] and a more benign disease course, including a lower incidence of renal disease, serositis, haemolysis and improved survival,[18,19] although a higher incidence of peripheral and central nervous system disease has been reported.[20]

RP is a prevalent feature of the idiopathic inflammatory myopathies (IIM), reported in 78% of those with anti-PM/Scl-75/100 antibodies in which features of SSc and myositis are found.[21] In the same series, the prevalence of RP was 39% in the anti-synthetase syndrome (ARS), 22% in dermatomyositis (DM), and 15% in necrotising myositis. Other skin signs are diagnostic of IIM, with mechanics hands a pathognomonic feature occurring in 80% of patients with anti-PM/SCl-75/100 antibodies, 58% of those with ARS and 28% with DM.[21] Thus the finding of co-existing skin signs including mechanics hands and the well described features of DM, such as Gottron's papules and a heliotrope peri-orbital rash, reveal IIM as a secondary cause of RP, and enable screening for muscle and lung disease.

✅ Autoantibodies are increasingly used to predict specific clinical phenotypes in CTDs.

✅ ANA is a useful screening test; when positive, further immunological tests and rheumatology referral should be considered.

SPECIALISED IMAGING FOR RAYNAUD'S PHENOMENON ASSOCIATED WITH CONNECTIVE TISSUE DISORDERS

NAILFOLD CAPILLAROSCOPY[4,22]

At the nailfold, the capillaries run in parallel to the skin surface enabling inspection of anatomical size and form. Nailfold capillaroscopy has become established as one of the most sensitive ways to screen for an associated CTD, especially SSc.[23] This technique uses 200–600 x magnification to directly visualise the capillaries at the nail fold. Lower magnification may be used by a variety of devices such as an ophthalmoscope or dermatoscope, with less detail visible. Very large abnormal capillaries can just be seen with the naked eye. Normal vessels are uniform in diameter and lie equi-spaced and in parallel with a 'hairpin' structure. Characteristic abnormalities in CTDs (Fig. 12.3), especially systemic sclerosis, include dilation, giant forms, distortion of shape, tortuosity, haemorrhage and regions of absence (drop-out).[24] The combination of abnormal nailfold vessels and autoantibodies has been shown to predict progression to CTD; studies suggest that RP patients with both abnormalities are up to 60 times more likely to go on to develop SSc than those with neither.[12,25] It should be noted that nailfold changes also occur with trauma and in diabetes mellitus.

✅ The diagnostic value of nailfold capillaroscopy is now validated with standardisation and algorithms developed to detect SSc[26,27]

INFRARED THERMOGRAPHY

Thermography uses a thermal imaging camera to measure skin surface temperature, as an indirect measure of cutaneous blood flow (Fig. 12.4). This can help distinguish SRP from PRP, given more severe disease in SRP, especially SSc.[22,28] This technique is yet to be routinely used in clinical practice, and requires specialised equipment and a temperature controlled room. It may also have potential as an indirect measure of response to therapy, though standardised protocols have not been established.

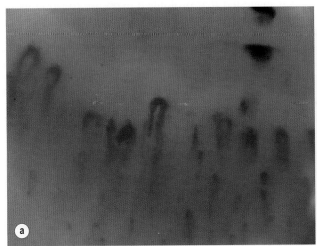
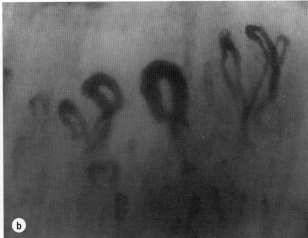

Figure 12.3 Nail-fold capillaroscopy changes in secondary Raynaud's phenomenon, showing drop out, abnormal architecture, dilated loops and giant forms. (Image courtesy of Dr Arvind Kaul, St George's Hospital, London, UK.)

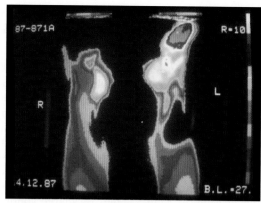

Figure 12.4 Thermography demonstrating Raynaud's phenomenon of the toes, worse on the right. The image shows a temperature gradient from the mid-foot to the toes on the left (L) and an absence of blood flow to the toes on the right (R), as detected by an infrared camera.

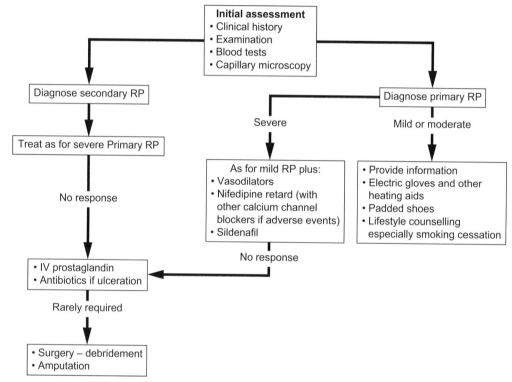

Figure 12.5 Flowchart for the management of Raynaud's phenomenon. *IV*, Intravenous; *RP*, Raynaud's phenomenon.

OCCUPATIONAL RAYNAUD'S PHENOMENON

Hand–arm vibration syndrome (HAVS, previously known as *vibration white finger*), is described in workers using vibrating tools such as chainsaws, pneumatic road drills and buffing machines. An estimated 4.2 million men and 667 000 women in Great Britain have occupational exposure to hand-transmitted vibration.[29] Vasospasm in HAVS has been described in the toes as well as the fingers and is likely related to vibration-induced damage of the endothelium.[30] The duration of exposure is important, as symptom severity and length of exposure are correlated.[31] The latency period between exposure and disease is usually more than 5 years of full-time work. Resolution of symptoms may occur in up to one-third of cases if there is a change of job early in the disease course.[32]

In the UK, HAVS has been a proscribed industrial disease since 1985. Patients may be eligible for industrial injuries disablement benefits if they fulfil certain criteria.[33] It has been suggested that prolonged exposure to vibrating computer game controls could also cause HAVS.[34]

Further examples of occupation-related RP include vinyl chloride disease, which is estimated to occur in 3% of exposed workers and can persist long after retirement,[35] and nitrate exposure related to ammunitions work, where habituation to vasodilatory nitrates means that RP can develop away from the work environment.

MANAGEMENT OF RAYNAUD'S PHENOMENON

A general approach to management of RP involves a hierarchy of intervention, starting with lifestyle measures, followed by pharmacological intervention (Fig. 12.5).[4,22] The evidence base for many of the pharmacological therapies used in routine practice is poor. In part this reflects difficulty in assessing efficacy as most treatment endpoints are subjective. Also, response may be affected by other factors, including seasonal changes in weather. The most recent systematic review and network meta-analysis of treatments available for SRP has concluded that only calcium channel blockers and phosphodiesterase-5 (PDE-5) inhibitors are effective pharmacological options, with moderate efficacy and low levels of evidence.[36] There was only very weak evidence for any benefit of oral prostanoids, selective serotonin reuptake inhibitors (SSRIs) and antioxidants over placebo.[36] Recent management guidelines from ESVM,[4] and the European Alliance of Associations for Rheumatology (EULAR) specifically for RP in SSc,[37] which predate this analysis, have broader recommendations reflecting changes in analysis methodology, and also the need for a practical approach in patients for whom several agents may need to be given to save digits.

GENERAL MEASURES

Scleroderma & Raynaud's UK (https://www.sruk.co.uk/) is a good source of information for patients. Education is vital to ensure patients are fully aware of the consequences of cold exposure and the wide range of protective measures available. Keeping the core temperature warm and specific protection of the extremities underpins this. For the hands and feet, double or multiple layers of clothing (gloves, socks) and warm shoes prevent heat loss from the digits. Pocket-sized thermochemical warming agents and electrically heated gloves and socks can supplement this. Cessation of smoking and where applicable drugs of misuse such as cocaine and amphetamines, is essential. Prescribed medications should be adjusted where possible to avoid those associated with RP (see Box 12.1). Vibration exposure should be avoided. Skin moisturiser is helpful in preventing skin cracks or breaks, which in SRP may be painful and often heal slowly. Secondary infection of such skin breaks or ulcers requires prompt use of antibiotics. Anecdotally, some patients get benefit from the use of surgical glue to enable skin breaks to heal.

For many patients, especially those with PRP, these measures are sufficient to control symptoms and a useful rule is that no more need be done if the re-warming time and full recovery of RP is less than 15 minutes.

PHARMACOLOGICAL THERAPY

This should be offered to patients not responding sufficiently to general measures, where the re-warming time is more than 15 minutes, if RP episodes are frequently induced by lifestyle or work (i.e., cold exposure, outdoor workers), or if there are features of ischaemic damage such as prolonged digital pain after re-warming, slowly healing skin cracks or ulcers. Most patients with SRP and some with PRP fall into this category. Oral pharmacological agents commonly used in the treatment of RP are shown in Box 12.3.

Calcium channel blockers

These drugs are vasodilatory. Nifedipine is recommended as first-line drug treatment for RP.[4,37] It may have additional antiplatelet activity and also suppress T cells.[38] Systematic reviews have shown that dihydropyridine calcium channel blockers (CCBs), nifedipine (the most widely studied), nicardipine, amlodipine, and felodipine can reduce the frequency and severity of attacks in PRP and SRP.[39]

Box 12.3 Oral drugs most commonly used in the treatment of Raynaud's phenomenon

Calcium channel blockers

Nifedipine (sustained release) 10–40 mg twice daily
Amlodipine 5–10 mg once daily

Phosphodiesterase-5 inhibitors

Sildenafil 25–50 mg three times daily
Tadalafil 10 mg alternate days – 20 mg daily

Other agents

Transdermal GTN '5' patch One patch (or portion) on 1 – 4 extremities
Losartan 25–100 mg once daily
Prazosin 500 µg – 2 mg twice daily
Fluoxetine 20 mg once daily
Iloprost intravenous, according to weight

Vasodilatory side-effects (flushing, headache and ankle swelling) are common, especially with immediate-release preparations, and may limit their use. Slow-release preparations are often better tolerated and should be up-titrated slowly to minimise side-effects.[4] Flushing and headache usually diminish over time. ESVM guidelines suggest amlodipine, lercanidipine and diltiazem as alternatives.[4] Nifedipine has no licence for use in pregnancy.

Other vasodilators

A 2012 Cochrane review examined the effect of vasodilators other than CCBs in the management of PRP.[40] These included captopril and enalapril (ACE-inhibitors), thymoxamine (alpha-1 antagonist), buflomedil (alpha-adrenoreceptor antagonist and weak CCB), beraprost (oral prostacyclin analogue), dazoxiben (thromboxane synthetase inhibitor) and ketanserin (serotonin 5 H-T and alpha adrenoceptor antagonist). Some benefit was seen for thymoxamine and buflomedil, though the studies were of low quality, and overall conclusions were of no benefit in PRP for these non-CCB vasodilatory agents.

EVSM guidelines[4] suggest losartan and fluoxetine as alternative vasodilators, though again evidence is limited. Fluoxetine, a selective serotonin receptor antagonist, has the advantage of not being associated with the same vasodilatory adverse effects as CCBs. An open-label cross-over study comparing fluoxetine with nifedipine in PRP and SRP demonstrated reduced frequency and severity of attacks.[41] EULAR guidelines indicate that fluoxetine might be considered in the treatment of SSc-RP.[37] Overall, naftidrofuryl oxalate (Praxilene), a mild peripheral vasodilator with a serotonin receptor antagonist effect, has some benefit in intermittent claudication but there is little evidence for effectiveness in RP.[42]

Phosphodiesterase-5 inhibitors

These drugs increase the availability or effect of nitric oxide, a potent vasodilator. Meta-analysis of six randomised controlled trials (RCTs) of phosphodiesterase (PDE)-5 inhibitors (sildenafil, tadalafil, vardenafil) showed a significant, modest benefit in RP secondary to SSc.[43] PDE-5 inhibitors have been shown to be the only agent effective in reducing the duration of SRP attacks.[36] EULAR guidelines indicate that they should be considered in the treatment of SSc-RP.[37] Larger studies are needed, but PDE-5 inhibitors offer a generally well tolerated alternative to CCBs, with a comparatively good evidence base, and are increasingly used second-line in the management of RP.

Prostanoids

Prostaglandin analogues of PGI_2 (prostacyclin) and PGE_1 have potent vasodilatory and antiplatelet effects. Older metanalyses suggested a definite benefit for intravenous iloprost (the most commonly used prostanoid in the UK) in SSc-RP.[44,45] It is recommended in EULAR guidelines for severe SSc-RP.[37] Despite recent updated and less favourable meta-analysis,[36] iloprost remains the agent of choice in cases of severe ischaemia or digital ulceration in SRP. It has the advantage of having a long-term benefit for many patients, sometimes for 6 months or more after an infusion. Side effects include nausea, headache and hypotension. Careful titration can help minimise these.

Other vasodilators

Topical nitrates, such as transdermal glyceryl trinitrate patches, are often used in clinical practice, placed on the volar surface of the wrist or dorsum of the foot. They appear effective for many patients and may be flexibly dosed by using up to 4 patches per day (one per hand and foot) or reduced to one extremity or cut to smaller sizes. This is particularly useful to minimise intolerance as, like CCBs, they can cause light headedness or headache.

Endothelin-1 receptor antagonists

Bosentan, an endothelin-1 antagonist, is licenced for the prevention of recurrent digital ulcers in SSc. It is therefore used for the prevention of ischaemic complications of RP but not for the management of RP per se alone. In trials, bosentan has been found to reduce new ulcers, but not to enhance healing of existing ulcers. The evidence base is well reviewed in EULAR guidelines.[37]

Antiplatelet therapies

This may be considered in SRP, particularly as there is evidence of platelet activation in SSc. Although there is no trial evidence of efficacy in SRP, the use of antiplatelet drugs may increase microcirculation and hence tissue perfusion.[22]

SURGICAL THERAPIES

Upper limb sympathectomy is no longer recommended. Digital sympathectomy, stripping the adventitia of affected digital arteries, is utilised in specialist centres. The evidence for this comes from observational small series in the literature, with no formal trials to date.[4,22]

For the complications of ischaemic damage in SRP, debridement of gangrenous tissue may be cautiously utilised. However, it is stressed that a general principle of SRP management complicated by gangrene is to maximise tissue perfusion with vasodilators and to provide adequate analgesia, allowing auto-amputation to occur in due course. Often, this leads to preservation of more viable tissue at the end of the affected digit, and hence function, than permitted by surgical amputation.

✅ Delay surgical amputation for severe digital ischaemia in SRP without a full trial of vasodilators, including prostanoids, and rheumatology review.

RAYNAUD'S MIMICS

Cold sensitivity

This is a commonly reported symptom, with the subjective experience of cold hands and feet, which may be accompanied by mild, poorly demarcated colour change. This reflects appropriate cold-induced closure of arteriovenous shunts in the skin, a thermoregulatory mechanism that decreases cutaneous blood flow and limits loss of body heat.

Chilblains (perniosis)

This condition is cold induced and characterised by tender, pruritic red or bluish swelling of the fingers, toes, ears and nose. The lesions present 12–24 hours after exposure to cold and usually resolve spontaneously in 1–3 weeks. Unlike RP, there is no sharp demarcation line, colour change is fixed, pruritis is common and there may be diffuse swelling of the digit. Biopsy reveals dermal perivascular lymphocytic infiltrates and fibrinogen deposition. Whilst many are idiopathic, chilblain lupus and other associations are described.[46,47] Chilblains may co-exist with RP, particularly in patients with CTDs and low body mass index.

Acrocyanosis

This is a benign, painless, symmetric discoloration of various shades of blue of the extremities, aggravated by cold and often associated with hyperhidrosis. It is distinguished from RP by lack of paroxysms of pallor, persistence of colour change for months and often years, and involvement of the entire hand or foot in some cases.[48]

Erythromelalgia

This condition is characterised by heat, tingling or burning pain and redness of the extremities, most commonly affecting the feet, but also the hands, ears, face and limbs. Unlike RP, it is triggered by an increase in temperature and relieved by cooling. Symptoms can be episodic and persist for days, and blotchy redness affects the entire foot or hand rather than the digits alone.[49] Primary erythromelalgia is caused by an autosomal dominant mutation of the *SCN9A* gene, coding for voltage-gated sodium channels. Secondary erythromelalgia is associated with myeloproliferative disorders.

Achenbach's syndrome

This condition is caused by haemorrhage from a dermal or subcutaneous digital vein or venule, also referred to as '*paroxysmal finger haematoma*'. Often a vessel crossing the distal or proximal interphalangeal joint is affected. The characteristic features are painful localised bruising and swelling originating from the palmar side of one finger, spreading around the digit, and resolving after a few days.[50]

CONCLUSION

RP is a common condition affecting around 5% of the population. Differentiation between PRP and SRP can be clinically difficult but crucial, as identification and treatment of underlying causes and disease associations, particularly

CTDs, improves long-term outcomes. In PRP, management hinges on education, and simple lifestyle interventions are often sufficient for most patients. Several guidelines support the use of CCBs, PDE-5 inhibitors, fluoxetine and prostanoids for more severe PRP and SRP, but individual response is unpredictable, and often several agents need to be trialled. Amputation is very much a last resort, and patients should have rheumatology review before this stage is reached.

VASCULITIS

Vasculitis means inflammation of the blood vessel wall. This can be primary or secondary. Primary vasculitis is caused by a group of overlapping systemic syndromes of unknown cause: the vasculitides. Secondary vasculitis is caused by a wide range of conditions, including infections, malignancy, drug reactions and systemic diseases (e.g., rheumatoid, sarcoid and SLE). The vasculitides are classified according to the size of the vessels affected, as shown in Table 12.4. As these are systemic inflammatory diseases, constitutional symptoms, such as malaise, fatigue, fever, night sweats, anorexia and weight loss are common features. Inflammation of the vessel wall can lead to aneurysm, stenosis and intraluminal thrombosis. Aneurysm rupture leads to haemorrhage, stenosis and thrombotic sequelae lead to ischaemia and ultimately tissue infarction, either of extremities or organ/s. Clinical manifestations reflect vessel size and site, and include for large vessel disease limb claudication, angina or abdominal pain (mesenteric disease), stroke and for small-vessel disease foot drop/mononeuritis multiplex (vasa nervorum), glomerulonephritis, pulmonary haemorrhage and skin ulceration. Diagnosis is made according to the pattern of clinical features, supported by serology, imaging and histology. Non-invasive imaging enables assessment of the extent and distribution of vascular disease. Techniques include ultrasound (US), computed tomography and magnetic resonance angiography (CTA and MRA) and [^{18}F]fluorodeoxyglucose positron emission tomography/computed tomography (PET-CT). The latter demonstrates the presence and distribution of metabolic uptake in vessel walls and can be used to monitor response to treatment. Biopsy allows histological confirmation and is always recommended, where possible.

QUICK CLINICAL TIPS. SIGNS CONSISTENT WITH VASCULITIS:

- splinter haemorrhages and/or nailfold infarcts
- palpable purpura
- foot drop
- blood or protein or urinalysis
- elevated eosinophil count
- elevated cardiac troponin I

LARGE VESSEL VASCULITIS

The term 'large vessel vasculitis' implies involvement of the aorta and its major branches. Two primary granulomatous conditions, separated by onset pre- and post-50 years of age are well described: Takayasu's arteritis (TAK) and giant cell arteritis (GCA, previously known as temporal arteritis). Non-granulomatous causes include inflammatory aortic aneurysm with or without retroperitoneal fibrosis, immunoglobulin (Ig)G4-related disease and Behcet's disease. Recognition of the inflammatory aetiology of these arteritides is essential, to ensure appropriate immune suppression for optimal outcomes. Particularly important is the prevention of blindness in GCA. Whilst immune suppression is the focus of therapy, surgical intervention may be a necessary adjunct, for example, endovascular prevention of aneurysmal rupture, and ureteric stents to avoid occlusion from retroperitoneal fibrosis.

✔ Three over-arching principles and 10 recommendations for management of large vessel vasculitis have been published by EULAR in 2020.[51]

TAKAYASU'S ARTERITIS

TAK is an idiopathic, chronic inflammatory, granulomatous arteritis. It primarily affects the large elastic arteries: the

Table 12.4 Relationship between vasculitis classification and vessel size

Type of vasculitis	Aorta and branches	Large and medium-sized arteries	Medium-sized muscular arteries	Small muscular arteries	Arterioles, capillaries and venules
Takayasu's arteritis	✓				
Giant cell arteritis (cranial and extra-cranial)	✓	✓			
Inflammatory aortic aneurysm, IgG4 disease	✓	✓			
Behcet's disease		✓	✓		
Polyarteritis nodosa, Kawasaki disease		✓	✓		
Buerger's disease			✓	✓	
AAV: GPA MPO, EGPA			✓	✓	✓
CTD & rheumatoid vasculitis				✓	✓
HSP, Cutaneous vasculitis					✓

AAV, Anti-neutrophil cytoplasm antibody –associated vasculitis; *CTD*, autoimmune connective tissue disorders; *EGPA*, eosinophilic granulomatosis with polyangiitis, previously known as Churg Strauss vasculitis; *GPA*, granulomatosis with polyangiitis, previously known as Wegener's granulomatosis; *HSP*, Henoch-Schonlein purpura; *MPO*, microscopic polyangiitis.

aorta, its major branches and the pulmonary arteries. The most common branches affected are the subclavian, common carotid and renal arteries. Chronic inflammation leads to arterial stenosis as well as occlusion and aneurysm formation.

TAK is a rare disease, most commonly described in Japan. The annual incidence in the UK is estimated at 0.8 per million. It has a striking female predominance, affecting women five to nine times more frequently than men. It usually occurs before the age of 50 years and most commonly in the second or third decades.[52]

Disease symptomatology can be divided into systemic features of inflammation and specific sequelae of ischaemia from impaired arterial vessel flow. Key symptoms are new onset or worsening of limb ischaemia accompanied by features of generalised inflammation including weight loss >2 kg, low grade fever, night sweats and fatigue. Other recognised features include arthralgia and myalgia, severe abdominal pain (mesenteric ischaemia), non-hypertensive stroke, seizures (cerebrovascular ischaemia), angina and myocardial infarction (coronary artery ischaemia), pulmonary hypertension (pulmonary artery stenosis) and acute visual symptoms such as amaurosis fugax or diplopia. Key clinical findings are diminished or absent arterial pulses, pulse inequality, bruits (e.g., over the aorta or subclavian artery), hypertension >140/90 mmHg, inequality of blood pressure between arms or between arm and leg and carotidynia. An elevated ESR and CRP are usually (but not always) seen. ANA and anti-neutrophil cytoplasm antibody (ANCA) are negative, and there are no specific disease markers or autoantibodies for TAK.

The American College of Rheumatology classification criteria for TAK (1990) are commonly used for diagnostic purposes; three of six clinical and imaging criteria are required, with 90% sensitivity and 98% specificity.[52]

Non-invasive imaging is essential to confirm a clinical diagnosis of TAK (Fig. 12.6). MRA is recommended by EULAR as the first-line imaging test to demonstrate mural inflammation and/or luminal changes.[53] PET, CTA or US may be used as alternatives, however, US is of limited value for assessment of the thoracic aorta. Conventional angiography is no longer recommended. Biopsy findings reveal inflammation in all arterial layers (panarteritis). There is thickening of the adventitia with nodule formation, leukocyte infiltration of the media with granulomas, and intimal hyperplasia, leading to progressive luminal narrowing. Over time, fibrosis of the intima and media ensues, resulting in stenosis or occlusion.

Induction of remission in TAK requires high-dose corticosteroid, usually prednisolone 40–60 mg per day, though lower starting doses may be appropriate for patients with localised disease.[51] Prednisolone is tapered to 15–20 mg daily within 3 months and to 10 mg daily or less by 1 year. In view of high relapse rates of 70%, the development of new vascular lesions and the inability of many patients to taper prednisolone to low doses, early administration of steroid sparing immune suppressants is recommended.[51] This includes azathioprine, leflunomide, methotrexate and mycophenolate mofetil, chosen on the basis of individual patient comorbidities and contra-indications. Tocilizumab and abatacept have been reported in RCTs and open label case series, and tumour necrosis factor (TNF) inhibitors also in case series. Overall, there is no high-quality evidence showing superiority of biological agents over conventional immune suppressing therapies in TAK.[51] Related comorbidities such as hypertension and diabetes should be treated aggressively. Assessment of response and monitoring for recurrence is difficult as there is no reliable assessment tool.[54] Long-term immune-suppression (ideally steroid-free) and specialist review for at least 10 years is advised, monitoring clinical signs and inflammatory markers.

Disease relapse is usually accompanied by a rise in CRP and repeat MRA or CTA is used to identify new or progressive vascular abnormalities. Management of relapse requires re-instatement of high-dose prednisolone and consideration of tocilizumab or a TNF inhibitor.[51]

Surgical intervention is reserved for selected complications and should be delayed until after remission. Indications include severe aortic coarctation, arterial stenoses causing critical limb ischaemia or cerebrovascular disease, renal artery stenosis causing accelerated hypertension, and unstable aneurysms. Upper limb claudication usually improves without intervention because of collateralisation. Outcome data are better for bypass grafting than percutaneous angioplasty.[55]

GIANT CELL ARTERITIS

GCA is an idiopathic, systemic, granulomatous large and medium vessel vasculitis. It is sometimes divided into two forms, cranial GCA affecting the cranial branches of the aortic arch, and extra-cranial GCA affecting the aorta and/or its proximal branches. The two forms may co-exist, in as many as 83% of cases overall.[56] Extra-cranial GCA may be accompanied by polymyalgia rheumatica in around 50% of cases.[57] Constitutional symptoms, such as low-grade fever, weight loss >2 kg, night sweats and fatigue, are common to all forms.

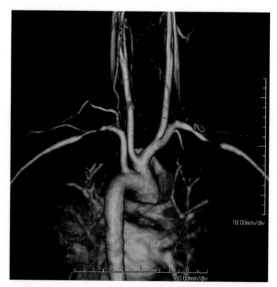

Figure 12.6 Posterior view of a three-dimensional volume-rendered thoracic aorta magnetic resonance angiogram showing severe bilateral subclavian artery stenoses in a 35-year-old woman who presented with chest pain. In addition, there were severe stenoses and occlusions of visceral and lower limb arteries. (Image courtesy of Dr John Bottomley, Sheffield Vascular Institute, UK.)

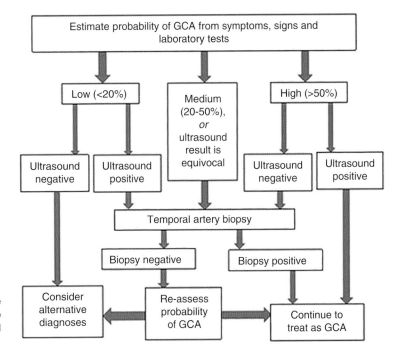

Figure 12.7 British Society for Rheumatology possible approach to using rapid-access vascular ultrasound to assist in clinical diagnostic decision making in suspected cranial giant cell arteritis (GCA).[56]

GCA occurs in people over 50 years of age, is commonest in Caucasians of northern European origin, and affects women two to three times more often than men. The overall incidence in people over 50 years is 17 per 100 000 per year, making it one of the most commonly occurring vasculitides. GCA has different epidemiological and clinical features to TAK, including age of onset, ethnic predominance, distribution of disease and speed of onset of symptoms.[58]

In cranial GCA, the most common symptom is new onset persistent localised headache, often in the temporal area, unresponsive to standard analgesia. Other key symptoms are scalp tenderness on combing the hair or resting the head on a pillow (superficial temporal and occipital arteries), jaw and/or tongue claudication (facial and maxillary arteries), amaurosis fugax, diplopia, sub-acute or acute visual loss (ophthalmic or posterior ciliary arteries) and stroke (carotid or vertebrobasilar arteries).[51,56]

✔ Risk factors for blindness in GCA include jaw claudication, older age and previous transient visual disturbance[56]

Key examination findings are temporal artery tenderness, beading or diffuse thickening, with or without reduced pulsation. There may also be scalp tenderness, bruits (particularly from the axillary artery) or reduced pulses or blood pressure in the upper limbs. Necrosis of the skin of the scalp or tip of the tongue is an extreme manifestation. Ophthalmic findings include a new deficit in visual fields or acuity, fundoscopic evidence of anterior ischaemic optic neuropathy, central or branch retinal artery occlusion, choroidal ischaemia and oculomotor cranial nerve palsy.

The diagnosis of GCA relies on clinical features, elevated CRP, specific US features of the temporal and axillary arteries and temporal artery biopsy. There are no specific serological tests, but inflammatory markers (CRP, ESR) are almost invariably raised. The CRP may be only mildly raised, and any level above 10 mg/L should be considered significant. Less than 3% of patients with positive temporal artery

biopsies will have both CRP and ESR in the normal range,[51] and CRP is considered more sensitive than ESR.[59]

Recent updates concerning the use of imaging in large vessel vasculitis have been published by EULAR.[51,53] They reflect recognition that US and temporal artery biopsy have similar sensitivities and specificities. However, US of bilateral temporal and axillary arteries is recommended as the first imaging modality, with a non-compressible peri-luminal 'halo' sign the most suggestive feature of GCA.[53] The 'halo' is a homogeneous, hypoechoic thickening of the wall of the artery, reflecting inflammation-induced oedema, with a 77% sensitivity and 96% specificity for GCA.[60]

✔ Temporal and axillary artery US is the first-line imaging modality in cranial GCA.[53,56]

✔ It has similar specificity and sensitivity to temporal artery biopsy.

If US is unavailable or inconclusive, high-resolution magnetic resonance imaging (MRI) of cranial arteries to investigate mural inflammation is a second-line alternative for GCA diagnosis.[53] PET-CT is not recommended for the assessment of cranial artery inflammation.[53]

A possible approach to diagnose cranial GCA is shown in Fig. 12.7, from the recent British Society for Rheumatology (BSR) guideline,[56] and is similar to EULAR recommendations.[53] In patients in whom there is a high clinical suspicion of GCA and a positive imaging test, the diagnosis of GCA may be made without an additional test (biopsy or further imaging).[53,56] In a patient with a low clinical probability of GCA and a negative imaging test, the diagnosis of GCA can be considered unlikely, however in all other situations temporal artery biopsy should be performed.[53,56] The hallmark histological finding is transmural granulomatous inflammation (Fig. 12.8). As inflammation occurs intermittently along the length of affected arteries (so called 'skip lesions'), temporal artery biopsies should be at least 1 cm in length to reduce the likelihood of a false negative result.[51,56] Neither US guidance nor biopsy of the

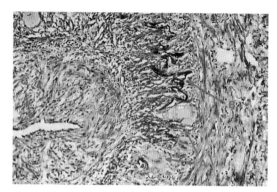

Figure 12.8 Temporal artery biopsy demonstrating granulomatous inflammation with giant cells (A), transmural mononuclear cell inflammation, disruption of the internal elastic lamina (B), and intimal hyperplasia with narrowing of the lumen (C).

contra-lateral artery are recommended, as they do not add significantly to the diagnostic yield.[51] Of note, biopsy or imaging performed after initiation of treatment may result in false negative findings.

Extra-cranial GCA has similar features to TAK and is histologically indistinguishable. The diagnosis can be difficult to make as there may be no vascular specific symptoms, such as limb claudication. Investigation of unexplained constitutional symptoms and an elevation of CRP in a patient over 50 years should include large vessel arterial assessment by imaging, such as MRI or PET, to identify mural inflammation.[53,56] The risk of later thoracic aortic aneurysm in GCA is doubled.[61] Long-term review of patients in remission is suggested, though the frequency of review and screening methods are not defined in guidelines.[56]

Because untreated active GCA carries a high risk of permanent visual loss, it is recommended that all patients 50 years or older with symptoms suggestive of GCA, and raised CRP with no other explanation, should be treated with glucocorticoids without delay, and before imaging or biopsy results are available.[53,56]

✓ GCA is considered a medical emergency because it can cause blindness.

✓ Start treatment with glucocorticoids immediately in suspected cases.

✓ Do not allow investigations to delay treatment,[53,56] but proceed with these as soon as possible to maximise diagnostic yield.

Patients should be started on 40–60 mg prednisolone per day, and intravenous methylprednisolone 0.25–1g for up to 3 days considered for those with visual symptoms.[51,56] The evidence that this is more effective than high-dose oral prednisolone at preventing blindness is limited. It is recommended that prednisolone be tapered to 15–20 mg daily within 2–3 months and then to 5 mg daily or lower by 1 year.[51] In routine care, patients are often maintained on prednisolone for 2 years. For some patients with a high risk of glucocorticoid adverse events, such as sepsis, osteoporosis, loss of diabetic control and glaucoma, the early use of a steroid sparing agent is desirable. In an RCT of tocilizumab (TCZ, an interleukin [IL]-6 receptor monoclonal antibody) given weekly or fortnightly,[62] placebo arms introduced a rapid

prednisolone taper to zero by 26 or 52 weeks, both shorter than usual practice, but desirable for steroid sensitive patients. This demonstrated high relapse rates in the placebo arms (86% and 82%, respectively) and a significantly lower relapse rate in the TCZ arms (53–56%), in which glucocorticoid was discontinued by 26 weeks. This provides evidence for the use of TCZ in GCA as a steroid sparing agent for selected patients.[56] Alternative steroid sparing agents to consider, with limited evidence, would be methotrexate, leflunomide or azathioprine,[56] and biological agents with a different mode of action, Abatacept and IL-12/23 inhibitors such as Ustekinumab.[63,64] More research is required to determine optimum use of these potential steroid-sparing strategies. Nonetheless, many patients remain relapse-free with glucocorticoid monotherapy, maintaining remission with low-dose prednisolone throughout the second year of treatment, and after complete withdrawal thereafter. This approach is endorsed first line by EULAR and BSR, with adjunctive use of TCZ or methotrexate only considered for refractory or relapsing disease, or in patients with a high risk of glucocorticoid adverse events.[51,56]

Given the long-expected duration of glucocorticoid therapy, osteoporosis prophylaxis should be started contemporaneously with calcium and vitamin D3, with bisphosphonate therapy for those with pre-existing osteopenia or osteoporosis. Low-dose aspirin is no longer recommended.[51,56]

CLINICAL VIGNETTE (EXTRA-CRANIAL GIANT CELL ARTERITIS)

A 76-year-old woman presents with an incidental finding of a thoracic aortic aneurysm following CT pulmonary angiogram. She has a history of GCA 5 years previously but was lost to follow-up. CRP is raised at 45 mg/L and she is noted to have a left subclavian bruit. A diagnosis of under-treated GCA with thoracic aneurysm is made. Her GCA is controlled with low-dose prednisolone, and she successfully undergoes repair surgery.

INFLAMMATORY AORTIC ANEURYSM AND IGG4-RELATED DISEASE

Inflammatory aortic aneurysms (IAA) account for 5–10% of all abdominal aortic aneurysms. Patients present with abdominal or back pain, and constitutional features associated with inflammation including anorexia, weight loss, low grade fever, malaise and an elevation of CRP. The anatomical site is almost always the infra-renal aorta extending to the iliac arteries, with marked thickening of the aneurysm wall and variable degrees of retro-peritoneal fibrosis. This consists of peri-aortic fibro-inflammatory tissue extending to the retroperitoneum, within which the ureters are prone to obstruction. These characteristic features are visualised on CTA, MRA and CT-PET imaging. The main associations are with male sex, smoking and a genetic predisposition, presenting 5–10 years younger than non-inflammatory atherosclerotic aneurysms. It is unclear whether IAA represents the most severe end of the spectrum of inflammation associated with atherogenesis or is caused by a different disease entity altogether. A report of histological findings in 10 cases of IAA revealed that IgG4-related disease (IgG4-RD) was the cause in four,[65] with eosinophilic rather than neutrophilic infiltrates in the peri-aortic tissue. Of 587 cases of IgG4-RD, peri-aortitis was a feature in 15%.[66] The most prevalent distribution of aortitis in IgG4-RD is the same as IAA, involving the abdominal aorta and iliac arteries (83%), with infrequent thoracic aortic involvement, involving 12.5%.[66] Whilst histologically different, atheromatous IAA and IgG4-RD aortitis are generally responsive to glucocorticoids, with shrinkage of the retroperitoneal tissue and suppression of CRP. Baseline serum IgG4 levels are not particularly helpful diagnostically, though can be used to help gauge response to treatment. Patients should be started on 0.5 mg/kg prednisolone daily, tapered to 5 mg daily over 6 months. If this fails to achieve or maintain suppression of inflammation, a range of steroid sparing agents may be considered including azathioprine, methotrexate, leflunomide and mycophenolate mofetil.[67] There are no controlled trials to guide optimal choice or duration of immune suppression, and pragmatic judgement should be used. In refractory or relapsing disease, rituximab may be considered for IgG4-RD. Where necessary, ureteric stents may be required to prevent hydronephrosis, and endovascular stenting of the aneurysm according to guidelines, usually once the diameter exceeds 5.5 cm or with rapid enlargement over 4.5 cm.

BEHCET'S DISEASE

Behcet's disease is a multisystem inflammatory disorder characterised by the triad of aphthous oral ulcers, genital ulcers and eye inflammation, especially uveitis. A range of other manifestations may occur including skin lesions, vasculitis, gastrointestinal and central nervous system disease. The vasculitis of Behcet's is distinctive because it involves arteries and veins of all sizes.[68] The highest prevalence is in men and those presenting with Behcet's at a younger age. Venous involvement is much more common than arterial, may be multi-focal, including superficial and deep veins of the legs, vena cava, hepatic vein and cerebral veins. In-situ thrombosis is common, rarely leads to embolism, and is treated with immune suppression over anticoagulation.

Arterial involvement is associated with aneurysm formation, with vasculitis in the vasa vasorum, non-granulomatous inflammation and minimal thickening of the arterial wall. The ascending aorta and femoral arteries are the commonest sites, but involvement of any site is recognised including coronary, mesenteric, splenic and limb vessels. The mainstay of management is aggressive immune suppression. Iatrogenic puncture of arteries may lead to aneurysm formation, so non-invasive imaging is preferred for diagnostic purposes. Arterial repair may be complicated by aneurysm at anastomotic sites and graft occlusion by thrombus. Synthetic graft over autologous vein grafting is recommended, as is endovascular repair. The unique challenges of this disease for surgical repair are well recognised, and adjunctive treatment with glucocorticoids and immune suppressive agents is recommended.[68]

MEDIUM VESSEL VASCULITIS

BUERGER'S DISEASE (THROMBOANGIITIS OBLITERANS)

Buerger's disease is a vasculitic syndrome characterised by segmental, non-atherosclerotic, inflammatory thrombotic occlusions of the small and medium-sized arteries and veins of the extremities. The lower limbs are most commonly affected.

Buerger's disease usually occurs in men less than 45 years of age, although disease in women and older people is recognised. The cause is unknown but smoking and/or tobacco use in any form is the most important risk factor and appears to be key in pathogenesis, to the extent that a smoking history is generally regarded as a prerequisite for diagnosis.[69,70] The presence of diabetes rules out the diagnosis.

Thrombus histology differs in acute and chronic disease. Acutely, thrombi are inflammatory and hypercellular, comprising neutrophils, giant cells and micro-abscesses. Later they become fibrosed ('organised thrombus') and inflammatory cells are absent. Throughout the disease process, there is sparing of the internal elastic lamina, and this is key in differentiating Buerger's disease from atherosclerosis and other vasculitides.

The symptoms of Buerger's disease are those of ischaemia to the affected limb/s, usually the foot or leg. Skin ulceration or distal gangrene of the digits can follow, and digital ischaemia may mimic Raynaud's phenomenon. Migratory superficial thrombophlebitis occurs in around 40% and manifests as tender nodules overlying veins. This is rare in the other vasculitides apart from Behçet's disease. Peripheral nerve involvement is seen in up to 70% of cases because of involvement of the vasa vasorum.

The diagnosis of Buerger's disease is clinical, supported by imaging. There are no specific tests, acute phase markers are not elevated and autoantibodies negative. Imaging reveals angiographically normal vessels, free of atherosclerosis, proximal to the popliteal arteries in the legs and brachial arteries in the arms. Distally, there are segmental occlusive lesions of the small and medium-sized arteries. Corkscrew collaterals may be seen around occlusions. It is wise to image all four limbs, even when symptoms are confined to one, as early disease may be detected in the others. Biopsy is only required in cases of diagnostic uncertainty and avoided in case the biopsy site fails to heal.

✓ Tobacco abstinence is the cornerstone of management for Buerger's disease. In patients who stop smoking, the appearance of new lesions and gangrene requiring amputation are unusual.

Tobacco cessation in any form is the only effective intervention. Immunosuppression is ineffective whereas aspirin and parenteral iloprost have been used to relieve rest pain and promote ulcer healing.[71] Major and minor limb amputation is fairly common (around 40% in one retrospective study[71] but rare after successful smoking cessation.

POLYARTERITIS NODOSA

Polyarteritis nodosa (PAN) is a rare necrotising vasculitis affecting the small and medium-sized muscular arteries. Variants include idiopathic generalised PAN, hepatitis (Hep) B-associated PAN and single-organ PAN, the commonest of which is cutaneous PAN. Hep B formerly accounted for one-third of cases, but now accounts for only 5%. The overall annual incidence in Europe has fallen to around 1 per million, owing to widespread vaccination against hep B. PAN is commoner in men with a peak incidence in the fifth and sixth decades, although children and older people are also affected. There is no ethnic predominance.

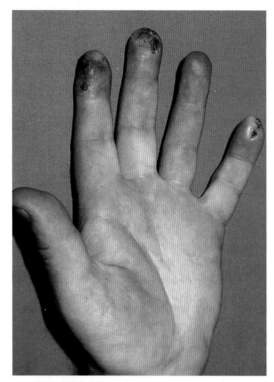

Figure 12.9   Digital infarct in polyarteritis nodosa.

The presenting symptoms are often indolent and constitutional, including malaise, weight loss, fever and myalgia. Further symptoms and signs depend on the organs affected. Any organ can be affected other than the lungs, the commonest being the skin and peripheral nervous system. Skin manifestations include nailfold infarcts, digital infarcts (Fig. 12.9), palpable purpura and livedo reticularis (Fig. 12.10). Peripheral nervous system manifestations include mononeuritis multiplex, which can present as wrist or foot drop, and polyneuropathy. The kidneys are often involved. Hypertension occurs secondary to renal artery disease, and renal infarcts can cause frank or microscopic haematuria with proteinuria. Glomerulonephritis does not occur. Gastrointestinal symptoms are common because of mesenteric ischaemia and range from non-specific abdominal pain, nausea and vomiting to life-threatening bowel infarction, perforation and haemorrhage.[72] Further manifestations include cardiac disease, orchitis secondary to testicular artery involvement, sensorineural hearing loss and eye involvement.[73]

Laboratory findings are non-specific. An elevated CRP is common. There is no serological test for idiopathic PAN, and ANCA is negative.[74] Screening for Hep B is imperative.

Diagnosis depends on imaging findings, the exclusion of related conditions such as small-vessel vasculitis and biopsy. Imaging of the renal, hepatic or mesenteric arteries characteristically shows multiple microaneurysms (classically described as *saccular* or *fusiform*) alongside stenotic lesions. Histology reveals a mixed inflammatory infiltrate with fibrinoid necrosis largely affecting arterial branch points. Muscle or nerve biopsy is preferred because of better diagnostic yield.

Life-threatening or severe disease is treated with high-dose corticosteroids and cyclophosphamide. Less severe disease is treated with corticosteroids alone. A steroid-sparing agent

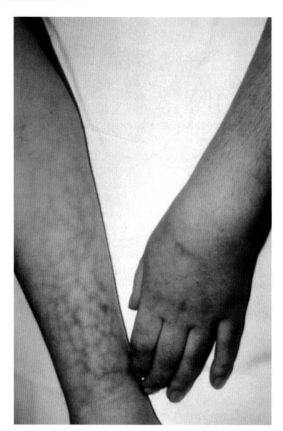

Figure 12.10   Livedo reticularis in polyarteritis nodosa.

such as azathioprine or methotrexate may be used to maintain remission. However, PAN is usually thought of as a monophasic disease, with only 10% relapse rate. The mainstay of treatment for Hep B-associated PAN is antiviral therapy.

SMALL-VESSEL VASCULITIS

The small-vessel vasculitides are a group of disorders characterised by inflammation of small intra-parenchymal and cutaneous arteries, arterioles, capillaries and venules. They are categorised as ANCA-associated vasculitis (AAVs) and immune complex-mediated vasculitis.[75]

ANCA-ASSOCIATED VASCULITIS

This is a group of systemic diseases associated with ANCA. The three subtypes are microscopic polyangiitis (MPA), granulomatosis with polyangiitis (GPA, formerly known as *Wegener's granulomatosis*), and eosinophilic granulomatosis with polyangiitis (EGPA, formerly known as *Churg–Strauss syndrome*). They are all characterised by necrotising vasculitis with an absence of immune complex deposition ('pauci-immune vasculitis'). The phenotypic expression ranges from single system or region (e.g., peripheral nervous system, or ear, nose and throat [ENT]) to multi-organ disease, with severity ranging from indolent to rapidly progressive and life-threatening consequences, and a high tendency to relapse over many years.

MPA has a European incidence of 2.4–10.1 per million with a usual age of onset around 50 years. Initial symptoms may be constitutional and non-specific, reflecting underlying inflammation. These include fever, malaise, weight loss, arthralgia and myalgia. Additional clinical manifestations depend on which organs or systems are involved, and the consequences of necrotising vasculitis and ischaemia. Skin involvement (dermal venulitis) results in palpable purpura, and peripheral nerve involvement (epineural arteritis) results in mononeuritis multiplex. Involvement of the renal glomeruli results in glomerulonephritis, which can be rapidly progressive and lead to renal failure. Alveolar capillaritis can result in pulmonary haemorrhage, which can be severe and diffuse. Gastrointestinal, cardiac, central nervous system and ocular disease are all recognised.

GPA affects a similar age group, with a European incidence of 2.1–14.4 per million. GPA has similar constitutional manifestations as MPA, and a predilection for midline structures, including the orbits, sinuses, upper and lower respiratory tract and kidneys. ENT symptoms include nasal crusting and bleeding with nasal septal perforation and nasal cartilage collapse (so called *saddle shaped deformity*). In the upper airway, subglottic stenosis is recognised and in the lower airway, cavitating parenchymal disease with potential alveolar haemorrhage is characteristic.[76] Ear involvement may present with otitis media. Eye involvement is more common than in MPA and includes conjunctivitis, uveitis and episcleritis.

EGPA is the rarest of the three, with a European incidence of 0.5–3.7 per million. It presents with severe, late-onset asthma, or allergic rhinitis with nasal polyps, and is associated with raised circulating eosinophils. The vasculitic phase occurs after a latency of up to 10 years, and any of the manifestations described for MPA can be seen. Granulomatosis in EGPA occurs as a result of infiltration of organs by eosinophils. The lungs ('eosinophilic pneumonitis') and heart are particularly susceptible. A raised cardiac troponin I is specific for myocardial injury.

The diagnosis of AAV is clinical, supported by serology and biopsy where feasible. The aim of investigations is threefold: to confirm the diagnosis of AAV, to screen for organ or system involvement and damage, and to exclude other conditions. Biopsy of skin or an affected organ is important in confirming a new diagnosis or relapse but should not delay urgent treatment where the clinical picture is convincing.[77] Findings of necrotising leucocytoclastic vasculitis, with or without granuloma, or pauci-immune glomerulonephritis, are confirmatory.

ANCA are believed to mediate vasculitis and vessel necrosis by activating circulating neutrophils and complement.[78] ANCA target a variety of autoantigens that originate within neutrophil granules and are expressed on the surface of activated neutrophils. First-line testing is for the presence of antibody reactivity to neutrophils, by indirect immunofluorescence (IIF). Two patterns are recognised, cytoplasmic and peri-nuclear, termed *cANCA* and *pANCA*, respectively. The pANCA pattern may be falsely positive in the presence of a strong positive ANA. Second-line testing identifies the presence of antibodies to one of two neutrophil granule enzymes, proteinase-3 (PR-3) and myeloperoxidase (MPO). In general, the cANCA IIF pattern is accompanied by PR-3 antibodies and this associates with GPA, whereas the pANCA IIF pattern is accompanied by MPO antibodies and associates with MPA and EGPA. The latter pattern is less specific, as conditions such as inflammatory bowel disease and primary sclerosing cholangitis can also give a positive MPO-ANCA. ANCA-negative disease is well recognised, particularly in EGPA and

single-organ GPA. Other neutrophil targets of ANCA are recognised, such as elastase (HNE) and bactericidal permeability-increasing protein, but their clinical significance is less well established.[79]

The differential diagnosis is wide as there are many causes of small-vessel vasculitis, especially infection and malignancy. Screening tests for other conditions include human immunodeficiency virus, Hep B, Hep C, human T lymphotropic virus Type I, ANA, RF, complement and cryoglobulins. A particular mimic is cocaine induced midline destructive lesions. This causes rapidly destructive ENT limited disease, with more widespread damage to the nasal septum, turbinates and maxillary structures than seen in GPA, and often an atypical ANCA association; pANCA with PR-3 antibodies or cANCA with MPO antibodies or an atypical ANCA such as HNE. An immune response to levamisole (added as a bulking agent to illicit cocaine) has been described. Rarer causes include atrial myxoma and cholesterol emboli.

EULAR recommendations for the treatment of AAVs[77] are comprehensive and informed by a large series of well conducted RCTs covering remission induction, maintenance of remission, relapsing disease and specific situations such as non-organ-threatening disease, rapidly progressive glomerulonephritis (RPGN), and diffuse alveolar haemorrhage (DAH). For organ-threatening disease, immune suppression with glucocorticoids and either cyclophosphamide or rituximab to induce remission, followed by azathioprine, methotrexate, mycophenolate or rituximab for maintenance for at least 2 years is the mainstay. Plasma exchange is recommended for RPGN, and DAH. New diagnoses and major relapses are treated in the same way. For non-organ threatening disease (e.g., skin, ENT), glucocorticoids with methotrexate or mycophenolate mofetil are recommended.

Disease activity is monitored by way of clinical assessment, aided by scoring tools such as the Birmingham Vasculitis Activity Score. The role of ANCA titres in monitoring disease activity is unclear, though PR-3 positivity and a failure to suppress ANCA by the end of remission induction are associated with a higher likelihood of relapse. Agents targeting complement C5a (e.g., Avacopan) and IL-5 (e.g., mepolizumab) provide new options for AAVs[80] and EGPA,[81] respectively.

CLINICAL VIGNETTE (MICROSCOPIC POLYANGIITIS)

A 63-year-old male smoker presents with a 6-month history of left sided leg claudication, and a 2-week history of malaise. He has three3 ischaemic toes on the left foot. eGFR has fallen to 57 mL/h from 85 mL/h. Angiography shows atheromatous non-critical stenosis of the left popliteal artery. He is noted to have splinter haemorrhages and blood and protein on urine dip. P-ANCA and MPO are positive. Renal biopsy shows crescentic glomerulonephritis. His renal function improves to baseline with high dose steroids and rituximab. The tips of three toes auto-amputate but he has good functional outcome.

IMMUNE COMPLEX-MEDIATED VASCULITIS

Deposition of immune complexes (immunoglobulins and complement) in the small-vessel walls results in activation of complement and inflammation. Examples include IgA vasculitis (Henoch–Schonlein purpura, HSP), cryoglobulinaemic vasculitis, anti-glomerular basement membrane disease and hypocomplementic urticarial vasculitis (anti-C1q vasculitis).[75] The course of these conditions is often benign, compared to AAVs, however, life-threatening organ based disease may occur. HSP is the commonest vasculitis in children and often self-limiting, whereas in adults may be more severe, more likely to relapse, and more likely to progress to renal failure with IgA nephropathy. The classic triad of presenting features is palpable purpura, arthralgia (without arthritis) and abdominal pain. Microscopic haematuria is an early indicator of glomerulonephritis. The disease course of HSP is variable; it is not possible to predict which patients will remit spontaneously, and which will progress to end-stage renal failure and require immunesuppression.[75]

Cryoglobulins are circulating immunoglobulins that precipitate in cool conditions. Type I cryoglobulinaemia is associated with B-cell lymphoproliferative conditions (e.g., multiple myeloma and Waldenstrom's macroglobulinaemia), whilst types II and III (mixed cryoglobulinaemia) are associated with hepatitis C virus (HCV) in around 80% of cases. Clinical features include fatigue, palpable purpura, peripheral nerve involvement (mononeuritis multiplex or polyneuropathy) and glomerulonephritis. Precipitation of cryoglobulins in the peripheries causes acrocyanosis and can mimic RP. The management of cryoglobulinaemia depends on identification and treatment of the underlying condition. Antiviral therapy is the mainstay of treatment in HCV-related disease and is associated with a good prognosis.[82]

PRIMARY CUTANEOUS SMALL-VESSEL VASCULITIS

Primary (or idiopathic) cutaneous small-vessel vasculitis is the term applied to small-vessel vasculitis affecting only the skin for which no secondary cause (e.g., drug reaction, infectious cause, systemic disease) is found. It usually manifests as palpable purpura occurring in the lower limbs. The lesions occur in crops, initially appearing as erythematous macules before progressing to purpura, and are usually symmetrical. It is typically self-limiting, with immunosuppressant treatment reserved for the most severe cases.[83]

Key points

- RP can be primary or secondary. Identification of SRP is important as it permits early detection of associated conditions. Management involves important general measures, CCBs and PDE-5 inhibitors. ANA is a simple screening tool for connective tissue diseases causing RP.
- The systemic vasculitides are a diverse group of conditions that can affect large, medium and small vessels. Consider vasculitis when vascular ischaemia unexplained by atheromatous disease is accompanied by constitutional symptoms and systemic inflammation.
- The presence of splinter haemorrhages, palpable purpura, blood and protein on urinalysis and blood eosinophilia are all signs of vasculitis.

References available at http://ebooks.health.elsevier.com/

KEY REFERENCES

[2] Maverakis E, Patel F, Kronenberg D, et al. International consensus criteria for the diagnosis of Raynaud's phenomenon. J Autoimmun 2014;0:605.
  Clear criteria for defining Raynaud's phenomenon.

[4] Belch J, Carlizza A, Carpentier PH, et al. ESVM guidelines – the diagnosis and management of Raynaud's phenomenon. Vasa 2017;46:413–23.
  Comprehensive international guidelines from the European Society for Vascular Medicine for the diagnosis and management of Raynaud's phenomenon.

[22] Herrick AL. Evidence-based management of Raynaud's phenomenon. Ther Adv Musculoskel Dis 2017;9:317–29.
  Comprehensive review of clinical trials and evidence for therapies for Raynaud's phenomenon.

[27] Smith V, Vanhaecke A, Herrick AL, et al. Fast track algorithm: how to differentiate a 'scleroderma pattern' from a 'non-scleroderma pattern'. Autoimmunity Rev 2019;18:102394.
  Expert based decision algorithm to differentiate 'non-scleroderma' from 'scleroderma patterns' on capillaroscopic images.

[36] Khouri C, Lepelley M, Bailly S, et al. Comparative efficacy and safety of treatments for secondary Raynaud's phenomenon: a systematic review and network meta-analysis of randomized trials. Lancet Rheumatol 2019;1:e237–46.
  SLR and network meta-analysis identifying evidence for efficacy of calcium channel blockers and phosphodiesterase-5 inhibitors in the treatment of secondary Raynaud's phenomenon.

[37] Kowal-Bielecka O, Fransen J, Avouac J, et al. Update of EULAR recommendations for the treatment of systemic sclerosis. Ann Rheum Dis 2017;76:1327–39.
  European League against Rheumatism (EULAR) recommendations for the management of Raynaud's phenomenon in systemic sclerosis.

[51] Hellmich B, Agueda A, Monti S, et al. Update of the EULAR recommendations for the management of large vessel vasculitis. Ann Rheum Dis 2018;79:19–30. PMID: 31270110.
  EULAR (European League Against Rheumatism) guidelines for the management of large vessel vasculitis.

[53] Dejaco C, Ramiro S, Duftner C. EULAR recommendations for the use of imaging in large vessel vasculitis in clinical practice. Ann Rheum Dis 2018;77:636–43. PMID: 29358285.
  EULAR (European League Against Rheumatism) recommendations for imaging in large vessel vasculitis.

[56] Mackie SL, Dejaco C, Appenzeller S, et al. British Society for Rheumatology guidelines on diagnosis and treatment of giant cell arteritis. Rheumatology 2020;59:e1–23.
  British Society of Rheumatology guidelines for the management of giant cell arteritis.

[66] Peng L, Zhang P, Li J, et al. IgG-4-related aortitis/periaortitis and periarteritis: a distinct spectrum of IgG4-related disease. Arthritis Res Ther 2020;22:103.
  Study clarifying the distinct clinical features of aortitis in IgG4-Related disease.

[69] Olin JW. Thromboangiitis obliterans (Buerger's disease). N Engl J Med 2000;343:864–9. PMID: 10995867.
  Review of thromboangiitis obliterans covering pathogenesis, clinical features and treatment.

[75] Lopalco G, Rigante D, Venerito V, et al. Management of small vessel vasculitis. Curr Rheumatol Rep 2016;18:36–46. PMID.
  Comprehensive review of clinical trials in ANCA associated and immune complex small vessel vasculitis.

[77] Yates M, Watts RA, Bajema IM, et al. EULAR/ERA-EDTA recommendations for the management of ANCA-associated vasculitis. Ann Rheum Dis 2016;75(9):1583–94. PMID: 27338776.
  EULAR recommendations for the management of ANCA-associated vasculitis.

[78] Jennette JC, Falk RJ, Gasim AH. Pathogenesis of antineutrophil cytoplasmic autoantibody. Curr Opin Nephrol Hypertens 2011;20(3):63–70. PMID: 21422922.
  Recent review outlining the detailed pathogenesis of ANCA-associated vasculitis.

Peripheral and abdominal aortic aneurysms

13

Andrew L. Tambyraja

INTRODUCTION

The normal diameter of the aorta varies with age, sex and bodyweight.[1] It decreases in size as it leaves the thorax and enters the abdomen, tapering to its iliac bifurcation. However, the infra-renal aorta enlarges progressively with age. An aortic aneurysm is a permanent localised dilatation of all three layers of the vessel wall of at least a 50% increase in diameter compared to the expected normal diameter of the aorta.[2] If the maximum normal diameter of the aorta is considered to be 2.1 cm, aneurysmal dilatation is said to occur when the diameter exceeds 3.0 cm.

The abdominal aorta is the most commonly affected artery and accounts for 90% of all aneurysms. Of these, 95% will originate below the level of the renal arteries. The aortic arch, thoracic aorta and thoracoabdominal aorta are involved in approximately 10% of aneurysms.

The morphology or shape of aneurysms may be classified as saccular or fusiform, although this description represents a continuous spectrum. Saccular aneurysms affect only a small portion of the aortic circumference while fusiform lesions involve the entire circumference of the vessel.

EPIDEMIOLOGY

The prevalence of abdominal aortic aneurysm (AAA) in men over 65 years is around 7–8%.[3,4] The condition is thought to be six times greater in men than in women.[5] In determining the prevalence of AAA, the frequently asymptomatic nature of the disease is a major confounding factor. Data on prevalence stem from four sources: autopsy surveys, routine mortality and hospital in-patient statistics and population-screening surveys. It should be noted that all of these sources have their limitations and potential for bias; screening surveys offer, potentially, the most accurate estimate of prevalence.

The prevalence of screen-detected AAA in men in England is reported to be between 1.3–12.7%.[6] This variation is accounted for by differing criteria for the definition of AAA and the age group screened. If the criterion of inner wall aortic diameter >29 mm is used as the definition for AAA, the prevalence in men aged 65 years within the UK screening programme in the year 2019–2020 was 0.9%.[7] These figures are in keeping with data from other European and North American series.[8,9] Interestingly, data from autopsy-based surveys yield similar results. The prevalence

of AAA at autopsy in the UK has been reported at 2.3% in men and 1.6% in women.[10]

Ruptured AAA accounts for around 3000 deaths each year in England or around 1.7% of all deaths in men aged 65 years and older.[11]

Cause-specific mortality data for England and Wales and Hospital Episodes Statistics for England have shown that AAA mortality and ruptured AAA admission have fallen in England and Wales by around one-third, while non-ruptured AAA admission has remained steady between 2001 and 2009.[12] A fall in the global incidence and prevalence of AAA has been shown, particularly in high-income countries.[13] National differences can be explained by variations in cardiovascular risk factors. Of these, the reduction in smoking prevalence correlates most closely with declines in AAA mortality.[14]

Epidemiological data on peripheral aneurysm are less readily available. However, the association with AAA is well recognised and approximately 25% of patients with AAA have synchronous femoral or popliteal aneurysms.[15] It is likely that peripheral aneurysm will have similar epidemiological trends to AAA.

PATHOPHYSIOLOGY

The cause of aneurysms remains unclear. Historically, aneurysmal change was thought to be underpinned by atherosclerosis. However, because of histological and epidemiological differences, it is now recognised that atherosclerosis is a co-existent phenomenon and the majority of AAA (90%) are thought to represent a degenerative or non-specific process.[16]

AAAs exhibit familial clustering. This raises the possibility of both genetic and environmental aetiological factors. Genes encoding for type III collagen, matrix metalloproteinases (MMPs) and protease inhibitors and plasminogen activator inhibitors have all been reported to play some role in AAA development or expansion.[17,18] However, no specific genes have been convincingly implicated to date and it is inferred that susceptibility to the development of AAA is an irreversible process with multiple genetic and environmental risk factors. Genetic influences are attributed to a few gene polymorphisms with large effects.[17]

North American and European data suggest that there is a fourfold increase in risk of having an AAA for the brother of a patient having an AAA.[19,20] Familial AAAs are more common when the index case is female and rupture is said to occur at a younger age and more often than with sporadic aneurysms.[21,22]

Established independent risk factors for AAA include male gender, age, hypertension, hyperlipidaemia and smoking.[5,23,24] In particular, the relationship between tobacco use and AAA development is striking. Aneurysms are four times more prevalent amongst smokers than non-smokers and the comparative relative risks of chronic cigarette smokers developing an AAA are threefold greater than their risk of developing coronary artery disease.[5,25] For these reasons, it is thought that smoking is the foremost environmental risk factor for aneurysm development and growth. Interestingly, diabetes is associated with a reduced risk; this may relate to glycated crosslinks in aortic tissue or metformin therapy conferring a protective effect.[26]

AAAs are characterised histologically by destruction of elastin and collagen in the tunica media and tunica adventitia, smooth muscle cell apoptosis with thinning of the medial wall, infiltration of lymphocytes and macrophages, and neovascularisation.[27] Four pathological mechanisms are thought to play central roles in AAA development: proteolysis of connective tissue, inflammation, biomechanical stress and genetic influences.[28]

PROTEOLYSIS

Macrophage and aortic smooth muscle cell derived MMPs and other proteases are secreted into the extracellular matrix and are integral to aneurysm formation.[29] Though MMPs are expressed and active during normal physiological aortic remodelling, they mediate degradation of elastin and collagen within the aortic media and internal lamina in AAA pathogenesis.[30] A shift in the balance between MMPs and their inhibitors moves away from normal remodelling activity towards pathological elastin and collagen degradation. Factors initiating and propagating proteolysis in the aorta remain unclear.[31]

INFLAMMATION

Transmural lymphocyte and macrophage infiltration is a histological characteristic of AAA.[27] An inflammatory cytokine cascade released by these cells is thought to stimulate protease activation leading to destruction of the aortic media and to vascular smooth muscle cell apoptosis and dysfunction.[26] The chemotactic trigger responsible for this cellular migration remains uncertain, although it has been proposed that aortic elastin degradation products, interstitial collagen or oxidised low-density lipoprotein, may be antigenic and chemotactic stimuli for macrophages.[31]

BIOMECHANICS

The aortic wall contains smooth muscle, elastin and collagen arranged in concentric layers to withstand arterial pressure. Elastin is the principal load-bearing element in the aorta while collagen provides tensile strength and helps maintain the structural integrity of the vascular wall.[32] The normal aorta displays a reduction in the elastin-to-collagen ratio as it passes from the thorax into the abdomen.[31] Thus, the abdominal aorta has less elastin and as a consequence, less load-bearing

potential than the aortic arch. Furthermore, the infra-renal aorta is exposed to high oscillatory shear stress.[26]

MMP-9 expression and activity is increased in the abdominal aorta compared with aortic arch and thoracic aorta. Activation of these proteases is also thought to be brought about by the disruption of normal laminar flow seen in the infra-renal aorta.[33] Furthermore, the attenuation of the vasa vasorum in the infra-renal aorta is proposed to contribute to relative hypoxia of the vessel stimulating MMP activity. These factors are all thought to contribute to the predisposition of the infra-renal aorta to develop aneurysmal change.[25]

GENETICS

As already discussed, though multifactorial genetic influences are involved in AAA development, the polymorphisms responsible for aneurysm pathogenesis remain elusive. A large genome wide association study identified eight single nucleotide polymorphisms that were individually associated with an increase or decrease in risk of AAA. Similarly, the phenotypic expression of these traits is uncertain. It is proposed that an abnormality of the primary structures of elastin and collagen or a mutation, directly or indirectly, affect matrix remodelling, immune function and lipid metabolism.[26]

CLINICAL FEATURES

About 75% of aortic aneurysms are asymptomatic and are discovered incidentally. A small proportion will present with symptoms related to pressure on adjacent structures (dysphagia, ureteric obstruction, caval obstruction).

A small subset of AAA cases may present with the triad of lower back pain, weight loss and raised erythrocyte sedimentation rate. This triad is characteristic of inflammatory AAA, which represents the most extreme end of the spectrum of chronic inflammatory change seen in degenerative aneurysms, and accounts for 10% of all AAAs. These cases are further characterised by a thickened aneurysm wall, retroperitoneal fibrosis that may cause obstructive uropathy and dense adhesions to adjacent viscera.

Most of the clinical symptoms caused by aortic aneurysm are related to aneurysm rupture or embolism of mural thrombus.

Aneurysm rupture is associated with an estimated overall mortality of 75–80% and a significant proportion of patients will not reach hospital. Of those that present, most will have a contained retroperitoneal haematoma causing tamponade and resulting in temporary haemodynamic stability. The characteristic triad of abdominal or back pain, hypovolaemic shock and a pulsatile abdominal mass is present in only a few patients and the symptoms may be vague, and an abdominal mass missed. Other symptoms and signs may include groin pain, syncope, paralysis, or flank mass. A ruptured aneurysm should be considered in any elderly patient with unexplained hypotension and abdominal symptoms. The diagnosis may be confused with renal colic, diverticulitis, pancreatitis, or disease affecting the lumbar spine. A small proportion of AAAs rupture into an adjacent structure causing a primary aortic fistula; rupture into the vena cava produces a large arteriovenous fistula. In this case, symptoms include tachycardia, congestive heart failure, leg swelling, abdominal thrill, abdominal bruit, renal failure and peripheral ischaemia. AAAs may rupture into the fourth part of the duodenum and presentation may be with a herald upper gastrointestinal bleed followed by massive haemorrhage.

Embolism: patients with embolisation of thrombus from an aortic aneurysm may also present with acute ischaemia of the lower limb because of occlusion of the femoral or popliteal artery. Small aortic aneurysms may also undergo acute occlusion because of thrombosis as the aortic lumen becomes progressively narrowed by the accumulation of mural thrombus; these patients may present with acute bilateral lower limb ischaemia.

SCREENING

Population screening for AAA is appealing for a number of reasons:

1. Most AAAs are asymptomatic.
2. The majority of patients who suffer rupture will die.
3. B-mode ultrasound is a highly sensitive and specific diagnostic tool for detecting AAA.
4. Elective aneurysm repair is an effective prophylaxis against rupture.

A meta-analysis of four randomised controlled trials of screening elderly men for AAA with 15-year follow-up, has shown a significant and substantial reduction in the risk of death from AAA and the need for emergency surgery with an associated increase in elective repair.[34–36]

A detailed analysis of the clinical benefits, harms and cost-effectiveness of screening women for AAA concluded that it was unlikely to justify costs.[37] Nevertheless, recent UK National Institute for Health and Care Excellence (NICE) guidelines do make a recommendation to consider screening in women aged >70 years with selected risk factors.[38]

The Multicentre Aneurysm Screening Study (MASS) trial has provided good statistical evidence to show that the prevalence of aneurysm-related death is reduced significantly in a screened male population aged 65–74 years, with a 53% reduction in those who attended for screening.[34] Because other causes of death overshadow those caused by ruptured AAAs, it has not been possible to demonstrate a statistically significant overall survival advantage for the screened population. Nevertheless, the case for extending population-based screening for AAAs is convincing.

In England, the National Health Service (NHS) AAA screening programme began in 2009. It offers all men aged 65 years an invitation for ultrasound screening. The same screening strategy is used in Sweden and the rest of the United Kingdom. Interestingly, both programmes have demonstrated an incremental cost-efficiency ratio of £7000 per quality-adjusted life-year (QALY).[39] Compared with existing screening programmes for breast and cervical cancer, AAA screening for men remains cost effective. Reassuringly, in over 3000 men referred for intervention from the screening programme in England, only 8% were turned down for medical reasons, and of those who underwent aneurysm repair, peri-operative mortality was 1.4%.[40]

The MASS trial data show that over 4 years, the mean incremental cost-effectiveness ratio for screening was £28 400 per life-year gained, equivalent to approximately £36 000 per QALY. It was estimated that this would fall to approximately £8000 per life-year gained at 10 years.[35]

Analysis of the 10-year Multicentre Aneurysm Screening Study (MASS) data shows that the NHS AAA Screening Programme (NAAASP) will prevent significant numbers of AAA ruptures and AAA deaths. It also proves that the number of lives saved will greatly outweigh the number of post-elective surgery deaths. The following figures use the 10-year MASS data and assume an 80% attendance for screening and a 5% post-elective surgery mortality: 240 men need to be invited (192 scanned) to save one AAA death over 10 years and each 2080 men invited for screening (1660 scanned) result in one extra post-elective surgery death. This means that over 10 years, for every 10 000 men scanned under the NAAASP, 65 AAA ruptures will be prevented, saving 52 lives. However, there will also be six post-elective surgery deaths involving men whose aneurysm is detected under the screening programme.[35]

DIAGNOSIS

Aortic aneurysms may not be detected by clinical examination alone. Calcification of the aneurysm wall may be apparent on plain abdominal or chest radiograph, but this method lacks sensitivity and is unsatisfactory for routine use.

B-mode ultrasound is the diagnostic investigation of choice for the detection of AAA, providing accurate assessment of the aneurysm diameter and some indication regarding site.

Computed tomography (CT) is the investigation of choice to delineate AAA morphology and relationship to the visceral and renal arteries (Fig. 13.1). CT or magnetic resonance imaging (MRI) will detect thoracic aortic aneurysms.

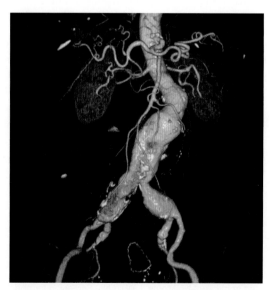

Figure 13.1 Reconstructed computed tomography aortogram of infra-renal aorto-iliac aneurysm.

PRINCIPLES OF MANAGEMENT

The principles of management in asymptomatic AAA are based on an assessment of the risk of aneurysm rupture weighed against the morbidity and mortality associated with surgical repair.

The size and growth of AAA are strongly associated with the amount and duration of smoking; smoking cessation can moderate this risk.[26] The association between hypertension and hypercholesterolaemia and AAA suggests that medical management of these conditions may have a benefit on aneurysm growth. However, several drugs have been investigated in randomised controlled and non-randomised trials – beta-blockers, angiotensin-converting enzyme inhibitors, angiotensin-receptor blockers and statins. None of these drugs has been shown to confer a benefit.[41] Nevertheless, given the strong association between atherosclerosis and AAA, it is recommended that aneurysm patients receive best medical therapy (BMT) to reduce the incidence of cardiovascular events.

The natural history of untreated asymptomatic AAA is considered to be one of expansion and potential rupture. Measurement of the maximum anteroposterior diameter of the aneurysm predicts the risk of rupture. Randomised controlled data on AAA of <55 mm diameter has demonstrated a mean risk of rupture of 1% per year.[42] However, there is little randomised evidence to inform the rate of rupture in large aneurysms. A multicentre study of 198 patients with AAA >5.5 cm for whom elective repair was not planned because of medical comorbidity or patient refusal, demonstrated a 1-year rupture risk for AAA of 5.5–5.9 cm of 9.4%, 10.2% for AAA of 6.0–6.9 cm and 32.5% for AAA of >7 cm.[43] Interestingly, the risk of rupture in the smallest AAA diameter cohorts was significantly greater than that reported in randomised controlled trials. This finding has been reported across other studies and it is likely that patients with significant co-existent morbidity are at a higher risk of rupture than their healthier counterparts. The projected annual rates of rupture for AAA from a meta-analysis of 13 studies are shown in Table 13.1.[44] However, some small aneurysms will rupture, and some large aneurysms will not.

Patients with asymptomatic AAA of 30–54 mm should be kept under regular ultrasound surveillance to monitor growth. Current recommendations for surveillance intervals are yearly for 30–44 mm, every 3 months for 45–54 mm.[45] Elective repair is only recommended in asymptomatic AAA of >55 mm diameter – this applies to both open and endovascular aneurysm

repair (EVAR). The operative mortality associated with elective infra-renal AAA repair is between 1% and 6%.[42,46]

✅✅ The Medical Research Council-sponsored UK Small Aneurysm Trial (SAT) randomised 1090 patients with asymptomatic AAAs of 4.0–5.5 cm diameter to either initial ultrasound surveillance (527 patients) or surgery (563 patients).[42] In the surveillance group, 321 patients eventually underwent surgery because of rapid expansion or growth to above the 5.5-cm threshold. In the early surgery group, the 30-day mortality rate was 5.8%. There was no difference in survival between the groups and the UK SAT concluded that early operative intervention for patients with AAAs of less than 5.5 mm diameter was not indicated. The rupture rate for untreated small aneurysms in this trial was less than 2% per annum. However, the rate was relatively higher in females, and this suggests that elective surgery may be indicated for smaller aneurysms in this group of patients. At present, the data are insufficiently robust to support this conclusion convincingly.

Symptomatic, intact AAA or rapid expansion (>1 cm/year) of an AAA >4 cm represents a relative indication for operative repair. It is thought that symptoms of pain attributable to an aneurysm are caused by acute expansion or imminent rupture and urgent repair is recommended.

Aneurysm rupture is usually an absolute indication for surgery because without repair, mortality is almost certain. Surgery in some patients may be futile because of comorbidity or poor pre-operative clinical condition (unconsciousness, cardiac arrest).

✅✅ The Canadian Aneurysm Study demonstrated an in-hospital mortality rate for open AAA repair of 4.7% with a 5-year survival rate of 68%. The UK Small Aneurysm Trial reported a 30-day mortality rate of 5.8% and the EVAR-1 trial, a 30-day mortality rate of 4.7% in patients fit for surgery. The 2019 UK National Vascular Registry reports an overall in-hospital mortality rate of 2.3%, with mortality from endovascular repair below 0.5%.[42,46–48]

PRE-OPERATIVE ASSESSMENT

Patients with asymptomatic AAAs >55 mm who are candidates for surgical repair require careful risk assessment of their general health and fitness to determine their suitability for surgery. The goals of assessment are: to identify patients in whom the balance of risk favours surgical intervention, to reduce peri-operative morbidity and mortality by identifying modifiable comorbidity; to determine suitability for either open or endovascular repair by assessing aneurysm anatomy; to determine patient preferences for management.

Thorough clinical assessment is necessary as it is recognised that peri-operative death is related to pre-existing physiological status. Most early deaths after AAA repair relate to cardiac events and if pre-existing cardiac disease is identified and treated before surgery, survival rates can be improved.

Pre-operative assessment often includes:

- Full blood count
- Serum urea and electrolytes
- Liver function tests
- Pulmonary function tests

Table 13.1 Annual abdominal aortic aneurysm rupture risk in relation to size

AAA size (cm)	Risk of rupture per year (%)
< 3.0	0
3–3.9	0.4
4–4.9	1.1
5–5.9	3.3
6–6.9	9.4
7–7.9	24

AAA, Abdominal aortic aneurysm.
Adapted from Law MR, Morris J, Wald NJ. Screening for abdominal aortic aneurysms. J Med Screening. 1994;1:110–15.

- Cardiac assessment with resting electrocardiogram (ECG) and echocardiography (ECHO)
- Cardiopulmonary exercise testing
- Multi-detector CT aortography.

Further cardiovascular assessment (exercise ECG, dobutamine-stress ECHO, or coronary angiography) may be indicated in patients with a history (or symptoms) of ischaemic heart disease.

In patients with significant and irreversible comorbidity, it is appropriate to continue ultrasound surveillance until aneurysm diameter reaches a size where the risk of rupture outweighs the increased risk of surgical mortality. It may be impossible to justify elective operative repair (regardless of size) in patients with overwhelming comorbidity and/or frailty.

REPAIR OF INTACT ABDOMINAL AORTIC ANEURYSM

There are two methods by which AAAs may be excluded – traditional open repair (OR) and EVAR. Open surgical repair of AAA is a durable and cost-effective procedure. EVAR is effective and safe in selected patients, with lower short- and medium-term morbidity and mortality rates than open surgery. Patients with AAAs have a markedly reduced life expectancy in comparison with age- and sex-matched controls. The 5-year survival of patients post open surgery varies from 62– 72% (compared with 83–90% in age- and sex-matched populations), with the majority of deaths caused by cardiovascular disease.[47,49] The introduction of endovascular solutions for AAA offers an option for patients in whom OR was unfavourable. Conversely, there are patients with aortic anatomical constraints that are ill suited for EVAR, and results of EVAR in adverse anatomies are worse in the medium and long term.

OPEN REPAIR

Under general anaesthesia and with peri-operative broad-spectrum antibiotic and thromboembolic (heparin [s/c]) prophylaxis, a transverse supra-umbilical or midline incision is used to allow a transperitoneal approach to the aorta. Alternatively, an oblique left-sided abdominal incision may be used to achieve an extra-peritoneal approach to the aorta. Epidural analgesia may also be used to improve post-operative respiratory function. The routine use of cell salvage for intra-operative autologous transfusion is a useful adjunct.

At laparotomy, the transverse colon is reflected upwards, and the small bowel reflected to the right. Division of the posterior peritoneum exposes the aneurysm. The left renal vein is identified and the neck of an infra-renal aneurysm will be identified. The common iliac vessels are also identified and exposed. Care should be taken to avoid damage to the hypogastric plexus of nerves to avoid post-operative sexual dysfunction.

A bolus of heparin is given intravenously (to reduce the risk of thrombosis in situ and peri-operative cardiac injury) after which aortic and iliac clamps are applied. If the aneurysm extends into the common iliac arteries, the vessels may be mobilised to the common iliac bifurcation and control obtained of the internal and external iliac arteries. The aneurysm sac is opened longitudinally, and mural thrombus removed. Back bleeding from the lumbar, median sacral and inferior mesenteric arteries may ensue and over-sewing these vessels controls this. The aneurysm may be repaired using a tube (60–70%) or bifurcated prosthetic aortic graft made from sealed or coated, knitted Dacron™. The graft is secured proximally and distally using an inlay technique and end-to-end anastomoses with a monofilament suture.

The lower limbs are re-perfused sequentially upon completion of the anastomoses. The anaesthetist should be warned before releasing the clamps of each limb because of the hypotension caused by limb reperfusion and the sudden release of anoxic metabolites from the lower limbs into the systemic circulation. The aneurysm sac is closed over the aortic graft to reduce the risk of late post-operative aorto-enteric fistulation. The lower limbs and left colon should be inspected to ensure adequate perfusion. Post-operatively, patients are extubated and managed in a high-dependency unit. Early procedure-specific complications are mainly cardiac and respiratory in aetiology although renal dysfunction, colonic ischaemia and lower limb problems caused by thromboembolism may also occur. The patient should be encouraged to mobilise early, and oral intake can be re-established within 24 hours. In-hospital stay is usually 7–10 days. The 30-day mortality rate has remained around 3–5% for the past 10 years.

Aortic aneurysmal disease extends above the renal arteries to involve a variable length of the thoracic aorta in 5–10% of patients. Transperitoneal supra-renal clamping may be possible for juxta-renal AAA, but more proximal aneurysms require supra-coeliac clamping performed by laparotomy with medial visceral rotation or thoracolaparotomy and replacement with a Dacron™ aortic prosthesis as well as re-implantation of the visceral and intercostal arteries. The results of surgery in specialist centres are good but complications such as paraplegia, organ dysfunction and death may occur. There is a strong relationship between open AAA repair outcomes and surgeon/centre volume.[50] For optimum results, open AAA repair should be performed by experienced surgeons in high volume centres.

A few centres have advocated the technique of laparoscopic aortic surgery. There is an absence of any randomised data to support its use outside of a clinical trial.

OPERATIVE REPAIR OF RUPTURED ABDOMINAL AORTIC ANEURYSM

Once a ruptured AAA is diagnosed, patients suitable for attempted repair should be transferred to the operating theatre immediately. In general, patients should receive cautious fluid resuscitation with permissive hypotension. Sudden overloading of the intravascular compartment (together with its associated increase in systemic blood pressure) may cause expansion and rupture of a contained retroperitoneal haematoma resulting in potential exsanguination.

In theatre, the patient is prepared and draped before the induction of anaesthesia; central venous access can be performed after induction. Rapid sequence induction is performed together with rapid entry into the abdomen (limiting the potential hypotensive effects of anaesthesia caused by the loss of tamponade from relaxation of the anterior abdominal wall). The neck of the aneurysm must be identified for clamping despite the significant distortion of anatomy that may be caused by a large retroperitoneal haematoma; iatrogenic injury in this period may prove fatal for the patient. If access to the infra-renal aortic neck is not possible, the aorta may be clamped at the diaphragmatic hiatus or control achieved by passing a balloon occlusion catheter up the lumen of the aorta. These techniques are associated with significant morbidity owing to the resultant visceral and renal ischaemia. When haemorrhage has stopped, aortic repair may be performed as for intact AAAs. Aggressive correction of haemostatic variables is recommended to limit the problems of coagulopathy caused by massive haemorrhage and transfusion. Despite improvements in perioperative care, the operative mortality rate from ruptured AAA remains high at around 40%.[51]

ENDOVASCULAR ANEURYSM REPAIR

EVAR was first described by Voldos and colleagues in 1986 and Parodi and colleagues in 1991.[52] The premise of EVAR is to exclude the aneurysm from the systemic circulation using a pre-operatively sized stent graft; this prevents further expansion and risk of rupture. This minimally invasive technique has resulted in a paradigm shift in the treatment of infra-renal AAA. Between 2000 and 2010, the use of EVAR increased from 5–74% of all AAA repairs in the USA.[53] It remains the predominant method of AAA repair in the UK accounting for 60% of repairs in 2019.[48]

INDICATIONS AND ELIGIBILITY FOR ENDOVASCULAR ANEURYSM REPAIR

In contrast to open aneurysm repair, suitability for EVAR depends on both aneurysm morphology and patient fitness. It is reported that up to 45% of patients will have an AAA that is morphologically unsuitable for conventional infra-renal endografting.[54] Traditional morphological variables that impact on suitability include length of infra-renal aortic (>10 mm), neck angulation (<60 degrees), neck diameter (<28 mm), smooth parallel neck without significant mural thrombus. In addition, the iliac arteries should be of a calibre wide and straight enough to deliver a stent graft. As endografts evolve, the capability to treat more challenging anatomy are expanding (Fig. 13.2). Treatment of aortic necks as short as 4 mm can now be achieved within manufacturers recommended instructions for use using mechanical endoanchors that provide additional fixation to the aortic wall, while neck angulation of up to 90 degrees can be accommodated with some conformable stent grafts. Long-term outcomes in these hostile anatomies and use of applied technologies, need careful study.

In general, there are four graft constructs for EVAR of infra-renal AAAs: straight aorto-aortic tube endografts, bifurcated systems, aorto-uniiliac systems and combined bifurcated grafts with iliac branch grafts to permit perfusion and sealing in the external and iliac arteries. All devices form their proximal seal in the infra-renal aortic neck with variation in the distal seal zone – aorta, common iliac, external iliac or both external and internal iliac arteries. Aorto-aortic stent grafts were the first described and have a very limited

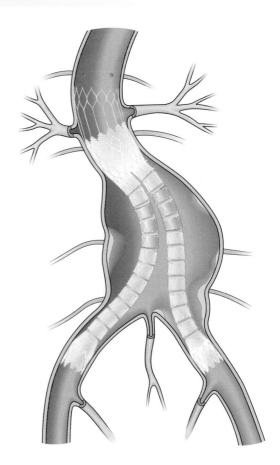

Figure 13.2 Schematic representation of abdominal aortic aneurysm repair using an aortic stent graft.

application in contemporary practice in short localised saccular aneurysms, post-operative pseudo-aneurysm and penetrating aortic ulcers. In conventional AAA, aorto-aortic endografts have an unacceptably high incidence of failure because of aneurysmal change in the seal zone.

Bifurcated grafts offer the most desirable solution by securing seal in vascular segments unlikely to be affected by aneurysmal change and preserving normal anatomical flow. These devices are suitable for around 50% of patients.[55] The remainder of EVAR-eligible aneurysms with more challenging anatomy require either an aorto-uniiliac or iliac branched stent graft. The former may be indicated where there are problems of unilateral iliac access because of tortuosity or stenoses and require occlusion of the contralateral common iliac artery with a plug and revascularisation of the limb with a femorofemoral cross-over graft. Iliac-branched grafts may be indicated in aneurysms that extend into the common iliac arteries and permit preservation of blood flow into the internal iliac arteries using a bifurcated iliac component.

PATIENT ASSESSMENT AND ENDOVASCULAR ANEURYSM REPAIR TECHNIQUE

The patient should be formally assessed, discussed within a multidisciplinary team and counselled for EVAR as for conventional open surgery. Multi-detector CT aortography should be obtained to enable multiplanar reconstruction and sizing of the entire abdominal aorta and iliofemoral segments and provide information regarding arterial access. Informed consent should include the routine morbidity and also the known EVAR-specific complications, including death, re-intervention, nephropathy, arterial injury, endoleak (see later) and open surgical conversion. Ideally, the theatre should be capable of endovascular and open procedures and equipped with fixed imaging capability. Mobile C-arm equipment may be used if necessary but affords poorer imaging capability and greater radiation dose exposure.

After anaesthetic induction, the patient is positioned, prepped and draped. A surgical cut-down to the femoral arteries permits catheterisation of the arterial circulation. A total percutaneous approach facilitated by the use of femoral closure devices is also now widely used. Evidence to justify this approach is emerging with claims of non-inferiority compared to surgical cut-down.[56] After femoral access is achieved, a soft wire and catheter are placed into the ascending aorta and a stiff guidewire is introduced through the catheter. Stiff guidewires are not intended to be 'working' wires and it is not sensible to try to negotiate tortuous iliac vessels with them. After systemic heparinisation, the stent graft body is introduced over the stiff guidewire and the renal arteries are imaged through a diagnostic catheter from the contralateral side. The image intensifier should be angled to optimise the view of the renal arteries, and this typically requires a small amount of cranio-caudal and oblique tilt.

The diagnostic catheter is left alongside the graft body as the top stents are released in stages. Further angiographic runs may be performed to ensure accurate positioning relative to the renal arteries. Modular devices require cannulation of the short leg of the main body of the device before introduction of the contralateral limb. This is generally performed by a retrograde approach from the contralateral femoral artery using angled catheters. Confirmation of successful cannulation is needed to avoid the error of inadvertently deploying the contralateral limb alongside rather than within the main graft. The iliac limbs are deployed close to the internal iliac origins, which are defined using oblique projections. Substantial overlap at the modular connections is essential to avoid late disconnections. Balloon moulding with a compliant aortic balloon can then be performed to optimise proximal and distal seal zones and junctions of the modular graft components.

Completion angiography is performed to confirm the aneurysm has been excluded and to ensure that there has been no encroachment by the fabric of the graft on the orifices of the visceral or internal iliac arteries (Fig. 13.3). Every effort must be made to resolve any significant primary type I endoleak before completion of the procedure.

ENDOVASCULAR ANEURYSM REPAIR–RELATED COMPLICATIONS AND DEVICE FAILURE

The physiological advantages of EVAR are reflected by the reduced requirement of post-operative critical care support and incidence of significant cardiac, pulmonary and renal complications. Some now advocate a day case approach to EVAR. However, in addition to the general causes of post-operative morbidity following AAA repair, EVAR carries some procedure-specific complications.

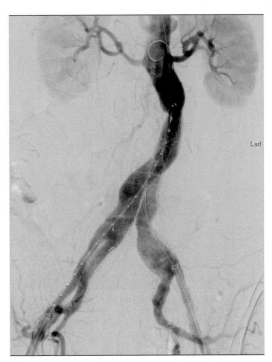

Figure 13.3 Completion angiogram of right iliac branched endovascular aneurysm repair showing satisfactory exclusion of aorto-iliac aneurysm and freedom from endoleaks.

Table 13.2   Endoleak classification

Endoleak type		Source
I	A: Proximal	Graft attachment site
	B: Distal	
	C: Iliac occluder	
II	A: Simple (single vessel)	Collateral vessel
	B: Complex (>2 vessels)	
III	A: Junctional leak	Graft failure
	B: Mid-graft hole	
	C: Other (e.g., suture hole)	
IV		Graft wall porosity
V	A: Without endoleak	Endotension
	B: With sealed endoleak	
	C: With type I or III leak	
	D: With type II leak	

Endoleak

Endoleak is defined as the persistence of blood flow outside the lumen of an endovascular stent graft but within an aneurysm sac or the adjacent vascular segment being treated by the stent. The leak may be described as primary, originating at the time of EVAR, or secondary, referring to a leak not seen at completion angiography but demonstrated on subsequent surveillance imaging. Endoleaks have been classified according to the source of aberrant blood flow, since this characterises the endoleak and the potential for aneurysm enlargement and eventual rupture (Table 13.2).[54] This is most often seen in type I (Fig. 13.4a) and type III (Fig. 13.4c) leaks that communicate directly with the aortic lumen, and re-intervention is almost always necessary in these patients.

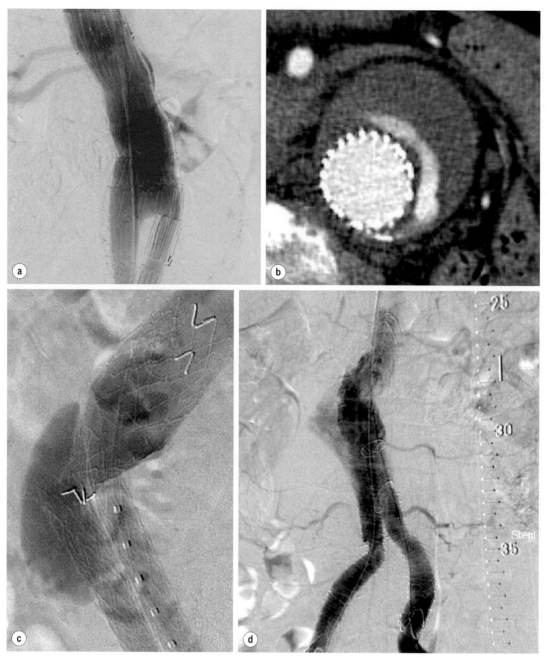

Figure 13.4   Images showing type I–IV endoleaks post–endovascular aneurysm repair (EVAR). (a) Completion angiogram showing a type I endoleak (proximal seal failure). (b) Post-EVAR contrast-enhanced computed tomography scan showing a type II endoleak. (c) Delayed angiogram showing a type III endoleak (junctional graft failure). (d) Completion angiogram showing a type IV endoleak (graft porosity).

Type II endoleaks (Fig. 13.4b) denote continued blood flow into the aneurysmal sac from refilling collateral vessels, typically the lumbar and inferior mesenteric arteries. The clinical significance of type II endoleaks is contentious and there is no standard treatment protocol. Increasingly, they are considered self-limiting and an expectant course of management is recommended, unless there is evidence of progressive sac expansion. There is some evidence that they are associated with an increased risk of re-intervention, but not aneurysm rupture or survival. At the very least, they should be kept under surveillance for signs of aneurysm sac enlargement.[57,58]

Blood flow across intact graft fabric within 30 days of EVAR defines the type IV endoleak (Fig. 13.4d). These leaks

typically seal spontaneously and may be seen more frequently with thinner and more porous stent grafts. Type V endoleaks are not true leaks but are defined as aneurysm sac expansion of >5 mm in the absence of a radiologically identifiable endoleak. They are considered to be resulting from a phenomenon of endotension caused by the accumulation of a transudate because of ultrafiltration of blood across the stent graft material.

Graft migration and dislocation

Successful EVAR depends on the generation of a blood-tight seal between stent graft and healthy native vessel for AAA exclusion. Failure at any attachment site renders the endograft insecure and prone to abnormal movement (migration) that is facilitated by systemic arterial blood pressure. Significant device migration at the seal zones predisposes the patient to endoleak (type I), whereas unwanted mobility of modular systems may lead to component dislocation and potential type III endoleak.

Device migration most likely results from the combined effect of patient and device related factors with a proximal attachment site failure most often described. In view of the significant risk of type I endoleak associated with distal migration of the proximal stent, remedial intervention is almost always indicated. This can usually be achieved with aortic cuff deployment to repair the proximal seal, but occasionally, stent revision is required.

Kinking and occlusion

Any distortion (kinking) of the endograft used in EVAR may result in stent stenosis, thrombosis and ultimately device (or limb) occlusion (Fig. 13.5). In a review of 4613 EVAR cases submitted to the EUROSTAR registry over an 8-year period, post-operative graft kinking was described in 3.7% cases.[59] Patent, symptomatic kinked stents can usually be treated by balloon angioplasty and adjunctive stenting, whereas occluded limbs typically require surgery.

Other endovascular aneurysm repair–related complications

Wire and stent manipulation within the aorta and aneurysmal sac during positioning and device deployment carries the risk of atheroembolisation with potential for organ infarcts and limb ischaemia. Introduction of guidewires, large-bore catheters and the endograft itself risks vessel injury such as rupture or dissection. Delayed presentations or iatrogenic arterial injury may occur, with pseudoaneurysm formation requiring prompt repair.

SURVEILLANCE AFTER ENDOVASCULAR ANEURYSM REPAIR

The modes of failure after aortic stent grafting are well documented. It is recommended that all patients be recruited onto a programme of systematic post-operative surveillance with the aim of detecting potential causes of late rupture. However, routine surveillance seldom identifies findings that require reintervention and lack of adherence to follow-up does not seem to affect long-term mortality or rupture rates.[60–62] The principal concerns are endoleak, aneurysm enlargement and migration of stents at the aortic or iliac landing zones or at the modular connections. Options for the method of surveillance include duplex ultrasound, CT, MRI and plain radiography.

It has been shown that ultrasound can be used to detect graft-related (type I) endoleaks reliably.[63] Ultrasound is less effective than CT for the detection of type II endoleaks, but since it is known that type II endoleaks without increased sac diameter are not associated with a significant risk of adverse clinical events, this may be regarded as an acceptable limitation. Plain radiography using a standardised protocol is an effective method for the detection of device migration. Stent fractures and separation of modular components are also relatively easy to identify. It is comparatively inexpensive and usefully complements ultrasound scanning. Used in combination, these two methods represent an acceptable alternative to CT for surveillance.

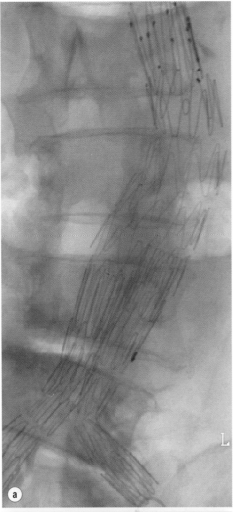

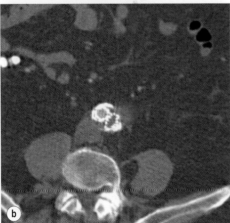

Figure 13.5 Post–endovascular aneurysm repair imaging showing graft kinking and occlusion in the same patient. (a) Plain film showing left iliac limb kinking. (b) Contrast-enhanced computed tomography scan showing consequent intraluminal occlusion.

Current 2020 recommendations from NICE and the 2019 European Society for Vascular Surgery (ESVS) guidelines advocate for surveillance protocols based on individualised risk of complications as determined by clinical features and early post-operative imaging; usually CT scan.[38,64] It is noteworthy that failure to adhere to manufacturer's instructions

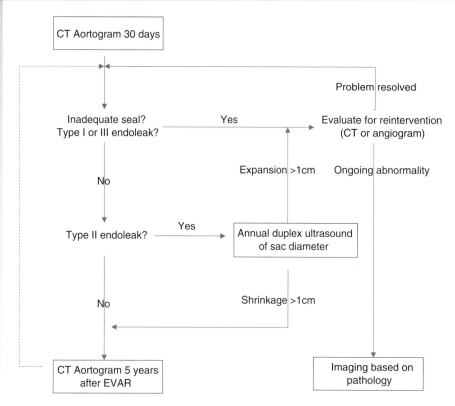

Figure 13.6 Proposed endovascular aneurysm repair surveillance (EVAR) protocol based on 2019 European Society for Vascular Surgery guidelines. *CT*, Computed tomography.

for use is associated with an increased risk of EVAR failure.[65] Early sac shrinkage has been shown to be a predictor of EVAR freedom from complication.[66] Conversely, sac diameter enlargement of 5 mm or more at 1 year, has been shown to be independently associated with late mortality regardless of the presence of an endoleak.[67] Based on these features, patients may be stratified for risk and the use of further surveillance investigations rationalised. Fig. 13.6 illustrates the proposed surveillance algorithm of the ESVS.[64] It is generally accepted that surveillance after EVAR should be indefinite.

OUTCOMES AFTER ENDOVASCULAR ANEURYSM REPAIR

There is now a good evidence base from randomised controlled trials in the UK, USA, Netherlands and France to support the use of EVAR in the normal infra-renal AAA population.[68–71]

✓✓ The UK EVAR-1 trial enrolled 1082 patients with suitable aneurysms (mean diameter 65 mm) that were considered fit enough for elective open AAA surgery and randomised them to either EVAR or conventional OR. Early outcome analysis revealed significantly lower 30-day mortality for the EVAR group (1.7%) compared to open surgical controls (4.7%). Medium-term study follow-up reported EVAR to be as effective as surgery in protecting from late aneurysm-related death, although there was a significantly higher rate of graft-related complications following EVAR (35% vs. 8%). In a smaller but similarly designed study, the Dutch DREAM trial compared outcome following EVAR and OR in 345 fit patients. A significantly lower operative mortality rate post-EVAR was confirmed (1.2% vs. 4.6%) with reduced incidence of early severe post-operative complications. At 4-year follow-up, however, there was no observed survival advantage after EVAR or OR.[68,70]

The UK EVAR-1 trial demonstrated a clear short-term benefit for EVAR compared with open surgery. Furthermore, EVAR was found to be associated with a shorter hospital stay. However, this survival advantage is eroded over follow-up. By 4-year follow-up, there are no differences in all-cause mortality between patients who had EVAR or open aneurysm repair. The latest 15-year results of the EVAR-1 trial have generated further debate; beyond 8 years follow-up, OR has a significantly lower all-cause mortality with an increased aneurysm and cancer mortality amongst EVAR patients. Potential explanations for this finding include poor compliance with EVAR surveillance protocols during the trial follow-up and whether endoleaks in the trial were managed to the level of contemporary standards.[72] Interestingly, this finding was not reproduced in late follow-up from the American OVER study; long-term overall survival was similar among patients who underwent endovascular repair and those who underwent OR.[73]

✓✓ The latest 15-year results of the EVAR-1 trial have shown that OR is associated with a long-term survival benefit when compared with EVAR. After 8 years of follow-up both total and aneurysm-related mortality were significantly higher in the EVAR group than in the OR group (adjusted hazard ratio [HR], 1.25; 95% CI, 1.00–1.56; $P = 0.048$ for total mortality; and 5.82, 1.64–20.65; $P = 0.0064$ for aneurysm-related mortality). After the first 6 months, the increased aneurysm-related deaths in the EVAR group were predominantly from secondary sac rupture (13 deaths [7%] in EVAR vs. 2 [1%] in OR). Re-interventions occurred in both groups during follow-up, including in patients who were free from re-intervention after 2 years or even 5 years. The rate of re-intervention was higher in the EVAR group at all follow-up timepoints. An increased cancer mortality was also observed in the EVAR group.[72]

Renal failure after EVAR is associated with an increased rate of mortality and its aetiology is probably multifactorial. Implicated factors include radiological contrast-associated nephropathy, renal artery trauma, stent-induced stenosis and aortic neck thromboembolism following vessel instrumentation and manipulation. It is rare for the renal ostia to be inadvertently covered by graft fabric, and careful planning and deployment decrease the risk of this occurring. There was concern that the introduction of supra-renal bare-stent fixation would lead to increased rates of renal failure, especially in patients with pre-existing renal impairment; however, studies have failed to demonstrate this.[74]

A large American observational study has also shown that EVAR patients are more likely to undergo AAA-related re-interventions during 4-year follow-up.[75] However, these were less likely to require in-patient hospitalisation compared to re-intervention following open aneurysm repair. Among patients who underwent EVAR in the randomised trials, 20–30% required a secondary re-intervention over the following 6 years. Cost-analyses from the EVAR-1 trial have shown EVAR to be associated with a higher cost than OR.[76]

These long-term results raise questions over the durability of EVAR. For the majority of patients, EVAR still provides short-term but no long-term benefits but it is clear that lifelong surveillance is necessary to prevent aneurysm-related death. For the very frail patient with multiple co-morbidities, if life expectancy is adequate, then EVAR after appropriate medical optimisation may bring some benefits; if life expectancy is short, EVAR is unlikely to bring any benefits.[77]

In 2019 ESVS released a Clinical practice Guideline for the Management of Aorto-iliac Aneurysms.[64] The UK NICE released their own guidelines for the diagnosis and management of AAA in 2020.[38] Despite similar objectives, fundamental methodological differences have resulted in some marked differences between the two documents. The methodological differences are centred on NICE adopting a strict protocol drawing heavily on randomised controlled trials to identify the most cost-effective care specifically for the UK NHS. In contrast, the ESVS utilises a more liberal search strategy, including recent observational data, and seeks clinical effectiveness across a range of European health economies. The outcome of these alternative approaches is that NICE recommend open surgical repair as the first-line treatment for patients with intact AAA, unless contraindicated by risk and comorbidity; while the ESVS recommend that EVAR should be the preferred treatment option in anatomically suitable patients with reasonable life expectancy. Expanding on these proposals, NICE does consider EVAR or conservative management an acceptable alternative for those in who open surgery may be unfavourable because of medical comorbidity, and EVAR for those with co-existent abdominal pathology, that is, hostile abdomen or horseshoe kidney. Similarly, the ESVS recommend OR as a first-line strategy for younger fit patients with a life expectancy of >10 years. Future work modelling the extent of any benefit in subgroups may help clarify these issues further. Patient preference is also important in terms of shared decision making. Sound clinical judgement remain of crucial importance in the management of patients with large aneurysms.

✔✔ The UK EVAR-2 trial randomised 338 medically unfit patients who were anatomical candidates for endovascular AAA repair (>55 mm) to either EVAR or 'BMT'. The early mortality in the EVAR limb was 9% and at a mean follow-up of 3.3 years there was no difference in the all-cause aneurysm-related mortality between the groups. Many clinicians have adopted these findings as justification not to offer EVAR in the higher-risk population. Caution is advised against this approach to management as closer scrutiny of the EVAR-2 results reveals some complicating issues. Firstly, there appeared to be an unacceptable delay from randomisation to treatment in the EVAR limb, so that nearly half (9 of 20) of the aneurysm-related mortality was explained by rupture before planned AAA repair. Operative (EVAR) mortality was surprisingly high (9%) and the rupture rate in the medically treated group (9 per 100 person-years) was significantly lower than expected, raising concern about disparate medical management between the two groups. Clearly, though, EVAR-2 demonstrates the poor long-term prognosis of the unfit AAA patient irrespective of treatment, with only 62–66% alive at 4 years.

The long-term follow-up of the EVAR-2 trial shows that after 8 years EVAR is associated with much improved aneurysm-related survival (86% at 6 years vs. 64% for no intervention), although no clear difference in all-cause survival was observed (30% at 6 years vs. 26%). The ability of EVAR to reduce aneurysm rupture (and aneurysm-related mortality) but not to improve survival is the sting in the tail for EVAR. However, after 8 years less than 20% of the patients remained alive, so that the long-term outcome for these patients might carry less weight than for those enrolled in the EVAR trial 1.[77]

THE FUTURE OF ENDOVASCULAR ANEURYSM REPAIR

RUPTURED ABDOMINAL AORTIC ANEURYSM

There is still some uncertainty whether the advantages of EVAR are reproducible in the case of AAA rupture, with several groups advocating its role. Avoidance of laparotomy confers a marked physiological advantage over OR in an already dire situation. However, the urgency associated with ruptured AAA repair results in little or no time being available to gather the required morphological information before EVAR. This is of particular importance since these aneurysms tend to have shorter and wider necks and are therefore more challenging for EVAR with current devices. Furthermore, the requirement of a permanently available on-call endovascular team with access to the appropriate facilities for EVAR is a significant obstacle in some centres. Nevertheless, there has been a paradigm shift towards pre-operative CT imaging for patients with suspected ruptured AAA in centres able to offer emergency EVAR.

The IMPROVE trial is the largest randomised controlled trial to determine whether endovascular repair improves the survival of all patients with ruptured AAA. This pragmatic trial randomised patients with an in-hospital clinical diagnosis of ruptured AAA. The trial showed no difference in mortality between EVAR and OR patients.[78] Similar findings were seen in two other contemporary European randomised controlled trials. Interestingly, the study did demonstrate shorter hospital stays, better quality of life and superior cost effectiveness for patients treated with EVAR.[79] The 2020 NICE AAA guideline recommends either OR or standard EVAR for ruptured AAA, with the caveat that for men >70 years and for women of any age, EVAR provide greater benefit whereas for men aged <70 years, OR is preferred. EVAR was felt to be cost effective in all women, but only men >70 years.[38] In contrast, the 2019 ESVS AAA guidelines recommend EVAR as first-line treatment in all those with suitable anatomy with no conditions on gender or age.[64]

✅✅ The UK IMPROVE trial enrolled 613 patients with a clinical diagnosis of ruptured AAA of whom two-thirds were randomised to either open or endovascular repair. Thirty-day mortality was 35% in the endovascular strategy group and 37% in the OR group. At 1 year, all-cause mortality was 41.1% for the endovascular strategy group and 45.1% for the OR group. The endovascular strategy group and OR groups had average total hospital stays of 17 and 26 days, respectively, $P<0.001$. Patients surviving rupture had health-related quality-of-life scores in the endovascular strategy compared to the OR groups at 3 and 12 months. There were indications that QALY were higher and costs lower for the endovascular first strategy.[78]

JUXTA-RENAL ABDOMINAL AORTIC ANEURYSM

More than 50% of patients have aneurysm morphology that is unsuitable for conventional endovascular repair.[54] Of these, a significant proportion will have an inadequate length of normal infra-renal aorta above the aneurysm within which to achieve a proximal seal, and account for up to 15% of AAA.[80] Fenestrated EVAR (FEVAR) was first described in 1999 as an endoluminal solution for patients with an inadequate infra-renal aortic neck.[81] Fabric fenestrations of the endograft, with or without bridging stents, permit perfusion of visceral branch vessels while achieving a secure proximal seal. Fenestrations may be one of three types: scallops, small or large circular fenestrations. Scalloped grafts have a U-shaped defect in the leading edge of the endografts for preserved patency of the most proximal visceral arteries. Both of the other types of fenestrations reside in the body of the device fabric. The bare-metal scaffold traverses large fenestrations, whereas small fenestrations lie between stent struts and require secondary stenting to achieve a seal and prevent occlusion (see Fig. 13.6). Observational data on the use of these devices has shown promise and these devices are now widely used in major vascular centres globally. An Achilles heel of these devices is their bespoke nature, which continues to necessitate a 6–12-week manufacture time for each graft.

Data from the United Kingdom have demonstrated that FEVAR can be performed with a high degree of technical success with good clinical outcomes[82] (Fig. 13.7). Although mortality rates of less than 5% were reported, the selected nature of these data and the lack of long-term follow-up make widespread application of this technique difficult to justify at present. Concerns about these devices include uncertainty regarding the long-term patency of stents in normal branch vessels, the increased number of modular connections and the possibility that the branches may kink if the aneurysm shrinks (Fig. 13.7). The technology is evolving rapidly and 'off-the-shelf' fenestrated grafts are now available.

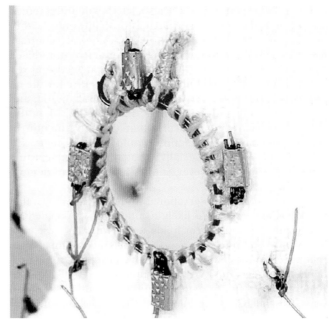

Figure 13.7   Fenestrated stent graft used for the treatment of perirenal aortic aneurysms. (Courtesy of Cook Medical.)

An alternative strategy for short-necked AAA is the use of parallel chimney grafts alongside conventional aortic endografts (Fig. 13.8). This technique has gained application as an off-the-shelf, less expensive alternative to custommade fenestrated graft. Again, promising results have been reported in observational studies and a systematic review reported a 5% 30-day mortality.[83] Nevertheless, concerns persist about the lack of randomised data and longer-term follow-up. Further concerns exist around the potential for endoleaks in the gutters between chimney and aortic grafts. The 2020 guidelines from NICE were concerned that FEVAR, parallel grafts and iliac branched devices were unlikely to be a cost-effective therapy within the UK NHS and recommend their use when undertaken within research or audit to explore the clinical and cost effectiveness compared to open surgery.[38] Once again, the 2019 ESVS guideline has a less restrictive view and recommends FEVAR as the preferred option for juxta-renal AAA when feasible. However, they make a strong recommendation for such repairs to be centralised to high volume centres that can offer both complex open and endovascular repair of complex aneurysms.[68]

More recently, polymer technology has been used to develop novel solutions for managing AAA. The main method modifies conventional aortic stent grafts to use inflatable polymer rings to create a seal at the neck of the aneurysm. It is argued that this method avoids the constant outward radial force, and potential for future dilatation, on the aortic neck that a conventional stent graft exerts.[84] A less successful application of polymer technology was seen in the technique of endovascular aneurysm sealing (EVAS). This procedure incorporated the use of two balloon expandable stents grafts with attached endobags, delivered up each iliac artery and deployed below the renal arteries. A biostable polyethylene glycol polymer was injected through the catheters into the endobags to fill the

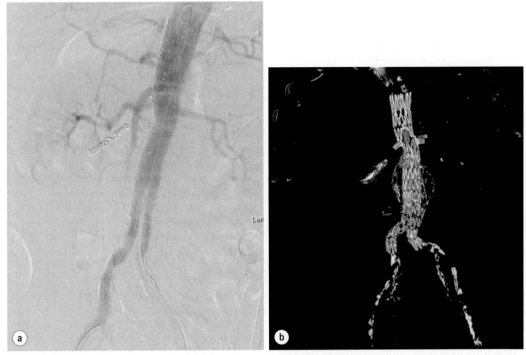

Figure 13.8 Three-fenestration stent graft with coil embolisation of accessory right renal artery and satisfactory exclusion of juxtarenal abdominal aortic aneurysm. (a) Completion angiogram. (b) Reconstruction of surveillance computed tomography aortogram.

aneurysm sac, sealing it off from the circulation and holding the stent graft in place. This technique was associated with an unacceptable rate of device failure and is no longer available for routine clinical practice in Europe.[85]

INFECTED ANEURYSMS

Although much less common than degenerative pathology, infected aneurysms remain an important subgroup of the disease. Since the introduction of antibiotic therapy and concomitant decline of endocarditis, true mycotic aneurysms are now uncommonly seen. Conversely, with increasing intravenous drug abuse, post-traumatic infected false femoral aneurysms are now a major clinical problem confronting the vascular specialist. These are discussed in more detail in the section on femoral aneurysms.

MYCOTIC ANEURYSMS

True mycotic aneurysm results when septic emboli lodge in the vasa vasorum of an artery. This is typically in the setting of infective endocarditis. Patients tend to be middle-aged and may have multiple aneurysms at differing sites. Both normal and abnormal vessels in any territory may be affected although there is a predilection of the aorta, intra-cranial, visceral and femoral vessels. The causative organisms are usually Gram-positive cocci, in particular *Streptococcus* spp. and *Staphylococcus aureus*.

MICROBIAL ANEURYSMAL ARTERITIS

With an ageing population with attendant increasing prevalence of atherosclerosis, microbial arteritis with aneurysm formation is now more common than true mycotic aneurysm. The pathological process involves blood-borne bacteria seeding into a diseased intima with subsequent suppuration, localised perforation and pseudoaneurysm formation. Unlike mycotic aneurysm, healthy native vessels are not affected. Aortic involvement is typical and pathology in this location is three times more common than in the peripheral circulation (Fig. 13.9). The classical infecting microorganisms are the *Salmonella* spp., but others have been reported, including *Escherichia coli*, *Staphylococcus* spp. and *Klebsiella pneumoniae*.

CLINICAL FEATURES AND MANAGEMENT PRINCIPLES OF INFECTED ANEURYSMS

The clinical presentation of an infected aneurysm depends both on the site of involvement and the underlying infective process. Usually, the patient presents with a pyrexia of unknown origin and little else; therefore a high index of suspicion is necessary. Supportive features include positive blood cultures, raised white cell counts, uncalcified aneurysms, vertebral erosion and a first presentation of aneurysm following an episode of bacterial sepsis. Classical radiological or appearances on angiography may or may not be present; and include saccular aneurysms, multilobulated and/or eccentric pathology with a narrow neck.

Following diagnosis, all patients should be commenced on appropriate antibiotics. Traditional management strategy for infected aneurysm has been one of open surgical repair. The principles of such surgery are generic, irrespective of the site and include: haemorrhage control, sepsis control (aneurysm resection, wide debridement, irrigation and drainage); confirmation of diagnosis (specimen

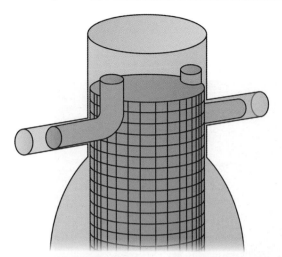

Figure 13.9 Schematic representation of chimney grafts/snorkels.

culture and sensitivity); and arterial reconstruction, usually with an autologous conduit, for example, superficial femoral vein for creation of a neo-aorta. In some instances, cadaveric or prosthetic grafts may be used in situ or routed away from the infected field. Post-operatively, the patient should be treated with long-term antibiotics that may be lifelong in some cases. Recently, increasing interest has centred on the use of endovascular stent grafts to treat infected aneurysms. The minimally invasive nature of this approach is appealing, with improved short-term outcomes, but balanced against uncertain long-term outcomes in terms of infection control.[86]

Despite improvements in diagnosis, surgical techniques and pharmacology, the early outcome for patients with infected aortic aneurysm remains poor, with a mortality rate of 23%. Infected post-traumatic false aneurysms are associated with better outcomes (5% mortality), but the lower limb amputation rate may be up to 25–33% if the femoral artery is involved.

PERIPHERAL ANEURYSMS

ILIAC ANEURYSMS

Up to 40% of iliac aneurysms occur in association with aortic aneurysms. Isolated iliac aneurysms are comparatively unusual, the prevalence having been estimated to be less than 2% of aorto-iliac aneurysms. They tend to be large (4–8 cm) and typically involve either the common or internal iliac arteries. Aneurysmal disease of the external iliac artery is extremely rare.

Generally accepted guidance is that elective open or endovascular intervention is indicated for asymptomatic iliac aneurysms greater than 3–4 cm in diameter.[87] Symptomatic and ruptured aneurysms require immediate surgical intervention. Once again, treatment may be performed with an open surgical repair with a Dacron™ graft or if anatomy permits, an endovascular stent graft for isolated common iliac aneurysm. Isolated internal iliac aneurysms are usually managed by open surgical ligation or endovascular embolisation.

COMMON FEMORAL ANEURYSMS

Femoral arterial aneurysms can be divided simply into true or false (pseudo) aneurysms. True aneurysms relate to a distinct pathological process involving all three layers of the femoral arterial wall. False aneurysms are caused by a traumatic breach of a vessel wall with an associated contained blood collection with flow out with the artery.

Both disease processes may be symptomatic or asymptomatic. Symptomatic femoral aneurysms can present as a pulsatile groin mass that may or may not be painful, leg swelling (because of femoral vein compression and deep vein thrombosis) or features associated with chronic ischaemia attributable to aneurysm thrombosis/embolisation. Rupture can occur but is rare. Asymptomatic pathology is usually discovered incidentally on clinical examination or imaging studies of a patient with an aneurysm elsewhere or with chronic ischaemia.

TRUE FEMORAL ANEURYSMS

True femoral aneurysms are the second commonest peripheral artery aneurysm after the popliteal artery. They occur in 2–3% of patients with aortic aneurysms and tend to be a disease of elderly men (male-to-female ratio 30:1). The condition is frequently bilateral and a co-existent generalised aneurysmal process may be manifest in other anatomical sites such as the aorto-iliac or popliteal arteries.

Small, asymptomatic true femoral artery aneurysms can be managed expectantly with clinical assessment at intervals. Surgical treatment is indicated for symptoms and probably for most aneurysms of 3.5 cm or more in size.[88] Usually, a short interposition or inlay tube graft anastomosed proximally at the level of the inguinal ligament and distal to the common femoral bifurcation is required. This is a relatively small operation with durable results.

FALSE FEMORAL ANEURYSMS

The common femoral artery is regularly used for catheterisation of the arterial circulation (e.g., angiography, cardiac catheterisation, EVAR, intra-aortic balloon pumps, etc.). As a consequence, iatrogenic injury leading to false aneurysm is a relatively common occurrence that complicates approximately 1% of transfemoral interventions. The diagnosis should be suspected in any patient with a pulsatile mass at the site of a recent arterial cannulation. Initially, a duplex scan should be obtained to both confirm the diagnosis and characterise the false aneurysm. If the pathology is small (<2 cm) and associated with minimal symptoms, simple observation with re-scanning may be justified, as most of these pseudo-aneurysms will thrombose spontaneously within 2–4 weeks. Other options include compression therapy (direct pressure and/or ultrasound guided) in an effort to seal the feeding arterial jet. Thrombin injection is an effective treatment with a reported success rate of over 95%. If these measures fail or in cases of tense swelling, threatened skin viability or neurology, open surgical repair is indicated. Unlike non-invasive methods, surgery has the advantage of combining both the arterial repair and field decompression. The former is usually a primary repair of the vessel with a Prolene suture, although formal graft reconstruction is sometimes required.

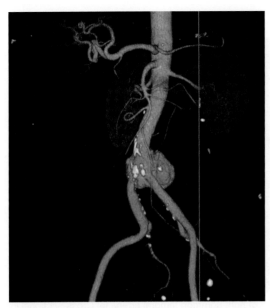

Figure 13.10 Reconstructed computed tomography aortogram of mycotic saccular aortic aneurysm.

Infected femoral pseudo-aneurysms are now the most common type of infected aneurysm observed in clinical practice, largely explained by increased intravenous drug abuse in recent years. Although the usual microorganism cultured is a *Staphylococcus* species, the infection may be polymicrobial and close liaison with the microbiology team is required for appropriate antibiotic therapy. The surgical strategy for infected femoral false aneurysms depends largely on its cause. For patients with no history of drug injection, arterial excision and reconstruction with autologous conduit (e.g., long saphenous vein and obturator bypass) following the operative principles for infected aneurysms outlined earlier is preferred. In those who do inject drugs, arterial excision with ligation alone (i.e., no reconstruction) is advised because of the unacceptable risk of subsequent graft infection with continued drug misuse and likelihood of exhausted superficial veins (Fig. 13.10). Ligation of the femoral artery does not necessarily mandate amputation if only one femoral segment is involved. If the femoral bifurcation is excised, however, the risk of limb loss is significant and reconstructive surgery may need to be considered, although this is contentious (Fig. 13.11).

POPLITEAL ARTERY ANEURYSMS

Popliteal aneurysms are the most commonly encountered peripheral aneurysm, accounting for more than 80% of all peripheral aneurysms. The ratio of popliteal aneurysms to AAAs is approximately 1:15. Half are bilateral, a third asymptomatic and 40% are associated with AAAs. Popliteal aneurysms are uncommon in women.

Although rupture is rare, 50% of cases present with peripheral limb-threatening ischaemia. In common with aneurysms at all other sites, laminated thrombus develops within popliteal aneurysms. The popliteal artery is continually subjected to flexion and extension, greatly increasing the risk of disintegration and embolisation of this thrombus. In many patients, microembolisation of the peripheral circulation occurs silently before main vessel occlusion or thrombosis of the popliteal aneurysm itself. For this reason, the viability of the limb may be seriously threatened. Furthermore, compromise of the run-off circulation can impact adversely on the outcome from emergency bypass surgery. The bigger the aneurysm, the more likely there is to be thrombus. The presence of intraluminal thrombus is therefore a more important indication for elective surgical intervention than the size of the aneurysm. Any thrombus detected by ultrasound, CT or MRI constitutes an indication for elective treatment. In the absence of laminated thrombus, it is generally accepted that aneurysms with a diameter of 2–3 cm or greater warrant consideration for elective surgical repair.

Traditionally, popliteal aneurysms are treated by proximal and distal ligation and bypass using autologous vein undertaken via a medial approach. However, recent studies have identified persistent flow within the popliteal aneurysm in 30% of patients treated in this way. Furthermore, there is a significant risk of continued expansion and even rupture caused by pressurisation of the sac resulting from backflow through geniculate branches. Therefore a posterior approach and insertion of an inlay graft is to be preferred.[89]

An acutely thrombosed popliteal aneurysm is a clinical emergency. Pre-operative or on-table thrombolysis has been used to open up the run-off vessels and thereby facilitate bypass surgery. There is some low-level evidence to suggest that this approach may improve the chances of successful limb salvage.

With the evolution of flexible endografts, endovascular repair is now a viable alternative to open surgery for the treatment of some popliteal aneurysms. Long-term follow-up suggests that in selected patients, this is a durable technique, capable of achieving excellent patency rates and limb preservation[90] (Fig. 13.12a–c). Further large-scale clinical trials are warranted to help define optimal candidates for this technique.

✓✓ Another important determinant of patient outcome following AAA repair is the ability and experience of the operating surgeon. A meta-analysis demonstrated a significantly lower mortality following AAA repair with higher volume surgeons and suggested a minimum caseload of 13 open AAAs per annum for continued practice. With further analysis, this number is likely to rise and, naturally, this has significant implications for the provision of vascular services and would support the argument for fewer, larger, regional vascular centres linked directly to a nationwide targeted AAA screening programme.[91]

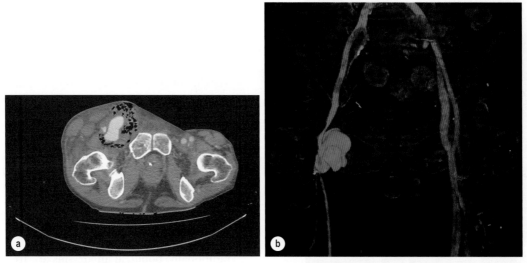

Figure 13.11   Computed tomography (CT) angiogram of mycotic false aneurysm of right common femoral artery. (a) Cross-sectional image of false aneurysm with gas in soft tissues. (b) Reconstructed CT of mycotic aneurysm at common femoral bifurcation.

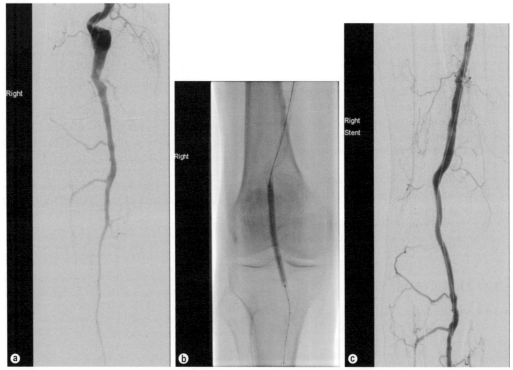

Figure 13.12   Angiogram of popliteal aneurysm. (a) Diagnostic angiogram. (b) Balloon moulding of popliteal stent graft. (c) Completion angiogram of popliteal stent graft.

Key points

- The prevalence of AAA appears to be declining, as does aneurysm rupture and mortality.
- There are good clinical and cost-effectiveness data to support targeted population-based screening programmes for AAA.
- The UK Small Aneurysm Trial supported a policy of surveillance rather than operation for patients with AAAs of less than 5.5 cm diameter.
- Three principal, randomised controlled trials for AAA have shown marked benefits of EVAR over open repair with respect to 30-day mortality.
- However, the total mortality benefit of EVAR was lost in these randomised controlled trials after 1–5 years.
- Beyond 8 years, open aneurysm repair was associated with better survival and durability than EVAR in the UK EVAR-1 trial.
- EVAR requires annual surveillance and has a crude annual reintervention rate of 4%.
- EVAR does not confer a survival advantage in patients who are unfit for open aneurysm repair as 50% will die within 5 years, mostly from cardiovascular comorbidity rather than aneurysm rupture.
- EVAR has not been shown to be superior, in terms of survival, to open repair in ruptured AAAs. However, it is associated with shorter hospital stay, better quality of life and cost-effectiveness.
- Technological advances have widened the endovascular treatment options for juxta-renal AAAs.
- Infected true aneurysms are associated with a poor prognosis, but their incidence is falling.

▶ RECOMMENDED VIDEOS

- EVAS – https://tinyurl.com/yaolz8ug
- EVAR – https://tinyurl.com/y7fyyvjl

🌐 References available at http://ebooks.health.elsevier.com/

KEY REFERENCES

[34] Ashton HA, Buxton MJ, Day NE, et al. The Multicentre Aneurysm Screening Study (MASS) into the effect of abdominal aortic aneurysm screening on mortality in men: a randomised controlled trial. Lancet 2002;360:1531–9. PMID: 12443589.

A UK multicentre population-based screening study of 67 800 men, aged 65–74 years, who were randomly allocated to be invited to attend for ultrasound assessment or not. The primary outcome measure was aneurysm-related death and there was a 42% risk reduction in the invited group.

[95] Multicentre Aneurysm Screening Study Group. Screening men for abdominal aortic aneurysm: 10-year mortality and cost effectiveness results from the Multicentre Aneurysm Screening Study. BMJ 2009;338:b2307. PMID: 19553269.

Cost-effectiveness analysis at 4 years showed that the cost per quality-adjusted life-year (QALY) was £36 000. It is projected that this value will fall to £8000 per QALY within 10 years.

[39] Wanhainen A, Hultgren R, Linné A, et al. Outcome of the Swedish nationwide abdominal aortic aneurysm screening program. Circulation 2016;134:1141–8. PMID: 27630132.

Outcome data on 302 957 men aged 65 years invited for AAA screening. There was a 1.5% prevalence and 29% had AAA repair. Screening was associated with a significant reduction in AAA-specific mortality. The number needed to screen, and the number needed to operate on to prevent 1 premature death were 667 and 1.5, respectively. Screening 65-year-old men for AAA is an effective preventive health measure and is highly cost-effective in a contemporary setting.

[42] The UK Small Aneurysm Trial Participants. Mortality results for randomised controlled trial of early elective surgery or ultrasono-graphic surveillance for small abdominal aortic aneurysms. Lancet 1998;352:1649–55. PMID: 9853436.

A multicentre randomised controlled trial of 1090 patients with asymptomatic aneurysms of diameter 4.0–5.5 cm who were randomly allocated to early elective surgery or ultrasound surveillance. There was no significant survival advantage at 6 years for those undergoing surgical repair.

[46] Greenhalgh RM, Brown LC, Kwong GP. Comparison of endovascular aneurysm repair with open repair in patients with abdominal aortic aneurysm (EVAR trial 1), 30-day operative mortality results: randomised controlled trial. Lancet 2004;364:843–8. PMID: 15351191.

A multicentre randomised controlled trial comparing open and endovascular repair in patients anatomically suitable for either. The 30-day mortality results show an initial survival advantage for patients treated with EVAR.

[47] Johnston KW. Non-ruptured abdominal aortic aneurysm: six-year follow up results from the multicentre prospective Canadian aneurysm study. Canadian Society for Vascular Surgery Aneurysm Study Group. J Vasc Surg 1994;20:163–70. PMID: 8040938.

A prospective analysis of 680 patients undergoing elective aneurysm surgery showed that cardiac-related death is the major peri-operative risk and cardiac and cerebrovascular events are the major causes of death at 6 years.

[68] The UK EVAR trial investigators. Endovascular versus open repair of abdominal aortic aneurysm. N Engl J Med 2010;362:1863–71. PMID: 20382983.

In this large randomised trial, endovascular repair of AAAs was associated with a significantly lower operative mortality than open repair. However, no differences were seen in total mortality or aneurysm-related mortality in the long term. Endovascular repair was associated with increased rates of graft-related complications and re-interventions and was more costly.

[72] The UK EVAR trial investigators. Endovascular versus open repair of abdominal aortic aneurysm in 15-years' follow-up of the UK endovascular aneurysm repair trial 1 (EVAR trial 1): a randomised controlled trial. Lancet 2016;388:2366–74. PMID: 27743617.

The 15-year follow-up data from this trial showed that after 8 years, open repair was superior to endovascular aneurysm repair in terms of all-cause mortality and aneurysm-related mortality.

[77] EVAR Trial participants. Endovascular aneurysm repair and outcome in patients unfit for open repair of abdominal aortic aneurysm (EVAR-2 trial): randomized controlled trial. Lancet 2005;365:2187–92. PMID: 15978926.

A multicentre randomised trial comparing EVAR and best medical therapy in 338 unfit patients with morphologically suitable AAAs; 30-day mortality was 9% in the EVAR group and at a mean follow-up of 3.3 years there was no difference in either the all-cause or aneurysm-related mortality between groups.

[78] Improve Trial investigators. Endovascular or open repair strategy for ruptured abdominal aortic aneurysm: 30-day outcomes from IMPROVE randomised trial. BMJ 2014;348:f7661. PMID: 24418950.

A multicentre randomised trial of 613 patients with ruptured AAA randomised to either an attempted endovascular strategy or open repair. Thirty-day mortality was 35% in the endovascular strategy group and 37% in the open repair group. A strategy of endovascular repair was not associated with significant reduction in either 30-day mortality or cost.

[82] British society for endovascular therapy and the global collaborators on advanced stent-graft techniques for aneurysm repair (GLOBALSTAR) registry. Early results of fenestrated endovascular repair of juxtarenal aortic aneurysm in the United Kingdom. Circulation 2012;125:2707–15. PMID: 22665884.

A registry study of 318 patients from 14 British centres undergoing fenestrated EVAR. Primary procedural success was achieved in 99%; peri-operative mortality was 4.1%. The early re-intervention (<30 days) rate was 7% (22/318).

[91] Young EL, Holt PJ, Poloniecki JD, et al. Meta-analysis and systematic review of the relationship between surgeon annual caseload and mortality for elective open abdominal aortic aneurysm repairs. J Vasc Surg 2007;46:1287–94. PMID: 17950569.

A meta-analysis involving 115 273 elective open AAA repairs demonstrating significantly lower mortality with higher caseload surgeons. The study suggested a critical case volume threshold of 13 open AAA repairs per annum.

14 | Thoracic and thoraco-abdominal aortic disease

Alexander Rolls | Ian Loftus | Peter Holt

INTRODUCTION

Diseases of the thoracic and thoraco-abdominal aorta are less common than infra-renal abdominal aortic aneurysms (AAAs) but their management should be familiar to vascular surgeons, as they often present acutely. This is partly because of the greater utilisation of cross-sectional imaging, which has in turn led to an apparent increase in the incidence of thoracic aortic conditions.[1]

Over the last two decades, endovascular repair has become the first-line treatment for most distal arch, descending and thoraco-abdominal aortic pathologies. Despite the move toward minimally invasive strategies, the increasing use of endovascular repair of the thoracic aorta (thoracic endovascular aortic repair [TEVAR]) has lacked the large randomised trials that underpinned the widespread adoption of standard infra-renal repair (endovascular aortic repair [EVAR]). Registry data, institutional case series and national routine data have suggested that endovascular procedures can be offered with low mortality and morbidity rates in comparison with open repair of thoracic pathology, and appear to be equally as effective in preventing aortic-related death.[2,3] Critics of the increase in the repair of thoracic pathology draw attention to the lack of accurate contemporary natural history data for untreated pathology, and also that newer and costly technologies lack data on their long-term durability.

In the case of aortic dissection, there is continuing controversy over the role of TEVAR in uncomplicated acute and chronic dissection and the ability of this procedure to prevent aortic-related death. The advance of fenestrated and branched stent-graft technology has allowed many patients that were previously not fit enough to undergo treatment by highly invasive open surgery of the thoraco-abdominal aorta to be offered complex TEVAR, although open repair is still recommended for those with connective tissue disorders.

This chapter reviews the contemporary treatment of thoracic and thoraco-abdominal aortic disease, excluding the ascending aorta.

IMAGING OF THE THORACIC AORTA

Computed tomographic angiography (CTA) is the investigation of choice to diagnose aortic pathology and plan subsequent repair. Modern workstations allow reformatting of images in multiple planes with the derivation of luminal centrelines. These techniques can be used to estimate lengths and diameters to a greater degree of accuracy than axial images alone and are essential if endovascular repair is planned[4] (Fig. 14.1). CTA is also the modality of choice when performing surveillance for patients that have had previous repair. The disadvantages of CTA are the relatively high dose of radiation required and the need for nephrotoxic intravenous contrast.[5,6] In younger patients, such as those with connective tissue disorders who are likely to require some years of surveillance, magnetic resonance angiography (MRA) may be more appropriate but offers less spatial resolution than CTA. MRA has been used in experimental applications for patients with aortic dissection to characterise flow in the false lumen and this may come to represent an important way to predict disease progression and success of treatment in the future.[7]

THORACIC AORTIC ANEURYSMS

CLASSIFICATION AND AETIOLOGY

The majority of thoracic aortic aneurysms (TAAs) are degenerative or atherosclerotic in nature, although approximately one-quarter are caused by a chronically dilating aortic dissection. Less frequently, aneurysms are related to connective tissue disorders such as Marfan syndrome or Ehler–Danlos syndrome. Mycotic or other inflammatory aneurysms of the thoracic aorta are relatively rare. False aneurysms can be caused by trauma and may present many years after the original precipitating event or may originate at the site of a previous surgical repair of the aorta. Aneurysms involving the descending aorta and the visceral segment are referred to as *thoraco-abdominal aortic aneurysms (TAAAs)*. The majority of aneurysms are fusiform in morphology. Saccular aneurysms are less common and are usually the result of infection or previous trauma.

INCIDENCE, CLINICAL PRESENTATION AND INDICATIONS FOR TREATMENT

The incidence of aneurysms of the descending thoracic aorta appears to have increased, and in the UK has doubled from 4.4 to 9 per 100 000 patients per year over the last decade.[1] The reason for this apparent increase is probably that thoracic aneurysms are most frequently discovered incidentally on routine chest radiography or cross-sectional imaging to investigate other conditions.

Thoracic aneurysms have a strong association with AAAs, and the conditions are concurrent in 23% of men and 48% of women with this condition.[8] Clinical presentations

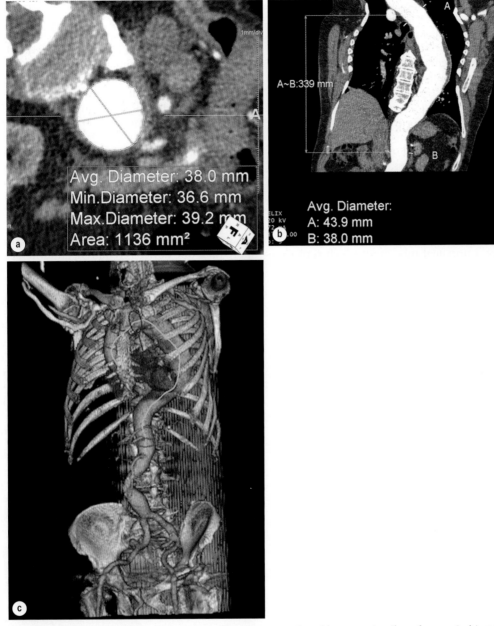

Figure 14.1 Planning thoracic endovascular intervention using images produced by reconstruction of computed tomography angiographic images of the thoracic aorta. This allows more accurate measurements of lengths and diameters, vital when selecting suitable devices (software shown produced by Terarecon, CA, USA).

include substernal, back or shoulder pain, superior vena cava syndrome, dysphagia, dyspnoea, stridor and hoarseness and rupture. The risk of rupture increases with the size of the aneurysm, but data regarding estimated annual rupture rates and aortic diameter are sparse and less robust than for the abdominal aorta.

The main indications for intervention are symptoms and size. There is controversy regarding the size criteria for treatment of TAAs, and the natural history remains poorly understood.[9] Juvonen et al. reported that the 2-year rupture rate for TAAs was 23% in aneurysms less than 7 cm,[10] whereas Elefteriades observed a 30% 5-year rupture rate when the aorta exceeded 6 cm.[11] A study of 257 patients with TAAs showed that event rates at 1, 3 and 5 years were $4.3 \pm 1.3\%$, $6.9 \pm 1.9\%$ and $9.7 \pm 2.6\%$ for definite aortic events and $6.6 \pm$

1.6%, $12.1 \pm 2.4\%$ and $16.5 + 3.1\%$ for possible events. Those with a starting aortic diameter of <50 mm experienced an event rate of less than 1%, but the rate of definite or possible event rates rose to 2.7 or 8.1% at aortic diameter between 50 mm and 60 mm and increased exponentially to 37.5 or 62.5% at >70 mm.[12] A more recent study of 907 patients conducted by the Yale-New-Haven Aortic Institute yielded several important findings. Firstly, the majority of ruptures and aortic deaths occurred above aortic diameter of 5 cm (71%). Secondly, two key hinge-points of 6 and 6.5 cm were associated with sharp increases in the combined endpoint of aortic rupture and death. In keeping with infra-renal disease, aortic growth rates increase with aortic diameter: Descending thoracic and thoraco-abdominal aneurysms 4 cm in size grew at a rate of 0.22 cm/year, whilst 8 cm aneurysms grew at 0.42 cm/year.[13] The American College of Cardiology/American Heart Association and European Society of Cardiology suggest considering open or endovascular repair in asymptomatic patients at a threshold of 6 cm.[14,15] Diameter thresholds should be reduced in patients with defined connective tissue disorders as rupture may occur at smaller aortic diameters.

TECHNIQUE OF SURGICAL REPAIR

The standard method of traditional open surgical repair of TAAs is a left thoracotomy for access, aortic clamping and inlay grafting. In cases involving the aortic arch, a two-stage approach may be used, which is known as an 'elephant trunk' procedure, and is usually performed in combination with cardiothoracic surgeons. This comprises open repair of the arch via a median sternotomy and is in itself comprised of two components; a proximal tube graft, which replaces the diseased arch, which is sutured to the origin of the descending aorta, and another length of unsupported graft, which is then inverted distally into the aneurysm beyond this point. In cases of more proximal disease extension, the supra-aortic trunks are managed by either incorporating them as an island or patch, which is anastomosed to the proximal component, or by "debranching", whereby multibranch inflow is taken from the ascending aorta and anastomosed end-to-end with the supra-aortic trunks. "Frozen elephant trunk" refers to more contemporary distal component, which is comprised of stent-supported fabric.

A second procedure can be performed through a left thoracotomy to continue the repair distally into the chest or an endovascular stent-graft can be deployed into it subsequently. In cases of more proximal disease extension, the supra-aortic trunks are managed by incorporating them as an island or patch, which is anastomosed to the tube graft used to replace the arch. The development of the more stable frozen elephant trunk has resulted in increasing numbers of second-stage procedures being completed endovascularly using TEVAR devices, with promising results.[16,17] These procedures are technically challenging and physiologically demanding for patients because of the need for aortic cross-clamping and organ ischaemia. Several adjuncts are available to achieve these aims, including the use of a Gott shunt, left heart bypass and distal aortic perfusion, selective intercostal shunting and cerebrospinal fluid (CSF) drainage.

ENDOVASCULAR REPAIR OF THORACIC ANEURYSMS

Successful endovascular repair is dependent on the presence of suitable access vessels with adequate sealing (or 'landing') zones proximal and distal to the aneurysm. Preoperative CTA is assessed to determine which endografts should be used and the mode of access. It is recommended that centreline image reconstruction is used using vascular-specific software to minimise error during planning.

The optimal proximal landing zones should be between 15 and 20 mm along the inner curvature of the aorta, depending on the specific stent-graft manufacturer instructions for use. If the landing zone is considered to be of inadequate length, surgical bypass may be performed to lengthen the effective sealing zone. The supra-aortic trunks that would

need to be covered by the endograft determine the Ishimaru zone of the repair (Fig. 14.2).[18] If left subclavian artery (LSCA) coverage for an aneurysm extending to Ishimaru zone 2 is required then a carotid subclavian bypass can be used (Fig. 14.3). If Ishimaru zone 1 extent coverage is required, a right-to-left carotid-to-carotid bypass must be used with or without left subclavian revascularisation. In zone 0 coverage, ascending aorta to innominate and left common carotid bypass via a median sternotomy is performed (Fig. 14.4).

Different commercially available stent-graft devices are available in different diameters, and these vary from 22–46 mm. A degree of oversizing is required with respect to the aortic diameter during device selection to ensure sufficient sealing, and it is recommended that this be 15–20%. As a result, the upper and lower limits of landing zone diameter are 40–42 mm and 18 mm, respectively. In many cases, more than one device is required, and when calculating the length of coverage then the overlap between adjacent devices recommended by manufacturers should be noted. A recent analysis has suggested that using endografts in unsuitable anatomy may significantly compromise durability.[19]

The TEVAR procedure is usually performed under general or regional anaesthesia, although stents can be inserted under local anaesthesia. Transfemoral access is most normally obtained using percutaneous closure technique. A 300-mm length of extra-stiff guidewire (e.g., Lunderquist guidewire, Cook, UK) is advanced so that the tip is placed in the ascending aorta. A pre-curved wire can be used to enhance conformation to the aortic arch. A pigtail

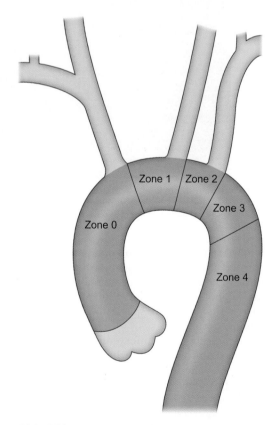

Figure 14.2 Ishimaru zones describing the proximal extent of the stent-graft landing zone required to achieve an adequate proximal seal.

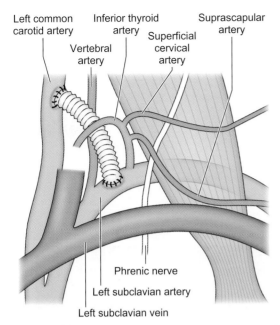

Figure 14.3 Carotid subclavian bypass performed selectively before thoracic endovascular aortic repair (TEVAR) where coverage of the origin of the vessel is required.

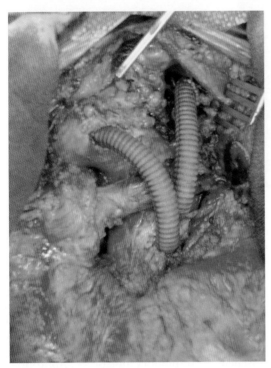

Figure 14.4 Operative photograph of ascending aorta to innominate and left common carotid. Surgery performed to create an adequate landing zone in a patient with a very proximal thoracic aneurysm.

angiographic catheter is placed alongside this, and the first device is advanced into position along the stiff wire. Angiographic images are obtained in the correct parallax to allow visualisation of the supra-aortic branches. This usually requires a steep left anterior oblique angulation of the imaging system. The systolic blood pressure should be reduced to below 100 mmHg peak systolic pressure to allow accurate deployment of the proximal endograft (Fig. 14.5). This can

be achieved by pharmacological means or overdrive pacing to reduce the cardiac output and a range of opinion exists as to what is required across the range of pathologies treated. Further endografts are placed as necessary with the required overlap between endografts. Angiographic imaging is then used to ensure correct positioning and seal.

NEUROLOGICAL COMPLICATIONS FOLLOWING ENDOVASCULAR THORACIC PROCEDURES

Neurological complications after TEVAR are not uncommon and are related to disturbance of flow in supra-aortic trunks or in the supply to the spinal cord. Stroke and paraplegia have devastating consequences for patients, and both are associated with a significant reduction in mid-term survival.[20] A number of risk factors for paraplegia has been suggested, including the length of aortic coverage, previous infra-renal aortic repair, and the coverage without revascularisation of the LSCA. Emergency surgery, blood loss and renal failure have also been cited. What appears to be most important is to support and allow development of the collateral network supplying the spinal cord. To protect against this, some centres advocate prophylactic drainage of CSF whilst others adopt a selective approach. Increasingly, the safest strategy that may obviate the need for CSF drainage, appears to be staging thoraco-abdominal aortic repair into a number of smaller procedures where feasible.

If signs of spinal cord ischaemia occur then cord perfusion pressure must be increased by reducing CSF pressure via the use of a spinal drain, ensuring a mean arterial pressure of 100 mmHg with the use of fluid boluses and inotropes, and enhancing oxygen delivery maintaining $PO_2 > 10$ and haemoglobin > 10.[21]

Regarding the management of the LSCA during thoracic endografting, consensus has determined that patients with a left internal mammary artery bypass graft or with a dominant left vertebral artery comprised a group where left subclavian revascularisation was considered mandatory. Where feasible, LSCA revascularisation is recommended in the management of atherosclerotic aneurysms, but the recommendation is weaker in the acute aortic syndromes including type B aortic dissection where paraplegia and posterior circulation stroke rates are lower.[20,22,23] Normally, LSCA revascularisation is performed surgically, although a number of novel techniques have been described to undertake this endovascularly, none are yet mainstream.

Recent investigation has focused on the investigation of "silent cerebral infarction" and its implications; The STEP registry evaluated 91 patients with diffusion-weighted magnetic resonance imaging (MRI) post-operatively; whilst there were no clinically apparent strokes in this cohort, 50% demonstrated new DW-MRI lesions. Whether this translates into cognitive decline or can be effectively reduced, remains to be clarified.[24]

OUTCOME OF TREATMENT

Results of open repair in centres of excellence have generally been good, with less consistent results reported by smaller institutions. Focus in the last decade has been on comparing the outcome of open and endovascular repair.

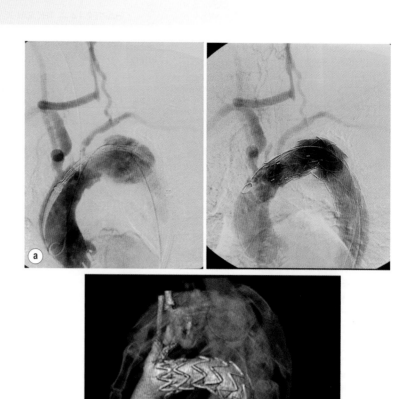

Figure 14.5 Angiogram demonstrating a large thoracic aneurysm with the landing zone involving the left common carotid artery. To enable endovascular aneurysm repair, a right-to-left common carotid bypass has been performed with ligation of the proximal left carotid artery.

The GORE TAG trial recruited 140 patients to undergo implantation of the GORE TAG (W.L. Gore & Associates, Flagstaff, Ariz, USA) device, retrospectively comparing outcomes with 94 patients undergoing repair of aneurysms in the descending or distal arch of the thoracic aorta. The 30-day mortality rate was 2.1% in the TEVAR group versus 11.7% in the open repair group.[25] The VALOR trial recruited 195 patients who had the Talent thoracic endograft (Medtronic, Santa-Rosa, CA, USA) implanted. An observed survival rate (OSR) control arm of 189 patients were matched retrospectively as a control group.[26] As with the TAG device, a lower 30-day mortality was noted in the TEVAR groups when compared to the OSR group (2% vs. 8%), and there were approximately half the number of major adverse events. The Cook TX2 pivotal trial recruited 160 patients to undergo treatment with the Cook TX2 thoracic endograft (Cook, Bloomington, USA), with 70 historical open surgical controls.[27] The rate of peri-operative adverse events was low in both groups, but there was a significantly lower rate of severe morbidity in the TEVAR group. The MOTHER registry included 670 patients who underwent TEVAR for aneurysmal disease from five Medtronic device specific trials reported an early death rate of 5%.[2]

Despite the protection that repair confers against aortic rupture, patients treated with TEVAR experience a high level of all-cause mortality that is often not related to the primary treated condition. This can be seen in comparisons with matched control groups of the same age and gender who do not have aneurysmal disease.[28] The MOTHER registry reported a 5-year survival rate of 56%, with most patients dying of cardiovascular causes or malignancy.[2] The Medicare and Health Episode Statistics studies study showed a similarly poor rate of survival, with many patients dying of cardiovascular or respiratory disease.[3,29] Appropriate patient selection is vital in maximising mortality benefits from TEVAR.[30] There are no randomised trials that compare TEVAR and endovascular arch procedures to open repair, but recent meta-analysis has demonstrated reduced 30-day all-cause mortality for endovascular repair, whilst open repair showed favourable longer-term survival.[31] In keeping with reports documenting outcomes in the visceral segment, the authors acknowledge that heterogeneous and inconsistent reporting, and differences in case selection, made meaningful data synthesis challenging.

Open surgical repair has remained the mainstay of management of more proximal lesions involving the aortic arch, given the need to preserve flow to the supra-aortic trunks, and requires cardiopulmonary bypass and deep hypothermic circulatory arrest. Even in centres of excellence, mortality rates approach 5%.[32–35] The last decade, however, has seen the development of arch branch and fenestrated stent-graft designs, opening the possibility of total endovascular repair of the aortic arch. In keeping with treatment for visceral segment disease, arch devices are customised according to patient anatomy, and can incorporate scallops as needed. Proximal deployment (zones 0 and 1), variable supra-aortic trunk and access vessel anatomy, arch tortuosity and the presence dissection flaps, and atherosclerotic disease can make accurate deployment challenging. Arch manipulation and cannulation of supra-aortic predisposes to risk of stroke. The available literature reflects this and is restricted to small case-series showing a 30-day mortality of up to 10%[36] with a contemporary meta-analysis yielding a stroke rate of 14%.[37] Some studies of multibranched devices have reported a stroke rate of up to 40%,[38] possibly as a result of wire manipulation in multiple supra-aortic trunks. Most of the studies report on a heterogeneous group of patients consisting of degenerative aneurysms, post-dissection aneurysms and connective tissue disorders, and this may, in part, account for the variability in outcomes.

Consistent findings are that the stroke rate generally exceeds mortality rate, and that retrograde type A dissections occur more frequently after arch repair in the post-dissection setting. Cook (Bloomington, USA) have more recently developed an inner branch device, which conceptually ought to reduce wire manipulation and shearing at the ostia of target vessels, with early reports showing promising lower stroke rates.[39,40] Whilst the mortality and stroke rates for endovascular arch treatments appear at face value to be comparable to open repair, it should be pointed out that most groups reporting this technique selected patients whose age and co-morbidities would have been prohibitive for open repair; a case-matched comparison is therefore not feasible. Going forward, total endovascular aortic repair comprised of staged fenestrated/branched arch and fenestrated/branched visceral segment intervention has been

shown to be achievable, with acceptable mortality and adverse neurological event rates.[41]

RECOMMENDATIONS FOR PRACTICE

Endovascular repair of TAAs is now first-line therapy for most thoracic aneurysms. The exceptions to this would be in patients with unfavourable anatomy in whom there is a likelihood of poor long-term durability, and elderly frail patients with a poor predicted life expectancy in whom the prevention of aneurysm-related death would not improve their overall survival.[19,30] The endovascular management of patients with connective tissue disease is controversial, but increasingly used. These patients are usually younger and fitter than patients with degenerative aneurysms and often have good outcomes from conventional surgery and poorer results from TEVAR.[42]

THORACO-ABDOMINAL AORTIC ANEURYSMS

CLASSIFICATION AND AETIOLOGY

Thoracic aneurysms that involve the visceral segment of the abdominal aorta are traditionally described as thoraco-abdominal aneurysms and are classified according to the extent of the aneurysmal disease (see Fig. 14.6 for a description of the Crawford classification). The aetiology of thoraco-abdominal aneurysms differs from infra-renal aneurysms, with medial degenerative disease and chronic dissection being particularly prevalent.[43] As with TAA, connective tissue disorders are a strong risk factor for the development of TAAAs.

INCIDENCE, CLINICAL PRESENTATION AND INDICATIONS FOR TREATMENT

The incidence of TAAA is poorly studied but is thought to be 5–10 per 100 000 per year. Relatively more patients with TAAAs are symptomatic than patients with other aortic aneurysms. The presence of back pain is particularly common,

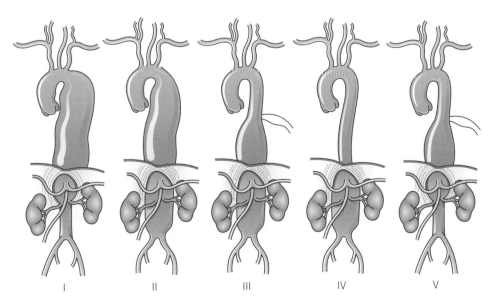

I   II   III   IV   V

Figure 14.6 Crawford classification of thoraco-abdominal aneurysms.

and this symptom may precede aortic rupture or intramural dissection. Recent European data suggests that the incidence of TAAA has increased over the last decade, with an ageing population and wider implementation of cross-sectional imaging suggested as the cause.[44] The rationale for treatment of TAAAs largely derives from a natural history study from Crawford and DeNatale, who reported a series of 94 patients unsuitable for surgery.[45] After 24 months' follow-up, only 24% of these patients were alive, which contrasted with the 59% 5-year survival of a concurrent cohort of patients who underwent operative repair. On the basis of these results, it was concluded that patients with significant thoraco-abdominal aneurysms should have an operative repair unless precluded by co-existent medical conditions. The advent of fenestrated and branched stent-graft systems has meant that many patients can now be treated by endovascular means. Despite being minimally invasive, this is a technically demanding procedure, and there is a relatively higher risk of morbidity and mortality in comparison with 'standard' infra-renal EVAR.

TECHNIQUE OF SURGICAL REPAIR

Before surgery can be considered, detailed imaging of the aorta must be obtained and examined using multiplanar reconstruction software. The physiological reserve of the patient should be comprehensively assessed and should include cardiac stress testing. Patients with significant coronary disease should be revascularised before TAAA repair, and severe aortic or mitral valvular disease should be corrected. Formal assessment of lung function should be undertaken. Pre-emptive CSF drainage is to be considered, especially for more extensive type I, II and III open repair, however, this will depend on unit policy and surgeon/anaesthetic preference.

The patient is placed in the right lateral decubitus position, with the left arm supported on a crossbar. A left thoracotomy is performed for extent of I–III aneurysms, with varying levels of incision chosen depending on the extent of aneurysm (sixth intercostal for type I and II, sixth or seventh for type III, eighth or ninth for type IV). Depending on the obliquity of the distal-most ribs and access for supra-coeliac clamping, it is possible to repair some type IV aneurysms via a totally abdominal approach, via a roof-top incision. The abdominal aorta is usually exposed by left medial visceral rotation and the diaphragm is partially divided with a circumferential incision preferred to preserve nerve supply. It is crucial to identify the left renal artery and ureter. For more proximal dissection within the thorax, the left phrenic, vagus and recurrent laryngeal nerves should be identified. Where necessary, the left crus can be divided to facilitate supra-coeliac clamping, avoiding the phrenic arteries.

After the dissection has been completed, the aneurysm is clamped at its proximal and distal extents, and an aortotomy made in the lateral aneurysm wall. It is important that the aortotomy is sited away from the visceral origins in the abdominal portion of the aneurysm. The proximal anastomosis is performed with a completely transected aorta to prevent aorto-oesophageal fistula. The proximal anastomosis is fashioned to include adjacent intercostal or visceral arteries, whilst any remaining intercostal arteries can be directly re-implanted into the graft as a patch or revascularised

by separate jump grafts. Preserving flow to the visceral and renal arteries can be achieved via two techniques; inclusion grafting, whereby a patch of native aorta containing these vessels is anastomosed onto the graft, or multi-branch grafting whereby each individual artery is supplied by an individual graft taken from the main aortic graft. The choice of technique depends on proximity of the visceral vessels to each other on the native aorta, and pathology being treated (e.g., connective tissue disorder), where subsequent patch aneurysmal degeneration has been reported to be 18%.[46] If possible, the coeliac, superior mesenteric and right renal arteries are taken on one patch. Anastomosing the distal graft to the aortic bifurcation or iliac arteries completes the reconstruction (Fig. 14.7).

During thoraco-abdominal aneurysm repair, prolonged visceral ischaemia is the main cause of post-operative renal dysfunction and can also contribute to multiple organ failure. For type I and II TAAA repair, partial left heart bypass with a centrifugal pump may be used to drain blood from the left atrium or upper pulmonary vein and return it via the femoral artery or aorta. This facilitates renal and visceral perfusion whilst the proximal anastomosis is fashioned as long as the distal aortic clamp remains proximal to the visceral vessels. Once this anastomosis is complete, the iliac clamps are applied, and the aorta is opened down its length, and, the coeliac trunk, superior mesenteric artery and both renal arteries can be selectively perfused with catheters that are connected to the left heart bypass.

Paraplegia may complicate thoraco-abdominal aneurysm repair in up to 20% of cases and is increased in more proximal aneurysms, with lengthy clamp time, renal impairment, advanced age and emergency presentations. Paraplegia results from damage to the spinal cord because of a combination of division of spinal cord arteries, prolonged spinal cord ischaemia during aortic clamping, reperfusion injury and post-operative hypotension. Maintenance of spinal cord blood supply may be achieved by re-implantation of patent intercostal arteries and by distal aortic perfusion. Moving the proximal clamp sequentially down the graft to incorporate the intercostal patch is valuable technique in this regard. CSF pressure increases during aortic clamping, and CSF drainage has been advocated to reduce paraplegia.[47] A functional approach to the problem of neurological deficit aims at intra-operative monitoring of the spinal cord function. Somatosensory-evoked potentials are widely used to detect spinal cord ischaemia during aortic cross-clamping and to identify vessels critical to spinal cord blood supply, which may then be perfused and re-implanted. An alternative

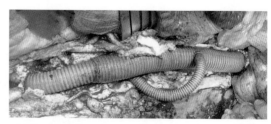

Figure 14.7 Operative picture of completed reconstruction of a thoraco-abdominal aortic aneurysm (TAAA). The visceral patch has been reinforced with Teflon pledgets. A separate graft has been anastomosed to a large intercostal.

approach is to use motor-evoked potentials, which have been reported to improve paraplegia rates.[48]

RESULTS OF SURGICAL REPAIR OF THORACO-ABDOMINAL ANEURYSMS

The mortality and morbidity rates following conventional repair of TAAAs are still significant, with specialised centres reporting mortality rates of 5–16%, with paraplegia rates of 4–11%.[49–53] Open repair in the United Kingdom is restricted to very few centres, with most recently published data reporting overall mortality rates of 6–11%.[54,55] The data in these reports are heterogeneous and include varying numbers of elective and urgent cases, connective tissue disorder patients, and varying aneurysm extent. Consistent findings are that age of patient and extent (type II TAAA) are predictors of mortality, and that results have generally improved over time. The latter is mostly likely a product of increasing centralisation, improved patient selection, and enhanced end-organ protection techniques (left heart bypass, hypothermia, CSF-drainage and spinal monitoring). However, these excellent results are not representative of outcomes outside of these centres, with national/community mortality rates exceeding 20% at 30 days and 30% at 1 year.[56]

ENDOVASCULAR REPAIR OF THORACO-ABDOMINAL AORTIC ANEURYSMS

Advances in stent-graft technology (Fig. 14.8) have allowed the manufacture of stent-grafts with fenestration (FEVAR) or branches (BEVAR) to treat thoraco-abdominal aneurysm. These seal above and below the diseased segment of aorta in a similar fashion to standard endografts but allow visceral branch perfusion via the placement of bridging stents between the main body of the stent-graft into the ostia of visceral vessels. Fenestrated stent-grafts are customised for each individual patient and require a period of weeks to months from ordering to being ready to use. Stent-graft systems with preformed branches can be used 'off the shelf' provided the necessary ancillary components are available. Anatomical suitability is important, and access problems, aortic tortuosity and target vessel morphology are some of the main reasons that patients are not suitable for this kind of repair. Initially, the application of this technology was limited, and the number of patients receiving this kind of repair was low and confined to a small number of super-specialised units. The results of these procedures have improved as technology and peri-operative care have developed, and now many centres are beginning to offer this as first-line therapy.

Both FEVAR and BEVAR require the partial deployment of an endograft in the visceral aorta through which the fenestrations or branches are cannulated. This is performed via access from the groin or the upper limb, and once secure access is obtained, the device can be fully deployed and the visceral stents can be advanced into position. When these are in position, the graft can be completed with a bifurcated section if necessary and a final angiographic run obtained to check that the aneurysm has been sealed and the visceral vessels are patent. A variety of devices are now commercially available in Europe and consistent design features include a main fenestrated or branched section to accommodate the visceral segment, and a bifurcated piece. These procedures can be combined with more proximal TEVAR to facilitate repair of more extensive aneurysms. In general, the use of branched or fenestrated technology is determined by the diameter of the aorta at the visceral segment, with increasing diameters at this level (e.g., type IV morphology), favouring the use branched devices.

RESULTS OF ENDOVASCULAR REPAIR OF THORACO-ABDOMINAL AORTIC ANEURYSM

Excellent early results have been reported in selected groups of patients treated at centres of excellence, although it is unclear to what extent these results are generalisable.[57] The largest modern institutional series reported the results of 354 procedures on type II and III TAAA, with a peri-operative mortality of 3.5–7%.[58] As with open repair, paraplegia remains a serious problem and complicated up to 4% of procedures. Long-term durability appeared to be good, with target vessel patency of 96% at mid-term follow-up, although re-interventions were reported in 19% for a variety of reasons. As previously discussed, staging of TAAA repair with endovascular techniques has considerably reduced the spinal ischaemia rate and the rate of permanent neurological deficit with improved recovery rates.

Longer-term all-cause mortality remains a concern, with this series reporting 57% freedom from mortality. The same group reported on long-term results in 610 patients in type IV and juxta-renal aneurysms, with an 8-year survival of 20%, and an aneurysm-related mortality of 2%.[59] Consistent with open TAAA repair, major adverse events and longer-term term survival are adversely impacted by the extent of disease and repair required.[60]

The UK GLOBALSTAR registry reported on 318 patients across 14 centres, showing a peri-operative mortality of 4.1%, consistent with the large single-centre experience documented earlier.[61] Many of these were short-neck infrarenal aneurysms rather than true TAAA, with expected good outcomes. There are no clinical trials that compare open surgery versus endovascular repair of TAAA, and it is widely acknowledged that patients selected for endovascular repair across multiple cohort studies are generally older, physiologically frailer and would not have tolerated open repair. Equipoise, in terms of co-morbidities, does therefore not exist, precluding a fair "like-for-like" comparison. Similarly, surgical techniques and outcome reporting, both in the endovascular and open surgical cohorts are heterogeneous, making understanding the true outcomes in the literature challenging.

RECENT TECHNOLOGICAL ADVANCES

Recent endeavour has focused on making endovascular solutions more broadly applicable, with a particular focus on 'off-the-shelf' devices for use in emergencies, and lower profile designs for use in post-dissection settings. Existing devices have been augmented by incorporating preloaded catheters and wires although adoption has been limited.

The success of complex endovascular repair relies on meticulous planning, and for customised devices entails a delay for device manufacture. Whilst rupture of elective cases

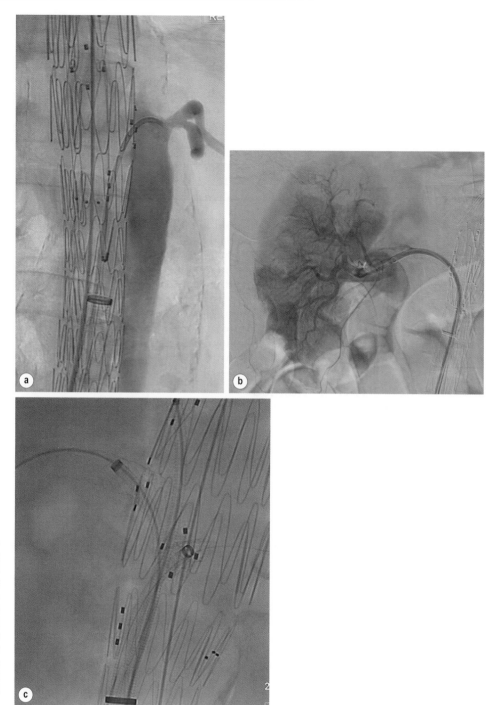

Figure 14.8 Intra-operative images of a fenestrated endograft being placed for a type IV thoraco-abdominal aneurysm: (a) shows a catheter being placed through the left renal fenestration and some contrast being injected before cannulation of the vessel; (b) shows a sheath advanced into the right renal artery with an angiogram to confirm correct positioning before the deployment of bridging stents; (c) shows stents deployed in both renal arteries.

during this waiting period is rare,[62] an immediate solution is required for symptomatic and ruptured cases. Surgeon-modified stent-grafts have been used in this setting, with acceptable early mortality of 0–16%.[63,64] Their use however, is characterised by the increased need for re-intervention, and the need for advanced endovascular planning and procedural skills.

A number of off the shelf thoraco-abdominal devices are now available from several manufacturers. The Cook T-branch (Bloomington USA), incorporates four pre-fashioned downward pointing branches. Each branch was positioned to accommodate 90% of patient anatomy for that given target vessel, with early estimates showing

that 88% of patients would be eligible for this device,[65] although this is lower when access vessel anatomy is accounted for.

Two meta-analyses that include a high proportion of emergent cases, show promising results: Silingardi et al. report on 73 patients across 13 centres, of which 44% were emergencies, and document a 30-day mortality of 4%, spinal cord ischaemia of 3% and a 7% re-intervention rate.[66] A more recent study documents outcomes in 197 patients, of which 64% were emergencies, with a 30-day mortality of 5.8%, major stroke rate of 4%, permanent paraplegia rate of 1.3% and a re-intervention rate of 5.7%.[67] Although the data are promising, longer-term data are required.

The use of the T-branch and custom-multibranch devices is limited in certain circumstances by a narrow visceral aortic lumen (<25 mm) such as in the management of some chronic aortic dissections. To circumvent this problem, an 'inner-branch' design is available for selected cases in which directional branches are manufactured to lie within the main body of the device.[68] Advantages of this configuration are generally those of branch design except that the device can be use in narrower aortas. The device can readily be accommodated in the narrower true lumen in post-dissection cases, and shearing of semi-stiff wires against fragile target vessel ostia is potentially reduced. In addition, target vessel angulation requirements are less stringent for inner branch grafts than for standard multi-branch devices. The mid-term and long-term results of this design are not known beyond early reports.

Jotec (Hechingen, Germany) and Gore (Flagstaff, AZ, USA) have also launched thoraco-abdominal grafts. Early feasibility studies demonstrate that the Jotec E-nside could be used in 43% of patients,[69] and the Gore TAMBE in 49% of patients with type IV and juxta-renal morphology, and 23% with more extensive pathology (types I, II, and III)[70] factoring in access and target vessels and aortic diameters. A single report documents the use of the TAMBE in 11 patients, with no early deaths, spinal cord injuries or need for dialysis.[71]

CHRONIC AORTIC DISSECTION

The optimal strategy for management of post-dissection aneurysmal degeneration remains a debated topic. Increasing detection and successful open treatment of type A dissection (TAAD) is resulting in higher numbers of patients presenting to vascular surgeons requiring complex repair of the residual dissected descending thoracic and visceral aorta.

Rylski et al. demonstrated that at 31 months, 76% of patients experience moderate or accelerated aortic growth after TAAD,[72] whilst data from the Internal Registry of Acute Aortic Dissection (IRAD) suggest that 73% of patients develop aneurysmal dilatation after medically managed type B dissection (TBAD).[73] Traditionally managed by open surgery, endovascular approaches are now being adopted. These procedures are technically demanding, given the frequently narrow true lumen, separate true and false lumen target vessel origins, and extension of dissection flaps into target vessels.

Despite this, early adopters of endovascular treatment in this setting report technical success of 86–100%, 30 day mortality of 0–9.6%, and permanent spinal cord injury of 0–5%. Re-intervention rates were high at 14–50%.[74–78] In these early reports, centres used a combination of fenestrated and branched devices and included a proportion of connective tissue disorder patients. Considering pooled mortality for open repair in this setting approaches 11%,[79] these results compare favourably, however, close surveillance is warranted given the high re-intervention rate.

CONNECTIVE TISSUE DISORDERS

Presentation of aortic emergencies, especially dissections, at younger ages (<50 years) should prompt consideration of the congenital collagenopathies. These patients are prone to extensive systemic cardiovascular anomalies and need to be managed carefully at centres capable of providing complex open and endovascular solutions in addition to cardiothoracic expertise, as required.

Acute type B aortic dissection in this context can be categorised as being associated with syndromic familial conditions, comprising predominantly of Marfan syndrome (MFS), Vascular Ehler-Danlos syndrome (vEDS) and Loeys-Dietz syndrome (LDS), or familial but non-syndromic (FT-BAD). In addition, a proportion of all-comers in this category (<50 years) will be sporadic. Data from the National Registry of Genetically Triggered Thoracic Aortic Aneurysms and Cardiovascular Conditions Consortium (GenTAC) found that acute type B aortic dissections in this cohort were MFS (in 45%), FTBAD (26%), LDS (3.8%), vEDS (1.3%) and sporadic in 22%.[80] Current European Society for Vascular Surgery guidelines advocate against the use of TEVAR as first-line therapy in this setting.[81] Traditionally, the domain of open surgery, procedures on the vasculature of these patients are characterised by increased blood vessel fragility, spontaneous rupture and thrombocyte dysfunction.[82,83] MFS patients are also at an increased risk of sudden cardiac death triggered by left ventricular arrhythmias and dysfunction.[84]

Concerns surrounding the fragility of tissues and the effects of radial forces at stent landing zones and subsequent aneurysmal degeneration have long deterred surgeons from using endovascular techniques in this setting. Many of the early endovascular device trials uniformly excluded these patients. Data for endovascular intervention are limited to a few selected centres, and in many instances are reported as a subset in a wider report on dissection patients. Technical success has been reported as 38–100%, with a peri-operative mortality of 0–14% and a paraplegia rate of 0–3.3%. Subsequent open conversion has been reported as ranging from 5–50% and endovascular re-intervention on the same segment as 5.8–38%.[85–87] By contrast, open surgical repair has shown a peri-operative mortality 0–14%, a paraplegia rate of 0–9%, and a re-intervention rate of 4–11%.[85,88,89] Given the high re-intervention rate and preliminary nature of these data, the role of endovascular repair in connective tissue disorders remains to be clearly defined. Survival of connective tissue disorder patients is gradually improving, as are outcomes for emergent type A repair in this setting; complex endovascular repair may have a place in revisional surgery in the latter stages of a patient's life where re-intervention rates may assume lesser importance.

HYBRID VISCERAL REVASCULARISATION AND ENDOVASCULAR REPAIR OF THORACO-ABDOMINAL AORTIC ANEURYSMS

A combination of open surgical and endovascular strategies has been suggested to reduce surgical insult by removing the need for thoracotomy and aortic cross-clamping, whilst reducing the duration of visceral and renal ischaemia. There are fewer technical considerations than for complex endovascular solutions as all that is required is sufficient length of proximal and distal landing zones in non-diseased or replaced aorta. In addition, visceral vessels must be able to be accessed for bypass from a healthy donor site, such as the iliacs. Most often, a transperitoneal retrograde visceral revascularisation is used to allow an adequate distal landing zone for placement of an endovascular stent-graft that extends from the thoracic to the distal abdominal aorta or iliac vessels. This approach may be combined with supra-aortic debranching to create a very proximal landing zone (Fig. 14.9). A collaborative paper reporting outcomes of 107 consecutive cases across three units described a 15% mortality and 8.4% permanent paraplegia rate in all-comers.[90] Superficially, these results do not appear to show a significant advantage over conventional surgery, but these patients tended to be older, have more comorbidity, and a higher proportion of type II and III aneurysms than comparable open series. As endovascular techniques have evolved, the role for hybrid aortic repair has diminished considerably and it is now an uncommon undertaking.

RECOMMENDATIONS FOR PRACTICE

Endovascular techniques have evolved significantly in recent years, and many centres would preferentially offer minimally invasive surgery as first-line therapy for patients with thoraco-abdominal aneurysms. Open surgery should be considered in younger patients with connective tissue disorders because of uncertain longer-term outcomes in these cases. Improvements in the delivery of FEVAR and BEVAR have rendered hybrid techniques less attractive in recent years.

THORACIC DISSECTION AND ACUTE AORTIC SYNDROME

PATHOLOGY, CLASSIFICATION AND CLINICAL PRESENTATIONS

The acute aortic syndromes are a group of conditions affecting the thoracic aorta that cause patients to present to hospital with chest pain and encompasses three main pathological entities: aortic dissection (Fig. 14.10a and b), intramural haematoma (IMH; Fig. 14.11) and penetrating aortic ulcers (PAUs; Fig. 14.12).[91] All three conditions may co-exist, and both IMH and penetrating ulcer may instigate a classical aortic dissection.

Aortic dissection is defined as a tear in the intima of the aorta that allows blood to form a pathological plane of cleavage between itself and the adventitia by disrupting the media. These two new channels are referred to as the *true* and *false lumens*. Typically, the pressure within the false lumen is higher than the true lumen, as the outflow is usually a small re-entry tear. This leads to compression of the true lumen, which can result in malperfusion of the viscera or

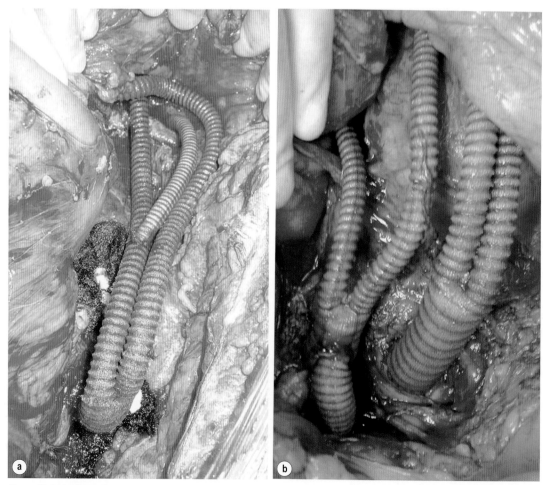

Figure 14.9 Operative pictures of two patients undergoing retrograde visceral revascularisation. Many different graft configurations are possible, with varying numbers of vessels requiring revascularisation.

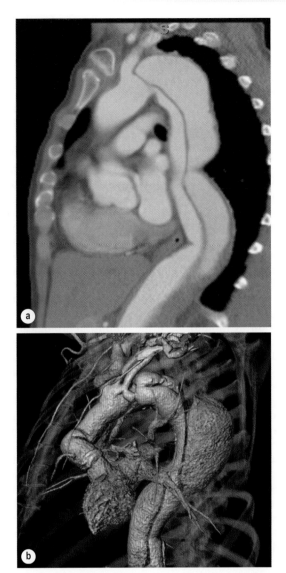

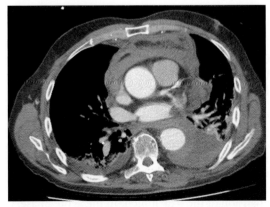

Figure 14.10   (a) Sagittal reconstruction showing the classic appearance of a type B aortic dissection. (b) A three-dimensional reconstruction of the same pathology.

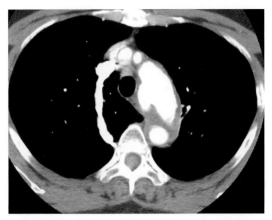

Figure 14.12   Axial computed tomography (CT) appearance of penetrating aortic ulcer.

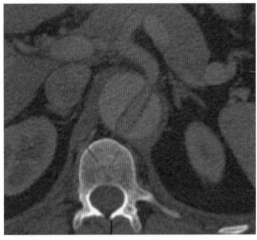

Figure 14.13   Patient with a type B thoracic aortic dissection showing compression of the true lumen causing malperfusion of the coeliac artery and therefore visceral ischaemia.

Figure 14.11   Axial computed tomography (CT) appearance of intramural haematoma. There is a relatively high-density crescentic rim of fresh blood in the wall of the aorta.

limbs, or rupture of the false lumen. Such branch vessel malperfusion may be described as 'dynamic', because of a mobile dissection flap intermittently 'shuttering' the ostia of vessels during systole, or static because of a relatively fixed flap (Fig. 14.13).

IMH is defined as clotted blood in the intramural space without an obvious intimal tear. This is thought to result from rupture of medial vasa vasora, and is often regarded as a precursor to dissection. IMH accounts for up to 5–15% of acute aortic syndromes and has a prognosis similar to classical aortic dissection.[92] PAU results from focal ulceration of an atherosclerotic plaque into the media and may be associated with haematoma within the aortic wall. Penetrating ulcers have a poorer prognosis than classical dissection, with higher rates of aortic rupture, but make up only 5% of acute aortic syndrome presentations. PAU is considered to be a disease of the intima, in comparison with dissection and IMH, which are considered to be diseases of the media.

Aortic dissections are classified by site, chronicity and presentation. The most crucial classification involves the site of dissection. Under the commonly used Stanford classification, type A dissection involves the ascending aorta whereas type B dissection originates distal to the LSCA. The DeBakey system is also used to classify site. DeBakey I dissections extend from the ascending aorta into the descending, DeBakey II involve only the ascending aorta and DeBakey

III originate from beyond the LSCA (IIIa do not extend below the diaphragm whereas IIIb do). Dissections are termed *acute* when they are less than 2 weeks after the onset of symptoms, and are *chronic* after this period. Many now recognise a third, subacute phase between 2 and 12 weeks.[93]

In addition, dissections may be complicated or uncomplicated. Complicated aortic dissections exhibit clinical or imaging findings such as impending or frank rupture, malperfusion, persistent pain and refractory hypertension.

A recent expert consensus suggested a more comprehensive way of classifying dissection using the mnemonic 'DISSECT', which stands for Duration of disease, Size of the aorta, Segmental Extent, Clinical complications and Thrombus within the lumen.[94]

Acute aortic syndromes often present with the sudden onset of sharp tearing or stabbing chest pain, which radiates to the neck and back. Pain is absent in 10% of patients, and asymptomatic presentation is more common in diabetics.[95] Acute rupture or malperfusion may lead to collapse and death, neurological deficits, symptomatic limb ischaemia, or visceral ischaemia. Hypotension is seen in patients with rupture or critical malperfusion, but hypertension is often present. Chronic dissection is often asymptomatic but can cause back pain or chronic visceral ischaemia.

INVESTIGATION OF SUSPECTED ACUTE AORTIC SYNDROME

Axial imaging to visualise the whole aorta must be undertaken if a diagnosis of acute aortic syndrome is suspected. Serum D-dimer levels can be raised, and concentrations above 500 ng/mL are often present in patients with acute dissection, although this has a relatively low specificity.[96] Multi-detector CTA is the preferred investigation and a meta-analysis of 1139 patients with aortic dissection found that CTA had a sensitivity of 100%, specificity of 98% and a diagnostic odds ratio of 6.5. The main disadvantage of CTA is the inability to assess functional aortic insufficiency in possible Type A aortic dissection.

Transoesophageal echocardiography (TOE) can visualise the entire thoracic aorta and despite the requirement for oesophageal intubation, can be performed at the bedside.[97] TOE can be an adjunct to endovascular repair because of the ability to see devices within the aortic lumen, and in graft sizing strategies.

MRA has a high sensitivity and specificity when used to diagnose aortic dissection. Gadolinium contrast agents are less nephrotoxic than iodinated substances used for CTA and there is no associated ionising radiation. Disadvantages include its limited use in patients with claustrophobia or metal devices, although it can be used in those with nitinol aortic stent grafts. Long acquisition times and limited availability reduce its usefulness in the emergency setting, for which CTA is ideal. The use of 'four-dimensional' cine MRI techniques may offer the potential for dynamic assessment of aortic dissection to determine the nature of blood flow within the true and false lumen. This information may be used to determine which patients are likely to benefit from earlier treatment because of an increased risk of subsequent aortic expansion but has not gained mainstream popularity.[7]

INITIAL MANAGEMENT OF ACUTE AORTIC DISSECTION

Management of aortic dissection involves rapid pharmacological control of blood pressure and left ventricular ejection velocity. The short-term goal of management is to resuscitate the patient and arrange definitive investigations to confirm the diagnosis. Persistent hypertension should be managed with intravenous beta-blockade using an agent such as labetalol to reduce aortic wall shear stress in the arch. A target heart rate of 60–80 beats/min. and systolic blood pressure of 100–120 mmHg should be the aim, taking into account the patient's normal blood pressure.

Glyceryl trinitrate should be avoided where possible as the reduction in diastolic blood pressure it causes may lead to a widened pulse pressure and a reflex tachycardia, which increases aortic wall shear stress. Invasive cardiovascular monitoring is required and transfer of the patient to a level II or III environment in a sufficiently experienced cardiovascular centre is mandatory. Whilst maintaining a low blood pressure is ideal, it is important to ensure adequate organ perfusion by monitoring urine output, neurological status checks and checking peripheral perfusion. Regular arterial blood–gas analysis and examination for trends in markers of tissue perfusion may provide clues that malperfusion is developing. Type A dissection has a 1% mortality per hour from aortic rupture, aortic regurgitation, pericardial tamponade or coronary ischaemia and is treated by emergency surgical graft repair of the ascending aorta, with or without aortic valve replacement.[98]

After the acute phase, the management of type B dissections is initially medical in those with acute uncomplicated presentations, with intervention reserved for those exhibiting signs of complications. Intravenous agents can be replaced by oral antihypertensives, and European, American and Japanese guidelines advocate beta-blockers with a target blood pressure of <130 mmHg, with the addition of vasodilators in refractory cases.[99] In connective tissue disorders, there is an increasing role for AII receptor blockers in addition to calcium-channel blockers, although the literature are mixed. For many years, this was thought to be adequate treatment in the longer term, but recent studies have shown failure rates exceeding 50% of medical treatment in the mid-term.[100,101]

ENDOVASCULAR MANAGEMENT OF COMPLICATED ACUTE TYPE B THORACIC DISSECTION

Endovascular therapy is now the first-line treatment for acute complicated type B thoracic dissections because of superior peri-operative results compared with open surgery.[2] The aim of treatment is to cover the primary entry tear with an endovascular stent-graft and to facilitate remodelling of the aorta through depressurising the false lumen and allowing expansion of the true lumen. In the acute phase, this reduces the probability of aortic rupture and alleviates dynamic branch vessel occlusion by allowing preferential perfusion of the true lumen (Fig. 14.14). The normal strategy on the basis of current evidence is to place endografts from the left common carotid artery to the coeliac axis to promote remodelling. In addition, other endovascular techniques

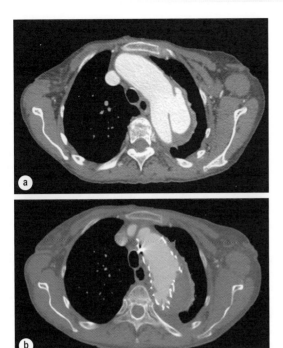

Figure 14.14 Patient with a subacute type B dissection who underwent treatment by endovascular stent-grafting. (a) Shows the pre-operative appearance and (b) shows complete remodelling of the false lumen following repair.

including visceral stenting or percutaneous fenestration may be required to treat malperfusion.

The early results of TEVAR of complicated type B dissections are significantly better than for open repair, with combined registry data suggesting a mortality rate of 13%, a stroke rate of 6% and a paraplegia rate of 2%.[2,102]

One critical technical aspect is to minimise graft oversizing, contrary to the strategy used for degenerative aneurysms. Graft oversizing is limited to 10% and balloon dilatation should be avoided. Some recommend avoiding stents with proximal bare stents, although the evidence for this highly conflicting and the characteristics of an ideal 'dissection stent' remain contested. These measures are designed to reduce the risk of retrograde dissection, and careful deployment of the proximal stent-graft with minimal manipulation in the dissected aortic arch is necessary.[103]

EARLY MANAGEMENT OF UNCOMPLICATED TYPE B DISSECTION

Given the high rate of failure of medical management observed at mid-term follow-up, patients with uncomplicated acute type B dissections are increasingly felt to benefit from early TEVAR to preventing acute and long-term complications. The rationale is that promoting aortic remodelling prevents the progressive degenerative changes that lead to late aortic events.

INSTEAD-XL was a long-term extension of a randomised trial that included 140 patients with a diagnosis of uncomplicated type B dissection a median of 3.5 weeks after diagnosis to be treated either by TEVAR and best medical therapy (72 patients) or by best medical therapy alone (68 patients).[100] In the intervention group, the peri-procedural mortality and morbidity was low, with two deaths, two serious intra-procedural technical complications and three serious neurological complications. A total of 14 patients crossed over from best medical therapy to intervention, with five of these performed as an emergency and four requiring open repair. Although the risk of mid-term all-cause death was similar in both groups (11.1% vs. 19.3%), aortic specific mortality was lower (6.9% vs. 19.3%) and disease progression was less frequent in the early TEVAR group (27% vs. 46.1%). These results in conjunction with other registry data have led to changes in treatment algorithms with uncomplicated type B dissection undergoing early TEVAR. The rationale for this is that the aorta has stabilised enough to reduce the risks associated with treating acute dissection, such as retrograde type A dissection, but still retains enough plasticity to allow remodelling of the aorta to take place. This remains a point of controversy and there is no conclusive evidence to support this viewpoint although many experts advocate this approach. Furthermore, newer data suggest that TEVAR can be safely undertaken hyper-acutely, in the first days after dissection with the maximum amount of remodelling being achieved. Future publications are required to confirm this.

Careful morphological studies and long-term follow-up will be required to define which subgroup of patients are at risk from late events and therefore may benefit from early TEVAR for uncomplicated disease. Many risk factors such as false lumen diameter of over 22 mm, entry tear located on the lesser curve of the aortic arch and partially thrombosed false lumen have been suggested.[104]

TREATMENT OF CHRONIC TYPE B DISSECTIONS

Uncomplicated chronic type B dissection is preferably managed conservatively, with regular surveillance scanning performed on an annual basis. Most published guidelines recommend the use of beta-blockers for blood pressure control, and findings from the IRAD support this by demonstrating a reduction in mortality. Calcium-channel blockers were shown to reduce mortality specifically in patients with type B dissection,[99] although there is no consensus algorithm for management of hypertension in patients with dissection. Despite medical management, many patients develop aortic dilatation that may eventually require intervention. Generally, patients are considered for surgery when the aorta measures over 5.5–6 cm, or when the false lumen diameter exceeds 4 cm.

Open surgical repair has the perceived benefit of completely replacing the diseased segment of aorta, therefore reducing the need for re-intervention in the future, but even modern series from specialised centres report high levels of debilitating peri-operative adverse events.[105] Endovascular treatment can be performed with a relatively low morbidity and mortality in comparison with open surgical repair, and protects against aortic-related death in the mid-term,[106] as discussed previously. The strategies are complex, but increasingly, total endovascular solutions are being used in a staged fashion to limit morbidity and mortality.

MANAGEMENT OF INTRAMURAL HAEMATOMA AND PENETRATING AORTIC ULCER

Management of these conditions closely resembles that of dissection in both the acute and chronic phase. There is a relative paucity of data to direct therapy in comparison with aortic dissection, and the most recent consensus guidelines for management incorporated mostly institutional series combined with expert panel opinion.[92] Medical management of both conditions appears safe in the early phase. However, in the setting of haemodynamic instability, persistent pain/hypertension, rapid aneurysmal expansion, signs of impending rupture or progressive peri-aortic haemorrhage, early endovascular intervention appears safe and effective.

Patients must then undergo surveillance to look for longer-term aortic changes that would indicate the need for repair. In both conditions, endovascular treatment is preferable to open surgery given the superior peri-operative and 3-year mortality reported in existing series.

RECOMMENDATIONS FOR PRACTICE

TEVAR is now considered to be the gold standard for complicated acute type B thoracic dissections and other acute aortic syndromes. Increasingly, patients with uncomplicated acute type B dissection appear to benefit from early TEVAR although there remain uncertainties in terms of ideal case selection and procedural timing. The indications for treatment and best interventional approach to chronic dissection, IMH and PAU require further study and refinement.

TRAUMATIC AORTIC INJURY

After head injury, traumatic aortic injury (TAI) is the second commonest cause of death in patients following blunt injury: 15–30% of deaths from blunt trauma have aortic transection at post-mortem. The mechanism of injury is usually caused by deceleration, creating shear forces at the aortic isthmus, where the relatively mobile arch joins the fixed descending aorta (Fig. 14.15). There is a spectrum of degree of injury to the aorta ranging from intimal haemorrhage through to complete transection (grade I: intimal tear; grade II: IMH; grade III: pseudo-aneurysm; grade IV: rupture). The surgical approach to treatment has changed considerably in the last decade. Previously, it was thought that emergency repair was mandatory because of the belief that there was a high risk of early rupture (79% within 24 hours) in immediate survivors, although procedural mortality rates of this approach were in excess of 30%. Pharmacological lowering of blood pressure and reduction in systolic ejection dynamics facilitate stabilisation of patients and the opportunity for delayed repair. Therefore surgery may be delayed until the immediate threat to life from other injuries is controlled.[107]

In many cases of low-grade injury, conservative management is now considered to be safe, and in those where intervention is necessary, TEVAR is now the mainstay of treatment for TAI.[107,108] It can be performed rapidly via percutaneous access under local anaesthetic and as a result causes very little in terms of additional morbidity to patients who often have multisystem injuries. Because of the focal

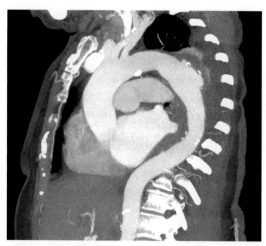

Figure 14.15 Blunt aortic injury shown in a patient with an unfolded arch in the classical location. In this case, there is a grade III injury with pseudo-aneurysm formation.

nature of the injury, only a short length of aorta requires covering with an endograft.

The peri-operative results reported in the literature are extremely good, and institutional case series have suggested that longer-term durability is satisfactory.[109] Peri-operative mortality across the available literature is reported to be 8% versus 19% for open repair, with lower rates of spinal cord injury.[61] The main disadvantage to TEVAR for TAI is that most devices are designed to treat dilated aortas with degenerative aneurysms or dissection. TAI occurs in a relatively young population with smaller aortas, more angulated aortic arches and smaller access vessels. Device conformability has improved over time, which has allowed greater confidence when placing them in cases of TAI, and has reduced the risk of so-called '*birdbeaking*' (where the aortic stent-graft does not conform to angulated aortic arch, seen especially in younger people, and the flow of the aorta conforms to the outer aspect of the stent-graft) resulting in endograft collapse and pseudo-coarctation.[110] In addition, there is a lack of availability of small-calibre endografts. This may cause problems in young patients.

RECOMMENDATIONS FOR PRACTICE

TEVAR is the gold standard for treatment of TAI requiring intervention irrespective of the age of the patient. In selected cases, serial imaging and conservative management is acceptable, but for more severe injury, it should be performed within 24 hours.

AORTO-OESOPHAGEAL AND AORTOPULMONARY FISTULA

Aorto-oesophageal fistula is a rare and highly lethal condition. Open surgical treatment is complicated by difficult access to the aorta, which is often surrounded by adhesions in the mediastinum, and the need for high thoracic aortic cross-clamping. TEVAR is therefore an attractive option, but concern exists regarding the risk of endograft infection. Most patients present with haematemesis and many have signs of hypovolaemic shock and sepsis. Causes of this condition include prior aortic surgery, malignant and benign disease of the oesophagus, primary pathology of the aorta and ingestion of foreign bodies. The peri-operative mortality rate for emergent open repair ranges from 45–55%, whereas a recent systematic review showed that for patients undergoing TEVAR this was 28%. Despite this, late infection rate was 15% in patients treated with TEVAR, and this led to death in a significant number of these patients.[111] In patients where a staged endovascular and open approach was taken, infection was less likely to be the cause of death and overall mortality at a mean of 6 months' follow-up was reduced. There is insufficient evidence to firmly recommend one treatment strategy for all, but it would appear that TEVAR is effective in preventing exsanguination but should probably be combined with open surgery after a suitable interval of targeted antibiotic therapy. Aortopulmonary fistula is rare and generally described after TEVAR, with cases caused by primary aortic pathology being very rarely described.[112] The mechanism of development is thought to be compression by the aneurysm sac and endoleak formation, and most patients develop clinical and radiological signs of pulmonary haemorrhage at presentation. Mortality was 61% over a 10-year period of study in a European-wide registry, although this was significantly better in patients fit for radical surgery (63% vs. 21% survival at 2 years).

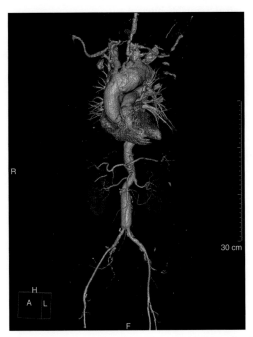

Figure 14.16   Proximal arch aneurysm (courtesy of Brendan Stanley, Fiona Stanley Hospital, Perth WA)

Case scenario

Two-vessel elective fenestrated arch branch graft for large asymptomatic arch aneurysm

A 54-year-old female was admitted for elective repair of a 6.3-cm aortic arch aneurysm (Fig. 14.16) in two stages. She was an ex-smoker, and co-morbidities included ischaemic heart disease, hypertension and asthma. Echocardiography revealed good left ventricular systolic function with no significant valvular disease. Pre-operative workup included carotid and vertebral duplex scanning, which showed no carotid disease, and MAG-3 scanning, which showed a broadly symmetrical split function (51% right, 49% left). She first underwent left carotid-subclavian bypass using a 6-mm PTFE graft and right iliofemoral bypass grafting with and 8-mm Dacron graft to form an iliac conduit for her subsequent definitive repair. The next day, 2-vessel fenestrated arch grafting performed using a custom-made Cook device (Bloomington, USA) under general anaesthesia. The right common carotid artery was exposed surgically and a bevelled 8-mm Dacron conduit was anastomosed in an end-to-side fashion. The left mid-brachial and right common-femoral arteries were exposed via open cut-down. The left common-femoral artery was punctured under ultrasound guidance. A temporary pacing wire was introduced via the right common-femoral vein and positioned in the right ventricle, and adequate capture was ensured. Five thousand units of unfractionated heparin were administered. A custom-made graft, main body measuring 46 mm proximally, 30 mm at the mid-graft, and 32 mm distally (Cook, Bloomington, USA) was positioned with visualisation in multiple planes, and after rapid overdrive pacing was deployed successfully. The left carotid fenestration was cannulated via the puncture of the carotid-subclavian bypass graft. The innominate artery fenestration was cannulated via the right carotid conduit. A 56-mm long TFLE (Cook reversed iliac leg stent) measuring 13 mm in diameter at the fenestration and flaring to 22 mm in the innominate artery was deployed. A 9x60-mm Fluency (Bard Peripheral Vascular, Tempe, AZ, USA) stent was deployed into the left carotid fenestration. The LSCA was occluded proximal to the left vertebral artery with a 16-mm Amplatzer plug (Abbott Cardiovascular, Chicago, IL, USA). Completion angiography demonstrated satisfactory exclusion of the aneurysm, with no endoleak and patent bridging stents. The patient was transferred to the intensive care unit (ICU). On the first post-operative day, she was noted to have bilateral arm weakness and a CT of the brain demonstrated watershed ischaemic changes in both hemispheres at the junction of vascular territories in the right frontal and both parieto-occipital regions. Over the course of the next week, the patient had fluctuating Glasgow Coma Scale levels and hypertension, which was judiciously managed with intravenous labetalol, however, improved steadily and was discharged from the ICU. The patient was transferred to a rehabilitation facility 3 weeks after her procedure. She made a complete neurological recovery, and the aneurysm remains excluded 9 years later, with patent bridging stents (Fig. 14.17).

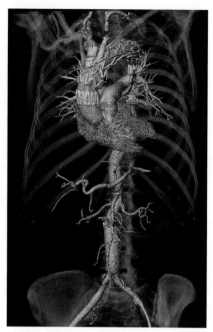

Figure 14.17 The arch aneurysm has been completely excluded, and flow to the innominate and left common carotid arteries remains preserved. The left subclavian is supplied by left carotid-subclavian bypass.

KEY REFERENCES

[2]   Patterson B, Holt P, Nienaber C, et al. Aortic pathology determines midterm outcome after endovascular repair of the thoracic aorta: report from the Medtronic Thoracic Endovascular Registry (MOTHER) Database. Circulation 2013;127(1):24–32. PMID: 23283856.

[13] Zafar M, Chen J, Wu J, et al. Natural history of descending thoracic and thoracoabdominal aortic aneurysms. J Thorac Cardiovasc Surg 2021;161:498–511. PMID: 31982126.

[25] Makaroun MS, Dillavou ED, Wheatley GH, et al. Five-year results of endovascular treatment with the Gore TAG device compared with open repair of thoracic aortic aneurysms. J Vasc Surg 2008;47(5):912–8. PMID: 18353605.

[49] Coselli JS, Bozinovski J, LeMaire SA. Open surgical repair of 2286 thoracoabdominal aortic aneurysms. Ann Thorac Surg 2007;83(2). S862–4 discussion S890–2. PMID: 17257942.

[59] Mastracci T, Eagleton M, Kuramochi M, et al. Twelve-year results of fenestrated endografts for juxtarenal and group IV thoracoabdominal aneurysms. J Vasc Surg 2015;61(2):355–64. PMID: 25619574.

Key points

- There are no prospective randomised controlled trials to guide practice with regard to diseases of the thoracic aorta, and current practice is driven by data from case series, registries, device-specific trials and consensus documents.
- Thoraco-abdominal aneurysm repair remains a technical challenge for surgeons and a physiological challenge for co-morbid patients, with a relatively high mortality and morbidity rate regardless of treatment modalities used. Advances in technology and surgical practice have meant that branched and fenestrated endovascular repair are now the treatment of choice in many centres, with a small number of specialist units performing a diminishing number of open surgical repairs.
- Endovascular repair is now the first-line treatment for most thoracic aneurysms, acute and chronic type B dissections, PAU, IMH and traumatic aortic injuries meeting the indications for intervention.
- The results of endovascular therapy in patients with connective tissue disorders are equivocal and open surgery should be considered in this patient group. Despite the increasing uptake of endovascular techniques in this setting, longer-term outcome data are required.
- Aorto-oesophageal and aortopulmonary fistula are rare conditions that often occur secondary to previous aortic surgery. TEVAR may be a bridge to definitive treatment, but radical surgery is associated with the best outcome if performed at a suitable interval.

 References available at http://ebooks.health.elsevier.com/

Renal and visceral arterial disease

15

Ramesh Kaushal Tripathi | Kirthi Bellamkonda | Martin Björck

PART 1 DISORDERS OF THE RENAL AND MESENTERIC CIRCULATION:

Kirthi Bellamkonda | Ramesh Kaushal Tripathi

INTRODUCTION

RENAL VASCULAR DISEASE

Vascular involvement of the renal artery and vein encompasses multitude of conditions and aetiopathologies; the treatment options for these are equally broad and evolve constantly. We present here a brief review of the traditional understanding of these diseases and the current evidence available in the management of a few specific conditions. Atherosclerotic renal artery stenosis (RAS) is the commonest symptomatic renal vascular pathology in the Western world. The renal arteries may also be affected in many other conditions, like aneurysmal disease, vasculitis, fibromuscular dysplasia (FMD), trauma and congenital hypoplasia. The renal veins may be affected by thrombosis from a variety of causes, including nephropathy, nutcracker syndrome, compression from mass effect, and coagulopathies.

ATHEROSCLEROTIC RENOVASCULAR DISEASE

PREVALENCE

Atherosclerotic renal disease is symptomatic in about 7% of elderly Americans, the incidence increasing with age. The prevalence of asymptomatic disease is higher, with autopsy studies showing renal vascular disease in over 40% of those aged 75 years or older. Atherosclerotic renal vascular disease (ARVD) and RAS are terms used interchangeably; however, the former may be a better term as a high-grade stenosis of the renal artery may not be present in all patients. ARVD is thus a manifestation of generalised atherosclerotic disease; concomitant disease in coronary, carotid and peripheral vascular fields is present in 15–45%. The correlation of ARVD and end-stage renal disease (ESRD) is complex and causality may be difficult to determine in this patient group: selective use of renal revascularisation also shows inconsistent associations with cardiovascular outcomes, renal replacement therapy and death.[1]

DEFINITIONS

ARVD occurs with between 50–75% renal artery diameter loss as diagnosed on conventional angiography (gold standard); however, lesions less than 50% may also be associated with significant (15 mmHg) pressure gradients.[2]

PATHOPHYSIOLOGY

A haemodynamically significant RAS will lead to a reduction in renal artery perfusion pressure and thus potentially an impairment of renal function simply because of a hydraulic effect, but only in a minority of patients. More commonly, there is a compensatory rise in renin and angiotensin levels in the post-stenotic kidney, constricting the post-glomerular efferent arteriole, which in turn helps to support glomerular capillary hydraulic pressure and filtration rate (Table 15.1). As glomerular perfusion in these patients is critically dependent upon angiotensin II, the risk of developing acute renal failure is significant, especially if the stenosis is bilateral or affects a solitary functioning kidney.

Studies in large cohorts of patients with ARVD have shown that there is often poor correlation between the degree of anatomical atheromatous stenosis, glomerular filtration rate (GFR) and overall renal function.[3,4] Patients with unilateral ARVD can have GFRs that range from normal to stage 5 kidney disease. Nuclear studies in patients with unilateral stenosis reveal that GFR may be the same or even lower in the non-stenotic kidney. This lack of correlation between the severity of renal ischaemic injury and kidney function may explain why renal function often fails to improve significantly after revascularisation despite restoration of renal artery patency. It should also be noted that 1–5% of patients with hypertension are diagnosed to have a significant RAS.

Patients with severe aortic atheroma undergoing arterial surgical or angiographic procedures, thrombolysis or anticoagulation are at risk of developing renal dysfunction secondary to cholesterol emboli.

CLINICAL PRESENTATION

The clinical index of suspicion remains essential in determining an appropriate diagnostic and therapeutic strategy in ARVD. Specific clinical pointers include:

- hypertension, often refractory to treatment; hypertensive crises;
- concomitant cardiovascular disease;
- angiotensin-converting enzyme-induced acute renal impairment;

Table 15.1 Pathogenesis of renovascular hypertension

Pathogenetic pathway progression	Stage of renovascular hypertension	Response to intervention
Renal artery occlusion Ischaemia Renin release Secondary increase in BP Conversion of angiotensin I to angiotensin II Severe vasoconstriction Aldosterone release (sodium and water retention)	Renin–angiotensin-dependent phase	Responds to correction of renal artery stenosis/occlusion
Functioning contralateral kidney → Pressure diuresis Previous volume retention Hypertension → Absence of pressure diuresis Volume retention Stimulus for renal renin production reduced Renal renin levels fall Renal parenchymal/vascular injury Persistent hypertension	Salt retention phase Renin–angiotensin- independent phase	Does not respond to correction of obstructions

- 'flash' pulmonary oedema (Pickering syndrome);
- vascular bruit, pulse deficit in a smoker;
- ischaemic nephropathy;
- secondary hypoaldosteronism.

DIAGNOSIS[5,6]

Laboratory investigations other than plasma renin levels are non-specific; their major role is in ruling out other conditions like Conn's syndrome or a pheochromocytoma. However, they may be used to evaluate the level of nephropathy present – for example, patients with advanced nephropathy indicated by >1 g/day proteinuria have poor outcomes from surgical intervention.[7] Functional studies such as captopril renography and selective renal vein renin sampling have a role in the detection of ARVD, with the potential to predict a blood pressure response to revascularisation or to document the functional significance of RAS.

Duplex scanning is a good initial diagnostic tool; however, problems with operator dependency and body habitus can hinder this. Significant lesions can be identified by measurement of peak systolic velocity (>200 cm/s) in the main renal artery and its branches, along with end diastolic velocity, parenchymal Doppler signals, the presence of post-stenotic turbulence, nature of waveforms, measurement of acceleration times, resistivity index, renal size and the ratio of renal artery to aortic peak systolic velocity of >3.5. Assessment protocols differ between institutions and a standardisation would be clinically useful.

The gold-standard for the imaging of RAS is digital subtraction angiography. One benefit is that intervention may be performed immediately upon diagnosis with this modality. However, given the invasive nature of the study, as well as the nephrotoxic potential of contrast agents, a number of other imaging modalities such as ultrasound, computed tomography (CT) and magnetic resonance imaging (MRI) exist with high sensitivity and specificity. CO_2 angiography also has a limited role in those in whom both MRI and CT angiography (CTA) are contraindicated.

CTA (Fig. 15.1a) provides information about the aorta and visceral vessels, neighbouring organs to exclude secondary causes or FMD and is of particular value in patients under consideration for open or endovascular revascularisation. The drawback of CTA is the risk of contrast nephropathy in a patient cohort that is already at risk for renal impairment. Other advances like fusion imaging or cone beam technology may become clinically useful in the future especially when considering endovascular therapy.

An alternative is MRI (Fig. 15.1b), but this requires long scan times with comparatively poor image quality. The risk of nephrogenic systemic sclerosis in RAS is significant; gadolinium should be avoided in patients with a GFR of less than 15 mL/min per 1.73 m^2.

MEDICAL MANAGEMENT

Medical management is twofold: to promote modification of atherosclerotic risk factors (aspirin, lipid-lowering drugs,

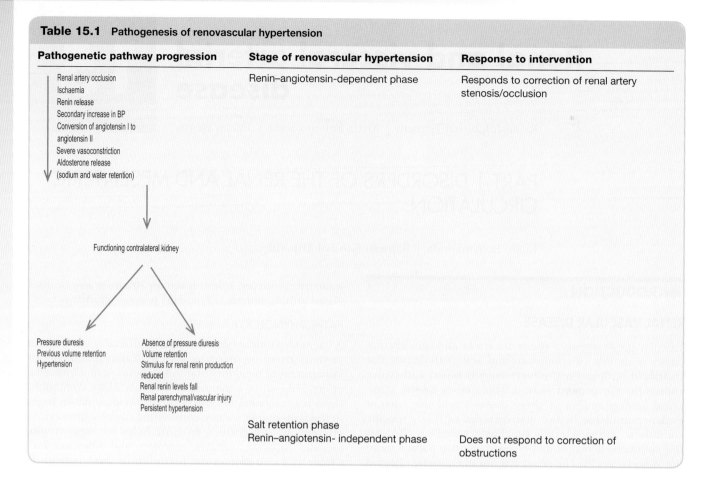

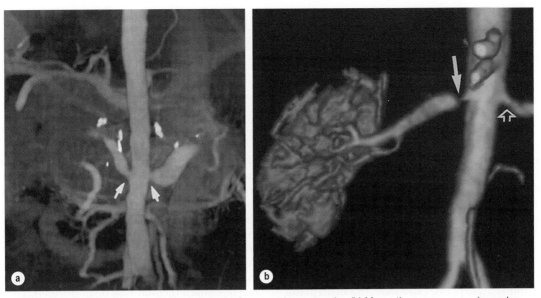

Figure 15.1   Bilateral renal artery stenosis. (a) Computed tomography; (b) Magnetic resonance angiography.

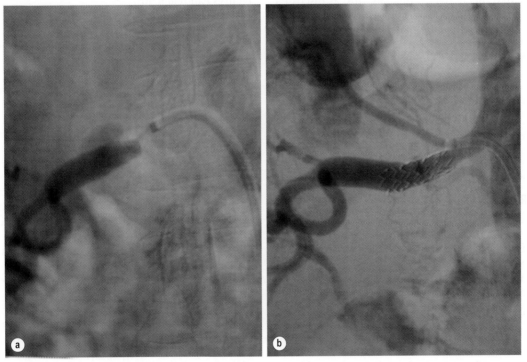

Figure 15.2   (a) Right renal artery stenosis caused by atherosclerotic renal vascular disease . (b) Post–renal artery stenting.

cessation of smoking, glycaemic control) and targeted management for hypertension.[7] Involvement of a nephrologist at an early stage is often necessary, as sudden drastic blood pressure reduction may be harmful. All imaging should be done with adequate hydration; the use of other renal protective agents (N-acetyl cysteine) is described but not universally accepted.

RENAL REVASCULARISATION

Endovascular treatment is the preferred mechanism of managing medically refractory RAS, although society guidelines detail a limited set of circumstances in which open surgery is indicated.

ENDOVASCULAR TREATMENT

Percutaneous transluminal renal angioplasty and stenting (PTRAS) is the current standard of care for renal revascularisation (Fig. 15.2a and b). Following initial reports of preventing renal vascular recoil in animal models by the use of stents, de Ven et al. demonstrated better patency with the use of stents compared to angioplasty in isolation.[8] A meta-analysis by Weinberg et al.[9] included the results of five studies

(HERCULES, SOAR, RENAISSANCE, RESTORE, ASPIRE) in patients with uncontrolled blood pressure, renal dysfunction and/or failed angioplasty and hypertension undergoing renal artery stent revascularisation were combined. Renal artery stenting resulted in significantly lower systolic and diastolic blood pressures at 9 months. An elevated baseline systolic blood pressure (SBP; > 150 mmHg) was predictive of therapeutic lowering of blood pressure in response to stenting. In contrast, the GREAT study randomised 105 patients to drug-eluting stents versus bare-metal stents and failed to demonstrate a benefit to using drug-eluting stents.[10]

While technical outcomes of PTRAS are excellent, and although clinical outcomes lag behind technical, some ~70% of patients experience some improvement. One in five patients experience sustained cure.[11] Despite promising short-term improvement, however, the most clinically significant complication is in-stent restenosis. Boateng et al. provide a detailed guide to the evidence surrounding management of this complication. The pathophysiology of restenosis is related to neointimal hyperplasia. Over time, this hyperplastic reaction may cause narrowing and even eventual thrombosis of the stent. Although in other areas of the body, drug-eluting stents have been able to mitigate this, as discussed earlier, they do not appear to significantly alter outcomes in PTRAS. A large variety of antiplatelet regiments are also used, per physician preference – commonly dual antiplatelet therapy, based on the cardiology literature. Zeller et al. provide a literature review of the rates on in-stent restenosis, which range widely, and appear dependent on vessel diameter, time of follow-up, and a variety of other factors.[12] When restenosis does occur, further endovascular interventions are required in patients with clinical deterioration. Angioplasty alone, or in combination with relining of the stent may be used. In rare, refractory cases, the patient may proceed to surgical bypass.

SURGICAL TREATMENT

A range of surgical options are available to treat renal artery disease (Box 15.1). Endarterectomy and bypass grafting are the two main surgical options for revascularisation. Current guidelines recommend surgery in patients with ARVD who have indications for revascularisation and have multiple small renal arteries or require aortic reconstruction near the renal arteries for other indications (e.g., aneurysm, severe aorto-iliac occlusive disease). The site of the lesion is also important, and if extra-anatomical bypass is considered, the condition of the donor visceral vessels must be optimal. In patients with renal artery occlusion, renal biopsy (performed either pre-operatively or peri-operatively) can indicate whether the kidney is viable and functionally salvageable on the basis of collateral vessels. However, this is not without risk of bleeding and potentially the loss of the kidney.

Nephrectomy is the oldest surgical procedure used in the treatment of ARVD, although rarely performed nowadays. In the presence of a normal contralateral kidney, it remains an option if the affected kidney measures less than 8 cm. In this situation measurement of renal vein renin levels is of value, with nephrectomy being indicated when the ratio of renal vein renins is greater than 1.5.

In the presence of aortic aneurysmal disease affecting the renal ostium, aortic graft and renal bypass may be indicated,

> **Box 15.1 Options for surgical revascularisation**
>
> Aortic graft and renal bypass
> Aortorenal bypass
> Aortorenal endarterectomy and patchplasty
> Extra-anatomical bypass
> Extracorporeal bench surgery

particularly if the aneurysm is not suited to endovascular aortic repair. Surgical options include a 6–8-mm limb of Dacron or polytetrafluoroethylene (PTFE) graft sutured onto the aortic graft with an end-to-end renal anastomosis and then bypass onto the affected renal artery in either an end-to-end (usually easiest) or end-to-side manner. Where bilateral RAS is present, an inverted bifurcated Dacron graft is preferred. When the pattern of aneurysm disease dictates that a supra-renal clamp is required for open surgery, transaortic endarterectomy may be performed. The ostial lesion is then carefully endarterectomised, and the procedure is completed with patch closure. Five-year patency in large centres can reach 90%.

Extra-anatomical bypass grafting is an attractive option for patients with unilateral RAS in the absence of significant aortic disease. Access is obtained via a subcostal incision, without the need for aortic cross-clamp or extensive dissection, and revascularisation is achieved using inflow from either the hepatic or splenic artery. An interposition saphenous vein graft may be used where there is insufficient arterial calibre and length for an end-to-end anastomosis. The inferior vena cava, the right renal vein and often the left renal vein must be fully mobilised. On the left side, the splenic artery is dissected from its midpoint from the pancreas. Splenectomy can be avoided, as there is a rich collateral supply and perfusion via the short gastric arteries. The Cleveland Clinic reports 175 extra-anatomical bypass procedures over a 12-year period, with 2.9% operative mortality. Graft patency reached 96%,[13–15] renal function improved in 40%[16–20] and hypertension was improved or cured in three-quarters of the series.[16,18–20]

Aortorenal bypass (Fig. 15.3) can be carried out using the long saphenous vein, PTFE, Dacron or rarely the internal iliac artery. The infra-renal aorta is preferred as an inflow site if it is relatively disease-free. If not, then a 'rooftop' incision is necessary to expose the aorta above the coeliac axis. The thoracic aorta can also be used as an inflow site. Where multiple small anastomoses are required, extracorporeal or bench surgery is performed for patients with disease affecting renal artery branches. Removal of the kidney, cooling and preservation as in renal transplantation surgery will allow multiple microvascular anastomoses to be performed before autotransplantation takes place. The internal iliac artery is commonly used for direct end-to-end anastomosis. The Cleveland Clinic again has the largest reported series of autotransplantation, with excellent long-term results.[17]

Surgical revascularisation is considered to be a high-risk option when compared to less invasive treatment methods. Results vary, with cure or improvement of hypertension and renal failure noted in 63–91% and 33–91%, respectively. Primary patency rates of 93–97% and mortality rates of 2–8% are reported.[16–22] These morbidity and mortality rates have

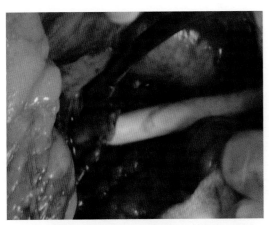

Figure 15.3   Aortorenal bypass with PTFE graft.

Box 15.2 Recommendations and guidelines for revascularisation

Percutaneous revascularisation is recommended in patients with haemodynamically significant atherosclerotic renal vascular disease (ARVD) and any of the following:[23–25]

Evidence class I

- Recurrent congestive heart failure or sudden unexplained pulmonary oedema

Evidence class II

- Unstable angina (class IIa)
- Accelerated, resistant, or malignant hypertension or hypertension with unexplained unilateral small kidney and intolerance to medication (class IIa)
- Asymptomatic bilateral or single functioning kidney; however, this treatment is clinically unproven in asymptomatic unilateral haemodynamically significant ARVD in a viable kidney (class IIb)

Box 15.3 Recommendations for percutaneous revascularisation

Percutaneous revascularisation is *reasonable* for patients with:[23–25]

- Progressive chronic kidney disease (CKD) and bilateral renal artery stenosis (RAS)
- RAS to a single functioning kidney
- Unilateral RAS with chronic renal insufficiency [23]
  Class I recommendation
- Renal stent placement recommended for ostial atherosclerotic renal vascular disease
- Balloon angioplasty with bailout stent placement recommended for fibromuscular dysplasia lesions, if necessary

Box 15.4 Contraindications for renal artery stenting

Patients with any of the following are typically *not good* candidates for renal artery stenting:[23]
- Mild or moderate stenoses (less than 70%)
- Long-standing loss of blood flow
- Complete occlusion of the renal artery

Box 15.5 Indications for surgical revascularisation

Class I recommendation[38]
  Atherosclerotic renal artery stenosis
  Multiple small renal arteries
  Early primary branching of the main renal artery
  Fibromuscular dysplasia, especially complex disease or macro-aneurysms

set the standards against which other treatment modalities can be compared. There have been no large trials to date comparing the outcomes of stenting with surgical revascularisation in ARVD. In young, fit patients, surgery may be preferred as it is cost-effective, and the long-term restenosis rate is reported to be 3–4%. The management of ARVD can be complex and certainly requires a multidisciplinary approach to maximise the therapeutic potential for each individual patient. Societal recommendations and guidelines form an effective template for evidence-based management of ARVD[23–25] (Boxes 15.2–15.5).

Revascularisation versus medical therapy

A review by Raman et al.[26] reports the results of management strategies for atherosclerotic RAS from 1993 to 16 March 2016. Fifteen comparative studies with a total of 4006 patients were identified; seven were randomised controlled trials (RCTs) and eight were non-randomised, comparative studies (NRCSs). Trial designs, interventions, endpoints, outcomes, follow-up and reporting were very variable. The ASTRAL, CORAL, STAR, RASCAD, NITER and RADAR trials remain the major trials on this topic to date. The meta-analysis demonstrated a low possibility of improvement of kidney function, with no difference

in blood pressure change, subsequent mortality, progression to need for renal replacement therapy, cardiovascular events and adverse events. However, the authors note that most of these studies exclude patients with high-grade lesions, presenting with acute decompensation. Patients with ARVD are at an overall threefold risk of cardiovascular and all-cause mortality to age-matched controls; the challenge remains in identifying the patient subset in ARVD who, if managed interventionally, will have improvement in renal function and mortality. Current evidence can justify intervention in patients with progressive, but not severe, chronic renal insufficiency and systolic hypertension with global high-grade stenosis, ARVD and rapidly declining kidney function or flash pulmonary oedema. It also has a role in the management of congestive heart failure. Efforts at developing predictors of clinical benefit from intervention (including high blood oxygen level-dependent MRI, brain natriuretic peptide levels) are under investigation but cannot yet be used generally.

Renal stenting during treatment of aortic aneurysmal disease

Advances in the endovascular treatment of aortic aneurysms with surgeon modified/fenestrated or branched devices have created a subgroup of patients who undergo renal

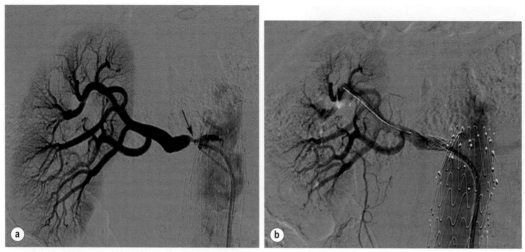

Figure 15.4   (a) Renal artery stenosis following endovascular aortic repair. (b) Adjunctive renal stenting performed to salvage as a planned procedure.

intervention when grafts cross the renal artery. Adjunctive renal stenting may be needed to salvage inadvertent coverage (Fig. 15.4a and b) or as a planned procedure when supra-renal fixation or endovascular repair of a thoraco-abdominal aneurysm or dissection is planned. Stent placement in these patients may be more challenging because of complex anatomy, technical risks and risk of atheroembolisation leading to a higher complication rate and reports of late decline in GFR.[27,28]

Renal artery denervation

Renal artery denervation (RDN) is an endovascular procedure for the treatment of resistant hypertension. This condition is thought to involve overactivity of the afferent and efferent sympathetic nerves that run in the adventitia of the renal arteries, the nerves running closest in the distal renal arteries and renal artery branches. Radical nephrectomy and surgical sympathectomy have been associated with the normalisation of blood pressure in patients with ESRD and hypertension. It has also been established that increased renal sympathetic nerve activity has an important role in the development of essential hypertension. Following positioning of a sheath within the renal artery, a probe is positioned with its tip in contact with the inner luminal surface of the vessel. Radiofrequency energy is then applied to disrupt the nerve fibres running in the renal artery adventitia. The procedure is repeated at several points in both arteries to interrupt the neurogenic signals thought to be involved in the maintenance of sympathetic overactivity and, hence, resistant hypertension.

In 2010 the Symplicity HTN-2 study demonstrated for the first time in humans that endovascular renal denervation is a safe and effective technique to reduce blood pressure in patients with resistant hypertension.[29] A total of 106 patients with uncontrolled blood pressure (systolic >160 mmHg) and taking at least three antihypertensive agents were randomised to renal denervation plus best medical therapy or best medical therapy alone. At 6 months, the group receiving renal denervation showed a significantly reduced blood pressure measurement. The larger Symplicity HTN-3 study included a total of 535 patients from 88 sites in the

United States, but this did not reveal a significant effect on SBP reduction. Pooled data from SYMPLICITY HTN-3 and the Global SYMPLICITY Registry revealed that reduction in blood pressure among patients with isolated systolic hypertension was less pronounced than the reduction in patients with combined systolic–diastolic hypertension.[30,31] Thus, this trial paradoxically did not provide the definitive proof in support of RDN that was expected. However, the results have been analysed in detail and have generated further insight into the location of the peri-renal sympathetics and there is still a need for further trials in this area.

OTHER RENAL VASCULAR DISORDERS

NUTCRACKER SYNDROME

Many types of thrombosis occurring in the renal vein are of non-vascular origin, such as coagulopathies resulting from liver disease or nephropathy. Nutcracker syndrome is unique in that primarily vascular interventions are available for treatment. The pathophysiology of nutcracker syndrome is caused by compression of the left renal vein between the aorta and the superior mesenteric artery (SMA).[32] Rarely, a retroaortic left renal vein may be compressed against the vertebral body. Because compression is so proximate to the vena cava, the typical venous collaterals that are relied upon during surgical transection, such as the adrenal veins and gonadal veins, are also occluded. While symptoms such as haematuria are typically mild, in rare cases, patients require intervention. Both stenting and open surgery are options, however, because of the rarity of this condition, further study is required to determine best practices.

RENAL ARTERY ANEURYSM

Renal artery aneurysms[33] are rare, with necropsy incidence of <0.1%. Coleman et al. extensively describe the characteristics of this condition. The annual growth rate is estimated to be 0.6 mm a year; the rupture rate being 3–5%, with a mortality of <10%. They are unique from other aneurysms in that patients are not typically vasculopathic and are not commonly smokers. It is not uncommon to have renovascular

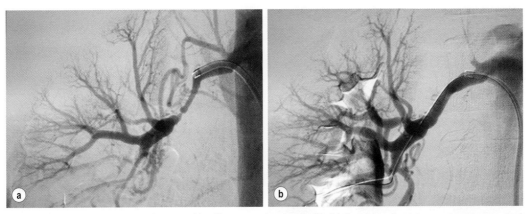

Figure 15.5 (a) Renal artery stenosis caused by fibromuscular dysplasia. (b) Good result post percutaneous angioplasty.

hypertension from areas of turbulence, stenosis, or embolisation from renal artery aneurysms. Treatment indications are the presence of clinical symptoms, thromboembolism, refractory hypertension, size >2 cm, female in reproductive age, dissection or rupture. Open, endovascular and robotic repair are reported with primary patency rates of 75–100%, re-intervention rates of 0–22% and overall mortality of 1%.

RENAL TRAUMA

Renal trauma[34] can be penetrating or blunt; concomitant renovascular injury is usually severe (American Association for the Surgery of Trauma grade 4 or 5) and associated with other injuries. Management options tend to be conservative unless complications occur; nephrectomy, open vascular repair, angioembolisation and endovascular repair have all been reported. The latter should not delay the management of other life-threatening injuries. Results of vascular salvage depend on the ischaemia time of less than 3 hours and the suitability of anticoagulation. The role of revascularisation is limited.

FIBROMUSCULAR DYSPLASIA

FMD[35,36] is a non-inflammatory, non-atherosclerotic disorder that may be observed in almost any arterial bed and can lead to arterial stenosis. Five different types are recognised and usually affect younger patients, with a female predominance, involving the distal main artery and/or the intrarenal branches. Rarely, FMD may be complicated by an aneurysm. Patients may be asymptomatic, but the most usual presentation is hypertension. Hypertension is commonly treated successfully with medication, but RAS and renal dysfunction may progress in up to one-third of patients. Occlusion and complete loss of renal function is exceptional. Magnetic resonance angiography (MRA) can detect FMD in the proximal vessels but is less sensitive for visualising the second- and third-order branches. The diagnosis will usually require conventional digital subtraction angiography and selective views may be necessary to detect subtle branch lesions. When treating FMD, the results of percutaneous angioplasty (PTA) are good (Fig. 15.5a and b), with 10-year cumulative patency rates of 87% and up to 50% of patients cured of their hypertension. The remainder often have a reduced drug burden and improved blood pressure control. Stenting is usually reserved for suboptimal PTA.[23–25]

POST-TRANSPLANT RENAL ARTERY STENOSIS

Post-transplant RAS[37] is another area that is being recognised to need further study. A meta-analysis by Ngo et al. included 32 studies with 884 interventions reporting the results of post-transplant stenosis managed with angioplasty or stenting. The overall patency rates were 42–100% with technical success in 90% but the diagnostic and reporting criteria were very heterogeneous and need further study.

MID-AORTIC SYNDROME

Mid-aortic syndrome[38,39] can be congenital or acquired secondary to neurofibromatosis or Takayasu's disease and may present with severe/resistant hypertension in a younger patient group. This group may require operative management with an emerging role of endovascular management. Concomitant medical management of systemic disease is crucial.

> ## Key points
>
> ### Renal disease
>
> - ARVD usually presents with hypertension, chronic renal failure, acute renal failure or pulmonary oedema. However, it is often asymptomatic and should be considered in patients with extra-renal vascular disease.
> - Angioplasty (PTA) is the procedure of choice for non-atheromatous lesions.
> - The improvement of blood pressure control in non-atheromatous lesions is good to excellent following PTA.
> - Stents have a higher technical success and patency rate compared with PTA in atheromatous ostial lesions.
> - Surgery gives the lowest restenosis rates but should be reserved for stent failures or young fit patients.
> - Improvement of blood pressure control in atheromatous lesions following stenting is marginal but may reduce the drug burden.
> - There is currently no consensus on the role of stenting in ARVD for hypertension or renal insufficiency. Further trials are under way.
> - Societal guidelines form an effective template for evidence-based management of ARVD (see Boxes 15.2–15.5).

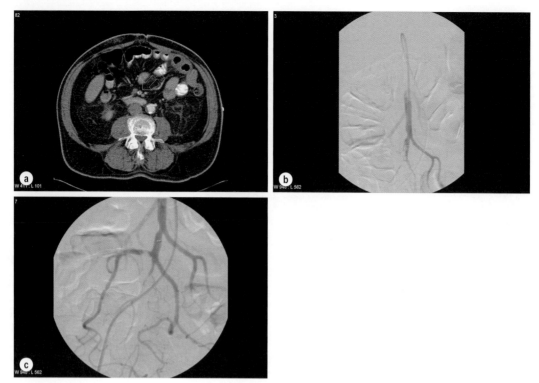

Figure 15.6   (a–c) Treatment of acute mesenteric ischaemia in an 85-year-old man. For details, see text.

PART 2 MESENTERIC VASCULAR DISEASE

Martin Björck

INTRODUCTION

The mesenteric arteries and veins are affected by a whole group of diseases. In the clinical situation, it is not always obvious if the ischaemia is acute or chronic, or acute-on chronic. It is also not always clear if the main disease is arterial or venous, nor if it is a result of embolus from the heart, local thrombosis because of atherosclerosis, an underlying aneurysm or a dissection. This was the rationale behind the European Society of Vascular Surgery (ESVS) guidelines on the 'Management of the diseases of the mesenteric arteries and veins', which cover all of these pathologies.[40] These Clinical Practice guidelines give 64 recommendations regarding diagnosis and treatment of the different clinical scenarios that are most commonly encountered. The North American Society for Vascular Surgery recently published another guideline, covering only chronic mesenteric ischaemia.[41] The recommendations of the two guidelines are quite similar, with the exception that the American guideline is more favourable to treat asymptomatic patients.[42]

ACUTE THROMBOEMBOLIC OCCLUSION OF THE SUPERIOR MESENTERIC ARTERY

This condition is more common than expected, and in most epidemiological studies, embolism is more common than primary thrombosis.[40] Without a high grade of clinical suspicion and targeted diagnostic tests, many patients are diagnosed too late, when the entire bowel is gangrenous and the patient beyond salvage. The classical clinical triad associated with acute embolic occlusion of the SMA consists of: (i) acute severe abdominal pain without signs of peritonitis ('pain out of proportion'), (ii) bowel emptying, most often both diarrhoea and vomiting and (iii) a source of embolus, most often atrial fibrillation or acute myocardial infarction.

Although a normal d-dimer can exclude the diagnosis,[40,43] it is not specific and in fact there is no specific laboratory test to detect acute mesenteric ischaemia (AMI). Lactate is effectively metabolised in the liver, explaining why it is elevated only late. It becomes diagnostic when the bowel is gangrenous and the patient has become septic and hypotensive,[40] explaining why the guidelines issued a strong recommendation not to use lactate to diagnose this condition early. Modern CTA is the mainstay investigation to diagnose an occlusion of the SMA, but it should be performed in all three phases and with thin slices over the SMA in the arterial phase.[40]

When treatment is discussed, one controversial issue is whether revascularisation should be performed before or after bowel resection (when needed). There are no RCTs, but cohort data suggesting that revascularisation should be performed before bowel resection.[40,44] Another controversial issue is whether open or endovascular revascularisation is the preferred approach. Here the data suggest that endovascular techniques are associated with better outcomes if the occlusion is thrombotic, but with an embolic occlusion, open or endovascular surgery have similar outcomes.[45,46]

There is consensus regarding the need for second look laparotomy, completion control (with angiography or flow measurements) and antibiotic treatment. The damage control strategy, first developed in trauma patients, should always be considered when treating patients with AMI. This may explain why treatment of a thrombotic occlusion with open surgery is less successful than stenting. The latter can be performed in local anaesthesia, resulting in an abbreviated laparotomy, if at all necessary. An alternative when antegrade stenting though the aorta is difficult, and in particular if there is also contamination because of bowel gangrene, is the retrograde open mesenteric stenting,[40,47] when the SMA is punctured through laparotomy.

A case example of how the damage control concept can be applied to a patient with AMI is illustrated in Fig. 15.6. The case involved an 85-year-old man who was admitted with atrial fibrillation and 2 days of abdominal pain. He had a slightly elevated troponin levels, was thought to have a myocardial infarction, and was admitted to the cardiology unit. Twelve hours later, the diagnosis was questioned, and a CTA showed an embolus in the SMA (see Fig. 15.6a). The patient had no peritonitis, but severe abdominal pain, and was taken to the hybrid operating room. An aspiration embolectomy was performed with a stiff 6-Fr introducer (see Fig. 15.6b), and the final angiography showed an almost complete revascularisation of the branches (see Fig. 15.6c). The procedure was performed under local anaesthesia and the patient experienced an almost complete and immediate relief of his abdominal pain, which prevented the need for an exploratory laparotomy. After 3 days of surveillance at the hospital, and initiation of warfarin treatment, the patient returned to his home. This case illustrates the potential benefit of endovascular therapy in these often elderly and frail patients.

CHRONIC MESENTERIC ISCHAEMIA

The typical clinical presentation of chronic mesenteric ischaemia (CMI) is post-prandial pain, weight-loss and diarrhoea. The typical patient is a smoking woman around the age of 60 years. In contrast to the patient with malignant disease, the patient's appetite is not affected. The patient refrains from eating, or eats very small meals, for fear of the pain that comes after the meal. This clinical history is the key to the diagnosis.

The patient usually has known cardiovascular disease and has often undergone multiple examinations for abdominal pain. One of the main problems is how to diagnose the condition, since asymptomatic stenosis and even occlusion of one of the mesenteric arteries is quite common, explained by the collateral network that is well developed in most people (Fig. 15.7). Duplex ultrasound is the recommended screening examination, when CMI is expected (in contrast to AMI when it is NOT recommended because of the risk of false negative findings[40]) and has the advantage of also including physiological evaluation of stenoses.[48]

If a single vessel is affected, the diagnosis of CMI is less likely and careful examination for alternative causes is warranted.[40,41] If, on the other hand, two or three of the mesenteric arteries are affected, and no other explanation was identified despite extensive gastroenterological examinations, CMI

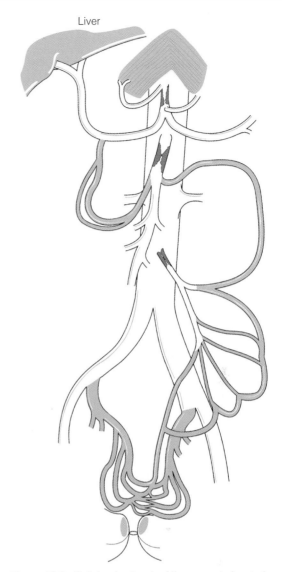

Liver

Figure 15.7 Collateral network of the mesenteric arteries.

should be considered the cause of the symptoms. Before treatment, the anatomy of occlusions and stenosis need to be mapped. CTA is most often used for mapping the disease before any intervention, although MRA is an alternative.

If there is severe CMI (defined as significant weight-loss, diarrhoea and/or continuous pain) treatment should not be delayed, since there is a risk of developing acute-on-chronic ischaemia with bowel gangrene. One controversial issue is if the patient with severe CMI should be given parenteral nutritional support before surgery. Data suggest that this is not advisable, since the delay may result in worsening ischaemia, and both guidelines issued strong recommendations not to delay treatment in this clinical scenario.[40,41]

When it is decided to treat the patient, a number of alternatives and controversial issues need to be addressed. Many vascular centres would consider endovascular treatment as the first alternative, but there are risk factors for a failed endovascular treatment that need to be considered. They include anatomical factors such as severe eccentric calcification, flush occlusions, and long lesions that extend into the middle segment of the SMA. In these cases, stenting may still be possible, but is not optimal since the risks of restenosis and of peri-operative complications are increased. The superior long-term results of open surgery should be balanced against a possible early benefit of endovascular intervention with regard to lower immediate mortality and morbidity.[40,41]

There are two other situations when an open arterial reconstruction may be preferred: after failed endovascular treatment and in young patients, often with non-atherosclerotic disease such as vasculitis or mid-aortic syndrome. A special case is also the median arcuate ligament syndrome, when the coeliac trunk is compressed by muscular fibres from the diaphragm. In this situation, primary stenting is contraindicated, but can sometimes be necessary and successful after prior open surgical release.[40,41]

Balloon angioplasty has been replaced by primary stenting in most centres because of the increased risk of elastic recoil and restenosis. The lesions are most often ostial, a result of atherosclerosis of the aortic wall. There are no RCTs comparing different treatment modalities, however, making the evidence base weak.

Another controversial issue is if a bare-metal stent or if a covered stent graft should be used. The SMA has multiple branches, some of which may be sacrificed with a covered stent, which should be balanced against the fact that data suggest that restenosis is less common after having used a stent-graft. This was shown in a large retrospective study on 225 patients.[49] A Dutch RCT is ongoing, randomising 42 patients in each group, and will hopefully give us more information in 2023.[50]

Another controversial issue is whether one or multiple vessels should be revascularised in the case of multi-vessel disease, and if the SMA or the coeliac trunk should be treated. The literature shows retrospective studies with diverging results: some have shown no significant advantage of two vessel stenting, others have reported better long-term results after two-vessel revascularisation.[40] Given the lack of proven benefit of the more extensive procedure, most centres would focus on the SMA, however, and treat only that vessel.

In the post-operative management, secondary prophylaxis and risk factor management are important, including antiplatelet therapy, statins, and smoking cessation. CMI is a life-threatening disease, and the patient benefits from a multidisciplinary approach. Since both diagnosis and treatment are rather complex, and the patients are uncommon, the patient should ideally be referred to specialised centres that can offer a multidisciplinary team, as well as both open and endovascular treatment.[40] Most patients do benefit from a routine follow-up assessing the clinical outcome, but it has not been shown that routine imaging adds benefit to the patient.[51] An asymptomatic patient probably does not need any imaging.[51]

ACUTE MESENTERIC VENOUS THROMBOSIS

Acute venous thrombosis of the superior mesenteric vein is the most common cause of acute venous ischaemia, also called *mesenteric venous thrombosis* (*MVT*). It is less common than arterial AMI by a factor of 7.[52] The condition is under-diagnosed, because of rather diffuse symptoms, and a less acute onset compared to AMI. It can also be over-diagnosed,

however, since many patients with abdominal symptoms undergo abdominal CT investigations, and old asymptomatic MVTs are identified incidentally. MVT was reported to be present in approximately 2% in one large post-mortem study.[53] This explains the great variations in incidence estimates, but a well conducted and population based Finnish study estimated it to be 0.5/100 000 inhabitants/year.[54] When bowel gangrene develops, its extension is usually less than in cases caused by arterial occlusion. Typically, the middle part of the small bowel is affected, and it is associated with oedema and ascites. The oedematous mesentery makes it technically demanding to perform both anastomosis and stoma.

When MVT is diagnosed, underlying prothrombotic conditions should be considered, since they may also need to be treated. Considering Virchow's triad is a systematic approach, including injury to the vessel wall, reduced flow and/or a procoagulant blood. The most common underlying risk-factors are venous thromboembolism (often inherited monogenetic disorders) and obesity.[40,52] Malignant disease, undiagnosed portal hypertension, intra-abdominal infections, or injury during surgery, should also be considered.

Anticoagulation with heparin is first-line therapy.[40] Most patients can be managed without laparotomy or bowel resection, but especially during the first days, this possibility needs to be considered. Bowel gangrene can develop late, however. The ischaemic injury is a product of the duration and the depth of ischaemia. This means that a low-grade ischaemic condition, such as MVT, can result in bowel gangrene after 1–2 weeks. Until resolution of abdominal pain, the risk of gangrene prevails.

This is the background to why unfractionated heparin is considered the best initial treatment, since it can be reversed more quickly, if a need of bowel resection develops. Later low-molecular-weight heparin may be used. The strong antiinflammatory effect of heparin is also an important therapeutic principle that explains why it is so effective in most cases.

Sometimes (approximately 5%) heparin treatment is not successful: the abdominal pain continues and the general status of the patient deteriorates.[40] In this situation, catheter delivered thrombolysis may be considered. Direct puncture of the liver and delivering the thrombolytic agent (usually r-tPA) directly to the superior mesenteric vein is associated with a rather high risk of bleeding complications, and since the outflow through the liver is compromised, significant clearance of the thrombus is seldom achieved. A solution to these problems is to puncture the jugular vein, perform a transjugular intra-hepatic portosystemic shunt (TIPS), and through that perform mechanical aspiration thrombectomy and direct thrombolysis.[55] This approach has the advantages of both reducing the bleeding risk and improving the outflow. The TIPS will usually thrombose spontaneously after some time.

After the acute episode, it is important to investigate if there is an underlying condition explaining the MVT. In patients with reversible causes (e.g., trauma, infection, or pancreatitis), anticoagulation for 3–6 months is recommended in the ESVS Guidelines.[40] Lifelong anticoagulation is recommended in case of proven thrombophilia, recurrent venous thrombosis or when progression or recurrence of thrombosis would have severe clinical consequences, such as in a patient with short bowel.[40,51]

NON-OCCLUSIVE MESENTERIC ISCHAEMIA

Finally, a few words about non-occlusive mesenteric ischaemia (NOMI), a term that was introduced by Ende in 1958.[56] In critically ill patients with low cardiac output, multiple interventions are often performed to save the life, but as a side-effect, the intestinal circulation may suffer.[57] The vasoconstriction can be caused by vasoactive drugs (in particular vasopressors, but also cocaine or crack-cocaine among drug addicts), as well as secondary to resuscitation leading to the abdominal compartment syndrome.[58] Other patients at risk are those with hypovolaemia during renal replacement therapy or after burn injury, as well as those who have undergone cardiac surgery.[40]

As in most cases of mesenteric ischaemia, clinical suspicion is the key to a timely diagnosis. In one study on patients who died from NOMI, 40% had a stenosis at the origin of the SMA.[59] Dilating and stenting such a stenosis may be lifesaving, as well as placing a catheter for selective intra-arterial administration of vasodilators into the SMA. This is why the ESVS guidelines recommend that a patient with life-threatening NOMI should be taken to a hybrid operating room, or an operating room with a C-arm, where both endovascular interventions and laparotomy (if necessary) can be performed.[40]

Key points

Mesenteric vascular disease

- **Patient history and clinical suspicion are important for diagnosing all kinds of mesenteric ischaemia.**
- Laboratory examinations are not helpful in diagnosing AMI.
- **Triphasic CTA is the most important imaging in AMI.**
- Endovascular surgery is associated with better survival if an acute occlusion of the SMA is thrombotic.
- An embolic occlusion can be treated with similar results with both techniques.
- **Most patients with AMI will need bowel resection, but that should take place after revascularisation.**
- Second-look laparotomy, completion control and antibiotics are recommended after revascularisation for AMI.
- **If a single vessel is affected, the diagnosis of CMI is less likely and careful examination for alternative causes is warranted.**
- In CMI, the superior long-term results of open surgery should be balanced against a possible early benefit of endovascular intervention.
- Primary stenting of the SMA is recommended in CMI.
- **Heparin treatment is first-line therapy in patients with venous mesenteric ischaemia.**

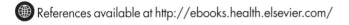 References available at http://ebooks.health.elsevier.com/

KEY REFERENCES

[7] Prince M, Tafur JD, White CJ. When and how should we revascularize patients with atherosclerotic renal artery stenosis? JACC: Cardiovasc Intervent 2019;12(6):505–17.

[8] Van de Ven PJ, Kaatee R, Beutler JJ, Beek FJ, Woittiez A-JJ, Buskens E, et al. Arterial stenting and balloon angioplasty in ostial atherosclerotic renovascular disease: a randomised trial. Lancet 1999;353(9149):282–6.

[23] Parikh SA, Shishehbor MH, Gray BH, et al. SCAI expert consensus statement for renal artery stenting appropriate use. Catheter Cardiovasc Intervent 2014;84(7):1163–71. PMID: 25138644.

[24] Anderson JL, Halperin JL, Albert NM, et al. Management of patients with peripheral artery disease (compilation of 2005 and 2011 ACCF/AHA guideline recommendations): a report of the American College of cardiology Foundation/American heart association Task Force on practice guidelines. Circulation 2013;127(13):1425–43. PMID: 23457117.

[25] Tendera M, Aboyans V, et al. ESC Guidelines on the diagnosis and treatment of peripheral artery diseases. Document covering atherosclerotic disease of extracranial carotid and vertebral, mesenteric, renal, upper and lower extremity arteries: the Task Force on the Diagnosis and Treatment of Peripheral Artery Diseases of the European Society of Cardiology (ESC). Eur Heart J 2011;32(22):2851–906. PMID: 21873417.

[40] Björck M, Koelemay M, Acosta S, Bastos Goncalves F, Kölbel T, Kolkman JJ, et al. Management of the diseases of the mesenteric arteries and veins. Clinical practice guidelines of the European Society of Vascular Surgery (ESVS). Eur J Vasc Endovasc Surg 2017;53:460–510.

[41] Huber TS, Bjorck M, Chandra A, Clouse WD, Dalsing MC, Oderich GS, Smeds MR, Committee ER, Murad MH. Chronic mesenteric ischemia clinical practice guideline from the society for vascular surgery. J Vasc Surg 2021;73:87S–115S.

[45] Schermerhorn ML, Giles KA, Hamdan AD, Wyers MC, Pomposelli FB. Mesenteric revascularization: management and outcomes in the United States, 1988e2006. J Vasc Surg 2009;50(2):341–8.e1.

[46] Block TA, Acosta S, Bjorck M. Endovascular and open surgery for acute occlusion of the superior mesenteric artery. J Vasc Surg 2010;52(4):959–66.

[51] Venermo M, Sprynger M, Desormais I, Björck M, Brodmann M, Cohnert T, et al. Editor's choice - follow-up of patients after revascularization for peripheral arterial diseases: a consensus document from the European society of cardiology Working group on aorta and peripheral vascular diseases and the European society of vascular surgery. Eur J Vasc Endovasc Surg 2019;58:641–53.

[57] Bjorck M, Wanhainen A. Nonocclusive mesenteric hypoperfusion syndromes: recognition and treatment. Semin Vasc Surg 2010;23(1):54–64.

16 Central venous and dialysis access

Julien Al Shakarchi | Andrew Garnham

INTRODUCTION

Access to the venous circulation is an almost universal requirement in hospitalised patients for intravenous fluid, medicine or blood products administration. This is most commonly achieved with an indwelling peripheral intravenous cannula, but central venous access may be required for central venous pressure monitoring, parenteral nutrition, haemodialysis (HD), haemofiltration, the administration of cytotoxic drugs or long-term antibiotics.

For acute HD, central venous catheters (CVCs) are the mainstay of access and provide high dialysis flows (>300 mL/min) but have high complication rates and are less suitable for chronic use. For long-term HD, an arteriovenous fistula (AVF) or graft (AVG) can provide sufficient flow (>300 mL/min) to allow dialysis via two needles inserted into the fistula or graft itself.

CENTRAL VENOUS ACCESS

INDICATIONS

In addition to central venous pressure monitoring, CVCs can be used to infuse large volumes of irritant solutions, such as antibiotics, blood products, parenteral nutrition and chemotherapeutic agents, particularly if required over long periods. In an emergency, CVCs allow the rapid administration of large volumes of fluid if peripheral access cannot be achieved. Depending on the indication and duration of access requirement, central catheters can also be inserted peripherally. Implantable injection ports, 'portacaths' (e.g., Bardport, Passport, Infuse-a-Port or MediPort), may be used for chemotherapy or long-term administration of other drugs.[1,2]

METHODS

CVCs are generally inserted under local anaesthetic through the internal jugular, subclavian or femoral veins, preferably using ultrasound guidance, by the Seldinger technique.[3] If short-term access is required, a multi-lumen catheter is inserted into the internal jugular vein (IJV) so that the tip lies in the superior vena cava (SVC). For long-term access, a catheter with an attached Dacron cuff is placed in a subcutaneous tunnel (e.g., Hickman line) for fixation and to act as a barrier to infection.

Implantable access ports are usually inserted into the jugular or subclavian vein in the operating theatre and tunnelled so that the port lies over the anterior chest wall. The subclavian route is discouraged because of the higher incidence of subclavian vein stenosis, access thrombosis and complication rates such as pneumothoraces. They contain a diaphragm that may be accessed repeatedly using a special side-hole needle. Central vein access can also be achieved using a peripheral intravenous central catheter inserted in the antecubital or long saphenous vein.

COMPLICATIONS

Air embolus can be avoided by placing the patient in the Trendelenburg position during insertion.

✅✅ Accurate placement under ultrasound guidance will reduce the incidence of arterial puncture, haematoma, haemothorax and pneumothorax.[4]

The long-term complications including infection and thrombosis are dealt later in this chapter.

RENAL REPLACEMENT THERAPY

CHRONIC KIDNEY DISEASE

Chronic kidney disease (CKD) is an important long-term condition caused by damage to the kidneys. It is initially without any specific symptoms and is detected incidentally on a routine blood test. In the later stages of the disease, patients might develop a number of signs and symptoms including hypertension, hyperkalaemia, fluid overload and anaemia.

The stages of CKD are based on the measured or estimated glomerular filtration rate (GFR), a measure of kidney function. There are five stages including stage 1 where kidney function is normal (Table 16.1). The stages of CKD are useful tool for physicians and aid in describing patient's renal failure and in planning management.

Renal replacement therapy (RRT) is provided to patients in end-stage renal disease (ESRD). It both prolongs survival and improves quality of life for these patients. RRT can take the form of HD, peritoneal dialysis (PD) or renal transplantation. In the rest of this chapter, we will focus on vascular access for HD.

Table 16.1 Stages of chronic kidney disease

Stage	Glomerular filtration rate	Description
1	>90	Normal renal function
2	60–90	Mildly reduced renal function
3	30–60	Moderately reduced renal function
4	15–30	Severely reduced renal function
5	<15	End-stage renal failure

TEMPORARY DIALYSIS ACCESS

About 75% of patients are known to have deteriorating renal function at least 90 days before dialysis is required so that permanent HD access can be created in advance. Unfortunately, this opportunity is frequently missed in UK practice, with only around half of patients starting HD with definitive access.[5] Over 96% of patients start HD on a CVC if presenting late (<90 days), with 75% still using the same modality 3 months after onset of dialysis. Referral to a surgeon before commencing dialysis leads to 70% of patients having an AVF, whereas 90% will start dialysis on a CVC if not seen by the surgical team before the onset of dialysis.[5] Urgent dialysis is required for hyperkalaemia, severe metabolic acidosis, uraemic symptoms or fluid overload.

For patients presenting as an emergency with ESRD, HD can start using a double-lumen CVC whilst awaiting a permanent access. However, CVCs have a high risk of infection,[6] lead to central venous stenosis or thrombosis,[7] compromising further access in the upper limbs, and have a higher morbidity and mortality than AVFs.[8] Therefore their use should be short term in the majority of patients. In addition, patients who start HD on a CVC have an overall reduced life expectancy than those who start on an AVF.[5]

✔ Temporary (non-tunnelled) catheters are used in patients who require short-term dialysis for transient renal failure or who present acutely with ESRD. They are also indicated after failure of a permanent access, whilst awaiting maturation of a new AVF or insertion of an AVG. Tunnelled catheters are preferred if dialysis is required for more than 2 weeks or for permanent access when the creation of an AVF or AVG is contraindicated or technically impossible.

The subcutaneous tunnel may reduce the rate of infection, but this has not been proven in a randomised trial.[9]

METHODS

Temporary femoral vein catheters are useful for acute dialysis but have a higher rate of infection than internal jugular CVCs[10] and should be replaced by a tunnelled (preferably jugular) venous catheter at the earliest opportunity. A median survival of 166 days has been reported for tunnelled femoral CVCs.[11]

The right IJV is preferred as this provides the most direct route to the SVC and right atrium (RA). The left IJV has a greater complication rate because the catheter has to traverse two 90-degree bends to reach the RA. As discussed earlier in the chapter with regard to CVCs, the subclavian route is discouraged because of the high incidence of subclavian vein stenosis and thrombosis that may compromise future access in the ipsilateral arm. When other routes have been exhausted, tunnelled catheters can be placed in the femoral vein or even the inferior vena cava (IVC) via a transhepatic or translumbar approach.

The catheter tip is usually placed at the SVC/RA junction. Atrial placement minimises recirculation and reduces the risk of migration on standing,[12] but may cause arrhythmias by stimulation of the sinoatrial node.

✔✔ The preferred site for a CVC is the right IJV. CVCs should be inserted under fluoroscopic or ultrasound guidance, without which there is a high malposition rate of 29%.[13]

COMPLICATIONS OF CENTRAL VENOUS CATHETERS

INSERTION

The complications related to catheter insertion are the same as for other CVCs described earlier and can be reduced by ultrasound guidance and a micropuncture technique.

CATHETER DYSFUNCTION

Catheter dysfunction occurs when an adequate extracorporeal blood flow of 300 mL/min cannot be achieved and therefore adequate HD is not achieved. Early dysfunction is usually caused by malposition or kinking and is corrected by repositioning. Later dysfunction is primarily caused by thrombosis or fibrin sheath formation. Rarely, tip migration demands repositioning with a snare or exchanging over a wire.

CATHETER-LOCKING SOLUTIONS

Catheter patency can be maintained between dialysis sessions using a catheter-locking solution. The standard procedure has been heparin instillation (1000–10 000 U/mL) into the catheter lumen in a volume sufficient to fill to the lumen tip. There is a risk of heparin loss because of diffusion into the bloodstream and unintentional systemic anticoagulation. Low-dose heparin (1000–5000 U/mL) seems as effective as high-dose.[14] Trisodium citrate, which also has antibacterial properties, is also an effective catheter lock and has been shown to be comparable to heparin lock in a recently published randomised clinical trial.[15]

A recent randomised clinical trial compared 270 patients on HD who had a CVC using a locking regime of heparin 5000 U/mL or a solution containing trimethoprim 5 mg/mL, ethanol 25% and Ca-EDTA 3%. The rate of central line associated bloodstream infection in the trimethoprim, ethanol and Ca-EDTA lock solution group was significantly reduced compared to the patients assigned to heparin and the rates of catheter removal did not differ.[16] It is important to avoid the use of dedicated dialysis catheters for other uses as the lock solution can cause significant systemic coagulopathy.

CATHETER LUMEN THROMBOSIS

Catheter thrombosis is the most common cause of poor long-term function and loss of access.[17] Prophylactic warfarin can be effective at reducing thrombosis.[18] There is a risk of bleeding and a need for regular monitoring with its use. The ideal target international normalised ratio range has not been established with conflicting evidence.

Catheter malfunction caused by thrombus can be treated by lytic agents such as recombinant tissue plasminogen activator (rTPA) or urokinase.

Urokinase has been withdrawn in the USA because of safety concerns.

Poor flow can be treated by a post-dialysis lock or intra-dialysis lytic infusion. Both seem to be effective methods but again there are no randomised trial data to guide clinical practice.

Lytic agents are also used for the treatment of catheter thrombosis. An instillation of rTPA 1 mg/mL for 30 minutes restored or maintained a flow rate of greater than 300 mL/min without line reversals in 36 of 50 (72%) patients, with a second instillation restoring patency for a further four patients (80%). The majority of patients required further thrombolysis or radiological intervention in the 4-month follow-up period.[19]

The optimal dwell times for lytic agents have yet to be determined. rTPA infusions are effective even when there is an associated fibrin sheath.[20]

Tenecteplase is a new lytic agent with increased fibrin specificity, greater resistance to plasminogen activator inhibitor 1 and a relatively long half-life. A randomised study showed a 1-hour dwell of 2 mg of tenecteplase more effective than placebo in restoring flow in dysfunctional HD catheters.[21] An extended dwell improves treatment success.[22]

CENTRAL VEIN THROMBOSIS

Mural thrombus is commonly seen in the SVC and RA with CVCs. If it compromises venous return, facial and arm oedema results, which is termed *superior vena cava syndrome*. Central vein thrombus can be identified by magnetic resonance, computed tomography (CT) or conventional venography. Infusion of a fibrinolytic agent can be successful, although organised thrombus may require angioplasty and stenting.

FIBRIN SHEATHS

Fibrin sheaths cause up to 43% of catheter dysfunction.[23] Contrast injection through the dialysis line may show a filling defect near the catheter tip or retrograde flow along the external surface of the catheter (Fig. 16.1). This may be treated by infusing a fibrinolytic agent over 6 hours, mechanical stripping using a snare from the femoral vein, or catheter exchange over a guidewire.

Stripping has a high technical success rate, but the fibrin sheath frequently recurs. In a randomised trial, there was no significant difference in additional patency between percutaneous stripping or urokinase.[24] In another randomised trial, 4-month catheter patency was significantly better after catheter exchange than percutaneous stripping.[25]

If the catheter is exchanged over a guidewire, the sheath must be mechanically disrupted with an angioplasty balloon, or the new catheter will be re-inserted down the existing sheath. There are no controlled trials comparing all three techniques.

CATHETER-RELATED INFECTION

Catheter-related infection is a major cause of morbidity and mortality and is related to the duration of placement. Gram-positive bacteria are the usual cause[26] and resistant organisms such as methicillin-resistant *Staphylococcus aureus* are increasing. Catheter-associated sepsis can result in infective endocarditis, osteomyelitis, septic arthritis, epidural abscesses and death. Infection spreads either through the lumen of the catheter or along the outside from the exit site.

Infections in non-tunnelled catheters should be treated by catheter removal and systemic antibiotics. In tunnelled catheters, 90% of exit-site infections respond to oral antibiotics but intravenous antibiotics and catheter removal may be necessary for more serious tunnel infections. Systemic infections associated with tunnelled catheters can be treated initially with antibiotics, but catheter removal is usually required. A new catheter should be inserted at a different site when the systemic sepsis has settled. Catheter exchange over a guidewire is controversial, but there is some evidence that infection-free survival is similar to that after removal and delayed replacement.[27]

The cornerstone of prevention is scrupulous asepsis with regular exit-site inspection and dressing changes. Chlorhexidine and alcohol 70% provide superior asepsis to povidone–iodine 10% as an exit-site cleaning solution.[28] Mupirocin

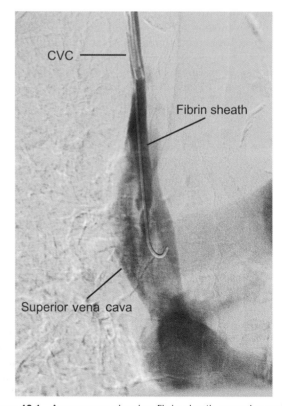

Figure 16.1 A venogram showing fibrin sheath around a partially withdrawn central venous catheter (CVC).

ointment is also effective,[29] but may increase colonisation by fungi and multi-resistant organisms. Antibiotic-coated catheters reduce line sepsis in intensive care patients[30] and temporary dialysis catheters[31] but there is no evidence of benefit for long-term dialysis as the antibiotic is washed off over time. Antibiotic catheter locks have also been used and are effective at reducing catheter infections but there is a danger of antibiotic resistance.[32] Antibiotic heparin and citrate heparin locks are superior to heparin alone but there are no randomised trials comparing antibiotic and citrate locks.[33,34]

PERMANENT DIALYSIS ACCESS

✓ An AVF should be constructed 16–24 weeks before the anticipated need for dialysis, when the creatinine clearance falls to 25 mL/min or the serum creatinine level rises above 400 μmol/L (4 mg/dL) to allow time for maturation or revision in the event of failure.[35–38]

Whereas CVCs are usually introduced on the ward or in the radiology department, peripheral arteriovenous (AV) access procedures require an operating theatre. However, most can be performed under local anaesthetic, usually as day cases.

✓ Dedicated access operating lists are an enormous advantage and one such list is required per week for every 120 patients on dialysis to prevent unacceptable waiting times and prolonged CVC usage.[5,38] Service organisation should include provision for regular interventional radiology lists to support such a service.[36,37]

ACCESS PLANNING

✓ In patients with chronic renal failure, it is essential that the cephalic and antecubital veins of both arms be reserved for dialysis access. Intravenous cannulae for other purposes should only be inserted into the back of the hand or the small veins on the anterior surface of the wrist, except in emergencies. A CVC, AVF or AVG should only be used for dialysis.[35–38]

An AVF should be created as distally as possible to preserve sites for future access. The non-dominant arm is preferred to allow greater freedom on dialysis or to facilitate self-cannulation for home dialysis patients. When upper limb access sites are exhausted, the lower limbs may be used.[35–38] Autogenous AVFs are preferable to prosthetic AVGs as they have higher patency,[39] lower infection rates, require fewer revisions[40] and are associated with a slightly lower mortality, especially in diabetics.[8,41]

Whereas a side-to-side radiocephalic AVF was originally described,[42] an end-to-side configuration is now preferred as there is less risk of peripheral venous hypertension. If a side-to-side anastomosis is used, the distal vein must be ligated to avoid venous hypertension. Some advocate an end-to-end anastomosis for distal radiocephalic AVFs, provided there is a good ulnar pulse, to reduce the small incidence of steal.[43] Autogenous AVFs require a period of maturation to allow arterialisation of the venous outflow whereas AVGs can be needled directly as soon as the wounds have healed.

PREOPERATIVE ASSESSMENT

✓ In many centres, patients proceed directly to primary AVF formation if there is a satisfactory radial pulse and suitable forearm veins. Opinion is divided on the need for preoperative imaging: the latest US National Kidney Foundation – Dialysis Outcomes Quality Initiative (NKF-KDOQI) clinical guidelines now recommend routine duplex imaging in all patients,[44] whereas the Vascular Access Society recommends a selective approach.[36]

There is an increasing trend for preoperative imaging to reduce primary failure, non-maturation and unnecessary surgery.[35–38,44] This remains untested by clinical trial.

Venography is advisable if central vein stenosis is suspected. In complex cases with unclear venous anatomy, particularly pre-dialysis patients in whom iodinated contrast could exacerbate renal failure, duplex ultrasound or magnetic resonance imaging may be preferable in the first instance. Angiography or arterial duplex is recommended if arterial pulses are diminished.

DUPLEX ULTRASOUND

Preoperative duplex ultrasound is particularly useful for obese patients with impalpable superficial veins or following previous access failure, but cannot assess central vein patency. In studies from the USA, where AVGs are more frequently used than in Europe, routine preoperative ultrasound significantly increased the prevalence, reduced early failure rate and increased primary patency of autogenous AVFs compared with historical controls.[45–47] Prosthetic AV access reconstruction and access complications also decreased significantly. In another study, duplex mapping changed the proposed procedure in a third of patients and almost doubled the proportion of AVFs constructed.[48] However, in a British study, duplex scanning rarely added any useful information except in those patients with poor vessels on clinical examination, when the proposed procedure was altered in 50%. This suggests that patients with good pulses and clinically adequate veins may proceed to surgery safely without preoperative ultrasound mapping.[49]

A radial artery luminal diameter of less than 1.6 mm is associated with early fistula failure,[50] and a minimum diameter of 2 mm is now usually advised.[36,38,44] Above this threshold, there seems to be no correlation between arterial diameter or flow and fistula success.

Venous diameter is an important determinant of outcome. In prospective studies, mean cephalic vein diameters are significantly smaller in non-functioning AVFs. Minimum venous diameters (with a tourniquet) of 2–2.5 mm have been advised for AVFs and 3.5–4.0 mm for synthetic grafts.[36,38,44]

Venous distensibility is another important predictor of success. Veins were found to dilate 48% with a tourniquet in successful fistulas compared with only 12% in fistulas that subsequently failed.[51]

VENOGRAPHY

✅ For many years, contrast venography was the gold standard and has the advantage of providing a venous map. It is mandatory in patients with prior ipsilateral central vein catheterisation, collateral vein development, oedema or arm swelling, indicating possible central vein obstruction.[36,38] Construction of a peripheral fistula in these patients can cause massive arm swelling. Previous radiotherapy to the shoulder area (e.g., for breast carcinoma) is a further indication for preoperative venography.

Iodinated contrast may precipitate acute renal failure and is relatively contraindicated in pre-dialysis patients. Duplex ultrasound is an alternative but is poor for assessing central vein stenosis. Contrast-enhanced magnetic resonance venography is promising, as the small volume of paramagnetic contrast agent used does not compromise renal function, but there have been concerns about the rare complication of nephrogenic systemic fibrosis. Imaging is likely to improve significantly with new pulse sequences and blood pool contrast agents.

Carbon dioxide venography is not nephrotoxic and is widely used in France but requires a costly injector, can cause local pain during injection, can overestimate the degree of venous stenosis and occasionally, cause acute right heart failure. New advances in technology (CO2MMANDER) have improved portability, reduced size and cost of the device.

PRIMARY ACCESS

The snuffbox AVF is the most distal access possible and gives the longest length of vein for needling. It is possible in about 50% of patients and, in the event of failure, a wrist AVF can still be performed in half of the cases[52] (Fig. 16.2).

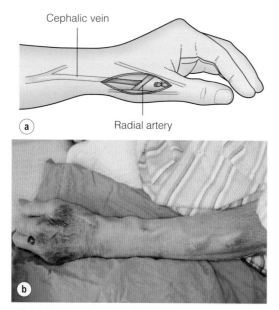

Figure 16.2 The snuffbox arteriovenous fistula. (a) Diagram showing position of anastomosis. (b) A mature snuffbox fistula showing the long length of available vein for needling.

The wrist radiocephalic AVF (Fig. 16.3) was the first to be described[42] and remains the standard access in most units. It has a low complication rate and gives a good length of available vein. Patencies of 65% at 1 year are usual.[53] If a wrist AVF fails, further forearm radiocephalic fistulas can often be created more proximally. In obese patients, the vein may remain difficult to needle so that it may be advisable to excise the subcutaneous fat overlying the vein through one or more transverse incisions. The incisions must be offset to avoid the line of the fistula as to not cause a needling challenge.

The brachiocephalic AVF is the next option, which can be performed in a variety of configurations (Fig. 16.4) and gives excellent flows at the expense of a greater incidence of steal (see later). To avoid this, some authors advocate anastomosing the cephalic vein to the radial artery 2 cm beyond its origin instead of the brachial artery itself.[54]

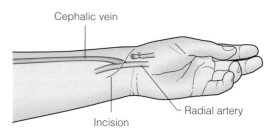

Figure 16.3 The radiocephalic arteriovenous fistula at the wrist.

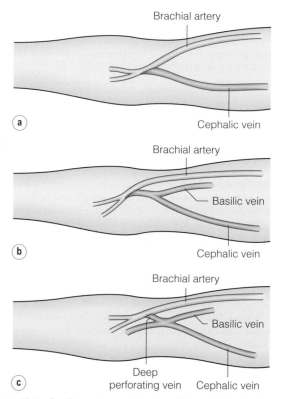

Figure 16.4 Configurations of the brachiocephalic arteriovenous fistula at the antecubital fossa. (a) Direct anastomosis between the cephalic vein and brachial artery. (b) Anastomosis including both median basilic and cephalic veins. (c) Gracz fistula between the deep perforating vein and the brachial artery.

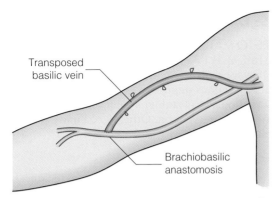

Figure 16.5 The basilic vein transposition arteriovenous fistula.

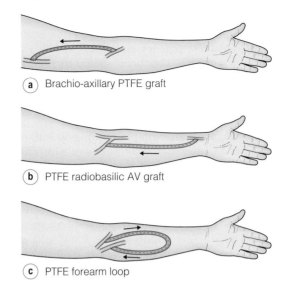

(a) Brachio-axillary PTFE graft

(b) PTFE radiobasilic AV graft

(c) PTFE forearm loop

Figure 16.6 Popular configurations for upper limb arteriovenous grafts: straight (a and b) and looped (c) brachio-axillary forearm grafts. *AV*, Arteriovenous; *PTFE*, polytetrafluoroethylene.

The ulnobasilic AVF is often possible after a failed brachial fistula but is more difficult to needle and seems to have a poorer patency than other upper limb AVFs.[55]

When the options are limited by venous thrombosis or arterial disease, an ulnocephalic or radiobasilic fistula may be possible in the forearm, but these require more extensive mobilisation and subcutaneous tunnelling of the vein across the forearm.[56]

SECONDARY AND TERTIARY ACCESS

When the cephalic vein is thrombosed, an antecubital brachio-basilic AVF may be possible but this leaves only a short length of vein for needling. Therefore the basilic vein is usually mobilised and re-routed superficially over the biceps muscle either in a single procedure or in a second stage after the vein has arterialised (the basilic vein transposition; Fig. 16.5).[57]

When an autogenous AVF cannot be performed, a prosthetic graft (AVG) can be used. A variety of graft materials are available, but polytetrafluoroethylene (PTFE) is the most popular. The graft can be used for needling after 2 weeks and may be used sooner though this can be associated with peri-graft haematoma formation. Prosthetic grafts have a higher rate of infection compared to AVF. Thrombosis is also more common than in AVF and is usually caused by intimal hyperplasia, at or just beyond the venous anastomosis. A wider graft,[58] a vein cuff[59] or an expansion of the venous end of the graft (Venoflo)[60] may reduce this and provide better patency. It is widely recognised that revision rates for grafts approach 80% annually compared to about 15% for AVF. Early cannulation grafts have now become the most popular choice as they allow grafts to be needled within 24–48 h with acceptable short-term patency rates and therefore reduce CVC usage.[61]

Biological grafts such as bovine mesenteric vein and bovine ureter are preferred in some units as they have greater resistance to infection, but they are prone to aneurysm formation.[62] A forearm AVG either in a looped or straight configuration allows a basilic vein transposition to be performed if it fails but has a poorer patency than a primary brachio-basilic fistula,[63] so which should be performed first is a matter of debate. If both cephalic and basilic veins are exhausted, an AVG can be created with the brachial veins (comitantes) being used as the outflow. A brachio-axillary AVG is the next option (Fig. 16.6).

Lower limb access is less popular but may be the only option when the SVC or both subclavian veins are occluded. An AVF at the ankle between the greater saphenous vein (GSV) and the posterior tibial artery is rarely possible because of underlying arterial disease. The GSV can be anastomosed to the popliteal artery above the knee or used as a subcutaneous loop from the femoral artery in the groin, but these are more difficult to needle and often fail to distend enough to be used for dialysis. Transposition of the GSV in the thigh is less popular as it is more difficult to needle but has fewer infective complications than synthetic thigh loop grafts.[64] The superficial femoral vein can be used in the same configurations (or transposed to the forearm) and gives an excellent fistula at the expense of a high incidence of steal. An alternative option to lower limb access is the HeRO graft. Comprising of two elements, a graft and venous outflow component, the graft is anastomosed to the ipsilateral brachial artery and tunnelled subcutaneously. The venous outflow component is placed percutaneously into the RA through the subclavian or IJV and SVC. This component is tunnelled subcutaneously towards the graft and the two elements are attached together via a titanium connector.[65]

In desperate cases, a variety of possibilities exist: axillofemoral, axillo-axillary, ilio-iliac or even aorto-IVC AVGs can be used. Where there are no available veins, the RA can be used as an outflow. Alternatively, an arterio-arterial graft, usually in the axillary position, is possible but risks distal embolisation to the arm.[66] Occlusion of arterial interposition grafts may precipitate acute limb ischaemia.

FACTORS AFFECTING ACCESS PATENCY

The following factors are known to affect access patency:

- **Vessel size.** Small arteries and veins have higher initial failure rates, more frequent failure to mature and poorer long-term patency.[50]
- **Fistula flow rate.** The flow rates the day after surgery correlates inversely with the risk of thrombosis, although

intra-operative flow rates are less reliable.[50] The hyper-aemic response of brachial artery blood flow is a strong predictor of access patency and maturation.[67] Infrared thermal imaging has also been shown to predict AVF maturation.[67]

- **Mode of presentation.** Patients presenting acutely with renal failure have poorer AVF patency, which may be linked to the need for temporary access via a CVC.[68]
- **Anastomotic method.** Non-penetrating vascular clips, which give an interrupted anastomosis with endothelial apposition and less bleeding, are quicker and have improved patencies compared with sutured anastomoses in randomised trials.[69,70] Recently, the RADAR technique whereby the radial artery is disconnected and anastomosed to the cephalic vein has shown promising results. The vascular supply to the hand and palmar arch must be imaged in detail before undertaking this technique.[71]
- **Access position.** More proximal AVFs have improved patency[70] but leave fewer options for access in the event of failure.
- **Anaesthesia.** A randomised controlled trial has shown improved primary 1 year patency rate with regional anaesthesia over local anaesthesia.[72]
- **Gender.** Patency of AVFs is poorer in women than men.[52,68,73,74]
- **Diabetes.** There is conflicting evidence as to whether diabetes is an adverse factor, with some authors suggesting that AVF patency is poorer[70] whereas others have found no effect.[52,75,76]
- **Age.** In a meta-analysis, access patency was found to be worse in the elderly.[77] Wrist fistulas may perform as well as more proximal AVF.[78]
- **Obesity.** Veins are more difficult to cannulate in obese patients, which may account for poorer patency reported by some authors.[79]
- **Smoking.** Smoking reduces AVF patency.[80]
- **Drugs.** Antiplatelet agents such as aspirin and dipyridamole prolong fistula survival and are used routinely.[81–83] A combination of aspirin and clopidogrel increased haemorrhagic complications without influencing patency in prosthetic AVGs in one study,[84] but clopidogrel alone significantly prolonged graft survival in another.[85] Warfarin reduces AVF thrombosis in patients with hypercoagulable states,[86] but routine use is best avoided because of the risk of haemorrhage. Surprisingly, warfarin was associated with poorer patency in the Dialysis Outcomes and Practice Patterns Study (DOPPS), but this may reflect its use in patients with a history of fistula thrombosis or known thrombotic disorders.[83] Calcium channel blockers are associated with improved primary patency.[83] Angiotensin-converting enzyme inhibitors did not affect primary patency in one study[87] but were associated with improved secondary patency in DOPPS.[82] Fish oil reduced AVF thrombosis in one randomised trial.[8,88] Erythropoietin does not reduce and may increase patency, at least in AVGs.[89,90] In a randomised trial, glyceryl trinitrate patches did not show to improve AVF maturation rate.[91]
- **Thrombotic tendencies and vasculitis.** Increased fibrinogen and vasculitis predispose to access thrombosis.[92]

ACCESS FAILURE

FAILURE TO MATURE

About 10% of AVFs remain patent but never achieve an adequate flow for dialysis. A duplex scan may reveal a proximal arterial or a venous stenosis, treatable by angioplasty or surgery. Occasionally, a fistulogram may be helpful in advance of planned re-intervention. Otherwise, a more proximal fistula will be required.

STENOSIS AND THROMBOSIS

Early thrombosis (10–15%) may result from technical error, unrecognised pre-existing arterial stenoses or thrombophlebitis in the outflow vein, usually from previous intravenous cannulation. Late failure can result from hypotension, dehydration and hypercoagulable states, 'blowout' after traumatic needling or inappropriate use for intravenous infusions, but the most common cause is juxta-anastomotic venous intimal hyperplasia in AVG. In AVF, failure may result from peri-anastomotic stenosis, but in long-standing AVF used for dialysis, mid-fistula stenosis between needling sites is also relatively common.

✔ Percutaneous angioplasty of stenoses in AVFs and AVGs preserves veins and may prevent access thrombosis. Stenting is controversial but probably offers little extra advantage. Endovascular thrombolysis or thrombectomy of occluded AV accesses is effective provided that any underlying stenosis is dilated.[35–38]

PREVENTION OF ACCESS FAILURE

To prevent damage, careful needling and the avoidance of inappropriate use of AVFs are essential. Attempts to prevent intimal hyperplasia pharmacologically (e.g., with drug-eluting wraps), have yet to lead to routine clinical application and no method can currently be recommended.[93,94] In a small industry sponsored trial, an external support device was found to be safe and achieved higher functional patency rate.[95]

ACCESS SURVEILLANCE

AVFs and AVGs may suddenly occlude without prior warning, resulting in hospitalisation and the need for a temporary CVC. Most of these will have unrecognised stenoses because of intimal hyperplasia. Detection by routine surveillance and treatment of such stenoses can prevent thrombosis and allow continuous use of the access.

Impending failure may be indicated by the loss of a palpable thrill, needling difficulties or a reduction in dialysis efficiency (e.g., reduced Kt/V [the volume cleared of urea/distribution volume], a reduced urea reduction ratio at each dialysis, a rising pre-dialysis serum potassium or evidence of re-circulation through the dialysis machine). Such monitoring is useful but does not identify all failing fistulas.

✔ Access surveillance is controversial but there is increasing evidence that access flow monitoring can identify stenoses in AVFs and AVGs and allow endovascular treatment to prevent access failure.

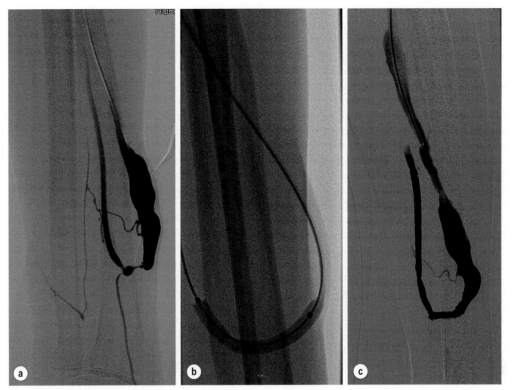

Figure 16.7   Fistulogram showing a stenosis adjacent to a radiocephalic arteriovenous fistula (a) successfully treated by angioplasty (b and c).

A variety of surveillance methods using static (with the pump turned off) or dynamic (at a standard pump speed) venous pressure measurements during dialysis have been proposed but are unreliable because the direction of any pressure change depends on whether the venous needle is upstream or downstream of the stenosis. Flow measurements are usually performed by an indicator dilution technique (e.g., ultrasound dilution).[96,97] A low flow (<500 mL/min) is a strong predictor of impending thrombosis in AVGs and is better than dynamic venous pressure.[98–100] The change in graft flow over time is a better predictor than a single value[101] and a 25% drop has been proposed as the trigger for further imaging and intervention.

Detection of stenoses is worthwhile, as intervention-free survival is better for grafts after pre-emptive angioplasty than after thrombectomy and angioplasty,[102] and vascular access flow monitoring reduces access morbidity and costs.[103] Reducing hospitalisation is an important element of providing high-quality care for renal patients.[104]

Surveillance using flow measurements also reduced thrombosis rates in AVFs in non-randomised[103,105] and randomised studies.[106] Others have failed to show improvement with surveillance but have been criticised on grounds of inadequate sensitivity[107] or inadequate angioplasty of detected stenoses.[108] Duplex surveillance also reduces thrombosis rates,[109] hospitalisation and CVC usage[110] in AVFs and AVGs.

ACCESS SALVAGE

Arteriovenous fistula stenosis

In radiocephalic fistulas, most stenoses occur close to the AV anastomosis (Fig. 16.7), with the remainder more proximally in the vein. In upper arm AVFs, they also occur at the cephalic/subclavian vein junction. Intervention is indicated for stenoses greater than 50% associated with flow reduction, compromised dialysis or arm oedema. Fistulography is usually performed through the draining vein, reserving brachial artery puncture for inflow and anastomotic lesions. The venous run-off and central veins should also be demonstrated.

Primary angioplasty is indicated for upper forearm and upper arm significant stenoses, with technical success rates of over 90% and 1-year primary patency of 51% for forearm and 35% for upper arm fistulas.[111] Secondary patencies of over 80% can be achieved but more frequent interventions are needed in the upper arm. Stents have not been shown to offer an advantage.

Stenoses in the upper arm cephalic vein (cephalic arch) are a common cause of failure in patients with brachiocephalic fistulas. These lesions respond poorly to angioplasty as they are resistant to dilatation, develop early restenosis and have high vein rupture rates. Primary patencies at 6 months and 1 year after angioplasty are 42% and 23%, respectively.[112] A small randomised trial of stent grafts versus bare-metal stents for the management of cephalic arch stenosis showed a 6-month primary patency of 81.8% for stent grafts and 39.1% for bare-metal stents.[113] There have been no randomised studies comparing angioplasty and stent placement. There is a danger of stent migration into the subclavian vein that could jeopardise future access in the whole ipsilateral limb. Surgical revision with cephalic vein transposition to the basilic or axillary veins can be considered if angioplasty fails, although this may be technically difficult in an extensively needled AVF. If recurrent stenoses are angioplastied in patients who have undergone surgical revision, secondary patency rates of 92% at 1 year can be achieved.[114]

If endovascular intervention fails, stenoses can also be repaired surgically using a vein or prosthetic patch. Alternatively, inserting a short PTFE graft segment appears to be as good as an autogenous patch.[115] Stenoses adjacent to a distal AVF are best treated by creating a more proximal fistula, which may have better patency than angioplasty.[116]

Arteriovenous graft stenosis

The most common cause for AVG dysfunction is a stenosis at or near the venous anastomosis. Indications for intervention are similar to those for AVFs, with similar high technical success rates. Restenosis is a greater problem and leads to poor primary patency rates of 23–44% at 1 year,[117] but 1-year secondary patencies of 92% can be achieved by repeated angioplasty.[111] Intra-graft stenoses from excessive ingrowth of fibrous tissue through cannulation defects can be treated similarly but may require surgical curettage or segmental replacement.

When angioplasty fails repeatedly, bare-metal stents can be considered but their primary patency is generally no better than angioplasty. There is an emerging role for covered stents in the treatment of angioplasty rupture and poor results from simple angioplasty. In one randomised trial, adding a covered stent after AVG angioplasty increased the 6-month patency from 23% to 51%.[118] However, there were similar access-assisted and cumulative patency rates at 6 months in both groups, and it remains unclear whether the high cost of stent grafts can justify their routine use.[119] There are no published randomised trials on the use of drug-eluting stents for this indication.

Unassisted graft survival after thrombectomy and angioplasty is significantly worse than after elective angioplasty of patent grafts. Graft survival after thrombectomy and angioplasty may also be improved by stent implantation,[120] but there are no prospective controlled data.

There is no evidence favouring surgical revision over endovascular repair, but revisional surgery by segmental replacement or a jump graft to bypass a venous outflow stenosis may be required for recurrent stenoses. A pragmatic approach of reserving surgery for resistant or rapidly recurring stenosis will minimise unnecessary surgical intervention.

Arteriovenous fistula and arteriovenous graft thrombosis

Percutaneous declotting of AVGs is well established and effective, but AVFs are also being increasingly referred for radiological salvage. A thrombosed access should be declotted as soon as possible, preferably within 48 hours, and the underlying stenosis treated by angioplasty (with or without stenting). Available techniques include thrombolysis, thromboaspiration and mechanical thrombectomy. None seems superior but the expertise and experience of the operator are paramount.

Thrombus in an AVF causes phlebitis. Keeping the inflammatory response to a minimum is a key component of successful intervention. Whilst AVG can be declotted up to several weeks after thrombosis, most AVF require intervention within 24–48 hours for success. The amount of thrombus can vary significantly. In some AVFs, only a short segment of vein thromboses because a side-branch just proximal to a peri-anastomotic stenosis maintains patency. These can usually be treated by simple angioplasty. In others, the large volume of thrombus in an aneurysmal draining vein has a risk of a significant pulmonary embolus unless it is aggressively aspirated or a mechanical clot-removing device is used.

Technical success is reported as 73–90%, with widely differing 1-year primary and secondary patencies of 9–70% and 44–93%, respectively.[121] Patencies are higher in the forearm than upper arm. There are no randomised trials of percutaneous intervention versus surgery for AVFs. Primary endovascular intervention has the advantage of preserving veins for needling, but surgical revision or a new AVF is often necessary.

AVGs thrombose more frequently than AVFs but are well suited to percutaneous intervention. Radiological declotting is less invasive than surgery and allows accurate treatment of the underlying cause, which is nearly always a venous outflow stenosis. No single device or declotting technique has been shown to be superior, and the success of treatment of the underlying stenosis seems to be the only predictive value for graft patency.[122] Thrombolysis or mechanical thrombectomy have clinical success rates of 74–94% but 6-month primary patencies are only 18–39%.[123] However, with repeated intervention, secondary patency rates of up to 83% have been reported.[124] Whilst there has been no prospective randomised multicentre trial, a meta-analysis found surgical intervention to have higher primary patency than endovascular intervention.[125] In many centres, endovascular declotting is preferred because of its low morbidity, preserving surgical revision for technical failures or repeated thromboses.[123]

The most common complication of endovascular declotting is distal arterial embolisation, which occurs in 1–9% of cases.[123] Others include vessel rupture (2–4%) and non-puncture site bleeding (2–3%). All methods of declotting, especially mechanical techniques, cause venous embolisation, but this is usually asymptomatic because of the small volume of thrombus displaced.

Surgical thrombectomy is usually easy if the access has failed recently. Any underlying stenosis must be corrected on table angioplasty, bypass or patch angioplasty at the same time. If surgery is delayed for 10 days or more, it may be best to abandon it and create a new access at another site.

OTHER ACCESS COMPLICATIONS

INFECTION

Infection is the commonest cause of hospital admission and mortality in dialysis patients. It is most frequent in patients with CVCs and commoner in patients with AVGs than AVFs. The most frequent organism is *S. aureus*. Bacteraemia or septicaemia may lead to endocarditis, mycotic aneurysms and septic arthritis.

Local needle-site infections may be controlled with antibiotics in the early stages but can lead to uncontrollable haemorrhage in autogenous fistulas, requiring emergency ligation or bypass of the infected area. AVGs with chronic needle-site infections or exposed segments (Fig. 16.8) may be salvaged by local excision and bypass of the area with appropriate antibiotic cover, but when the whole graft is infected, it requires total excision with insertion of a temporary CVC for dialysis. A further graft may be inserted once the wounds have healed.

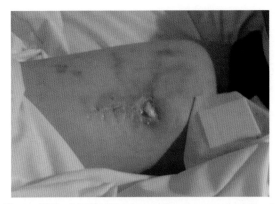

Figure 16.8   A PTFE thigh loop with an exposed segment.

Table 16.2	The stages of access steal syndrome
Stage	**Clinical features**
Is	Pale/cyanosed and/or cold hand without pain
II	Pain on exercise and/or dialysis
III	Rest pain
IV	Ulcer/necrosis/gangrene

HAEMORRHAGE

Traumatic cannulation leads to localised haematomas. Prosthetic grafts can be destroyed by repeated punctures in the same area. This may necessitate local graft explantation and replacement.

ISCHAEMIC MONOMELIC NEUROPATHY

This condition needs to be differentiated from Steal because of its long-term effects if not treated promptly. Awareness among clinical staff, along with very early recognition, diagnosis and management are essential. Usually, patients will develop acute severe hand pain in the recovery area following their access creation. The underlying aetiology is likely to be acute neuronal ischaemia. While a rare complication, the impact can be devastating. Prompt surgical ligation of the access is required to avoid permanent disability.

STEAL

An AVF tends to reduce digital arterial pressures[126] by lowering the peripheral resistance and may cause ischaemia (high-flow steal). The presence of a proximal arterial stenosis will amplify the reduction in finger pressures on AVF creation by limiting the increase in inflow (low-flow steal).

Mild steal symptoms, such as coldness, pain, cramps, diminished sensation or reduced grip strength, are common in patients with AVFs. At least one symptom is present in 80% of brachial AVFs, 50% of those with forearm AV loops and 40% of radiocephalic AVFs,[127] but clinically significant steal with rest pain or tissue loss occurs in only 1–8% of patients.

Four grades of steal are recognised (Table 16.2). Grades 1 and 2 can usually be managed conservatively, but grades 3 and 4 require surgical intervention.

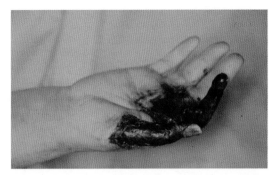

Figure 16.9   Severe steal with digital gangrene after a brachial arteriovenous fistula.

Predisposing factors include proximal AVF, diabetes mellitus, cardiac ischaemia, peripheral vascular disease[128,129] and low preoperative finger pressures.[126] Steal is the most likely cause of unilateral hand or finger ischaemia occurring after AVF creation (Fig. 16.9).

The clinical diagnosis can be made by a clear history of steal associated with the finding of an absent radial pulse that returns when the fistula is occluded. If in doubt, the diagnosis is confirmed by a digital pressure of 60 mmHg or less, with a significant increase on AVF occlusion.[130] A digital:brachial pressure index of less than 0.4 is also associated with steal. A duplex scan will demonstrate any proximal stenosis, quantify AVF flow and show reversed flow in the artery distal to the AVF (although this is not diagnostic). Fistulography is rarely required.

Steal syndrome should be treated promptly to avoid permanent neurological sequelae. These rarely recover completely if allowed to persist for any length of time.

AVF ligation cures steal syndrome and may be the sensible course of action in severe cases with rapid onset. Clinicians should undertake this only if they are confident that alternative access can be safely provided. As the majority of patients have similar arterial and venous pathologies in all of their limbs, attempting new access in the contralateral limb may simply reproduce steal in a new site. Steal syndrome associated with arterial inflow stenosis can usually be corrected by angioplasty or surgical bypass. There are a variety of effective treatment options for steal.[131] At the wrist, radial arterial ligation distal to the fistula to prevent reversed flow is usually successful in those AVFs with an intact ulnar artery and palmar arch.

Distal arterial ligation may also be sufficient in brachial AVFs when associated with a bypass from the proximal brachial (at least 8 cm proximal to the AV fistula anastomosis) or the axillary artery to the brachial artery distal to the ligature. This will increase the distal pressure enough to relieve symptoms in most cases. This is the so-called *distal revascularisation interval ligation* (*DRIL*) procedure[132] (Fig. 16.10).

Another technique to prevent distal reversed flow is 'proximalisation of the arterial inflow' in which a brachial AVF or AVG is taken down and a prosthetic graft is led from the axillary or proximal brachial artery and anastomosed to the outflow vein or the arterial end of the AVG[133] (Fig. 16.11). This preserves fistula flow but transfers the inflow to a larger, high-flow artery capable of adapting to

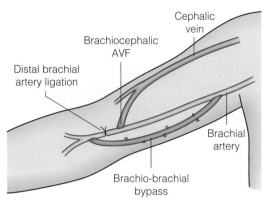

Figure 16.10 The DRIL (distal revascularisation interval ligation) procedure. *AVF,* Arteriovenous fistula.

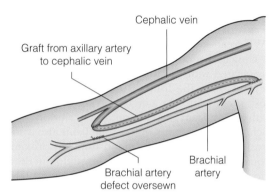

Figure 16.11 Proximalisation of the arterial inflow.

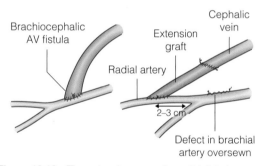

Figure 16.12 The extension procedure. *AV,* Arteriovenous

the reduction in peripheral resistance without distal flow reversal. This may be useful in patients where a diseased run-off might compromise the distal revascularisation of a DRIL procedure.

An alternative flow-reduction method is the 'extension procedure',[134] which is also known as the '*revision using distal inflow*' (*RUDI*),[135] in which the cephalic vein or AVG is detached from its origin on the brachial artery and extended onto the radial artery 2–3 cm from its origin using a vein or prosthetic graft. This narrows the inflow and permits hand perfusion through the ulnar artery (Fig. 16.12). The choice of procedure depends on experience and personal preference.

Fistula flow can be reduced by narrowing the outflow vein ('banding') but achieving the appropriate degree of stenosis is difficult. It is not uncommon to either narrow the outflow

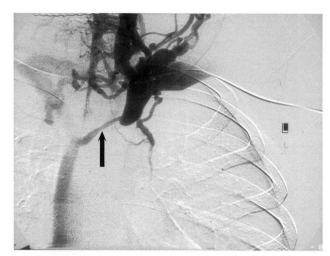

Figure 16.13 Venogram showing an innominate vein stenosis.

sufficiently to cause thrombosis, or to fail to reduce flow and relieve the steal. However, in a recent report, the degree of stenosis was successfully controlled by tightening a polyester band in stages whilst monitoring the flow rate, digital pressures and subclavian venous oxygen saturation.[136] In another report, banding was accomplished by a spindle-like suture and a PTFE strip during intra-operative flow monitoring.[137]

CARPAL TUNNEL SYNDROME

The incidence of carpal tunnel syndrome is increased by the presence of an AVF, possibly owing to mild oedema because of venous hypertension.[138]

CARDIAC FAILURE

High-output cardiac failure is a rare complication, occurring occasionally with proximal AVFs with fistula flows in excess of 1.5 litres per minute. Underlying heart disease and anaemia are important predisposing risk factors. Bramham's sign (slowing of the heart rate on AVF compression) confirms the diagnosis. Treatment is either by fistula ligation or flow reduction by the extension procedure or controlled banding.[136]

VENOUS HYPERTENSION AND CENTRAL VEIN OBSTRUCTION

Venous hypertension with oedema, venous collateral formation, or ulceration and tissue loss can occur with side-to-side AVFs but is more commonly associated with central venous obstruction (Fig. 16.13). If venous hypertension occurs with a side-to-side AVF, ligation of the distal vein draining the AVF is easy to perform and usually curative.

An AVF distal to a central obstruction is likely to exacerbate venous hypertension and may precipitate symptoms. This will develop over a short period of time after AVF formation as the fistula matures. Treatment of central vein obstruction by endovascular means or, as a last resort, surgical bypass will preserve the AVF, but sometimes the access must be ligated and created elsewhere, usually in the lower limb.

Subclavian stenosis or thrombosis is usually caused by a previous subclavian CVC. IJV catheters are now preferred to avoid this complication but there is still a significant

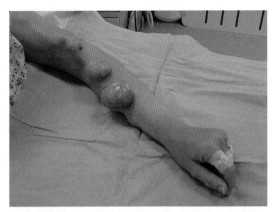

Figure 16.14 An aneurysmal wrist arteriovenous fistula.

incidence of innominate and SVC stenosis (see Fig. 16.13) or thrombosis. Endovascular treatment of these lesions is ideal, but simple angioplasty has a disappointing primary patency rate at 1 year of less than 40% in most studies.[7] Primary assisted or secondary patency rates are more encouraging at 35–97%.[139] Drug-eluting technology has shown some promise but more research is required to advocate its routine use.[140] Stents have a major role and can either be routinely placed at the initial intervention or reserved for early and frequent re-stenosis. There are no randomised trials of stents versus standard angioplasty. There is no evidence at present advocating covered stents.

Surgical bypass gave a similar primary patency rate (70–80%) at 1 year to primary angioplasty and stenting in one study,[141] but has significant morbidity and mortality and is therefore rarely performed. Isolated subclavian vein occlusions may be repaired surgically by direct patch angioplasty, an axillo-jugular venous bypass or the jugular turndown operation.

SVC obstruction is best treated endovascularly, often requiring stent insertion to achieve patency. The symptomatic relief for the patient is immediate. Surgical bypass is a major undertaking with significant morbidity and should be regarded as a last resort in younger patients. Surgical incisions in an engorged neck can be associated with significant venous bleeding.

ANEURYSM

The AVF outflow vein usually hypertrophies but sometimes reaches aneurysmal proportions (Fig. 16.14). In general, such aneurysms can be observed, as rupture is rare. Indications for intervention are rapid or persistent enlargement, skin breakdown with or without bleeding and patient request. The psychological effects of large and unsightly access in younger patients should not be underestimated. Surgical aneurysmorrhaphy can significantly reduce the bulk of AVF whilst excising damaged skin and preserving the AVF for use.

There is debate as to whether mesh wrapping of the aneurysmorrhaphy is required, but this has not been formally tested.[142,143] A recently published systematic review has shown that patency rate was similar for aneurysmorrhaphy performed with a stapler and without.[144]

There is interest in the use of covered stents for exclusion of pseudo-aneurysms, but this has not been formally tested in a clinical trial. However, this method has proven to be both safe and the results have been encouraging so far.

CANNULATION

Cannulation of AVFs should be performed by adequately trained staff under strict aseptic conditions. A new autologous AVF is usually rested for at least 6 weeks before needling, to allow the vein wall to thicken, although early cannulation did not appear to be a risk factor in the DOPPS.[145] There may be cultural differences, with a tendency to earlier needling in Japan. An experienced dialysis nurse should always perform the first cannulation and ultrasound guidance can be useful. Prosthetic grafts are needled directly and are usable for dialysis once the post-operative swelling and seroma have settled usually at around 2 weeks.

There are three major strategies:

- The buttonhole technique, where the same site is needled at each dialysis, which is less painful and causes less aneurysm formation but is less suitable for grafts because it can cause local graft destruction.
- Area puncture, where the vein or graft is needled over a specific area for each of the withdrawal and re-infusion sites, results in venous dilatation over an area but can also cause stenoses between aneurysmal sections. Area puncture has been shown to be associated with a high risk of access failure and therefore should be avoided.
- The rope-ladder technique, where needles are inserted for each dialysis by moving along the vein or graft in a sequential pattern. This is probably most suitable for AVGs as the damage of repeated needling is distributed over a larger area and delays the need for revision.

ACCESS IN CHILDREN

The small calibre of the vessels has discouraged many surgeons from constructing AVFs in small children. Alternative methods such as continuous ambulatory peritoneal dialysis are therefore preferred in many units, but when HD is unavoidable, CVCs are commonly used. However, excellent results of radiocephalic or brachial AVFs constructed by microsurgery in small children have been reported from experienced units.[146] There are technical challenges, which include small vessel size and the paediatric tendency for vessels to go into spasm.

NEW DEVELOPMENTS

Early results with newly approved devices to create percutaneous AVFs suggest that they have adequate patency rates without compromising conventional surgical sites for future dialysis access creation.[147]

ACCESS FOR NON-RENAL INDICATIONS

It is also important for vascular surgeons to be aware that AVFs can be created for non-renal indications, these include plasmapheresis, parenteral nutrition and long-term vascular access for patients requiring recurrent infusions.

ACKNOWLEDGEMENT

This text is based on the earlier chapter by Peter W.G. Brown and David C. Mitchell in the sixth edition of this volume.

Key points

- The veins of the dorsum of the hand should be the preferred site for intravenous cannulation. The cephalic and antecubital veins should be reserved and protected for dialysis access in patients with renal failure.
- The right IJV is the preferred site for central venous cannulation, which should be performed under ultrasound control with a Seldinger technique.
- The use of CVCs for acute or short-term dialysis should be minimised because of the risks of septic complications, central venous thrombosis and a higher morbidity and mortality than AVFs.
- Tunnelled CVCs should be used for dialysis if required for longer than 2 weeks but should only be used long term when an AVF or AVG cannot be constructed.
- Permanent vascular access should, wherever possible, be constructed 16–24 weeks before the anticipated need for dialysis.
- For permanent dialysis access, an autogenous AVF should be constructed as distally as possible, preferably in the non-dominant arm.
- AVGs should be used only when the construction of an autogenous AVF is not possible.

References available at http://ebooks.health.elsevier.com/

KEY REFERENCES

[13] Mallory DL, McGee WT, Shawker TH, et al. Ultrasound improves the success rate of internal jugular vein cannulation: a prospective, randomised trial. Chest 1990;98:157–60. PMID: 2193776.

In this prospective randomised trial, ultrasound was shown to increase the success rate and reduce the complications of internal jugular cannulation.

[39] Huber TS, Carter JW, Carter RL, et al. Patency of autogenous and polytetrafluoroethylene upper extremity arteriovenous hemodialysis accesses: a systematic review. J Vasc Surg 2003;38:1005–11. PMID: 14603208.

A review and meta-analysis comparing 34 non-randomised studies of upper limb AV access showing a significantly better primary patency for autogenous AV fistulas at 6 months (72%) and 18 months (51%) than PTFE AV grafts (58% and 33%, respectively).

[40] Hodges TC, Fillinger MF, Zwolak RM, et al. Longitudinal comparison of dialysis access methods: factors for failure. J Vasc Surg 1997;26:1009–19. PMID: 9423717.

A large retrospective single-centre study showing similar secondary patency for autogenous and prosthetic access but a much higher revision rate for AV grafts.

[41] Astor BC, Eustace JA, Powe NR, et al. Type of vascular access and survival among incident hemodialysis patients: the Choices for Healthy Outcomes in Caring for ESRD (CHOICE) Study. J Am Soc Nephrol 2005;16:1449–55. PMID: 15788468.

A large non-randomised multicentre study on the outcome of different forms of AV access, showing a relative mortality for CVCs of 1.5 and prosthetic access 1.2 in comparison with autogenous AV fistulas.

Varicose veins 17

Manjit S. Gohel

INTRODUCTION

Varicose veins are extremely common and part of a spectrum of chronic venous disorders. The management of venous disease is a major cause of healthcare expense in the UK National Health Service (NHS) and worldwide.[1,2] The enormous impact of venous disease, including varicose veins on patient quality of life is widely acknowledged.[3,4] As venous disease may present in many different ways, a variety of clinical teams may be involved in the management of patients with chronic venous disorders and associated complications, including vascular surgeons, dermatologists, plastic surgeons, primary care teams, tissue viability staff and other specialists. A widespread appreciation of the growing prevalence and importance of chronic venous disease has driven a wave of research and innovation in venous diagnostics and treatment modalities.

Optimal patient management involves a detailed holistic patient assessment, evaluation of patient expectations and minimally invasive, multimodal therapy to address underlying haemodynamic abnormalities and reduce venous hypertension.

PATHOPHYSIOLOGY

NORMAL VENOUS FUNCTION

The venous system of the legs returns deoxygenated blood from the capillary beds to the right atrium via low-pressure, high-capacity venous channels. Muscle pumps located in the calf and foot promote venous flow towards the heart, which is maintained by unidirectional valves throughout, predominantly the peripheral venous system. Retrograde flow (away from the heart) is termed *venous incompetence* or *reflux* and is usually secondary to damage to the venous valves.

CHRONIC VENOUS HYPERTENSION

The underlying cause of venous disease is chronic venous hypertension. Persistent high venous pressure causes pathophysiological changes leading to the clinical manifestations of chronic venous disease. A common cause is superficial venous reflux secondary to vein valve incompetence, but other factors contributing to chronic venous hypertension may include deep venous reflux, venous outflow obstruction (post-thrombotic, non-thrombotic or extrinsic compression), calf

muscle pump failure (usually because of ankle stiffness or poor calf muscle bulk), leg dependency or patient obesity.[5] The clinical consequences of venous reflux depend not only on the severity of reflux, but also on other factors contributing to venous hypertension (Fig. 17.1) and the effectiveness of measures that reduce venous hypertension (elevation, compression, calf muscle pump activity). The dogma that venous skin changes and ulceration are caused by deep venous disease, whereas superficial venous reflux causes varicose veins has been disproved in recent years; anatomical studies have clearly demonstrated that patients with chronic venous ulceration often have superficial reflux only.[6]

DEVELOPMENT OF VARICOSE VEINS

Varicose veins are usually caused by superficial venous reflux affecting the great saphenous vein (GSV) (Fig. 17.2), small saphenous vein (SSV), accessory saphenous or non-truncal veins.[7] Whether the valve failure is a primary phenomenon or secondary to vein wall dilatation is debatable.[8] Two theories have been proposed to explain the development of superficial venous reflux leading to varicose veins. The 'descending theory' was popularised by Trendelenburg in the 19th century and suggests that superficial venous incompetence begins at the saphenous junctions and progresses distally, with sequential failure of valves. The 'ascending theory' advocates the proximal progression of distal venous incompetence and is supported by the observation that superficial venous incompetence often occurs with a competent saphenous junction.[9] Although both explanations have merits and proponents, the development of varicose veins is likely to be multifactorial.[10] Tortuous, dilated veins seen in patients with deep venous obstruction are often important collateral vessels and should not be confused with varicose veins.

EPIDEMIOLOGY AND NATURAL HISTORY

The incidence of venous disease in the population has been evaluated by several large European population studies.[11–14] These observational studies demonstrated that most adults have reticular or thread veins (CEAP C1), whereas varicose veins or more severe stages of venous disease (CEAP C2–C6, see Box 17.1) are present in 25–40% of the population. Venous disease is more common in more industrialised countries, possibly because of higher life expectancies and differences in lifestyle and activity. Interestingly, deep reflux

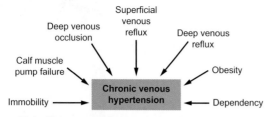

Figure 17.1 Factors contributing to chronic venous hypertension.

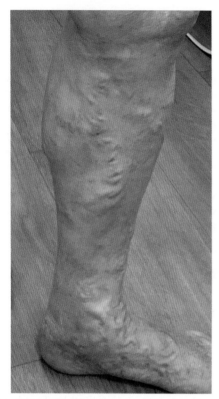

Figure 17.2 Typical varicose veins secondary to reflux in the great saphenous vein (CEAP C2).

was more common in men, whereas superficial reflux had a higher incidence in women.[12,15] Overall, the incidence of venous disease was similar in males and females, which is contrary to most clinical studies, where a female preponderance of 3–4:1 is commonly reported. This discrepancy may reflect gender differences in symptoms experienced, or in the threshold to seek medical advice. The prevalence of chronic venous ulceration (CEAP C6) is 0.3–1.0% in the adult population and venous skin changes (CEAP C4–C5) were present in 5–10%. Although the progression of venous disease is poorly understood, between 3% and 7% of patients with venous skin changes (CEAP C4) are thought to progress to venous ulceration per annum. In general, the greater the patient age, the higher the prevalence and the more advanced the chronic venous disease.[11]

CLINICAL PRESENTATION

Patients with venous disease may seek medical help for a variety of reasons. In the Edinburgh Vein Study, patients reported an inconsistent and gender-dependent association between lower limb 'venous' symptoms (heaviness/tension, feeling of swelling, aching, restless leg, cramps, itching, tingling) and the presence and severity of thread, reticular or varicose veins. Although there may be considerable discordance, venous symptoms correlate with severity of venous reflux on duplex imaging.[15,16] The CEAP classification was devised in 1994, revised most recently in 2020. It offers a useful classification tool to describe a patient using Clinical, aEtiological, Anatomical and Pathophysiological criteria (see Box 17.1).[17] The clinical component of the CEAP classification is often used in isolation. It should be noted that the CEAP classification is a descriptive tool and is not intended for monitoring progression of disease or response to treatment. Other recognised scoring systems include the venous clinical severity score (VCSS)[18] and venous disability score (VDS). In recent years, there has also been a growing interest in patient reported outcomes and quality-of-life scores, which are likely to be most useful for evaluating success after venous interventions.[19]

THREAD VEINS AND RETICULAR VEINS (CEAP C1)

These small, superficial veins may be highly visible and can cause cosmetic concern (Fig. 17.3) or symptoms. Thread veins (also known as *spider veins, telangiectasia, venous flare*) are <1 mm, whereas veins of 1–3 mm are termed *reticular veins*. Superficial, tortuous veins >3 mm are considered varicose veins. Although not usually funded by state healthcare systems, these veins can be effectively treated using injection sclerotherapy or laser techniques. In general, significant underlying superficial reflux should be addressed before treating thread veins.

VARICOSE VEINS (CEAP C2)

Varicose veins are superficial, dilated and tortuous veins usually caused by superficial venous reflux (see Fig. 17.2). They are usually seen below the knee, but are also common in the thigh, with the precise location depending on the anatomical distribution of the underlying venous reflux. Most varicose veins are caused by an incompetent GSV, although SSV reflux is the cause in around 20% of patients.[9] Up to a quarter of patients have had previous varicose vein intervention, with the new veins either truly recurrent veins, residual veins not treated in the previous intervention or de novo varicose veins arising in a new distribution. Some patients may have varicose veins because of an incompetent perforating vein, refluxing pelvic/abdominal or other, unnamed, veins. It should be noted that in thin patients, or those with an athletic physique, superficial veins may be very prominent. However, these veins are usually straight and physiological, rather than abnormal.

OEDEMA AND SKIN CHANGES (CEAP C3–C4)

Venous oedema occurs secondary to increased hydrostatic pressure from chronic venous hypertension. The lymphatic system is unable to adequately drain the increased volume of interstitial fluid. This usually occurs around the ankle but may involve the foot and leg. Swelling is often worse after prolonged standing and towards the end of the day. Isolated oedema because of venous disease is unusual, in the absence of other signs of venous disease. Non-venous causes of oedema, including lymphoedema and cardiac failure, should be considered and may co-exist with venous disease.

Box 17.1 CEAP classification

Clinical classification

C0: no visible or palpable signs of venous disease
C1: telangiectasias or reticular veins
C2: varicose veins
C3: oedema
C4a: pigmentation or eczema
C4b: lipodermatosclerosis or atrophie blanche
C5: healed venous ulcer
C6: active venous ulcer
s: symptomatic, including ache, pain, tightness, skin irritation, heaviness and muscle cramps, and other complaints attributable to venous dysfunction
a: asymptomatic
r: recurrent

Aetiological classification

Ec: congenital
Ep: primary
Es: secondary (post-thrombotic)
En: no venous cause identified

Anatomical classification

As: superficial veins
Ap: perforator veins
Ad: deep veins
An: no venous location identified

Pathophysiological classification

Pr: reflux
Po: obstruction
Pr,o: reflux and obstruction
Pn: no venous pathophysiology identifiable

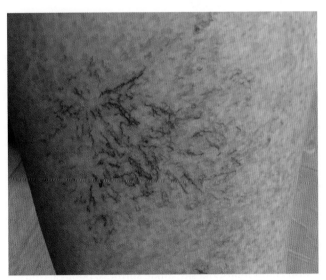

Figure 17.3 Typical reticular and thread veins.

Chronic venous hypertension is associated with a number of skin changes (Fig. 17.4), including:

- **Venous eczema (also known as 'venous stasis dermatitis').** Itchy, dry and scaly skin is a common early skin change caused by venous hypertension. As with most venous skin changes, eczema often occurs on the medial aspect of the lower leg (the 'medial gaiter area'). While symptoms may be improved with topical creams, eczema is likely to persist or deteriorate unless the underlying causes of venous hypertension are addressed.
- **Haemosiderinosis and skin pigmentation.** Chronic venous hypertension may lead to extravasation of red blood cells, resulting in pigmentation because of haemosiderin deposition in the subcutaneous tissues. There may be an associated inflammatory response, which can mimic cellulitis (see section on Lipodermatosclerosis later). Once the inflammation has settled, pigmentation is usually permanent, despite subsequent venous treatment.
- **Lipodermatosclerosis.** Chronic venous hypertension and inflammation may result in fibrosis and thickening of the skin and subcutaneous fat in the lower leg, with the classic 'inverted champagne bottle' appearance. Acute inflammation caused by venous hypertension may be referred to as '*acute lipodermatosclerosis*'. As with haemosiderinosis, chronic skin and subcutaneous changes are generally considered irreversible. The primary aim of venous treatment is usually to reduce symptoms, improve patient quality of life and prevent disease progression.
- **Corona phlebectatica.** Also referred to as '*malleolar flare*' or '*ankle flare*', this refers to a leash of prominent intradermal veins, located around the medial malleolus. The skin is often fragile, and patients may progress to venous ulceration.
- **Atrophie blanche.** Literally translated as 'white atrophy', this refers to a pale, smooth scarring, often associated with telangiectasia that may occur at the site of previous ulceration. Patients with atrophie blanche have a high risk of developing venous ulceration.

CHRONIC VENOUS ULCERATION: HEALED OR ACTIVE (CEAP C5–C6)

Venous ulceration is the commonest cause of leg ulceration and is considered the worst extreme in the spectrum of chronic venous disorders. Venous ulcers are distressing for patients, expensive to manage and challenging to treat. The estimated prevalence is 0.3–1% of the adult population in Western countries, with an increased prevalence in patients >65 years.[20,21] A chronic venous ulcer may be defined as a full-thickness defect of the skin, occurring primarily because of chronic venous hypertension, of >4 weeks' duration, but where there are clear signs of venous hypertension, treatment should be commenced as soon as a wound is present. The medial aspect of the lower leg (the medial gaiter area) is the most common location and other signs of chronic venous hypertension are frequently present, helping to differentiate chronic venous ulcers from other causes of leg ulceration. Ulcers are usually superficial and although a healthy granulating base is commonly seen, healing times are generally protracted, with the median healing duration of 4–6 months. As venous ulcers often affect elderly and frail patients, other factors contributing to poor wound healing (medication, comorbidity, poor nutrition) are frequently present in addition to chronic venous hypertension.

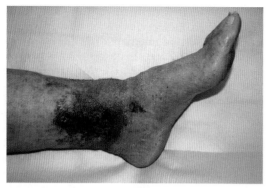

Figure 17.4   Advanced skin changes secondary to chronic venous hypertension.

✓ Varicose veins are part of a spectrum of venous disease caused by chronic venous hypertension.

✓ The CEAP classification is an important descriptive tool for patients with venous disease.

COMPLICATIONS OF VARICOSE VEINS

In addition to the clinical manifestations described earlier, there are specific complications of varicose veins that are important to recognise.

Bleeding varicose veins

Superficial varicosities may be a cause of significant bleeding either spontaneously or after minimal trauma. Initial care should consist of first aid measures such as elevation and direct pressure. However, fatalities caused by haemorrhage from varicose veins have been reported, often in elderly and vulnerable patients with poor mobility who are unable to bend down to apply direct pressure to the bleeding point. Bleeding varicose veins should be considered an emergency and intervention should be planned urgently. A localised sclerotherapy procedure may be useful as a primary procedure.

Superficial vein thrombosis

Patients may present with pain, redness and hard swelling over varicosities or truncal superficial veins. Traditionally, superficial vein thrombosis (SVT, previously referred to as 'phlebitis' or 'thrombophlebitis') has been considered a benign pathology and managed in primary care with analgesia or antibiotics. However, in recent years, it has become clear that the natural history of SVT is much more aggressive than previously appreciated. At the time of diagnosis, around a quarter of patients with SVT have deep vein thrombosis (DVT) or pulmonary embolism (PE, often remote from the site of SVT) and recurrent venous thromboembolism (VTE) events are common. It is clear that the presence of SVT probably signifies a more prothrombotic tendency. Recent guidelines have focussed specifically on the diagnosis and management of SVT[22] and anticoagulation (either prophylactic dose or therapeutic dose, depending on the extent of the SVT) if often indicated. Residual superficial venous reflux should be treated (see treatment section) once the acute inflammation has resolved, after 3 months.

CLINICAL ASSESSMENT

HISTORY

When assessing patients with venous disease, a detailed history of the presenting symptoms should be recorded and potential non-vascular causes should be excluded (particularly orthopaedic, spinal and arterial disorders). It is important to describe the impact of symptoms on patient quality of life as the decision to treat, choice of treatment modality and funding approval may all be guided by these considerations. Cosmetic appearance is a common concern and should always be a consideration when planning intervention, although this is rarely enough for treatment to be approved in state-funded healthcare systems. Other common symptoms include heaviness, aching, burning, itching, swelling, restless legs, cramping or 'tingling'. The correlation between the size of veins and the severity of symptoms reported by the patient is often poor. This patient group accounts for a significant proportion of medicolegal claims in surgical specialties.[23] Unhappiness after treatment is often caused by recurrent/residual varicose veins or neurological symptoms.

Patients should be asked specifically about the following:

- history of DVT;
- history of thrombophilia or major risk factors for previous DVT;
- use of oestrogen-containing medications (combined oral contraceptive pill, hormone replacement therapy or tamoxifen);
- details of previous venous interventions (open or endovenous).

PATIENT EXAMINATION

Patients should be evaluated in the standing position to allow filling of varicosities. Most of the required clinical information can be elucidated from inspection alone. Both legs should be examined, in addition to the groins and lower abdomen. The following features should be specifically assessed and documented:

- distribution and extent of varicosities (the examiner should specifically document the presence of a saphenovarix and other particularly large or troublesome varicosities);
- presence of skin changes of chronic venous disease (oedema, pigmentation, lipodermatosclerosis, ulceration);
- arterial status (presence of pulses, ankle–brachial pressure index or toe pressures);
- scars and evidence of previous venous interventions;
- other factors potentially contributing to venous hypertension (immobility, obesity, ankle stiffness, poor calf muscle bulk);
- general patient status and suitability for an intervention (fitness, mobility);
- Chronic venous skin changes and ulceration may be present without visible varicose veins, but where chronic venous hypertension is evident, appropriate venous investigations should be performed to detect potentially treatable superficial or deep venous disease.

HAND-HELD DOPPLER AND OTHER BEDSIDE TESTS

The accuracy and widespread availability of colour venous duplex scanning has meant that hand-held Doppler assessment of veins should not be used to guide venous interventions and are rarely used in modern practice. Other bedside tests, such as the Trendelenburg test or tourniquet test, are well described in clinical textbooks, but rarely used in routine practice.

VENOUS INVESTIGATIONS

The primary goal of venous investigations is to identify treatable superficial and deep venous disease, although in some atypical cases, investigations may help to make the diagnosis of venous disease. A wide range of tests are available, but clinicians should adopt a pragmatic, stepwise approach starting with cheap, non-invasive investigations and avoiding radiation where possible.

COLOUR DUPLEX ULTRASOUND SCANNING

Colour duplex ultrasound scanning (DUS) is the first-line and gold standard investigation for patients with venous disease.[24] In trained hands, use of this non-invasive imaging modality can accurately identify the presence of reflux or occlusion in deep and superficial veins, and assess for arterial disease. Increasing availability and reducing cost of duplex machines has meant that appropriately trained vascular surgeons are able to perform scans in the outpatient clinic and during interventions to improve outcomes. Routine duplex imaging before venous intervention should be considered mandatory.[25]

DUS is increasingly considered an almost routine extension of the clinical examination (Fig. 17.5) and modern vascular training programmes include specific duplex ultrasound components. For the assessment of venous disease, specific advantages include:

- accurate evaluation of pattern of superficial reflux (including incompetent perforating veins);
- identification of deep venous disease (obstruction and reflux);
- assessment of suitability of superficial veins for endovenous intervention and assistance in identifying the best modality for treatment (see 'Treatment' section);
- accurate evaluation of recurrent varicose veins;
- identification of anatomical variants.

There is good justification for the use of DUS post-intervention for quality control and prognostication (higher risk of recurrent symptoms with residual reflux). However, economic considerations have meant that routine follow-up with DUS after superficial venous intervention is uncommon in the UK.

✔ All patients being considered for superficial venous intervention should undergo colour venous duplex imaging performed by an appropriately trained professional.

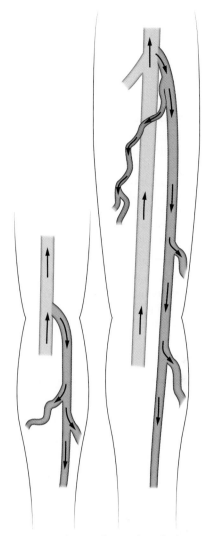

Figure 17.5 Example of report from colour duplex scan for patient with varicose veins. Reflux is present in the great saphenous vein (GSV) and small saphenous vein (SSV) arising from saphenofemoral and saphenopopliteal junctions.

OTHER VENOUS INVESTIGATIONS

While DUS is often the only investigation needed to plan intervention for varicose veins, other diagnostic modalities may be useful in specific circumstances.

Computerised tomography or magnetic resonance venography

Cross-sectional imaging techniques can accurately visualise iliac veins, the inferior vena cava and may help identify sources of pelvic vein incompetence.

Transvaginal ultrasound

In patients with varicose veins with a possible pelvic source, or in patients with pelvic pain, transvaginal ultrasound may supplement conventional DUS and provide additional information about the presence of pelvic vein reflux (in ovarian or internal iliac veins). Currently, this has a limited role as the technique is highly user-dependent, more invasive than conventional DUS and, most importantly, the clinical significance of pelvic or ovarian vein reflux is unclear.

Diagnostic venography (or phlebography)

Traditional diagnostic venography for the assessment of superficial veins has virtually no role in modern clinical practice. However, venography may have a role in the assessment of patients with suspected pelvic venous reflux or deep venous outflow obstruction.

Haemodynamic assessments

Tools to assess venous haemodynamics may be able to assess the level of physiological venous dysfunction. Ambulatory venous pressure monitoring is considered the gold standard, but is invasive and generally limited to research use. Potential clinical benefits of digital photo-plethysmography, air plethysmography and other minimally invasive assessments of venous hypertension have been reported, but these techniques are rarely used in routine practice.

Intra-vascular ultrasound

Intra-vascular ultrasound (IVUS) is an excellent tool for the evaluation of venous outflow obstruction and is commonly used to guide deep venous stenting procedures.[26] IVUS may be helpful in some complex cases with mixed deep and superficial disease, but there is no role in the assessment of superficial veins.

TREATMENT

There have been significant advances in the treatment of varicose veins since 2000 and a wide range of intervention options are now available. An individualised management strategy should be considered for each patient. This may involve using multiple treatment modalities and/or more than one treatment episode, with procedures often performed under local anaesthesia in an ambulatory setting. For patients with bilateral varicose veins, opinion varies regarding the optimal approach (one-stage or multistage intervention). Patient preference should be considered, and the treatment strategy adapted accordingly. The CEAP classification is commonly used as a tool for rationing treatment and identifying which patients may get the greatest benefits. This approach is likely to be suboptimal, as CEAP is a descriptive tool only and significant quality-of-life improvements are seen after superficial venous intervention in patients with all classes of venous disease.

CONSERVATIVE OPTIONS, MEDICATIONS AND COMPRESSION

Conservative measures or compression may be the most appropriate therapy in some patients, particularly those unsuitable for or unwilling to undergo a procedure, those where the benefit of intervention may be limited or risks may be high. Specific groups where conservative therapy or compression may be preferred include:

- pregnant patients;
- elderly patients with significant co-morbidity;
- patients with mild symptoms, or symptoms that may not be caused by venous disease;
- where previous varicose vein treatments have not been beneficial;

- patients unwilling to accept the risks of surgical or endovenous interventions.

CONSERVATIVE OPTIONS

Conservative measures such as weight loss, limb elevation and reduced periods of standing may improve symptoms but may be difficult to achieve for patients in full-time employment or those with young families. Exercise should be encouraged and may have a role in improving calf muscle pump activity.

VENOACTIVE DRUGS AND PHARMACOTHERAPY

Several venoactive drugs have been studied in patients with chronic venous disease.[27] Commonly studied medications include micronized purified flavonoid fraction and suledoxide, with some promising clinical results. However, these drugs are not available in the UK or North America. Small studies have suggested potential benefits with rutins and horse chestnut seed extract, although their use is limited.

COMPRESSION STOCKINGS AND GARMENTS

Compression therapy has been used for the treatment of venous disease for centuries and remains a key component of management for patients with venous ulceration.[28] For patients with healed venous ulceration (CEAP C5), the use of elastic compression stockings has been shown to reduce the risk of recurrent ulceration. For patients with CEAP C2–C4 disease, stockings are prescribed frequently, but the evidence for benefit is less clear.

POTENTIAL BENEFITS OF COMPRESSION THERAPY INCLUDE:

- improvement of venous symptoms and patient quality of life;
- prevention or slowing of disease progression;
- aiding clinical assessment in patients where there may be uncertainty about the extent to which the symptoms are attributable to venous disease;
- concealment of visible varicosities.

Compression stockings may be classified by the subbandage pressure applied at the ankle. Using the British Standard system for classification, class I stockings apply 14–17 mmHg, class II 18–24 mmHg and class III 25–35 mmHg. In practice, patients are often unable to tolerate stockings greater than class I and many patients find class III stockings impossible to don. Before commencing compression therapy, arterial disease should be excluded (by clinical assessment ± ankle–brachial pressure index measurement). Care should be taken to fit stockings correctly and to avoid rolling down of the stocking, as this may cause pressure damage to the skin or create a tourniquet effect.

Patient compliance remains a major problem with compression stockings, as they may be itchy, hot (particularly in summer months) and difficult to don or doff, despite the availability of applicator devices. Moreover, any benefit from compression stockings only exists while they are worn, and they need to be replaced regularly. Studies have suggested that compliance may be as low as 50% overall and probably much lower with class III stockings.[29] There have been recent advances in compression therapy, with the increasing availability of adjustable compression garments or 'Velcro wraps'. These garments may be easier to wear and promote more patient independence in managing their compression.[30]

In a systematic review and meta-analysis assessing the efficacy of compression stockings, the paucity of high-quality evidence was highlighted.[31] Although many prospective studies were identified, there was significant heterogeneity in patient populations, type of compression and outcome measures evaluated. The authors concluded that wearing compression stockings improved patient symptoms, although selection bias could be a confounding factor. Compression was also found to reduce oedema, but the suggestion that wearing compression can slow the progression or reduce recurrence after intervention was not supported by the published literature.

Compression therapy is the mainstay of treatment for patients with chronic venous ulcers and may reduce symptoms of varicose veins in other patients.

PRINCIPLES OF ENDOVENOUS AND SURGICAL INTERVENTIONS

In patients with symptomatic superficial reflux requiring treatment, the underlying principle of intervention is to remove, close or obliterate the incompetent superficial venous channel. The choice of treatment modality is often based on the personal experience of the treating physician. Before undertaking any superficial venous intervention, the clinician should have strong evidence that the superficial reflux is significantly contributing to symptoms of venous hypertension. In patients with mixed superficial and deep venous reflux, superficial venous intervention is usually safe and beneficial. Some studies have shown that the refluxing deep veins may even become competent after superficial venous intervention (possibly because the incompetent venous reservoir is removed).[32]

However, residual deep venous reflux may cause significant ongoing venous hypertension. The treatment of superficial veins in patients with venous outflow obstruction is usually not advisable, as these channels may be contributing to venous drainage, even if incompetent.

INFORMED CONSENT

Varicose vein interventions are notorious for the relatively high number of medicolegal claims following procedures.[23] Therefore the importance of informed consent is worthy of specific mention. Patients should be specifically warned of common complications and should also understand that veins may (and often do) recur. Other, modality-specific risks should also be explained (see later), both verbally and using written information. In patients with visible varicosities, they should appreciate that some residual veins may be present and their legs will not be cosmetically perfect. Specific consent forms may be useful and discussions with the patient should be clearly documented in the medical records. Patient distress and complaint after intervention is commonly driven by a disappointing clinical outcome from intervention. Therefore the patient's expectations from

treatment should be clarified before intervention and ideally match those of the treating clinician.

Varicose vein treatments are a common cause of medicolegal claims. Patient expectations from interventions should match those of the surgeon.

ENDOVENOUS THERMAL ABLATION

Endovenous procedures have largely superseded traditional, surgical interventions for varicose veins in many units and thermal ablation is widely considered the 'gold-standard' intervention for superficial venous reflux. Walk-in walk-out interventions, performed using only local anaesthesia, are feasible and expected. Perceived potential advantages of these procedures include:

- avoidance of the risks of general anaesthesia;
- improved early morbidity (no groin dissection or vein stripping) with earlier return to normal activity/work;
- ability to perform procedures in outpatient or 'office-based' settings with significant potential cost savings;
- Ability to perform procedures without stopping anticoagulation medications;
- lower risk of complications such as wound infection, nerve injury, bruising and recurrence.

Despite the drive towards endovenous treatments, surgical stripping operations are still commonly performed and critics of endovenous ablation would highlight potential disadvantages, including:

- expense of the generators, endovenous catheters and consumable items;
- learning curve associated with the new procedure;
- some patients may be unsuitable (tortuous or superficial veins);
- lack of long-term follow-up data.

The most commonly used endovenous thermal ablation techniques are endovenous laser ablation (EVLA) and radiofrequency ablation (RFA).[33] With both techniques, a fibre is used to deliver thermal energy to the incompetent superficial vein to be ablated. Devices from several different manufacturers are available and the choice of thermal ablation modality is usually down to clinician preference and cost. EVLA procedures must be performed in an appropriate clinical area complying with laser safety regulations and protective goggles must be worn during periods of activation.

SETTING AND ANAESTHESIA

Both EVLA and RFA are ideal for outpatient or 'office-based' therapy as procedures can be performed using only 'tumescent' anaesthesia. This refers to a very dilute mixture of local anaesthesia (0.1% lidocaine) with epinephrine (1:2 000 000), which is injected under ultrasound guidance to surround the truncal vein to be ablated. The use of sodium bicarbonate to neutralise the mixture reduces pain during injections.[34] The anaesthetic allows the ablation to be performed without pain, but also provides a heat buffer to protect surrounding nerves, tissues and skin. Early procedures were performed in operating theatres, but outpatient treatment rooms are commonly used for endovenous procedures.

TECHNIQUE

Accurate, colour venous duplex assessment is essential to plan and perform endovenous ablation procedures.[24] Suitability for treatment should be evaluated using duplex, ideally by the specialist performing the procedure (see Fig. 17.5). Although specific eligibility criteria vary between clinicians, veins should be straight, >3 mm in diameter and in the saphenous fascia, or deep enough to be >1 cm from the skin after infiltration of tumescent anaesthesia. The patient should be positioned in the supine position for GSV ablation and prone for SSV procedures. The stages of the procedure are summarised here:

- With the patient in the reverse Trendelenburg position, the vein to be treated is cannulated under ultrasound guidance (Fig. 17.6). The site of cannulation should ideally be at the distal point of reflux. A sheath appropriate for the catheter to be used can then be inserted.
- The endovenous ablation catheter is positioned 2 cm from the saphenofemoral (SFJ) or saphenopopliteal (SPJ) junctions under ultrasound guidance. The bed is tilted to move the patient to the Trendelenburg position.
- Tumescent anaesthesia is injected around the vein under ultrasound guidance, with the aim of creating a 'halo' of infiltration surrounding the circumference of the vein to be ablated (Fig. 17.7). Care should be taken to infiltrate between the proximal GSV and CFV and to ensure that the vein is at least 1 cm from the skin along the entire length. Tumescent injection may be facilitated by using local anaesthetic cream (to reduce the pain of injection) and an injection pump. Volumes of tumescent anaesthesia injected may vary between patients and practitioners but are typically around 75–100 mL per 10 cm of vein.
- Thermal ablation should be performed as per the instructions for use of the specific EVLA or RFA fibre being used. With experience, it is common to adapt the ablation depending on anatomical factors (such as the size and depth of the vein).
- After ablation, access site haemostasis is secured with direct pressure, successful closure of the superficial vein and patency of the deep vein should be verified with duplex and documented.

✓ During endovenous thermal ablation procedures, the vein should be cannulated at the distal point of reflux.

COMPLICATIONS

In general, the rate of complications after endovenous interventions is low. Many of the complications after EVLA and RFA are comparable to those seen after traditional surgery and other modalities.

1. Bleeding/bruising: In general, the incidence of early complications is significantly lower after endovenous procedures in comparison to traditional surgery. Significant

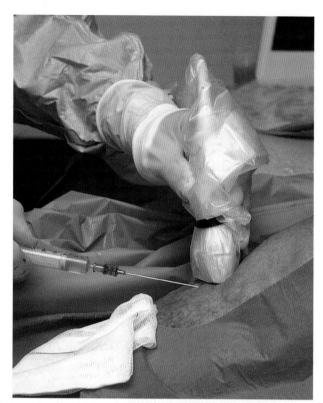

Figure 17.6   Ultrasound guided cannulation of the truncal vein to be ablated, ideally at the lowest point of reflux.

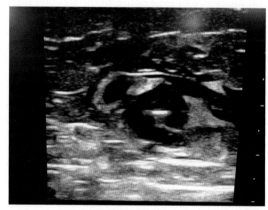

Figure 17.7   Duplex image demonstrating 'halo' of tumescent anaesthesia around truncal vein to be ablated.

discomfort or bruising is uncommon, but is probably more likely after EVLA than RFA. Pain using the newer radial laser fibres may be reduced compared to the older fibres.

2. Thromboembolic events: The incidence of DVT after RFA and EVLA is very low (<0.5%).[35] However, thrombus is sometimes seen at the SFJ or SPJ at the level of or protruding into the deep vein. This phenomenon has been termed *endovenous heat-induced thrombosis* (EHIT) and four classes have been described:[36]
   - Class 1: thrombus to the level of the deep vein, without protrusion;
   - Class 2: protrusion into the deep system, with <50% luminal occlusion;
   - Class 3: protrusion into the deep system, with >50% luminal occlusion;

- Class 4: protrusion into the deep system, with total deep venous occlusion.
3. Skin burns: Thermal injury to the skin is a complication unique to endovenous thermal ablation modalities. This usually occurs after ablating a superficial vein after inadequate tumescent anaesthesia. This may result in an area of pigmentation, although frank ulceration may also occur. This complication may be more common when treating extrafascial saphenous veins. Use of the ultrasound probe for compression during ablation may alert the operator to infiltrate more tumescent anaesthesia if the vein is too close to the skin.
4. Phlebitis: Phlebitis can occur after any venous intervention, either in the treated vein, or in associated varicosities. After endovenous thermal ablation, phlebitis is most frequently seen in varicosities, where flow may have diminished after ablation of the truncal vein.
5. Nerve injury: Although less common than in traditional surgery, areas of abnormal sensation are common after endovenous ablation. This is often an area of paraesthesia over the ablated truncal vein. Thermal injury to saphenous, sural or other nerves may occur, although the generous and accurate use of tumescence should reduce this risk. An added advantage of treating the awake patient is that they may feel pain when an EVLA or RFA catheter is near a nerve, alerting the operator. Most areas of abnormal sensation recover with conservative management.

ULTRASOUND-GUIDED FOAM SCLEROTHERAPY

Sclerotherapy is a type of chemical ablation, where the sclerosant acts on the vein wall to induce fibrosis and closure of the lumen.[37] Three broad categories of endovenous sclerosant are available: detergent (sodium tetradecyl sulphate [STS], polidocanol), osmotic (hypertonic saline, used in Europe and the USA), chemical irritant (chromated glycerine). In the UK, STS and polidocanol are in popular use, although the latter is unlicensed. In general, larger veins require a stronger concentration of sclerosant. The conversion of liquid sclerosant into foam by mixing it with air or carbon dioxide (Tessari method) has gained popularity in recent years. This approach has the advantage of increasing the potency and volume of the sclerosant, as well as making it echogenic. Ultrasound-guided foam sclerotherapy (UGFS) is an outpatient procedure usually performed without any anaesthetic.

✔✔ For the treatment of truncal veins (such as GSV or SSV), foam sclerosant is superior to liquid sclerosant.

TECHNIQUE

More than most other venous treatments, UGFS is associated with a significant learning curve. The ability to modify almost every component of the treatment (cannulation sites, volume and concentration of sclerosant) means that good training is imperative, and techniques usually evolve and improve with increasing personal experience.

- It is worth noting that sclerosant activity is reduced in contact with blood, so multiple access sites are preferable to a single injection point.

- Foam sclerosant is created by combining liquid sclerosant with air in a 1:3 or 1:4 ratio using the 'Tessari' technique (Fig. 17.8).
- With the leg elevated (to empty the veins), foam should be injected, and movement of the foam should be monitored using ultrasound.
- The patient should be encouraged to move the ankle to promote deep venous flow.

COMPLICATIONS

Thromboembolic complications and phlebitis of the treated vein may occur after UGFS. Early aspiration of painful thrombosed varicosities may be helpful. Despite being the least invasive of endovenous treatment modalities, case reports of major neurological events after UGFS have raised safety concerns.[38] There is anecdotal evidence that adverse events may be more common with larger volumes of foam injection and neurological events may be more likely in patients with regular migraines. The volume injected will depend on the specific case, but most experts would suggest that 10–12 mL (of foam) should be considered a maximum for a single session. Pigmentation or staining of the skin may occur (to varying degrees) in a significant proportion of patients. Pigmentation usually fades over 3–6 months but may be permanent in some cases.

✔ Neurological events after foam sclerotherapy have been described but are rare. The incidence of adverse events is likely to be related to the volume of foam injected and may be higher in patients with migraines.

NON-THERMAL, NON-TUMESCENT ENDOVENOUS MODALITIES

The development of non-thermal, non-tumescent endovenous interventions has been the latest innovative advance for superficial venous interventions.[39] Although not currently in widespread use, many believe that these procedures are the future for varicose vein treatment.

MECHANOCHEMICAL ABLATION

The mechanochemical ablation (MOCA) catheter is positioned within the vein to be treated. A rapidly rotating fibre

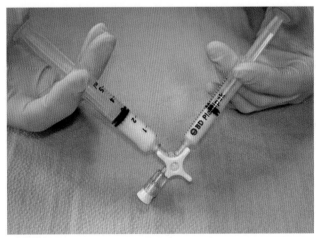

Figure 17.8 Creation of foam by mixing liquid sclerosant with air (1:4 ratio) using 2 Luer-lock syringes and a three-way tap (Tessari technique).

is activated, and the catheter is slowly withdrawn while injecting liquid sclerosant. The combination of mechanical damage to the vein wall and chemical ablation deep into the damaged wall is purported to lead to fibrosis of the vein.

CYANOACRYLATE GLUE CLOSURE

Cyanoacrylate glue has been used for a variety of medical indications for decades. In recent years, specific n-butyl cyanoacrylate preparations and customised catheters have been developed to permit endovenous use for varicose veins. Long-term evidence is awaited, but advocates believe that this offers enormous potential for virtually pain-free superficial venous treatments for the future.[40]

TRADITIONAL SURGERY FOR VARICOSE VEINS

Trendelenburg described ligation of the proximal GSV in 1890 and modifications of this technique have remained the mainstay of treatment for varicose veins for over a century. The proportion of patients treated with surgical stripping has declined, but traditional surgery remains popular in parts of Europe and lower income countries where adoption of endovenous interventions has been limited.

SETTING AND ANAESTHESIA

Traditional varicose vein operations are usually performed in a sterile operating theatre, with virtually all varicose vein operations potentially performed as day case procedures. Although most procedures are performed using general anaesthesia, regional or local techniques may also be used. Epidural/spinal anaesthesia or femoral nerve blocks can facilitate surgery, but the motor block may persist for several hours, potentially hindering same-day discharge. The routine use of prophylactic antibiotics has been shown to reduce the risk of wound complications in one randomised study.[41]

TECHNIQUE

GSV stripping is performed with the patient in the supine position, with legs in a slightly abducted position, whereas SSV surgery is usually carried out with the patient prone. A 'head down' or Trendelenburg position can reduce venous bleeding during the procedure and while a detailed description of surgical technique is beyond the scope of this chapter, some important technical principles are listed subsequently:

- In the modern era, all superficial venous interventions (including traditional surgery) should be guided by intra-operative ultrasound imaging to ensure appropriate location of incisions and technical success.
- Stripping of the GSV after groin tributary ligation and flush SFJ disconnection reduces varicose vein recurrence (compared to ligation alone).[42] Most surgeons would avoid stripping below the knee (to avoid the risk of nerve damage) and the use of tumescent anaesthesia is advisable.
- Ligation of the SSV should be performed at a safe level (not flush with the SPJ) and stripping of the SSV is controversial.
- Significant varicosities should be pre-marked in agreement with the patient and concomitant phlebectomies

should be performed (with tumescent anaesthesia) with GSV or SSV surgery.

Stripping of the GSV is an essential component of traditional varicose vein surgery.

COMPLICATIONS

Adverse events of specific relevance after traditional superficial venous surgery include:

1. Bruising/bleeding: Bruising is a very common early complication after surgery, particularly along the tract where the truncal vein (GSV or SSV) has been stripped. Bleeding requiring a return to the operating theatre is usually caused by persistent venous bleeding in the groin but is rare. Anecdotally, bruising may be reduced by using epinephrine-soaked swabs or tumescent anaesthesia with epinephrine infiltrated in the tract of the stripped vein.
2. Thromboembolic events: The incidence of DVT after traditional varicose vein surgery ranges from 0.5–5.3% in the literature. The risk of PE has been estimated at one in 60. Duplex studies have identified that many patients have small, below-knee DVTs of questionable clinical significance.
3. Nerve damage: A degree of sensory abnormality may be present in up to 40% of patients after traditional surgery, although this is rarely troublesome. True saphenous nerve injury after GSV stripping (to the knee) is likely to be <10%. The risk of sural nerve injury during SPJ disconnection is unknown but is likely to be higher. Disabling motor nerve injury may occur, particularly involving the common peroneal nerve at the head of the fibula. This may be injured during stab phlebectomy in this area.
4. Recurrence: Poor results after traditional varicose vein surgery have often been attributed to poor surgical technique by inexperienced operators. While technical failure was certainly a problem, it has become clear that even with 'technically' successful surgery, performed by experienced operators, recurrence is common. Reported recurrence rates range from 20–80% at 5–20 years, although most patients remain satisfied with surgery.

TREATMENT OF RECURRENT VARICOSE VEINS

Up to a quarter of patients presenting with varicose veins have had previous superficial venous surgery. These patients present a unique management challenge as the patterns of venous reflux may be significantly more complex than for patients with primary venous disease. Patients with more advanced clinical stages of venous disease are more likely to have recurrent varicose veins. Patients should undergo detailed clinical assessment and comprehensive colour duplex imaging to map the pattern of superficial and deep venous disease. Attention should be paid to sites and reasons for recurrent superficial reflux (such as neovascularisation, incompetent perforating veins or pelvic sources of reflux).[43] In reality, incomplete initial surgery is a common finding. Re-do groin surgery or popliteal fossa surgery is associated with an unacceptable risk of complications, including infection, seroma, DVT and nerve damage. Therefore even for enthusiastic open vascular surgeons, endovenous interventions are widely considered the first line in the treatment of patients with recurrent varicose veins, particularly in the popliteal fossa.

✓ Endovenous interventions should be considered the first line for patients with recurrent varicose veins.

EVIDENCE FOR VARICOSE VEIN INTERVENTIONS

The rapid expansion in available treatment modalities for superficial venous reflux has resulted in a confusing landscape for patients and clinicians. However, this expansion in treatments has been accompanied by a large volume of randomised and prospective clinical studies. Most comparative trials include two modalities, meaning that comparison between treatments often relies on inference.

ENDOVENOUS THERMAL ABLATION

Many studies have been conducted using EVLA and RFA interventions. A common criticism of these trials was that follow-up periods were short and outcome measures did not include patient-reported outcomes. However, there are now studies with reliable data to 5 years or longer, allowing clinicians to have greater confidence in the longer-term durability of these procedures.[44] For thermal ablation procedures, early outcomes have proved to be an accurate surrogate marker for long-term treatment success. As a result, endovenous thermal interventions have largely superseded traditional surgery as the gold standard treatment for superficial venous reflux. Based on published studies, the following broad conclusions can be drawn regarding the effectiveness of endovenous thermal ablation procedures:

- The early post-procedure outcomes (pain, bruising, time to mobilise, return to normal activity) are better after EVLA and RFA in comparison to traditional surgery.
- EVLA procedures performed using radial fibres using favourable laser wavelengths (such as 1470 nm) are probably less painful and associated with less bruising than previous generation forward-firing fibres.
- Target vein occlusion rates of >90% can be expected using RFA and EVLA procedures. Thermal ablation procedures are at least as effective as traditional surgery.
- It is difficult to distinguish between different types of RFA or EVLA devices in terms of technical success.

✓✓ Early outcomes (pain, bruising and return to normal activity) after endovenous procedures are superior to traditional varicose vein surgery.

ULTRASOUND-GUIDED FOAM SCLEROTHERAPY

UGFS has unique advantages over other modalities, as it is probably the least invasive intervention and extremely versatile. In general, the efficacy and safety of foam sclerotherapy has been clearly demonstrated by studies published over many decades. However, most comparative studies have suggested lower GSV occlusion rates in comparison to traditional surgery and thermal ablation treatments.[45,46] The use of foam sclerosant has been shown to be superior to liquid sclerosant,[47] although comparative treatment success rates for different types or concentrations of sclerosants remain unclear. Although the reported incidence of visual disturbance is <1%, there have been reports of major neurological events after UGFS resulting in some unease, not least because the mechanism of neurological adverse events is unknown.

MECHANOCHEMICAL ABLATION AND CYANOACRYLATE GLUE CLOSURE

As non-thermal, non-tumescent ablation procedures have not been available for as long as other endovenous modalities, the evidence base is less extensive. However, published randomised studies have demonstrated that both MOCA and cyanoacrylate glue have comparable technical, clinical and patient-reported outcomes in comparison to RFA.[48,49]

VARICOSE VEIN INTERVENTIONS FOR PATIENTS WITH VENOUS ULCERATION

As varicose veins are commonly seen in patients with healed or active ulceration, several trials have specifically assessed the role of superficial venous treatment in this group. In the ESCHAR trial, 500 patients with healed or active venous ulcers and varicose veins were randomised to compression therapy alone, or compression with surgical stripping of varicose veins. The study showed that surgery in addition to compression therapy significantly reduced ulcer recurrence rates (31% vs. 56% at 4 years).[6] No benefit in terms of ulcer healing was seen in this trial and a criticism was that modern endovenous modalities were not assessed.

More recently, the Early Venous Reflux Ablation (EVRA) trial evaluated the role of early (within 2 weeks of randomisation) endovenous interventions in patients with active venous leg ulcers. The results were entirely supportive of an early intervention strategy as ulcer healing rates were improved (85.6% vs. 76.3% at 24 weeks), there were fewer ulcer recurrences and the early intervention approach was not only cost-effective, but associated with cost savings.[50,51] The benefits were seen irrespective of the treatment modality used, indicating that the timing of intervention is likely to be the most important factor.

✓✓ Patients with leg ulceration should undergo early duplex ultrasound assessment and ablation of superficial reflux to accelerate ulcer healing and reduce the risk of recurrence

CHOOSING BETWEEN TREATMENT MODALITIES

The increased choice for varicose veins treatments is welcomed by patients and doctors but has led to significant confusion and heterogeneity in practice. The regular addition of new modalities, such as MOCA, cyanoacrylate glue and others, potentially compounds the confusion. Most of the available modalities are highly effective and choosing between interventions is likely to be driven by other factors such as cost, patient comfort, clinician preference and skill as well as unique advantages that specific modalities may have to suit individual circumstances. The modern treatment of varicose veins may involve several different modalities, potentially performed at the same time.

There have been large randomised studies comparing multiple treatment modalities. In the CLASS trial, 798 patients were randomised to either traditional surgery, UGFS or EVLA. The authors concluded that UGFS was associated with lower ablation rates and slightly worse disease-specific quality of life.[45] In another randomised study of 500 patients comparing EVLA, RFA, UGFS and surgical stripping, 3-year results demonstrated that re-canalisations and re-interventions were more likely after UGFS (in keeping with other studies).[52] However, UGFS is associated with improvement in patient quality of life and may be a particularly suitable modality for the often elderly and frail leg ulcer population.[53]

✔✔ Based on large randomised trials, technical success rates are likely to be best after EVLA/RFA and worst after UGFS.

To aid the decision-making of clinicians and commissioners, numerous guidelines (from the UK, Europe and the USA) have been published for the treatment of venous disease.[25,54] Some key messages are summarised subsequently:

- Treatment of varicose veins is cost-effective for symptomatic patients and those with venous skin changes or venous ulceration (active or healed).
- For the treatment of GSV reflux, endovenous thermal ablation is recommended as the first-line treatment, in preference to traditional surgery or UGFS.
- When performing EVLA or RFA, concomitant phlebectomies should be considered.
- For the treatment of recurrent varicose veins, endovenous treatments should be considered in preference to open surgery.

✔✔ Traditional surgery and endovenous interventions are likely to be cost-effective in the treatment of patients with varicose veins.

AREAS OF CONTROVERSY

MANAGEMENT OF VARICOSITIES

Many patients with varicose veins have troublesome superficial varicosities. When traditional open surgery was the dominant treatment option, superficial varicose veins were usually treated (by phlebectomy) at the time of surgery. However, the growing use of endovenous interventions, performed under local/tumescent anaesthesia in outpatient settings, has meant that treating the varicosities at the same time as truncal ablation may be less convenient or not feasible. This development has raised the question whether varicosities need to be treated at all (after saphenous ablation). Several authors have suggested that varicosities regress after truncal vein ablation and phlebectomy may be unnecessary,

particularly if the refluxing superficial truncal vein is ablated to the lowest point of reflux. However, randomised studies suggest that synchronous treatment of varicosities may also have benefits, primarily by reducing the risk of further interventions.[55] The strategies for treating varicosities are:

1. Treat at the time of truncal vein intervention.
2. Do not treat varicosities at all.
3. Review the patient after truncal vein treatment and treat varicosities if required.

Local circumstances (type of treatment room, staff skill mix, reimbursement policies) are likely to influence the management approach to varicosities as much as clinician preference. Many clinicians prefer a selective policy for treating varicosities, as part of a shared decision-making process with the patient. Once a decision to treat varicosities has been made, options include:

- Phlebectomy: This is performed via a small incision using a specific hook to deliver the varicose vein through the incision (Fig. 17.9). Care should be taken to avoid nerves and other structures, particularly around the lateral knee (common peroneal nerve), the medial malleolus (posterior tibial vessels) and the regions of the saphenous and sural nerves. Ambulatory phlebectomy, performed under local anaesthesia in an outpatient setting, is feasible and gaining in popularity. Ligation of the distal end of the vein to be resected (rather than simple 'avulsion') is an important technical tip to minimise post-operative bruising.
- UGFS: Sclerotherapy may be used to treat varicosities and can be performed in an outpatient setting. For more superficial veins, a lower concentration of sclerosant may be preferable to reduce the risk of phlebitis and skin pigmentation.

✔✔ When performing endovenous ablation procedures, concomitant phlebectomies should be considered.

TREATMENT OF INCOMPETENT PERFORATING VEINS

Perforating veins connect the deep and superficial systems in the leg. Incompetent perforators (with flow from deep to superficial veins) are seen in many patients with varicose

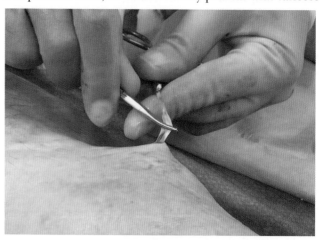

Figure 17.9 Phlebectomy of superficial varicosities.

veins, particularly in those with more advanced venous disease and leg ulceration. The optimal management of incompetent perforators is unknown. Several studies have reported favourable outcomes when incompetent perforators are treated in combination with refluxing superficial veins. Conversely, there are numerous studies that have demonstrated that incompetent perforators may become competent after GSV or SSV treatment. Therefore the additional value of perforator treatment over and above truncal vein ablation alone is unproven. Although each case should be considered individually, a pragmatic approach adopted by many is to treat the refluxing truncal vein as an initial intervention and reserve perforator treatment for patients with residual/recurrent disease clearly attributable to an incompetent perforator. If perforator treatment is deemed necessary, options include endovenous thermal ablation (endovenous thermal ablation), open surgical ligation or UGFS.[56]

✅ The routine treatment of incompetent perforating veins is not justified for patients with primary varicose veins.

SAPHENOUS PRESERVING INTERVENTIONS

CHIVA (French acronym for Ambulatory Conservative Haemodynamic management for Venous Insufficiency) and ASVAL (French acronym for Ambulatory Selective Ablation of Varicose veins under Local anaesthesia) are alternative techniques for the surgical management of superficial venous reflux.[57,58] Both popularised in parts of Europe, CHIVA aims to redistribute superficial venous flow into deep veins by strategically ligating tributaries and/or the SFJ and ASVAL involves the selective ligation of specific incompetent tributaries, with the aim of restoring competence in the saphenous trunk. The aim of such 'saphenous-preserving' approaches is to maintain the venous drainage of GSV and to preserve the option of using the vein as a future vascular conduit. Prospective studies and randomised trials from enthusiastic units have reported favourable results in comparison to surgical stripping, but these techniques have not gained widespread acceptance. This may be because of the excellent results that can be achieved using less esoteric and more reproducible ablation options.

THROMBOPROPHYLAXIS AFTER ENDOVENOUS PROCEDURES

Although VTE is a recognised complication after superficial venous procedures, the approach to VTE prophylaxis varies dramatically between hospitals and clinicians. The rare occurrence of VTE events in this group makes it difficult to conduct trials to guide practice. However, high-profile fatal VTE events have occurred after varicose vein interventions, suggesting that there is a role for appropriate thromboprophylaxis in selected patients.[35,59] Although precise stratification models are yet to be defined, there is growing consensus that patients undergoing endovenous procedures should undergo some form of modified VTE risk assessment. High-risk patients should be prescribed pharmacological prophylaxis (such as low-molecular-weight heparins). The optimal duration of treatment is unknown, but as the VTE risk exists for several days after intervention, a course of 2 weeks or longer may be reasonable for selected high-risk patients.[60]

COMPRESSION AFTER SUPERFICIAL VENOUS INTERVENTIONS

There is uncertainty regarding the use of compression therapy after superficial venous interventions. Compression bandages or stockings have been used commonly after open surgical procedures (stripping and/or phlebectomies), where there may be a role in reducing bruising and pain. However, the case for the routine use of compression after endovenous interventions alone is less clear. There are theoretical benefits after sclerotherapy treatments, as a compressed and empty vein may be less likely to develop thrombophlebitis (Fig. 17.10). However, evidence to support this assumption is lacking and the use of compression after UGFS is not universal. In practice, many patients have advanced venous hypertension and therefore may be in long-term compression already. In the UK, most practitioners recommend compression after interventions, with a maximum duration of 7 days suggested in the NICE guidance. However, advocates of newer modalities such as cyanoacrylate glue closure, suggest that compression is usually not necessary.

RATIONING OF VARICOSE VEIN TREATMENTS

The cost and cost-effectiveness of venous treatments has always been under great scrutiny, not least at the current time with the additional strain placed on healthcare systems by the CoViD-19 pandemic. There is a widely held (and false) perception that varicose vein treatments are largely cosmetic and should be considered as low priority. In the UK NHS, commissioning guidance has become increasingly stringent, making it more difficult to treat superficial venous disease even in the presence of significant complications of chronic venous hypertension. This real-world commissioning landscape is in stark contrast to the published advice, including National Institute for Health and Care Excellence guidance for varicose veins, which recommends that patients with symptomatic varicose veins, skin changes, phlebitis, bleeding or ulcers should be offered treatment.[25]

Many consider rationing to be inevitable and the optimal approach is controversial. In many healthcare settings, the CEAP clinical grade is used to decide whether patients should be treated. However, this is a flawed strategy, as patients with severe, disabling symptoms may only be CEAP C2, whereas patients with a higher CEAP clinical grade may

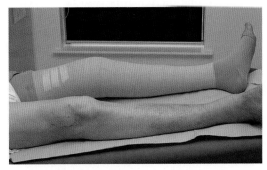

Figure 17.10   Class II compression stocking and bandage applied after ultrasound guided foam sclerotherapy procedure.

be totally asymptomatic. Vein diameter and patient-reported quality-of-life scores have also been proposed as rationing tools, without support. Further work is needed to help define precisely which patients benefit most from varicose veins interventions.

ATYPICAL VARICOSE VEINS VULVAL AND PELVIC VARICES

In some cases, female patients may have perineal or leg varicose veins from ovarian or internal iliac venous tributary incompetence. Varicose veins of pelvic origin may extend along the medial thigh and join the GSV, which may also be incompetent. Pelvic causes of venous disease should be considered in all patients, particularly those with recurrent varicose veins after GSV intervention. Duplex scanning can often identify an incompetent vein arising from the pelvis that is feeding the visible varicosities. Magnetic resonance venography or venography may be needed to identify the source of the pelvic reflux.

There remains considerable controversy over whether pelvic venous reflux needs to be treated aggressively. Where the primary clinical symptoms relate to leg varicose veins, treatment of the visible veins (without pelvic vein treatment) is an accepted strategy. Where patients have pelvic pain and symptoms suggestive of pelvic congestion syndrome, there may be a greater role for endovenous coil embolisation of the incompetent pelvic veins, under fluoroscopic control. The use of foam sclerotherapy in addition to coils has also been described.

CONGENITAL CAUSES OF VARICOSE VEINS

Patients commonly state that other family members have also suffered with varicose veins. The published evidence does suggest a hereditary or genetic contribution to the disease process in some cases, although specific genetic causes of varicose veins have not yet been identified.[61] In one study, patients with varicose veins were over 20 times more likely to report a positive family history in comparison to controls. Varicose veins may also be part of some inherited disorders, such as Klippel–Trenauney syndrome. Patients may present with a combination of cutaneous capillary malformations (port wine stains), limb hypertrophy/overgrowth and varicose veins. Most patients have varicose veins, which are commonly located on the lateral aspect of the leg. Although incompetent superficial veins may be treated, clinicians should be aware that there may be associated deep venous abnormalities, including atresia. Detailed venous mapping with colour duplex, with supplementary venous imaging in selected cases, is essential before considering intervention.

CONCLUSIONS

The management of patients with varicose veins has evolved rapidly in recent years. Our understanding of the significance of SVT has advanced significantly. The importance of early endovenous treatment of varicose veins in patients with leg ulcers has also been demonstrated in recent trials. Endovenous thermal ablation procedures such as endovenous laser and RFA are considered the gold standard and have largely replaced traditional surgery. Non-thermal endovenous procedures such as ultrasound-guided foam sclerotherapy, mechanochemical ablation and cyanoacrylate glue closure may also have a role. After a century of open surgery and vein stripping, the modern management of varicose veins involves the routine use of colour duplex imaging and delivery of a range of minimally invasive, effective and well-tolerated treatments, under local anaesthesia in an office-based setting, with the primary goal of improving patient quality of life.

Key points

- Varicose veins are common, associated with significant quality-of-life impairment and part of a wide spectrum of disorders caused by underlying chronic venous hypertension.
- Interventions for symptomatic varicose veins result in significant clinical, quality-of-life and health-economic benefits.
- All patients should undergo venous duplex imaging before planning intervention.
- Careful discussion of the risks and documented informed consent are essential in view of the risk of medicolegal consequences of adverse outcomes.
- Endovenous treatment modalities including endovenous thermal ablation (using laser or radiofrequency) and ultrasound-guided foam sclerotherapy (UGFS) have become the treatment modalities of choice, ahead of traditional surgery.
- Endovenous modalities are associated with lower early morbidity in comparison to surgical stripping.
- In a rapidly evolving area, non-thermal, non-tumescent options such as mechanochemical ablation or cyanoacrylate glue closure are the latest advances.
- Each of the endovenous treatments has advantages and disadvantages, but the technical success rates are likely to be greatest after EVLA or RFA.
- For patients with venous ulceration, early endovenous ablation has been shown to accelerate ulcer healing, reduce the risk of recurrence and is associated with cost savings
- For the treatment of recurrence varicose veins, open surgery has been superseded by endovenous interventions.

 References available at http://ebooks.health.elsevier.com/

KEY REFERENCES

[2] Onida S, Davies AH. Predicted burden of venous disease. Phlebology 2016;31(Suppl. l):74–9.
[6] Gohel MS, Barwell JR, Taylor M, et al. Long term results of compression therapy alone versus compression plus surgery in chronic venous ulceration (ESCHAR): randomised controlled trial. BMJ 2007;335(7610):83.
[16] Ruckley CV, Evans CJ, Allan PL, Lee AJ, Fowkes FG. Chronic venous insufficiency: clinical and duplex correlations. The Edinburgh Vein Study of venous disorders in the general population. J Vasc Surg 2002;36(3):520–5.
[17] Lurie F, Passman M, Meisner M, et al. The 2020 update of the CEAP classification system and reporting standards. J Vasc Surg 2020;8(3):342–52.
[20] Guest JF, Fuller GW, Vowden P. Venous leg ulcer management in clinical practice in the UK: costs and outcomes. Int Wound J 2018;15(1):29–37.
[22] Kakkos SK, Gohel M, Baekgaard N, et al. Editor's choice - European Society for Vascular Surgery (ESVS) 2021 clinical practice guidelines on the management of venous thrombosis. Eur J Vasc Endovasc Surg 2021;61(1):9–82.
[25] Marsden G, Perry M, Kelley K, Davies AH, Guideline Development G. Diagnosis and management of varicose veins in the legs: summary of NICE guidance. BMJ 2013;347:f4279.

[31] Shingler S, Robertson L, Boghossian S, Stewart M. Compression stockings for the initial treatment of varicose veins in patients without venous ulceration. Cochrane Database Syst Rev 2013;12:CD008819.

[32] Gohel MS, Barwell JR, Earnshaw JJ, et al. Randomized clinical trial of compression plus surgery versus compression alone in chronic venous ulceration (ESCHAR study)–haemodynamic and anatomical changes. Br J Surg 2005;92(3):291–7.

[45] Brittenden J, Cooper D, Dimitrova M, et al. Five-year outcomes of a randomized trial of treatments for varicose veins. N Engl J Med 2019;381(10):912–22.

[46] Brittenden J, Cotton SC, Elders A, et al. A randomized trial comparing treatments for varicose veins. N Engl J Med 2014;371(13):1218–27.

[51] Gohel MS, Heatley F, Liu X, et al. A randomized trial of early endovenous ablation in venous ulceration. N Engl J Med 2018;378(22):2105–14.

[57] Guo L, Huang R, Zhao D, et al. Long-term efficacy of different procedures for treatment of varicose veins: a network meta-analysis. Medicine (Baltimore) 2019;98(7):e14495.

18 Chronic leg swelling

Prakash Saha | Stephen Black

There are various conditions that can cause chronic lower limb swelling (Box 18.1). The three most common are chronic venous insufficiency (CVI), lymphoedema and dependent oedema, which may be associated with inactivity and obesity. This chapter explores these three conditions further.

CHRONIC VENOUS INSUFFICIENCY

CVI encompasses disease of the lower limb veins in which venous return is impaired over a number of years, by reflux, obstruction or calf muscle pump failure. This leads to sustained venous hypertension and ultimately clinical complications including oedema, eczema, lipodermatosclerosis and when severe, ulceration.

CLINICAL FEATURES

The clinical features of CVI include skin changes, varicose veins, swelling, pain and ulceration and pain.

SKIN CHANGES

Varicose eczema presents as dry, scaly and itchy skin. The skin becomes friable and may become infected following scratching. Pigmentation, caused by the deposition of haemosiderin in the tissues, produces a brown discoloration characteristic of CVI, which together with fibrosis leads to the clinical picture of lipodermatosclerosis around the ankle (Fig. 18.1). There may also be loss of pigmentation resulting in pale skin changes called *atrophie blanche*.

VARICOSE VEINS

Varicose veins may be present and a history of previous varicose vein treatment should be sought. The absence of visible varicose veins does not exclude the presence of significant superficial reflux. Varicose veins on the lower anterior abdominal wall are a sign of inferior vena cava or iliac vein obstruction and the patient should be examined standing to identify these.

PAIN

The patient may complain of a general ache and heaviness in the leg after long periods of standing. This is worse towards the end of the day but improves with elevation or bed rest.

A history of deep vein thrombosis (DVT) should be sought. Venous claudication is an uncommon symptom that is usually caused by iliofemoral vein occlusion or a significant stenosis. The symptoms differ from arterial claudication because the increase in arterial inflow during exercise combined with decreased outflow results in distension of the limb, giving rise to generalised pain and a severe bursting sensation in the leg. The pain often requires elevation for 10–20 minutes for relief after cessation of exercise.

SWELLING

Swelling is caused by an accumulation of oedematous fluid, which is initially pitting, but as the disease progresses subcutaneous fibrosis and induration occur. If there is any break in the skin, this can lead to copious exudation of fluid.

ULCERATION

Ulceration is often precipitated by minor trauma and venous ulcers occur predominantly on the lower leg, more commonly around the medial aspect of the ankle. There may be surrounding eczema or pigmentation and frequently exudation of fluid can cause maceration of the surrounding skin. In patients presenting with lower limb ulceration, approximately 80%[1,2] will have evidence of venous disease and 10–25%[3] of limbs will have Doppler-verified arterial disease. Approximately 12% will have co-existing diabetes or rheumatoid arthritis.[4] Immobility is often a contributory cause and can also cause stasis ulceration in isolation. As with pain a history of DVT should be sought as ulcers are a common feature of post-thrombotic syndrome (PTS).

EPIDEMIOLOGY

The prevalence of CVI in the adult population lies between 2% and 9% and may be higher in males than females.[5,6] The most serious feature of CVI is ulceration, which is a distressing and debilitating condition. Leg ulcers affect approximately 1% of the adult population in developed countries, with 50% of ulcers having been present for more than 12 months, and 72% are recurrent.[7] Within the UK, Australia, Sweden and Italy, overall rates for active ulceration range from 0.15–0.5% and increase with age.[8–12] In the UK, the current total cost to the National Health Service is estimated to be around £1 billion a year.[13]

AETIOLOGY

To understand CVI, the changes that occur in both the larger veins (macrocirculation) and the capillary bed (microcirculation) must be considered.

Box 18.1 Differential diagnosis of chronic leg swelling

Venous disease

Primary varicose veins
Primary deep venous incompetence
Post-thrombotic syndrome
Arteriovenous malformations

Lymphoedema

Primary
Secondary

General disease

Lipidema
Congestive cardiac failure
Pre-tibial myxoedema
Nephrotic syndrome
Hepatic failure

Tumours

Pelvic tumours causing extrinsic compression

Drugs

Dependency

Box 18.2 Causes of venous hypertension

Superficial venous reflux

Long saphenous vein reflux
Short saphenous vein reflux

Deep venous reflux and occlusion

Primary (idiopathic)
Secondary to deep venous thrombosis or injury

Perforating vein reflux

Abnormal calf pump
Neurological
Musculoskeletal
Combination of the above

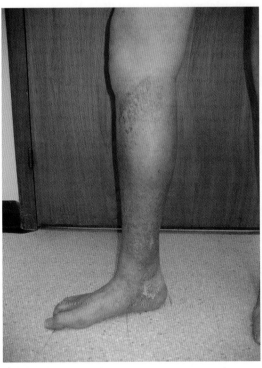

Figure 18.1 Chronic venous insufficiency with pigmentation and severe lipodermatosclerosis resulting in the typical 'inverted champagne bottle' shape.

MACROCIRCULATION

During exercise in the normal individual, effective contraction of the calf muscles combined with vein patency and valvular competence aids venous return and reduces venous pressure in the lower leg from about 90 mmHg to 30 mmHg. Failure of any of these mechanisms can result

in post-ambulatory venous hypertension, which is accepted as the underlying haemodynamic abnormality in CVI. The recognised causes are outlined in Box 18.2.

Deep and superficial reflux

Most venous ulcers were thought to be secondary to a previous DVT but duplex scanning has demonstrated that some patients have primary deep venous reflux. Isolated superficial venous incompetence without deep venous incompetence occurs in between 31%[14] and 57%[15] of patients with venous ulceration.

Perforating vein reflux

The contribution of incompetent perforators to the development of CVI remains controversial. Isolated perforator incompetence occurs in only 2–4% of limbs with skin changes, and perforator incompetence is usually associated with reflux in the superficial or deep systems. However, the prevalence of incompetent perforators increases linearly with the clinical severity of CVI.[16] There has been a recent trend towards treatment of incompetent perforating veins with laser or radiofrequency ablation (RFA), but the indications for this remain uncertain. In those cases where superficial and perforator reflux coincide, treating only the former results in healing rates of 95%.[17]

MICROCIRCULATION

The pathophysiology is still not fully understood but the following two hypotheses exist:

1. **White cell trapping hypothesis.** Increased venous pressures lead to white blood cell plugging of capillaries, adherence of white cells to the endothelium and release of proteolytic enzymes. This leads to increased capillary permeability and tissue damage causing ulceration.[18–21]
2. **Fibrin cuff hypothesis.** A rise in venous pressure causes widening of the pores between endothelial cells.[22] This results in leakage of fibrinogen out of the intravascular compartment into the tissues, which polymerises to form fibrin. A defective interstitial fibrinolytic system may also contribute to the build-up of fibrin.[23] Fibrin 'cuffs' form around the capillaries, which acts as a barrier to oxygen, resulting in local tissue ischaemia and cell death, producing ulceration.[24]

Matrix metalloproteinases help remodel the extracellular matrix by protein degradation, and enhanced matrix metalloproteinase activity has been demonstrated in lipodermatosclerosis.[25] This may also contribute to the development of ulceration.

CLASSIFICATION

CVI involves a variety of anatomical and physiological abnormalities and so a standardised system is required to allow uniformity of reporting.

✅✅ A classification was developed in 1994 by an international consensus conference under the auspices of the American Venous Forum and recommendations for change were made in 2004 and updated again in 2020.[26]

This includes clinical signs (C), aetiology (E), anatomical distribution (A) and pathophysiological condition (P) and is therefore known by the acronym CEAP. This system is helpful in comparing limbs for the purposes of research, although it is rather unwieldy for everyday use (Box 18.3).

INVESTIGATION

Patients often present with mixed arterial and venous disease and so ankle–brachial pressure indices must be recorded if foot pulses are weak or absent and when compression therapy is being considered. The investigation of the venous disease is discussed later.

HAND-HELD DOPPLER

Continuous-wave hand-held Doppler using an 8-MHz probe is a useful outpatient tool in screening for arterial and venous disease. Its limitations are that the exact vein being insonated is unknown, it is operator dependent and the significance of reflux of short duration may be uncertain.

DUPLEX SCANNING

Duplex is an important investigation of lower limb venous disease and is now first line. Modern equipment allows easy identification of normal and abnormal venous anatomy, along with the presence of venous reflux. It is also extensively used for the diagnosis of DVT.

✅ An international consensus document recommends duplex scanning as an essential investigation for patients with CVI.[27]

VENOGRAPHY

Venography is invasive and to a large extent has been superseded by duplex scanning for the investigation of venous disease of the lower limb. Venography still has a place in the diagnosis of upper limb DVT when ultrasound is inconclusive and clinical suspicion persists and in patients with post-thrombotic limb where an obstruction in the iliac veins and inferior vena cava, is not readily visualised by ultrasound. With the increased use of deep endovenous therapy, however, to treat such lesions, axial imaging with either computed tomography (CT) or magnetic resonance (MR) venography is often used for pre-operative planning.

Box 18.3 CEAP classification

Clinical signs (C$_{0-6}$)

Limbs are placed into one of seven clinical classes according to objective signs as follows:
- Class 0: no visible or palpable signs of venous disease
- Class 1: telangiectases, reticular veins, malleolar flare
- Class 2: varicose veins
- Class 3: oedema without skin changes
- Class 4a: pigmentation or eczema class 4b, lipodermatosclerosis or atrophie blanche
- Class 5: skin changes as aforementioned with healed ulceration
- Class 6: skin changes as aforementioned with active ulceration

Each limb is further classified as asymptomatic (A) or symptomatic (S)

Aetiology (E$_{C,P,S,N}$)

This classification refers to congenital (C), primary (P; unknown cause but not congenital), secondary (S; acquired) and no aetiology identified (N). These groups are mutually exclusive

Anatomical distribution (A$_{S,D,P,N}$)

This refers to superficial (S), deep (D), perforating (P) veins and no venous location identified (N). More than one system may be involved

Pathophysiological condition (P$_{R,O,N}$)

This refers to reflux (R) or obstruction (O), or both may be present. P$_N$ implies no venous pathophysiology identified

---

COMPUTED TOMOGRAPHY VENOGRAPHY

Computed tomography venography (CTV) can be used to image thrombosis affecting the abdominal and pelvic veins. A contrast agent injected either directly into the dorsal veins (direct) or in the antecubital veins (indirect) is required. Extra-vascular anatomical structures can be visualised, and the lungs can be imaged at the same time for the detection of pulmonary embolism. The main disadvantages of this technique are the use of ionising radiation, risk of contrast nephropathy and cost. CTV is mainly therefore only used when interventions are being considered.

MAGNETIC RESONANCE IMAGING

Magnetic resonance imaging (MRI) techniques can be used for the assessment of the deep veins, particularly when intervention is being considered. It uses non-ionising radiation, which is beneficial to the younger patient cohort and by applying a number of different sequences both anatomical and functional information can be obtained. There are a number of limitations to the use of MR, however, including cost. Nevertheless, it is likely that this imaging technique will become first line for the assessment of patients with iliofemoral venous pathology before intervention is considered.

INTRAVASCULAR ULTRASOUND

Intravascular ultrasound (IVUS) is an invasive technique that can be used to visualise the vessel lumen and surrounding wall in real time. It complements venography and is a useful aid in measuring and deploying venous stents precisely. It is also more reliable than venography when assessing stent characteristics intra-operatively and is a vital adjunct to deep endovenous procedures.

FUNCTIONAL MEASUREMENTS

Various investigations may be used to examine the function of the venous system in the lower limb.

Ambulatory venous pressure measurement

This provides direct measurement of the superficial venous pressure at the ankle. This is achieved by cannulation of a vein on the dorsum of the foot connected to a pressure transducer, amplifier and a recorder. The pressure changes recorded in the long saphenous vein in the foot during and after 10 tiptoe exercises are shown in Fig. 18.2. This investigation is an indicator of overall lower limb venous function including calf muscle pump function.

Plethysmography

There are many different types of plethysmography, which measure either alterations in calf volume directly or parameters that indirectly reflect volume change. These include photoplethysmography, strain gauge plethysmography and air plethysmography. The utility of these is largely confined to research and they are rarely used in routine clinical practice.

TREATMENT

The management of patients with CVI may be divided into either the prevention of or the treatment of clinical complications such as lipodermatosclerosis and ulceration. Correcting the underlying cause can help to stop or reverse these complications. In addition, vigorous treatment of conditions known to lead to CVI, particularly acute DVT, may reduce the incidence of this problem in the long term. Management of patients with ulcers of mixed aetiology will require treatment aimed at each specific cause but this section deals predominantly with the treatment of isolated venous disease.

GENERAL MEASURES

These should include elevation of the legs at rest above the level of the heart. This helps to reduce oedema, decrease exudate from ulcers and accelerate regression of skin changes.[4]

Immobility, occupation, obesity and co-existing disease may also influence the development of skin complications and should be addressed. Placing the patient in bed reduces the venous pressure at the ankle to about 12–15 mmHg and can help lead to ulcer healing. However, this is not a treatment enjoyed by most patients and may increase the risk of DVT. It is therefore generally reserved for ulcers that have failed to heal by all other methods.

GRADUATED ELASTIC COMPRESSION

Compression therapy remains the primary treatment for the majority of patients with CVI. It provides symptomatic relief, promotes ulcer healing and helps in preventing ulcer recurrence. Applying a sustained graduated compressive force that is highest at the ankle and decreases proximally has been shown to reduce venous pressure at the ankle, increase femoral vein blood flow and increase venous refilling time. This improves venous function and can heal up to 93% of venous ulcers.[28] Graduated elastic compression may be applied using either bandages or stockings, but this is dependent on factors such as levels of exudate, amount of oedema and leg shape. It is important that these are applied by experienced staff as inexpertly applied compression can cause skin damage. Compression can also be used to treat mixed arterial and venous ulcers, but this requires specialist assessment.

In the healing of leg ulcers: (i) compression is more effective than no compression; (ii) elastic compression is more effective than non-elastic compression; (iii) multi-layered high compression is more effective than single-layer compression; and (iv) there is no significant difference between four-layer bandaging and other high-compression multi-layered systems.[29]

In the prevention of ulcer recurrence, there are no randomised trials comparing recurrence rates with and without compression.

A review of trials comparing different grades of compression stocking concluded that higher grades of compression are associated with lower recurrence rates, but at a cost of lower patient compliance.[30] Approximately one-third of patients do not comply with the long-term use of compression hosiery.[31]

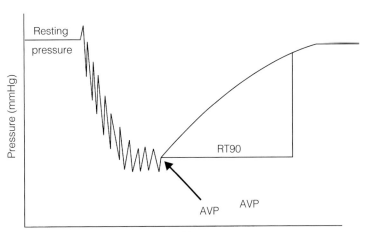

Figure 18.2 Venous pressure trace recorded from a superficial vein on the dorsum of the foot during 10 tiptoe exercises and return to the resting value after exercise. *AVP*, Ambulatory venous pressure; *RT90*, time for 90% refilling.

Stockings are classed according to the pressure they exert at the ankle and are designed to provide a linear graduated decrease in pressure above this, although in practice this may not always be the case. Pressures of up to 60 mmHg may be produced by elastic stockings, and conventional pressure classes and indications are given in Table 18.1.

For the majority of patients with CVI or mild lymphoedema, a knee-length compression stocking designed to apply compression of 25–35 mmHg is ideal, but this will be influenced by how well they tolerate the stocking and their ability to apply them. Thigh-length stockings seem to confer little benefit over knee-length ones and as shorter stockings are easier to put on, compliance with these tends to be better. Stocking applicators may also aid patient compliance.

INTERMITTENT PNEUMATIC COMPRESSION

There is some evidence that intermittent pneumatic compression may provide accelerated ulcer healing when used either alone or in combination with elastic compression, although there is a need for further trials in this area.[32]

LASER AND ELECTROMAGNETIC THERAPY

A review of low-level laser therapy for venous leg ulcers has not found any benefit in healing rates.[33] Similarly, there is no high-quality evidence that electromagnetic therapy increases the rate of healing of venous leg ulcers.[34]

PHARMACOTHERAPY

Dressings

For those patients with venous ulceration, there are a wide variety of topical dressings available.

The type of dressing applied beneath compression has not been shown to affect ulcer healing, although dressing choice has an impact on pain, frequency of dressing change, maceration and odour. Decisions regarding which dressing to use should be based on local costs and practitioner or patient preference.[35]

Additional factors to consider in choosing a dressing are exudate, odour and patient comfort. Whatever dressing is chosen should be used in conjunction with treatment of the underlying venous insufficiency, usually by adequate graduated elastic compression. Simple non-adherent dressings are all that is required for many ulcers. Vacuum-assisted closure dressing systems are sometimes useful for deep ulceration and can be used under compression. There is recent evidence that they reduce time to healing at a lower cost when compared to conventional dressings.[36] The Vulcan trial suggested that silver dressings made no impact on ulcer healing when compared to any other dressing, although this has been questioned as many of the ulcers treated with silver within the trial would not have had silver applied in clinical practice.[37]

Emollients

These soothe, smooth and hydrate the skin and are indicated for all dry or scaling disorders such as varicose eczema. Their effects are short-lived and frequent application is necessary. Preparations containing an antibacterial should be avoided unless infection is present.

Oxpentifylline (pentoxifylline)

There have been several randomised controlled trials of oxpentifylline compared with placebo, with or without compression, in the healing of venous leg ulcers.[38] These have demonstrated that this drug is more effective than placebo in ulcer healing.

Nutrition

Adequate nutrition is important for ulcer healing; protein, vitamins A and C, zinc and other trace elements are all important. It may be appropriate to consider dietary supplements if these are deficient.

SUPERFICIAL VENOUS INTERVENTION

Superficial venous surgery

Superficial surgery may be of benefit in healing ulcers in situations of isolated superficial venous incompetence or combined superficial and deep venous incompetence. Surgery for isolated superficial venous incompetence may also reduce long-term recurrence rates. With the advent of minimally invasive techniques, it may be possible to treat some patients who previously were not fit for conventional varicose vein surgery. These techniques include RFA, endovenous laser ablation (EVLA) and foam sclerotherapy, and are discussed in Chapter 17.

A randomised controlled trial comparing superficial venous surgery plus elastic compression with compression alone for venous ulceration has demonstrated no difference in initial healing rates but a reduction in recurrence rates at 12 months in the surgical group (12% vs. 28%). The authors concluded that most patients with chronic venous ulceration will benefit from addition of simple venous surgery.[39]

Perforating vein surgery

There has been renewed interest in medial calf-perforating vein incompetence with the advent of subfascial endoscopic perforating vein surgery, and more recently with minimally invasive techniques such as EVLA and RFA. The evidence for the benefit of treatment of incompetent perforating

Table 18.1 Conventional pressure classes of compression stockings

Class	Pressure at ankle (mmHg)	Indications
I	<25	Mild varicosis, venous thrombosis prophylaxis
II	25–35	Marked varicose veins, oedema, chronic venous insufficiency
III	35–45	Chronic venous insufficiency, lymphoedema, following venous ulceration to prevent recurrence
IV	45–60	Severe lymphoedema and chronic venous insufficiency

veins by any of these methods is weak and the precise indications and benefit of perforator treatment remain unclear.

Deep venous valvular reconstruction

Worldwide experience of deep venous valvular reconstruction is limited as most patients with CVI can be managed adequately with superficial venous surgery and the conservative measures described earlier. Therefore it is usually reserved for those patients with severe symptoms that prove resistant to conservative treatment.

The benefit of deep venous valvular reconstructive surgery is unclear as many of the published series have included ancillary procedures such as high saphenous ligation and stripping, and in the few series where the influence of these procedures has been excluded, the numbers involved tend to be small or the follow-up short. A number of different procedures have been described and these are shown in Box 18.4.

✅✅ A Cochrane review[40] has found no evidence for benefit (or harm) of valvuloplasty in the treatment of patients with CVI secondary to primary valvular incompetence. The individual trials included in the review were small and of poor quality and the benefit of valvuloplasty remains uncertain.

Skin grafting

Large ulcers may be treated with a split-skin graft or pinch grafts, which if successful, may reduce the healing time. Before this is undertaken, it is important that the ulcer bed is clean and free from infection (particularly β-haemolytic streptococci, *Pseudomonas* and *Staphylococcus aureus*). However, unless the underlying venous abnormality is also treated, failure of the graft and subsequent recurrence is inevitable.

Endovascular management of venous outflow obstruction

Following DVT, a degree of re-canalisation can occur in affected venous segments usually by 90 days.[41] Many patients are, however, left with functional outflow obstruction and deep venous reflux. When the iliofemoral vein is affected and there is persistent venous outflow obstruction, symptoms tend to be severe resulting in a swollen leg, skin changes and venous claudication, which leads to a poor quality of life. Until recently, the majority of these patients were treated conservatively with compression hosiery, however, the development of endovascular treatments in recent years has led to the use of endoluminal stenting to treat iliac venous occlusions. These interventions have been shown to

---

Box 18.4 Procedures for correction of deep venous valvular incompetence

Valvular repair

Valvuloplasty
Valve transposition
Valve transplantation

External support of vein wall

Dacron cuff
Vein wall plication

---

be of benefit in selected patients and Raju et al.[42] have reported treating long iliac venous occlusions, with primary and secondary patency rates at 2 years of 49% and 76%, respectively. Further studies have reported patency rates in the region of 90% at 1 year for stenting of iliac venous stenoses (non-thrombotic iliac vein lesions).[43,44] This refers to the chronic pulsatile compression of the proximal left common iliac vein by the overlying right common iliac artery or aortic bifurcation, resulting in an intra-luminal venous spur, web or membrane – and has been known as *May-Thurner/Cockett syndrome*. This common lesion (20% of the adult population) is an increasingly well-recognised cause of left iliac vein thrombo-occlusive disease, particularly in young patients. The clinical picture is of left leg venous hypertension or DVT and is likely to explain the preponderance of left-sided DVT. The development of dedicated nitinol venous stents is likely to increase the use of these interventions, which show promise in the short term and long-term data are awaited.

Venous bypass

Surgical bypass of an obstructed vein may be possible, but this should be reserved for those patients in whom there is measured evidence of outflow obstruction, endoluminal interventions have been exhausted, and there are severe symptoms. Two principal surgical procedures have been described:

1. The femorofemoral crossover graft for iliac obstruction (Palma operation; Fig. 18.3).[45] Only a small number of patients are suitable for this procedure, but in these patients' long-term patency and relief of symptoms may be achieved in up to 70% of cases.[46] The long saphenous vein on the unaffected side is used as a crossover graft.
2. Limbs with functional outflow obstruction caused by stenosed or occluded deep thigh veins may be suitable for saphenopopliteal bypass, which uses the long saphenous vein as a bypass channel. The theoretical difficulty with this procedure is that the long saphenous vein may already be acting as a collateral channel and to interfere with this may make matters worse should thrombosis occur.

PREVENTING THE POST-THROMBOTIC LIMB

CVI developing secondary to previous DVT is commonly referred to as PTS or post-phlebitic syndrome. The management of DVT has historically been directed at preventing thrombus extension and pulmonary embolus in the acute phase. There has been little focus on long-term treatment to prevent the development of PTS. However, 30% or more will develop features of mild or moderate PTS.[47–49] This risk increases with more proximal DVT and recurrent episodes of thrombosis. Even with isolated calf vein thrombosis, there is a risk of development of PTS.

✅✅ The risk of developing severe CVI with ulceration following DVT is of the order of 2–10% at 10 years.[47,50]

The causes of PTS related to previous DVT are either valvular incompetence or residual outflow obstruction with eventual calf muscle pump failure. Treatment of

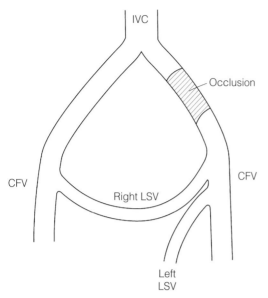

Figure 18.3 Femorofemoral crossover graft using the long saphenous vein (LSV) to bypass unilateral iliac obstruction. *CFV*, Common femoral vein; *IVC*, inferior vena cava.

the primary DVT should be aimed not only at preventing thrombus propagation and pulmonary embolism, but also at preventing venous damage and preserving or restoring venous function. This may include anticoagulation, limb elevation, and elastic compression therapy. Increasingly, thrombolysis and catheter thrombectomy are being used in the management of acute iliofemoral DVT and should be considered first-line therapy in young patients without contraindications. Patients who have had a DVT should be encouraged to wear lifelong elastic compression hosiery, in particular those patients with residual reflux and who are on their feet all day or travel long journeys.[46] They should be encouraged to take regular exercise to stimulate the calf muscle pump and maintain ankle mobility. These simple measures are often recommended for life but there is controversy as to their success in preventing PTS.

SUMMARY

Investigation and treatment must be tailored to the individual patient, but a simplified everyday management plan is shown in Fig. 18.4.

DEPENDENCY AND INACTIVITY

Patients who sit for long periods are exposed to a raised venous pressure at the ankle for longer periods of time. Normal daily activity includes activation of the calf muscle pump by walking, thereby decreasing the venous pressure, but without this pressure reduction, the effects on the lower limb are similar to those seen in venous reflux because of prolonged venous 'hypertension'. As a result, inactive patients, for example those confined to a wheelchair, can develop venous-type leg swelling in the absence of any true

venous pathology. Those with a stiff or fused ankle may also be affected. The use of prophylactic compression therapy should therefore be considered in these patients. Morbid obesity adds to this problem and is becoming a major aetiological factor in lower limb ulceration. The management of obesity is an important component of treatment in these patients and whilst this may be done in primary care in the majority of cases, some may require referral for gastric banding or bypass.

LYMPHOEDEMA

Lymphoedema is a progressive, chronic and debilitating swelling that can affect any part of the body, most commonly the limbs, leading to distortion in shape, size, reduction of mobility and impaired function.

AETIOLOGY

Lymphoedema can be caused by intrinsic factors (primary) or extrinsic factors (secondary).

PRIMARY

The traditional classification of primary lymphoedema is shown in Box 18.5. Congenital lymphoedema occurs at or soon after birth and in some rare cases, it is autosomally inherited (Milroy's disease). Lymphoedema praecox presents up to the age of 35 years and is more prevalent in females. Typically, this is not familial, although lymphoedema–distichiasis syndrome, which develops at puberty, is familial and is linked to the *FOXC2* gene mutation.[51] Lymphoedema tarda presents over the age of 35 years. It is likely that these three groups represent different parts of the same spectrum of disease, which has been attributed to aplasia, hypoplasia or hyperplasia of the lymph vessels during development. A fibrotic obstruction in the lymph nodes has also been described.[52]

In addition to this, a functional classification more orientated to the treatment of these conditions may be used. This type of classification was first described by Browse.[53]

- Obliterative (80%): the distal lymphatics undergo progressive obliteration. This occurs predominantly in females and is often bilateral.
- Proximal obstruction (10%): proximal occlusion occurs in the abdominal, pelvic or inguinal lymph nodes. This is predominantly unilateral.
- Lymphatic valvular incompetence and hyperplasia (10%): development of the valve system is incomplete and lymphatic dilatation and hyperplasia occur. This is usually bilateral.

SECONDARY

Secondary lymphoedema develops following extrinsic damage to part of the lymphatic system. The lymphatic channels distal to the obstruction become dilated and the valves secondarily incompetent. The commonest cause worldwide is filarial infestation but in Europe the commonest cause is neoplasia and its treatment, for example post-mastectomy lymphoedema. The causes of secondary lymphoedema are also listed in Box 18.5.

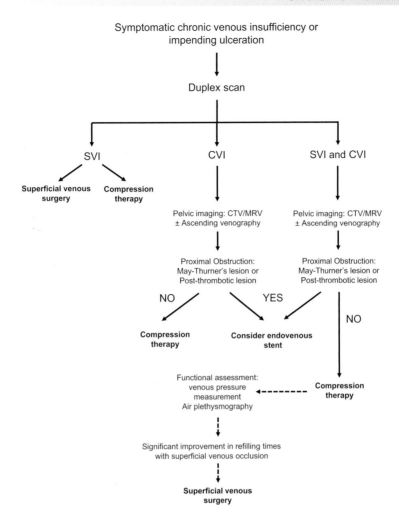

Figure 18.4 Flow diagram for the management of chronic venous insufficiency. *CTV*, Computed tomography venography; *DVI*, deep venous incompetence; *MRV*, magnetic resonance venography; *SVI*, superficial venous incompetence.

Box 18.5 Causes of lymphoedema

Primary

Congenital (age <1 year)
- Familial (Milroy's disease)
- Non-familial

Praecox (age <35 years)
- Familial
- Non familial

Tarda (age >35 years)

Secondary

Malignant disease
Surgery
- Radical mastectomy
- Radical groin dissection

Radiotherapy
Infection
- Parasitic (filariasis)
- Pyogenic (β-haemolytic streptococci, *Staphylococcus aureus*)
- Tuberculosis

Impairment
- Arterial surgery
- Venous disease and venous surgery

PRESENTATION

Initial presentation is with peripheral oedema. History and examination will usually differentiate lymphoedema from other causes of limb swelling and may distinguish between primary and secondary causes.

HISTORY

The patient complains of a slowly progressive swelling of the whole or part of the limb, which typically does not reduce overnight with elevation. Limb swelling usually commences distally and may progress during the day, particularly on standing for long periods. The patient may describe the limb as heavy and up to 50% will complain of pain requiring analgesia.[54] There may be a history of recurrent lymphangitis. The age of onset and a history of previous surgery, malignancy or radiotherapy should be sought.

Lymphoedema can also occur secondary to lipoedema. Lipoedema is abnormal symmetrical swelling caused by excess deposit and expansion of fat cells. It is always bilateral, occurs from the waist down and spares the ankles. It cannot be lost through diet and exercise, and often causes pain, particularly surrounding the tibial area. It occurs almost exclusively in women and can occur in women of all sizes and can be inherited. The expanding fat cells interfere with the lymphatics so many lipoedema patients develop lymph-oedema, which is difficult to treat because of the inability to tolerate compression caused by pain.

EXAMINATION

Examination reveals swelling of the limb, which may be unilateral or bilateral. Initially, it will pit like other types of oedema, but with time, the swelling becomes non-pitting because of hypertrophy of adipose tissue and increasing subcutaneous fibrosis. The swelling is uniform and as it progresses, the leg becomes like a tree-trunk (Fig. 18.5). The skin develops a 'peau d'orange' appearance with hy-perkeratosis of the toes and skin fissuring with secondary fungal infection. The skin gradually thickens, becoming less elastic until it is not possible to pick up a fold in the lower leg. This inelasticity produces a positive Stemmer sign (the inability to pinch the skin of the dorsum of the second toe between the thumb and forefinger). The dor-sum of the foot is usually involved, producing the charac-teristic 'buffalo hump' appearance, and chylous vesicles may occur on the pre-tibial area.

Ankle ulceration is unusual with lymphoedema as the skin remains more elastic than in venous disease, allow-ing expansion to occur without increased tension.[55] The presence of surgical scars or skin telangiectasia fol-lowing radiotherapy may indicate a cause of secondary lymphoedema.

CLINICAL STAGING

There is no consensus on a universal clinical staging system for all forms of lymphoedema, but the consensus document of the International Society of Lymphology suggests the staging system in Table 18.2.[56,57] Within each stage, severi-ty based on volume difference can be assessed as minimal (<20% increase) in limb volume, moderate (20–40% in-crease) or severe (>40% increase).

INVESTIGATION

The diagnosis of lymphoedema can usually be made clinical-ly. Investigation is needed when the diagnosis is uncertain, to exclude sinister underlying causes or, if surgery is being considered, to confirm the diagnosis and plan treatment.

DUPLEX ULTRASONOGRAPHY

This is useful to exclude CVI. The B-mode image will also detect the changes in the dermis and subcutaneous layers and can therefore be used as a means of monitoring the disease.

LYMPHANGIOSCINTIGRAPHY (ISOTOPE LYMPHOGRAPHY)

This is now one of the most frequently performed in-vestigations as it provides an overall assessment of lym-phatic drainage by demonstrating isotope flow up the lymphatics, and in the majority of cases avoids the need for conventional lymphangiography (Fig. 18.6). Radiola-belled (usually technetium) colloid is injected into the

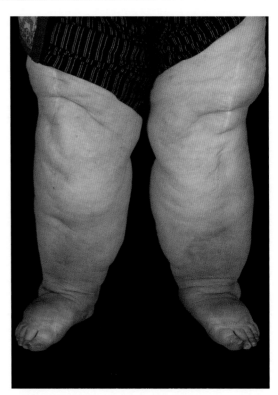

Figure 18.5 Chronic lymphoedema of the leg with tree-trunk ap-pearance and 'buffalo hump' of the foot.

Table 18.2   Clinical staging of lymphoedema

Stage 0	Latent or subclinical condition where swelling is not evident despite impaired lymph transport
Stage I	Early accumulation of fluid that subsides with limb elevation. Pitting may occur
Stage II	Limb elevation alone rarely reduces tissue swelling and pitting is manifest Late in stage II, the limb may or may not pit as tissue fibrosis supervenes
Stage III	Lymphostatic elephantiasis where pitting is absent and trophic skin changes such as acanthosis, fat deposits and warty overgrowths develop

interdigital space between the second and third toes on both sides and gamma-camera pictures are taken at 5-minute intervals to assess transit through the lymph channels. Scintigraphy has been demonstrated to have a sensitivity of 92% and a specificity of 100% for the diag-nosis of lymphoedema.[58] A negative scintigram effectively excludes the diagnosis.[59]

COMPUTED TOMOGRAPHY

CT may show the presence of dilated lymphatic channels, thereby aiding the diagnosis of obstructive lymphoedema and lymphatic valvular incompetence.[60] It will also provide evidence of lymphoedema by the presence of a honeycomb appearance of fluid in the subcutaneous tissues and has been used to monitor the response to compression therapy by measuring the cross-sectional area of limb compartments. Patients with a previous history of pelvic or abdominal

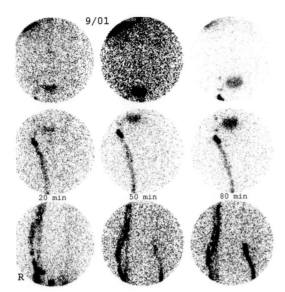

Figure 18.6 Lymphoscintigram confirming left-sided lymphoedema. On the right, the isotope is travelling up the lymphatics of the leg with concentration in the ilioinguinal nodes (normal). On the left the isotope has remained in the leg.

malignancy should be scanned for recurrent disease to diagnose enlarged lymph nodes or pelvic masses that may be compressing the lymphatic channels.

MAGNETIC RESONANCE IMAGING

In patients with chronic lymphoedema, MRI has been shown to demonstrate circumferential subcutaneous oedema, thickening of dermis and a honeycomb pattern of fibrosis between the muscle and subcutis, increased subcutaneous fat and variability in lymph node size and appearance.[61,62]

INTERSTITIAL MAGNETIC RESONANCE LYMPHANGIOGRAPHY

Interstitial MR lymphography involves intra-cutaneous injection of a paramagnetic contrast agent for the visualisation of lymphatic vessels.[63] Dilated lymphatic channels are a common finding and collateral vessels along with dermal backflow indicate proximal obstruction.[64,65] Dynamic MR lymphangiography is more sensitive and accurate than lymphoscintigraphy in the detection of anatomical and functional abnormalities in the lymphatic system.[66]

FLUORESCENCE MICROLYMPHANGIOGRAPHY

Fluorescence microlymphangiography involves visualisation of the superficial network of lymphatics with a fluorescence microscope following intra-cutaneous injection of fluorescein isothiocyanate–dextran. It can confirm the clinical diagnosis of lymphoedema and can distinguish various forms of oedema.[56,67] Emanating from the fluorescent spot, the surrounding network of microvessels is filled and becomes easily visible and is recorded by photography or video. In Milroy's disease, a lack of microlymphatics (aplasia) is typical, while in other primary and secondary lymphoedema the network remains intact, but

the depicted area is enlarged. In lipoedema, lymphatic microaneurysms are seen.

CONTRAST LYMPHANGIOGRAPHY

This investigation is now used only rarely in the diagnosis of lymphoedema and has been largely replaced by scintigraphy. It is for patients being considered for microvascular lymphatic reconstruction.

TREATMENT

The aim of treatment is to reduce limb swelling, reduce the risk of infection and improve function. If management begins early in the disease process when pitting oedema is present, conservative measures should be successful. Once achieved, the improvement must be maintained. Surgical options are available in a few centres for resistant and severely symptomatic cases.

GENERAL MEASURES

Once the diagnosis is made, a clear explanation of the condition and its non–life-threatening nature should be given to the patient, along with referral to a specialist service.[51] The treatment is improved by empowering the patient to manage their own condition, and the earlier education and treatment are instituted the better the outcome, hence information leaflets can be helpful. In the early stages elevation of a lymphoedematous limb while resting and at night can reduce oedema by increasing venous return and reducing the production of interstitial fluid. Exercise, such as on an exercise bicycle, encourages movement of lymph along non-contractile vessels and increased contractility of collecting lymph vessels. Managing obesity is also important.

MANUAL LYMPHATIC DRAINAGE

This involves manipulating the leg by squeezing just above the most proximal area of oedema and then working from proximal to distal. This enhances lymphatic flow.

GRADUATED ELASTIC COMPRESSION

Compression stockings need to exert a pressure of approximately 50 mmHg or higher. The stockings can be used for maintenance of the limb after oedema reduction, but compliance is low in the summer months, and the elderly and frail find them difficult to apply. Multi-layer bandaging is an essential stage of the intensive phase of management. Inelastic bandages are applied to the limb, providing a low resting pressure but high exercise pressure. This is used to reduce severe swelling and improve limb shape and skin condition before fitting compression hosiery.

✔✔ If graduated elastic compression is used initially followed by a stocking for maintenance, a greater and more sustained limb volume reduction is achieved than if stockings alone are used throughout.[68]

INTERMITTENT PNEUMATIC COMPRESSION

Intermittent pneumatic compression (IPC) involves placement of the limb in a multi-compartmental sleeve. Each compartment consists of air cells that are sequentially inflated to a pressure of about 80 mmHg and deflated from distal to proximal, thus massaging the lymph centrally. Patients use this for 4 hours a day and it can be done at home. If the lymphatic system is obliterated or obstructed more proximally, massaging the lymph centrally can precipitate collections elsewhere, such as the genitals, and high pressures may injure peripheral lymphatics. Reports combining IPC with stockings quote figures of 90% for immediate benefit and long-term maintenance.[69] The poor responders have usually had oedema for more than 10 years. In these chronic patients, compression using the hydrostatic pressure of mercury has had some effect.[70] The leg is placed in a cylinder and is covered by two membranes, which are filled and emptied with mercury in cycles. Pressures of up to 80 mmHg are generated at the foot and this linearly decreases towards normal atmospheric pressure at the surface. This is well tolerated, and improvement is even seen in those with fibrosclerotic oedema. Despite its theoretical simplicity, the application and safety precautions are complex.

THERMAL TREATMENT

Hyperthermia of the leg is produced by microwave heating or immersion in hot water. There is no change to the flow of lymph, but it does reduce the local inflammatory infiltrate and extracellular protein matrix.[71] A reduction in limb volume follows, along with a decrease in the rate of recurrent infections.

COMPLEX DECONGESTIVE PHYSIOTHERAPY (COMPLEX PHYSICAL THERAPY)

Complex decongestive physiotherapy generally involves a two-stage treatment programme over 2–4 weeks. The first phase consists of skin care, light manual massage, range of motion exercise and compression, typically applied with multi-layered bandage wrapping. Phase 2 aims to conserve and optimise the results obtained in phase 1. It consists of compression by a low-stretch elastic stocking or sleeve, skin care, continued 'remedial' exercise and repeated light massage as needed. With good compliance, a 65–67% reduction in limb volume can be achieved, with 90% of the reduction being maintained at 9 months.[72] As an added benefit, the incidence of infection almost halves and quality of life is improved.[73]

PREVENTION OF INFECTION

The lymphatic system transports lymphocytes, enabling rapid response to foreign antigens. Stagnation of lymph prevents this and so increases the risk and severity of infection. The common pathogens are β-haemolytic streptococci and S. aureus. With each attack of cellulitis or erysipelas, the organisms further obliterate the lymph channels, making the oedema worse. Well-fitting comfortable shoes prevent small cracks in the skin that may act as a portal of entry. Meticulous skin care is essential, and the patient should develop a routine that includes washing followed by thorough drying of the limb, application of an emollient, and monitoring the skin for any problems that develop into cellulitis. Any early signs of infection should be treated aggressively with antibiotics. Recurrent infection can be managed by long-term low-dose prophylactic antibiotics such as amoxicillin, flucloxacillin or a cephalosporin.

Current guidelines recommend that antibiotics be taken for at least 14 days after signs of clinical improvement are observed.[74]

DRUGS

Benzopyrones are thought to reduce oedema by reducing vascular permeability and thus the amount of fluid forming in the subcutaneous tissues. Advocates for this treatment method believe that the drugs have some beneficial effect on pain and discomfort in the swollen areas. Proponents also claim that these drugs increase macrophage activity, encouraging the lysis of protein, which in turn reduces the formation of fibrotic tissue in the lymphoedematous limb. A Cochrane review in 2009 concluded that it is not possible to draw conclusions about the effectiveness of benzopyrones in the management of lymphoedema from the current available trials.[75] Diuretics are not recommended in the management of lymphoedema as there is no evidence that they improve lymphatic drainage.[51]

SURGICAL TREATMENTS

Surgical options are available in some specialist centres. They should be reserved for severely symptomatic patients (e.g., lymphorrhagia or recurrent lymphangitis) in whom all conservative methods have failed. The patient must have realistic expectations of the likely outcome and will need long-term compression therapy after treatment. Surgical procedures can be divided into debulking operations (for obliterative causes) and bypass procedures (for lymphatic obstruction).

Debulking operations

These procedures aim to excise variable amounts of the excess skin and subcutaneous tissue from the affected limb. The techniques range from removal of ellipses of tissue and primary closure (Homan's operation; Fig. 18.7) to the radical Charles operation, which excises all the skin and subcutaneous tissues of the calf down to and sometimes including the deep fascia. Primary skin grafting is then required. Good functional results have been obtained with this method but cosmesis is poor and it may be complicated by warts, resistant ulceration, lymph weeping and pantalooning of the thigh. Suction lipectomy, which has good results in the post-mastectomy arm,[76] has been advocated to overcome these problems but only in the less severe situation because there is a tendency for greater fibrosis in the lower limb. Modern liposuction devices along with the use of tumescent solution and power-assisted cannulae are thought to improve efficacy.[77]

Bypass procedures

These are very rarely performed and are reserved for regional blockage of the lymphatics, because of either primary obstructive or secondary causes. If an iatrogenic secondary cause is suspected, a period of 6 months should elapse to allow any procedural swelling to subside before embarking

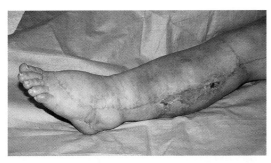

Figure 18.7 Homan's operation. A long ellipse of skin and subcutaneous tissue has been excised from the lateral side of the leg after a previous procedure on the medial side. Poor wound healing is common.

Box 18.6 Bypass procedures for lymphoedema

Skin and muscle flaps
Omental bridges
Enteromesenteric bridges
Lymphatico-lymphatic anastomosis
Lymphatico-venous anastomosis

---

on a lymphatic bypass. The bypass procedures are listed in Box 18.6.

Skin, muscle and omentum have been used to bypass regional obstructions, but these tissues tend to have a paucity of lymphatics and as the technique relies on the development of new channels, high levels of success have not been reported. The technique of enteromesenteric bridging was designed to overcome this problem. A 10-cm segment of ileum is resected on its mesentery and opened along its antimesenteric border. The mucosa is dissected off, leaving a submucosal area rich in lymphatics and blood vessels. The uppermost normal nodes are identified and bisected. The submucosal patch is then stitched in place over the top. Investigation has shown the early development of a lymphatic bridge and follow-up for 6 years has demonstrated a maintained improvement in 75% of legs, but the numbers are very small.[78]

Autologous lymphatic vessels harvested from the contralateral normal limb are used to perform lymphatico-lymphatic anastomoses and bypass obstruction. A suitable conduit is identified after the injection of patent blue dye into the interdigital spaces. The anastomoses are technically demanding. Limb volumetry reveals initial improvements in 66% of cases but this falls to about 50% at 1 year. Recent studies show that lower limb bypasses maintain improvement for up to 10 years.[79]

Lymphatico-venous anastomosis is physiological if one considers the termination of the thoracic duct at the subclavian vein. Excellent long-term results have been published, with volume reductions on average of 67% lasting more than 7 years in the 85% of patients followed up, along with an 87% reduction in the incidence of cellulitis.[80]

Key points

- CVI is the commonest cause of chronic leg swelling.
- The risk of mild to moderate chronic venous insufficiency after DVT is 30% at 10 years.
- The risk of severe CVI after DVT is 2–10% at 10 years.
- Superficial venous reflux alone may cause CVI.
- Graduated elastic compression is effective in healing ulcers and preventing recurrence.
- Superficial venous surgery may be of benefit in isolated superficial venous incompetence and combined superficial and deep venous incompetence.
- Deep venous reconstructive surgery with endovascular stents are playing an increasingly important role in the treatment of patients with PTS, though long-term data are awaited. In young patients with an iliofemoral DVT, thrombolysis should be considered as first-line therapy.
- Lymphoedema may be classified as primary or secondary.
- A further functional classification of obliterative, proximal obstruction, and valvular incompetence and hyperplasia may be used.
- The commonest cause of lymphoedema worldwide is filariasis but in Europe the commonest cause is malignancy and its treatment.
- Oedema is initially pitting but becomes non-pitting because of subcutaneous fat deposition and fibrosis.
- Ulceration is rare in lymphoedema.
- Diagnosis is usually confirmed by isotope lymphangioscintigraphy.
- Satisfactory treatment can usually be achieved by conservative measures, including manual drainage, elastic compression, complex decongestive therapy and prevention of infection.

References available at http://ebooks.health.elsevier.com/

KEY REFERENCES

[4] The Alexander House Group. Consensus paper venous leg ulcers. J Dermatol Surg Oncol 1992;18:592–602.
   A condensed consensus report summarising the status of various aspects of epidemiology, diagnosis and treatment of venous ulcers. Various investigational and treatment approaches are summarised and recommendations given. Level II evidence.

[26] Lurie F, Passman M, Meisner M, et al. The 2020 update of the CEAP classification system and reporting standards. J Vasc Surg Lymphat Disord 2020;8(3):342–52. 40.
   This is an international consensus document produced under the auspice of the American Venous Forum that provides a classification for CVI.

[29] O'Meara S, Cullum NA, Nelson EA. Compression for venous leg ulcers. Cochrane Database Syst Rev 2009;1:CD000265.
   This is a meta-analysis of 39 randomised controlled trials reporting 47 comparisons of compression versus no compression or versus other types of compression in the healing of venous leg ulcers.

[30] Nelson EA, Bell-Syer SEM, Cullum NA, et al. Compression for preventing recurrence of venous ulcers. Cochrane Database Syst Rev 2000;4:CD002303.
   This is a review of two randomised controlled trials, one of which compared class III stockings with class II stockings and the other compared two different makes of class II stocking in the prevention of ulcer recurrence. Higher grades of compression are associated with lower recurrence rates. Also, not wearing stockings is strongly associated with ulcer recurrence.

[32] Nelson EA, Mani R, Thomas K, et al. Intermittent pneumatic compression for treating venous leg ulcers. Cochrane Database Syst Rev 2011;2:CD001899.
   This is a review of seven randomised controlled trials; four compared IPC plus compression with compression alone. One of these found increased ulcer healing with IPC, while three found no evidence of benefit. One trial compared IPC without additional compression with compression alone

and found no difference, and in one trial more ulcers healed with IPC than with dressings. One trial found that rapid IPC healed more ulcers than slow IPC.

[33] Flemming K, Cullum NA. Laser therapy for venous leg ulcers. Cochrane Database Syst Rev 2000;1:CD001182.

Four trials were available, two randomised controlled trials compared laser therapy with sham, one with ultraviolet light and one with red light. Neither of the two randomised controlled trials found a difference in healing rates and there was no significant benefit for laser when the trials were pooled.

[34] Aziz Z, Cullum NA, Flemming K. Electromagnetic therapy for treating venous leg ulcers. Cochrane Database Syst Rev 2011;3:CD002933.

This is a review of three randomised controlled trials comparing electromagnetic therapy (EMT) with sham treatment. One small trial of 44 patients reported significantly more ulcers healed in the EMT group, one reported no difference, and one reported a greater reduction in ulcer size in the EMT group.

[35] Palfreyman SSJ, Nelson EA, Lochiel R, et al. Dressings for healing venous leg ulcers. Cochrane Database Syst Rev 2006;3:CD001103.

This is a meta-analysis of 42 randomised controlled trials evaluating various types of dressings in the treatment of venous leg ulcers. In none of the comparisons was there evidence that any one type of dressing was better than others in terms of the numbers of ulcers healed.

[38] Jull AB, Arroll B, Parag V, et al. Pentoxifylline for treating venous leg ulcers. Cochrane Database Syst Rev 2007;3:CD001733.

This is a meta-analysis of 12 trials, 11 of which compared pentoxifylline (oxpentifylline) with placebo or no treatment. Pentoxifylline is more effective than placebo in terms of complete ulcer healing or significant improvement. The relative risk of ulcer healing with oxpentifylline compared with placebo is 1.70.

[39] Barwell J, Davies C, Deacon J, et al. Comparison of surgery and compression with compression alone in chronic venous ulceration (ESCHAR study): randomized controlled trial. Lancet 2004;363:1854.

This is a randomised controlled trial of 500 consecutive patients with chronic venous ulcers randomly assigned to compression alone or in combination with surgery to assess the role of superficial venous surgery in the healing and prevention of recurrence of leg ulcers. There was no difference in initial healing rates but a reduction in recurrence at 12 months in the surgical group (12% vs. 28%).

[40] Goel R, Abidia A, Hardy SC, Surgery for deep venous incompetence, et al. Cochrane Database Syst Rev 2015;2:CD001097.

[47] Janssen MC, Haenen JH, van Asten WN, et al. Clinical and haemodynamic sequelae of deep venous thrombosis: retrospective evaluation after 7–13 years. Clin Sci 1997;93:7–12.

In this study, 81 patients with venographically confirmed lower-extremity DVT were clinically and haemodynamically re-examined 7–13 years after DVT (mean 10 years) to assess PTS; 7–13 years after DVT, 31% of the patients had moderate and 2% had severe clinical PTS, while 57% of the patients had abnormal haemodynamic findings. Level II evidence.

[68] Badger CM, Peacock JL, Mortimer PS. A randomised, controlled, parallel-group trial comparing multilayer bandaging followed by hosiery versus hosiery alone in the treatment of patients with lymphedema of the limb. Cancer 2000;88:2832–7.

This is a randomised, controlled, parallel-group trial in which 90 women with unilateral lymphoedema (of the upper or lower limbs) underwent 18 days of multi-layer bandaging followed by elastic hosiery or hosiery alone, each for a total period of 24 weeks. The reduction in limb volume caused by multi-layer bandaging followed by hosiery was approximately double that from hosiery alone and was sustained over the 24-week period. The mean overall percentage reduction at 24 weeks was 31% (n=32) for multilayer bandaging versus 15.8% (n=46) for hosiery alone, with a mean difference of 15.2% (95% confidence interval, 6.2–24.2, P=0.001). Level I evidence.

The acutely swollen leg

Cees H.A. Wittens | Rob H.W. Strijkers

19

INTRODUCTION

The acutely swollen leg is a common presenting complaint in the emergency room. It may represent a sudden presentation of an underlying chronic disease, or it may be the manifestation of a new acute problem, in particular deep vein thrombosis (DVT). A number of diseases can be associated with swelling of the lower extremity. It is important to identify the cause of the swelling, as treatment differs greatly depending on the underlying pathology. The underlying diagnosis may be life-threatening and make immediate action necessary and will also influence long-term prognosis and follow-up.

This chapter will help in the evaluation of the acutely swollen leg and will present up-to-date information on the treatment of DVT.

PATHOPHYSIOLOGY OF OEDEMA

Acute swelling of the leg is caused by tissue oedema. Oedema formation is caused by excess water accumulation in the interstitial space of the tissue. Reasons for accumulation of water in the interstitial space are increased hydrostatic pressure, decreased colloid osmotic pressure, increased capillary permeability and lymphatic obstruction. These factors cause rapid fluid shifts in the body. There are also chronic states that cause oedema, but these are beyond the scope of this chapter. The mechanisms causing the shift in fluids are described later.

Increased hydrostatic pressure forces fluid out of the intravascular space. This is usually seen with any process that increases venous pressure. Central causes for increase of hydrostatic pressure include congestive heart failure, right heart failure and tricuspid insufficiency. Focal or unilateral oedema is often the result of DVT causing venous outflow obstruction.

Decreased colloid osmotic pressure allows passive transfer of intravascular fluid to the interstitial compartment. This is generally the result of reduction of intravascular protein content (i.e., hypoalbuminaemia). This mechanism causes generalised oedema and is rarely acute.

Increased capillary permeability removes the barrier to water moving from the intravascular space to the interstitial space. This is observed with focal trauma, burns, infection, ischaemia and immunological injury. This can cause rapid oedema forming in a single leg or it can present as a generalised oedema.

Lymphatic obstruction (lymphoedema) may be the result of hereditary hypoplasia, acute infection, or a consequence of lymphatic ablation following surgery, trauma or radiation. The trigger is usually identifiable, and presentation is rarely acute.

MEDICAL HISTORY

A good medical history from the patient will often raise suspicion regarding the underlying pathology. A previous history of operations on the leg, trauma or a history of DVT may be useful, along with an overview of the patient's general health. There are often several differential diagnoses despite an accurate history. The correct diagnosis, or exclusion of DVT, is essential to prevent potentially life-threatening complications. Consequently, several decision tools have been developed, including the Wells score.[1] It is important to ascertain the precise time point when symptoms began, as this can influence both treatment and prognosis.

PHYSICAL EXAMINATION

Upon examination of the leg, specific features should be identified. The swollen leg may be accompanied by redness, tenderness in the calf and increased temperature. An entry point may be found in cases of erysipelas. Swelling around a specific muscle or muscle compartment may increase suspicion of muscle rupture. Despite a good medical history and thorough physical examination, additional investigations are usually required to confirm a diagnosis. If DVT is suspected, additional imaging may be necessary. Severe pain and loss of sensory and motor function may point towards a compartment syndrome. Skin changes, varicose veins and ulceration of the leg may point towards a chronic venous insufficiency.

DIFFERENTIAL DIAGNOSIS

There are a few differential diagnoses for the acutely swollen leg. The most frequent cause is a DVT. If DVT is suspected, it should be ruled out before any other diagnosis is considered. Other possible causes for acute leg swelling include a ruptured Baker's cyst, erysipelas, cellulitis, fasciitis, muscle rupture or lymphoedema. These causes are mostly limited to one leg. If the patient has swelling of both legs, then alternative causes should be considered, in particular systemic causes such as chronic heart failure, renal failure or sepsis.

MUSCULOTENDINOUS RUPTURE

Sudden intense pain of the calf usually suggests a musculoskeletal aetiology. If associated with sudden dorsiflexion of the foot, rupture of the musculotendinous portion of the medial head of the gastrocnemius muscle or the plantaris muscle (tendon) should be suspected. Localised pain in the medial or mid-calf area and swelling at the ankle level is common. Ecchymotic discolouration at the ankle level often follows 2–5 days later because of blood tracking down the fascial planes when the leg is dependent. Excluding DVT with a venous duplex examination is appropriate.

Treatment consists of symptomatic and supportive care until symptoms resolve. Leg elevation, ice early followed by heat, analgesics and reduced weight bearing may be necessary until symptoms resolve, usually within a month.

BAKER'S CYST

Patients presenting with sudden, instantaneously severe calf pain and swelling of the leg may suffer from a ruptured Baker's cyst. A Baker's cyst forms as a result of overproduction of synovial fluid secondary to an underlying cause such as degenerative arthritis, meniscal tears, gout or rheumatoid arthritis. It is common among adults but can occur in children.[2] A Baker's cyst is usually located on the dorsolateral side of the knee. If the cyst bursts, immediate pain occurs, with swelling of the leg and redness, often mimicking a DVT.[3] The Baker's cyst is usually easily identified with duplex ultrasound.[4] Treatment consists of anti-inflammatory medication, leg elevation and application of cold packs.[5]

CELLULITIS AND ERYSIPELAS

Sudden swelling of the leg, combined with redness, pain and increased warmth, is seen in patients with erysipelas or cellulitis. Accompanying complaints can be nausea, vomiting, headaches and fever. The terms erysipelas and cellulitis are both used. There is, however, a small distinction between the two diagnoses. They differ in that erysipelas involves the upper dermis and superficial lymphatics, whereas cellulitis involves the deeper dermis and subcutaneous fat. This manifests in a different presentation in erysipelas, where there is a clear line of demarcation of the redness and the skin involved. In cellulitis, there is no clear demarcation visible. Upon physical examination, it is important to look for a break in the skin as a portal for entry of bacteria. Common skin barrier breaks are abrasions, insect bites or tinea pedis. Any fluid coming from the wound should be cultured. The most likely causative bacteria are *Staphylococcus aureus* and Group A streptococci.[6] Treatment comprises antibiotics targeted towards Gram-positive bacteria, rest and elevation. Duplex ultrasound should be considered to exclude DVT. Patients treated for erysipelas or cellulitis should experience symptom improvement within 24–48 hours.

NECROTISING FASCIITIS

Fasciitis is a very serious condition with a high morbidity and mortality. While this may present as excruciating pain,[7] other clinical signs may be absent. Possible clinical signs include erythema, crepitations caused by gas formed by subcutaneous bacteria, fever, nausea, vomiting, local oedema, blisters and necrosis of the skin and underlying structures. The underlying mechanism is a bacterial colonisation of *S. aureus* or Group A streptococci. The microorganisms produce endotoxins, which cause a severe inflammatory reaction, with destruction of the deep fascia and surrounding structures. Patients with a compromised immune system are more susceptible to infection with opportunistic bacteria. If this situation is left untreated, the destruction of the fascia will spread and eventually lead to the death of the patient. Treatment of necrotising fasciitis consists of aggressive surgical debridement of the infected tissues. Broad-spectrum antibiotics should be given to include coverage for Gram-positive, Gram-negative and anaerobic organisms.[8] Additional intensive care support is vital to improve the chance of survival. Even with optimal treatment, the mortality rate is over 30%.[9]

LYMPHOEDEMA

Although lymphoedema usually presents as a chronically swollen leg, it can occasionally present acutely. Lymphoedema is the result of impaired lymphatic drainage caused by obstruction or destruction of lymphatic tissue. The major causes of lymphoedema can be classified as primary (hereditary) or secondary (acquired). Causes of primary lymphoedema are congenital lymphoedema, lymphoedema praecox and lymphoedema tarda. These causes manifest themselves in childhood (congenital lymphoedema), puberty (lymphoedema praecox) or early adulthood (lymphoedema tarda). Secondary lymphoedema can be caused by malignancy, surgery with lymph dissection, radiation therapy, infection of lymph nodes, recurrent cellulitis or a connective tissue disease. The management of lymphoedema is discussed in Chapter 18.

BILATERAL SWELLING

Swelling of both legs is usually a sign of a systemic problem, such as heart failure, renal failure, liver failure, sepsis, pulmonary hypertension or drugs (non-steroidal anti-inflammatory drugs [NSAIDs] and calcium-channel blockers), but it is essential to rule out bilateral DVT or vena caval obstruction. History and examination will usually guide further investigation.[10] If the patient has a bilateral swelling caused by a systemic disease, treatment should focus on the primary cause. If the patient uses calcium-channel blockers or NSAIDs, alternatives for these medications can be considered.

DEEP VENOUS THROMBOSIS

DVT is very common in the Western world, with an incidence of 1.6 per 1000 persons per year.[11] The incidence of DVT increases exponentially over the age of 70 years. In people under 18 years of age, DVT is very uncommon, with an incidence of 0.07 per 10 000 per year.[12] In the 19th century,

Table 19.1   Risk factors for deep vein thrombosis

Risk factor	Hypercoagulability	Stasis	Venous injury
Age	X	X	
Immobilisation		X	
Surgery	X	X	
Trauma	X	X	X
Malignancy	X		
Primary hypercoagulable states	X		
History of DVT	X		
Family history	X		
Oral contraceptives	X		
Oestrogen replacement	X		
Pregnancy and puerperium	X	X	
Antiphospholipid and anticardiolipin antibody	X		
Central venous catheters			X
Inflammatory bowel disease	X		
Obesity		X	
Myocardial infarction/congestive heart failure		X	
Varicose veins		X	

DVT, Deep vein thrombosis

Virchow postulated the mechanisms for clot formation. The three main mechanisms are stasis of blood, vessel wall damage and hypercoagulability. Once the clot has formed, it has the tendency to extend. Thrombosis in calf veins does not usually elicit much in the way of symptoms. Once the clot has propagated in the popliteal vein, symptoms may become more apparent. If the clot further propagates to the femoral vein and common femoral vein, obstructing venous outflow from the leg, more severe symptoms are likely. At the most severe end of the spectrum is phlegmasia cerulea alba or phlegmasia cerulea dolens (Fig. 19.1). These conditions require immediate attention from the physician, because of possible limb ischaemia and loss of the leg.

PATHOPHYSIOLOGY OF DEEP VEIN THROMBOSIS

DVT should be viewed as a dynamic condition, and often results from a combination of risk factors that shift the balance of coagulation to a hypercoagulable state. A number of risk factors have been identified, which can be categorised relating to Virchow's triad (Table 19.1).[13] Thrombus usually forms around valves on the endothelium. In 80% of cases, one or more risk factors can be determined in the patient.

CLINICAL DECISION RULES

Because clinical signs are not very specific for DVT, clinical decision tools have been developed to aid patient management. The Wells score is the most widely used and validated clinical decision tool.[14,15] The patient's risk for having a DVT is assessed by the criteria shown in Table 19.2. The patient is then categorised into either a high- or low-risk group. A Wells score of 2 or more indicates that the patient has a high risk of DVT.[1] A Wells score of 0 or 1 puts the patient in the low-risk group. The Wells score combined

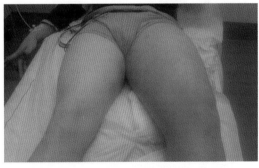

Figure 19.1   Leg with phlegmasia cerulea dolens.

with a D-dimer test can guide the clinician with regard to the need for a duplex scan. A patient with either a Wells score of 2 or more and/or positive D-dimer test will need a duplex scan to look for a possible DVT. Conversely, a Wells score of 0 or 1 with a negative D-dimer almost entirely rules out DVT and the patient does not require a duplex scan. Studies show the negative predictive value for this combination of findings to be 99% for excluding DVT.[16] The clinical decision flow chart is shown in Fig. 19.2. An alternative clinical decision rule has been proposed dividing patients in three groups. Similar to the Wells approach, a negative Wells score and a negative D-dimer safely rules out DVT. The patient with either an elevated Well score or elevated D-dimer qualifies for limited compression ultrasound. Whole leg ultrasound is suggested in patients with both high clinical suspicion and elevated D-dimer levels. This approach was tested by Ageno et al., but has yet to be confirmed to find widespread adaptation.[17]

✓✓ If the patient has a low Wells score combined with a negative D-dimer, DVT can safely be ruled out without the need for a duplex scan.

Table 19.2　Wells score for deep venous thrombosis

Score	Clinical factor
1 point	Active cancer <6 months or palliation
1 point	Paralysis, paresis or recent plaster immobilisation of the lower extremities
1 point	Recently bedridden for more than 3 days or major surgery within 4 weeks
1 point	Entire leg swollen
1 point	Calf swelling by more than 3 cm when compared with the asymptomatic leg
1 point	Pitting oedema
1 point	Collateral superficial veins (non-varicose)
1 point	Previously documented DVT
– 2 points	Alternative diagnosis more likely or greater than that of deep vein thrombosis
Total score	
<2	Low risk of DVT
≥2	High risk of DVT

DVT, Deep vein thrombosis

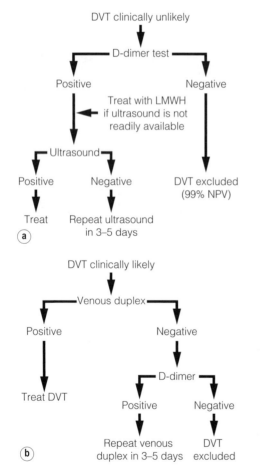

Figure 19.2　Clinical decision flow chart. *DVT*, Deep vein thrombosis; *LMWH*, low-molecular-weight heparin; *NPV*, negative predictive value.

IMAGING TECHNIQUES

The current standard for diagnosing a DVT is a two-point duplex scan.[18] The non-invasive two-point ultrasound examination looks at the popliteal vein and the common femoral vein. The physician will compress the vein at these two points. If the vein is non-compressible, the presence of thrombus is proven. Thrombus may also be visible on sonography and venous flow may be absent. Alternative diagnoses, such as a Baker's cyst, may also be identified on ultrasound. If the duplex scan is inconclusive, but the suspicion of DVT is still high, a conventional venogram or other imaging may be considered. Conventional venography is still the gold standard, but duplex ultrasound is much more accessible, less invasive and easier to perform. In cases of recurrent DVT, it may prove difficult to differentiate between newly formed thrombus and old residual thrombus. Standardised documentation of the previous thrombus location may be helpful. The size of the vein and the identification of scarring may help guide the clinician, with small, scarred veins most likely to represent chronic changes. In experienced hands, it is also possible to estimate thrombus age based on homogeneity. A thrombus with a homogenous aspect is more likely to be fresh. It should also be recognised that fresh thrombus may form within a re-canalised area of old thrombus. Fig. 19.3 shows a duplex scan of the common femoral vein with intraluminal thrombus.

Other techniques are becoming more readily available for imaging of the venous system, including computed tomography, magnetic resonance venography and magnetic resonance direct thrombus imaging. These techniques can be used to identify DVT but are especially useful in determining the precise extent of the thrombus and any underlying stenosis. In particular, the iliac vein segment and the inferior vena cava can be assessed in a simpler manner than with duplex ultrasound.[19,20] These techniques will become very important in identifying patients suitable for more aggressive intervention than standard anticoagulation therapy. Reporting standards have been developed to standardise the scoring of venous disease with different imaging techniques (LOVE score). With these standardised reports, it is possible to identify and report DVT systematically and stratify patients into different treatment groups (LET score).[21,22] This will become more important as treatment options advance further. Fig. 19.4 shows a magnetic resonance venograph with a DVT present in the popliteal vein and femoral vein of the left leg. Magnetic resonance direct thrombus imaging can be used in case of suspected recurrent ipsilateral deep DVT.[23]

INVESTIGATION OF MALIGNANCIES

There is an association between occult malignancies and unprovoked DVT. Between 4% and 12% of patients with an unprovoked DVT will be diagnosed with cancer during treatment for their DVT. Guidelines suggest limited screening for malignancy consisting of a medical history, physical examination and basic blood test with additional sex specific tests.[24]

TESTING FOR THROMBOPHILIA

There are many hereditary and acquired thrombophilia factors associated with DVT. Routine testing for these factors is not recommended. Testing for thrombophilia factors should be considered in patients with unprovoked venous thromboembolism (VTE) and a family history of VTE in the first degree.[24]

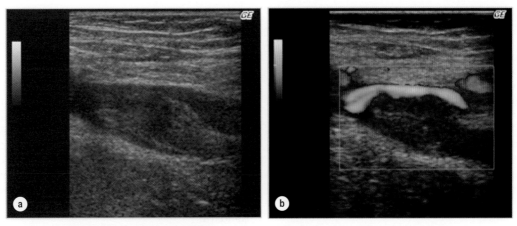

Figure 19.3 Duplex scan of the common femoral vein with intraluminal thrombus.

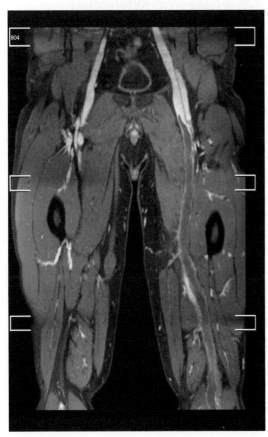

Figure 19.4 Magnetic resonance venography with a deep vein thrombosis (DVT) present in the popliteal vein and femoral vein of the left leg.

TREATMENT OF DEEP VEIN THROMBOSIS

DVT needs to be treated immediately to prevent potentially lethal pulmonary emboli and to stop thrombus propagation. Standard treatment of DVT as formulated by the American College of Chest Physicians (ACCP) guidelines consists of three aspects, namely oral anticoagulation, compression therapy and mobilisation.[25]

Anticoagulation treatment prevents extension of thrombus and pulmonary embolism. Treatment should be started as soon as the diagnosis has been confirmed or in a patient with a Wells score of 2 or more and/or a positive D-dimer test while awaiting duplex scan confirmation. Anticoagulation is achieved by immediate subcutaneous administration of therapeutic levels of low-molecular-weight heparins (LMWHs). Oral anticoagulation with vitamin K antagonists (VKAs) can be started simultaneously. Treatment with the LMWHs can be stopped after the international normalised ratio (INR) has reached the therapeutic range for 2 consecutive days. The INR range for a first-time DVT should be between 2 and 3.[26] Since 2012 new oral anticoagulants (NOACs) are available as alternatives for treatment with VKAs. Drugs like rivaroxaban, dabigatran, apixaban and edoxaban have been tested extensively on their effectiveness and safety. The NOACs have shown to reduce the risk of recurrent VTE complications equal to that of VKAs and are equally safe in regard to bleeding risk.[27–30] Anticoagulation should be given for at least 3 months. Depending on the balance of risk of bleeding and further DVT, the physician can choose to prolong the anticoagulation to 6 or 12 months.[31] Patients with malignancy should be treated with LMWHs for 3–6 months. Patients with a recurrent episode of DVT should be treated with lifelong anticoagulation. Hospitalisation for anticoagulation therapy is not necessary and treatment can be performed safely in the community.[32] Anticoagulation has no effect on the existing thrombus, resolution of which depends on the patient's own lytic system.[25,31]

✅✅ Patients with DVT should be treated with anticoagulation therapy for at least 3 months.

For a long time, compression therapy was given for 2 years routinely to patients with DVT in order to prevent post-thrombotic syndrome (PTS). However, recent trials have changed this approach and international guidelines now recommend using compression stockings for 6 months. After evaluation of the leg with the Villalta scale, compression therapy is either stopped, continued for another 6 months or recommended indefinitely. In the acute phase with leg oedema, compression therapy can be achieved with short stretch bandages. Once this has reduced the acute swelling, the patient can be switched to therapeutic elastic compressive stockings. The stockings should be to the knee and effect a minimum pressure of between 30 and 40 mmHg. Current guidelines still advise to wear compression stockings for 2 years based on trials, which show a 50% reduction in post-thrombotic morbidity.[33] However, the randomised controlled sox-trial by Kahn et al. showed no reduction at all in PTS in the group of patients with compression stockings compared to patients wearing sham stockings.[34] Despite encouragement, patient compliance for compression hosiery is low. The ideal-study by Ten Cate et al. compared 6 months of compression therapy to 2 years of compression therapy in acute DVT. The trial showed no difference in occurrence of PTS after 2 years between the two strategies.[35]

✓✓ The use of compression stockings should be patient tailored. Based on the Villalta score, compression therapy ends after 6 months, is prolonged to a year or is recommended indefinitely.

Finally, immediate mobilisation is proven to be safe and does not increase the risk of pulmonary embolism.[36,37]

Thromboprophylaxis is discussed in Chapter 2 of *Core Topics in General and Emergency Surgery* in this Companion to Specialist Surgical Practice series.

PROGNOSIS

If patients are treated according to the ACCP guidelines, the risk of recurrent DVT is 30% within 5 years of the initial DVT.[38] More worrisome is the high incidence of PTS, affecting between 20% and 50% of patients with DVT within 2 years,[39,40] because the variability in reported incidence relates to the use of different scales to assess PTS.[41] Patients with iliofemoral DVT have a twofold increased risk of developing PTS compared with patients with a below-knee DVT.[42] The CaVenT study showed that 56% of patients after iliofemoral DVT develop PTS within 2 years.[43]

ILIOFEMORAL DEEP VEIN THROMBOSIS

In iliofemoral DVT, the thrombus is located proximally, having extended from the common femoral vein segment or commenced within the iliac veins or inferior vena cava. Thrombus in the common femoral vein obstructs outflow of the superficial and deep femoral vein, usually resulting in marked leg swelling and pain. Severe venous obstruction can result in phlegmasia cerulea dolens. This is a dangerous condition, where the circulation is compromised and may lead to amputation. Current ACCP guidelines suggest that immediate clot removal may be considered in specific patients with low bleeding risks. In all other cases of iliofemoral DVT, anticoagulation is still considered the gold standard.[25]

POST-THROMBOTIC SYNDROME

PTS is a chronic disease following DVT, with significant impacts on patient quality of life and healthcare burden.[3] PTS incorporates a range of patient complaints and physical signs of venous disease. The severity of PTS can be recorded using the validated Villalta–Prandoni scale[44] (Table 19.3). The precise aetiology is unknown, though there are identified risk factors that increase the risk of developing PTS. Obstruction of the venous outflow tract together with insufficiency, residual thrombus and recurrent DVT are significant risk factors correlating with the development of PTS.[40,45] In particular, poor re-canalisation of iliofemoral DVT causes outflow obstruction and a state of venous hypertension, which in turn causes inflammation and vein wall damage.[46–48] The re-canalisation process and inflammation also cause valves to be destroyed, resulting in

Table 19.3 Villalta–Prandoni scale for post-thrombotic syndrome (also incorporates the presence or absence of venous ulceration)

Symptoms and clinical signs	None	Mild	Moderate	Severe
Symptoms				
Pain	0	1	2	3
Cramps	0	1	2	3
Heaviness	0	1	2	3
Paraesthesia	0	1	2	3
Pruritis	0	1	2	3
Clinical signs				
Pre-tibial oedema	0	1	2	3
Skin induration	0	1	2	3
Hyperpigmentation	0	1	2	3
Redness	0	1	2	3
Venous ectasia	0	1	2	3
Pain on calf compression	0	1	2	3
Venous ulcer	Absent	Present		
Total score	<5	5–9	10–14	≥15 or venous ulcer
PTS classification	No PTS	Mild PTS	Moderate PTS	Severe PTS

PTS, Post-thrombotic syndrome.

venous insufficiency. Successful early thrombus removal or lysis should avoid these complications and thus lower post-thrombotic morbidity.[49] The concept of lysis is not new. Reports and case series from the 1980s stimulated interest in systemic thrombolytic therapy. While results of clinical trials showed that systemic thrombolysis slightly improved complete clot lysis, the high incidence of major bleeding complications has rendered the technique obsolete.[50,51]

✓✓ Systemic thrombolysis should not be given to patients with DVT, because of high major bleeding risk.

However, the severity and chronicity of symptoms is still well recognised,[52] stimulating interest in lysis delivered locally. Catheter-directed lysis has been shown to improve patient quality of life without the high rate of bleeding complications associated with systemic treatment.[53]

CATHETER-DIRECTED THROMBOLYSIS

Catheter-directed thrombolysis (CDT) involves the placement of a catheter directly into the thrombus and local administration of the thrombolytic agent. The drug activates tissue plasminogen, which is converted into plasmin, which in turn can dissolve the fibrin strands of the clot.[54] Local administration in the thrombus enhances the thrombolytic effects but reduces the bleeding complications, because of the lower dosages needed. Retrospective studies have shown that successful lysis directly correlated with improved health-related quality of life.[55]

Three randomised controlled trials evaluated the use of CDT. The CaVenT study showed that patients with iliofemoral DVT treated with CDT had an absolute risk reduction of 14% in developing PTS compared to patients treated with standard therapy after 2 years. After 5 years of follow-up, the absolute risk reduction increased to 28%, but quality of life did not differ between the intervention and conservative treatment group.[56]

There was a 3% incidence of major haemorrhage. This is the first randomised controlled trial showing the benefits of early clot removal in iliofemoral DVT with an acceptable bleeding risk.[43]

The American Attract-trial randomised 692 patients to either pharmaco-mechanical CDT and anticoagulation or anticoagulation alone. The addition of CDT did not result in a lower incidence of PTS in patients with proximal DVT after 2 years. It did however, increase the risk of major bleeding.[57] The Dutch CAVA trial randomised 184 patients with an iliofemoral DVT to either CDT or anticoagulation alone. After 1-year median follow-up, no difference in the occurrence of PTS was observed.[58] Post-hoc analysis of the CAVA-trial showed a reduction of PTS severity in patients with successful CDT intervention. However, no reduction in PTS was shown.

A systematic review and meta-analyses in 2021 showed no statistical difference in PTS occurrence between CDT and anticoagulation in iliofemoral DVT with the pooled data from Cavent, Attract and CAVA.[59]

The European Society for Vascular and endovascular Surgery developed guidelines for the use of CDT and other clot removal techniques (see later). The guidelines advise to consider early thrombus removal in selected patients with iliofemoral DVT and low bleeding risk. In femoral or popliteal DVT, early thrombus removal is not recommended. Meta-analysis of four randomised controlled trials showed lower incidences of PTS in the early thrombus removal treatment group. After early thrombus removal therapy, routine anticoagulation should be started.

A number of CDT studies have demonstrated underlying iliac vein stenosis as a potential contributing factor for further DVT.[60,61] May–Thurner syndrome is the most prevalent of the stenotic lesions in the left common iliac vein. This syndrome is a condition where the left common iliac vein is compressed by the overlying right iliac artery, as demonstrated in Fig. 19.5.[62] Treatment of the underlying stenosis with balloon venoplasty, stenting or both, can be performed to relieve venous outflow obstruction, though the role of these interventions remains ill-defined.[63,64] As more data become available regarding CDT for iliofemoral DVT, we will obtain greater understanding of the role and appropriate management of underlying iliac vein stenoses.

✓✓ Patients with iliofemoral DVT and low bleeding risk should be considered for CDT to reduce the severity of PTS.

NEW TREATMENT MODALITIES

Although the results of lysis in the CaVenT study are good, the mean treatment time of 2.4 days is considered long. Future techniques will focus on shortening the treatment time, lowering bleeding risk and avoiding the need for expensive intensive care hospitalisation. Therefore the addition of a mechanical component has been suggested to speed up clot removal. This technique is called pharmaco-mechanical thrombolysis (PMT). Different PMT catheters are commercially available. A number of them are discussed in the next section.

EKOS ENDOWAVE

The EKOS endowave catheter combines the standard CDT with ultrasound elements. These elements emit high-frequency, low-energy ultrasound waves that enhance the penetration of the thrombolytic drug into the thrombus,

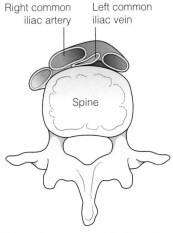

Figure 19.5 Schematic overview of the May–Thurner syndrome.

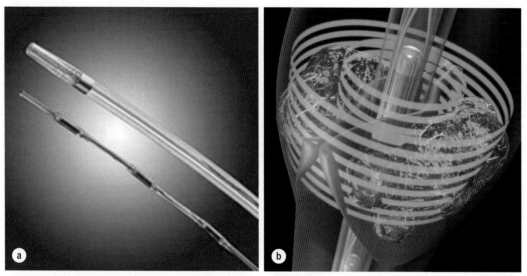

Figure 19.6 EKOS device.

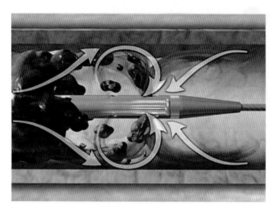

Figure 19.7 Angiojet device.

enhancing the lytic effect. In vitro studies have shown better permeability of the agent in the thrombus and reduced treatment time. Retrospective case series have shown that thrombolysis with the EKOS catheter is feasible and safe. The ongoing randomised controlled Dutch CAVA trial is further investigating the role of the EKOS endowave system in patients with iliofemoral DVT (Fig. 19.6).[65]

ANGIOJET

The Angiojet Power Pulse system (Fig. 19.7) uses a complex mixture of rapid fluid streaming and hydrodynamic forces to fracture the thrombus, allowing extraction at the catheter tip as a result of negative pressure (the Bernoulli effect). The catheter infuses normal saline through an infusion port while simultaneously suctioning through the effluent port. If the effluent port is clamped, the infusion port acts as a mechanical 'pulse spray' that delivers the pre-loaded thrombolytic drug to the thrombus. This is the only device that can be solely used as a mechanical thrombectomy device. Safety and feasibility of the Angiojet have been demonstrated in retrospective case series only.[66]

OTHER PHARMACO-MECHANICAL DEVICES

The AngioVac Cannula (AngioDynamics, Latham, New York) (Fig. 19.8) is a mechanical suction device that is designed for removal of intravascular material such as thrombus, tumour, foreign bodies and vegetation, while maintaining flow during extra-corporeal circulation. The suction cannula is a 22-Fr device that can be advanced over a wire using an internal dilator. The device has an expandable tip that opens up to 48-Fr. This tip serves as the suction end of a veno-venous non-oxygenating bypass circuit that filters removed blood and returns it to the venous system via a separate re-infusion cannula or sheath. The patient requires general anaesthesia to perform this procedure. Maximum anticoagulation is given to keep the bypass circuit open and a perfusionist monitors it. Evidence for this procedure is limited.

The Aspirex®S 10 F system (Straub medical AG, Wangs, Switzerland) is a new PMT device. The device has a corkscrew-shaped wire on the tip of the catheter, which fragments and aspirates fresh thrombus out of the veins. A close-up view of the tip of catheter is shown in Fig. 19.9. Data on this device are limited to case reports.

THE FUTURE

A more aggressive approach to the treatment of iliofemoral DVT will reveal underlying venous anomalies in approximately 50% of patients.[67]

Additional treatment of the underlying stenosis may enhance patency and improve the prevention of PTS. Dedicated thrombus removal devices and venous stents may further enhance clot lysis and long-term patency, but randomised clinical trials are essential to define their precise role in clinical practice.

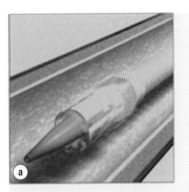
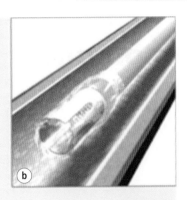
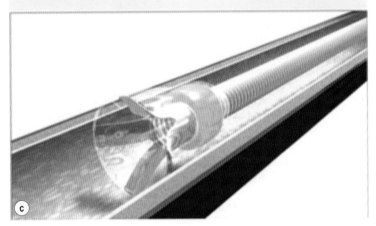

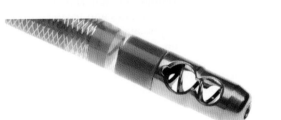

Figure 19.8 AngioVac device.

Figure 19.9 Aspirex device.

Key points

- Acute leg swelling can indicate a number of diseases. An important differential diagnosis is DVT, which needs to be treated immediately to prevent potentially lethal pulmonary emboli.
- A low Wells score combined with low D-dimer levels is safe for ruling out DVT.
- Duplex sonography is the standard modality to confirm DVT.
- Standard treatment for DVT is oral anticoagulation, compressive stockings and mobilisation.
- Patients with iliofemoral DVT are associated with severe post-thrombotic morbidity and should be considered for additional CDT therapy.

References available at http://ebooks.health.elsevier.com/

KEY REFERENCES

[16] Wells PS, Anderson DR, Rodger M, et al. Evaluation of D-dimer in the diagnosis of suspected deep-vein thrombosis. N Engl J Med 2003;349(13):1227–35. PMID: 14507948.
   This randomised controlled trial evaluates the value of D-dimer testing in combination with the Wells score in evaluating the chance of the patient having DVT and the ability to safely exclude DVT.
[25] Kearon C, Akl EA, Ornelas J, Blaivas A, Jimenez D, Bounameaux H, et al. Antithrombotic therapy for VTE disease: CHEST guideline and expert panel report. Chest 2016;149(2):315–52.
   These guidelines extend a level 1a recommendation for treating DVT with anticoagulation for at least 3 months. These guidelines have been composed after an exhaustive search of multiple studies carefully selected by authorities in the field.
[34] Kahn SR, Shapiro S, Wells PS, et al. Compression stockings to prevent post-thrombotic syndrome: a randomised placebo-controlled trial. Lancet 2014;383(9920):880–8. PMID: 24315521.
   This randomised controlled trial compares treatment of DVT with and without compression therapy and the impact on incidence of PTS on both groups.
[59] Broderick C, Watson L, Armon MP. Thrombolytic strategies versus standard anticoagulation for acute deep vein thrombosis of the lower limb. Cochrane Database Syst Rev 2021;1:CD002783.
   Systematic review reporting on the effects of CDT for acute DVT. No statistically significant difference in PTS occurrence was found between CDT and anticoagulation for acute iliofemoral DVT.

20

Vascular anomalies

Ian McCafferty

INTRODUCTION

Vascular anomalies are a complex broad group of developmental abnormalities that present significant challenges in diagnosis and management. The rarity and diverse presentation of vascular anomalies often mean patients are seen by multiple specialists, before a correct diagnosis and treatment can be instigated. Accurate and timely diagnosis are crucial, and a multidisciplinary team approach is essential for their appropriate evaluation and management. The exact make-up of the multidisciplinary team varies but vascular surgery, interventional radiology and plastic surgery typically play a central role, along with other specialities, for example, maxillofacial surgeons, dermatologists and laser specialists.

Mulliken and Glowacki[1] originally proposed a new way of classifying vascular anomalies in 1982, based on the biological and pathological differences of lesions. The classification broadly separates vascular anomalies into two groups: proliferative vascular tumours and vascular malformations. In 1992 Mulliken and Young founded the International Society for the Study of Vascular Anomalies (ISSVA) and the classification was adopted by the society. The classification has been modified over the years as the understanding of vascular anomalies developed. Vascular malformations are caused by errors in development at various stages of vasculogenesis or angiogenesis and are further classified on the basis of the main vessel involved: capillary, lymphatic, venous, arterial or combined.

CLASSIFICATION

One of the original aims of ISSVA was to achieve a uniform classification for the understanding and management of vascular anomalies. Following the proposed biological classification by Mulliken and Glowacki in 1982, and adoption by ISSVA in 1992, the system has become widely accepted, helping to resolve the confusing terminology in the field of vascular anomalies. In 2013 a group of experts within ISSVA met to update the classification to include new understanding, and elements of other classification systems, for example, the Hamburg classification system. This system, described in 1988, separates malformations based on the timing of arrested development of the vascular system. Extra-truncal lesions are defects at an early stage of angiogenesis, with immature amorphous vascular tissue and truncal lesions arising from pre-existing mature vascular structures. The updated ISSVA vascular anomalies classification was published in 2014 at the 20th ISSVA workshop. The new classification has updated the proliferative vascular tumour section into benign, locally aggressive or malignant, and the vascular malformation section into simple, combined, named vessel and association with defined syndromes (Table 20.1).

VASCULAR TUMOURS

INFANTILE HAEMANGIOMA

These are the most common benign tumours in children, occurring in 2.5% of all neonates and having a distinct life cycle. Infantile haemangiomata (IH) are not present on the day of birth but usually appear within days to weeks after birth. They are characterised in early infancy (<10 months) by an initial proliferative phase, which can be rapid, followed by an involutional phase leading to spontaneous complete regression in most patients. IH occur in 5–10% of Caucasian infants and are three times more common in females. Some 10% have a history of an affected family member and they are more common in prematurity, multiple births and low birth-weights. In 30–50% of individuals, a premonitory mark 'herald spot', that is, focal area of pallor, is present. The precise pathogenesis is unknown; however, IH have a unique phenotype, which closely resembles placental vasculature rather than mature cutaneous vasculature, and as such is glucose transporter-1 (GLUT-1)-positive. Cellular markers of angiogenesis, for example, vascular endothelial growth factor, are also increased, especially during the proliferative phase.

The diagnosis is clinical, with lesions having a typical natural history and being warm to palpation, because of the fact that they are high-flow lesions. IH involving the superficial dermis produce lobulated, bright red lesions that are commonly referred to as '*strawberry birthmarks*' (Fig. 20.1), whereas deep dermal involvement produces a swelling with either no discolouration or a blueness of the skin. Anatomical location plays a critical role in determining whether complications may occur. IH can occur anywhere, although 60% occur in the head and neck region, with their distribution typically along facial developmental subunits.

The proliferative phase of an IH varies in its duration, but rapid growth will usually occur during the first 6–10 months of life, followed by gradual involution of the IH. This process is complete in 50% of individuals by 5 years, in 70% by 7 years, 90% by 9 years and virtually all by 12 years. Residual skin changes following complete involution are common; in the majority they are mild and inconspicuous, but 20–50% have significant changes of skin distortion and a fibro-fatty remnant.

DIAGNOSIS AND IMAGING

The diagnosis of IH is straightforward based upon the clinical history and examination; imaging is often unnecessary unless there is a concern about associated underlying structural anomalies. It may occasionally be difficult to differentiate deep haemangiomata from other vascular anomalies or tumours; in such instances, further investigation, and occasionally biopsy, may be necessary. GLUT-1 positivity on the pathological specimen is pathognomonic.

The imaging features during the proliferative phase are usually characteristic; ultrasound demonstrates a well-defined, reflective lesion that is highly vascular, with central feeding vessels. Magnetic resonance imaging (MRI) will demonstrate a well-defined lobulated tumour that is iso-intense or hypointense when compared with normal muscle on T1-weighted images and hyperintense on T2-weighted images. If intravenous contrast is given, the tumour will enhance avidly and homogeneously.

COMPLICATIONS AND STRUCTURAL ASSOCIATIONS

The majority of complications of IH occur when growth is most rapid in the first 6 months. These include ulceration, bleeding, infection, compromise to vital organs and in rare instances cardiac failure. Cutaneous ulceration is the most common complication, occurring in 10%, and is often when the lesions become painful. Significant bleeding is very uncommon.

- **Amblyopia:** Is a complication of peri-ocular haemangioma. Closure of the eye can lead to occlusion of the visual axis, which will prevent light stimulation and result in loss of vision. Close ophthalmic review and early intervention is essential in these cases.
- **Subglottic haemangioma:** Infants with large segmental haemangiomata of the neck and 'beard area' require careful follow-up during the first 12–16 weeks of life as they have a 60% risk of associated airway haemangiomata. These tumours may be life-threatening.
- **PHACE syndrome:** PHACE syndrome[2] (an acronym for: Posterior fossa; Haemangioma; Arterial anomalies; Coarctation of the aorta and other cardiac defects; Eye abnormalities) describes the association between large segmental facial haemangiomata and several structural abnormalities. Affected individuals are nearly always female and the haemangioma most commonly involves the upper face and forehead, but this is not invariable. A child with such a lesion should be carefully examined for signs and symptoms of the syndrome and appropriate investigations should be performed to exclude associated anomalies, especially heart and aorta.

Table 20.1 Vascular malformations associated with other anomalies/syndromes

Syndrome	Associated vascular malformation
Klippel–Trenaunay syndrome (KTS)	CM + VM ± LM + limb overgrowth
Parkes–Weber syndrome	CM + AVM + limb overgrowth
Servelle–Martorell syndrome	Limb VM + bone overgrowth
Sturge–Weber syndrome	Facial + leptomeningeal CM + eye ± bone and soft tissue
Maffucci syndrome	VM ± spindle cell haemangiomata + enchondroma
Proteus syndrome	CM + VM ± LM + asymmetrical somatic overgrowth
Macrocephaly and microcephaly	CM
CLOVES syndrome	LM + VM + CM ± AVM + lipomatous overgrowth
Bannayan–Riley–Ruvalcaba syndrome	AVM + VM + macrocephaly + limb overgrowth
Rendu–Osler–Weber syndrome	CM
Blue rubber bleb naevus syndrome	VM
Gorham–Stout syndrome	LM

Malformations: AVM, *Arteriovenous;* CM, *capillary;* LM, *lymphatic;* VM, *venous.*

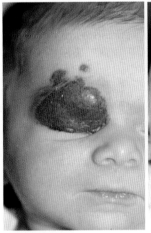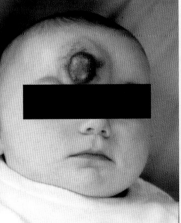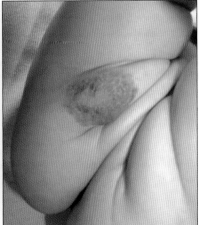

Figure 20.1 Typical infantile haemangioma with a 'strawberry-like' appearance, a rapidly growing infantile haemangioma and a non-involuting congenital haemangioma.

MANAGEMENT

Haemangiomata are extremely heterogeneous in location, size and growth characteristics. The majority of the smaller lesions can be treated conservatively with parent information and clinic visits to wait for resolution after the involuntary phase. Intervention is indicated when a lesion causes significant mass effect or disfigurement, when it involves the airway and when it obstructs the visual axis or in the presence of secondary complications. The mainstay of management is medical, with treatment with beta-blockers the preferred first-line therapy.[3] Bleomycin injections have also been used to treat complications of ulceration and vision as first-or second-line therapy.[4] Occasionally, in visceral haemangioma, particulate embolisation techniques are required to treat severe bleeding or cardiac failure.

The surgical management of haemangioma can be divided into two main areas. Early surgery, during the proliferative phase, is generally reserved for lesions obstructing the visual axis when more conservative measures have failed, following partial or complete involution, between the ages of 3 and 5 years, and may be considered for persistent cosmetic deformity or when a large haemangioma persists and is having a detrimental effect on the child's social development because of its appearance. The surgical scar that is likely to result from such an operation should, however, be weighed against the likely outcome if the haemangioma were allowed to involute completely.

CONGENITAL HAEMANGIOMA

These haemangiomata differ in their natural history and prognosis when compared with infantile haemangiomata.[5] They are rare, with an estimated incidence of 0.3%. They are present and fully grown at birth and often regress rapidly before 1 year of age, remain stable or partially involute. On this basis, they have been divided into two main distinct groups: rapidly involuting congenital haemangiomata (RICH) and non-involuting congenital haemangiomata, (NICH) (Fig. 20.2). Both types are histologically and immunophenotypically distinct from infantile haemangiomata; they are high-flow lesions composed of capillary lobules where endothelial cells do not express GLUT-1 positivity and are associated with large extralobular veins, arteries and lymphatics. RICH may be associated with transient thrombocytopenia and consumptive coagulopathy.

TUFTED ANGIOMA

Tufted angiomas (TAs) appear as brown or erythematous plaques in children and young adults. Occasionally, they are present at birth and can be associated with hyperhidrosis or hypertrichosis. TAs are composed of small tufts of capillaries characteristically surrounded by a crescentic slit-like vessel dispersed throughout the dermis in a cannonball pattern.

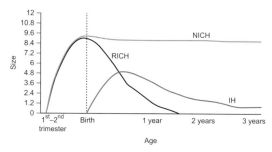

Figure 20.2 Evolution scheme of natural history of untreated infantile haemangioma (IH) and congenital haemangioma (CH) (non-involuting congenital haemangiomata [NICH] and rapidly involuting congenital haemangiomata [RICH]). IH appears after birth and grows rapidly before stabilising. CHs are fully-grown at birth, with RICH involuting rapidly and NICH persisting.

KAPOSIFORM HAEMANGIOENDOTHELIOMA

Kaposiform haemangioendotheliomas (KHE) are rare lesions that may affect the skin but often affect deeper tissues and organs, for example, the liver. They are high-flow lesions and can occur as a focal abnormality or as diffuse organ involvement. The majority present in early infancy. Histologically, KHE resembles a TA with larger and tumour lobules in a more infiltrative pattern.

Both TA and KHE tumours express lymphatic endothelial markers and are GLUT-1 negative. Many authors consider the two tumours to be part of a spectrum rather than distinct entities. Both may be associated with the life-threatening Kasabach–Merritt phenomenon (KMP), which is characterised by profound thrombocytopenia and a severe consumption coagulopathy and is associated with a high mortality. KMP is not a complication of the common infantile haemangioma[6] and should not be confused with the less profound coagulopathy that may be associated with large venous malformations.

VASCULAR MALFORMATIONS

Vascular malformations are believed to be present at birth, but they may not become evident clinically for many years. They are sporadic and persist for life, never spontaneously regress and commonly may undergo periods when they increase in size and become painful.[7] This is most common during puberty or pregnancy or following trauma or spontaneous thrombosis (a triggering event is not always recognised). They can be localised or diffuse lesions, which do not respect anatomical boundaries, and their clinical presentation and prognosis is often dependent on the degree of anatomical involvement. They are most conveniently divided into low-flow and high-flow subsets, a differentiation that is usually evident on clinical examination (see in later subsections). Low-flow malformations are further subdivided into capillary, venous and lymphatic subtypes, which may exist as a single entity, combined or associated with other anomalies in syndromes as described in updated 2014 ISSVA classification. High-flow malformations are termed *arteriovenous malformations* (AVMs) and are further subdivided on the basis of the predominant level of fistulous communication.

CAPILLARY MALFORMATIONS

Capillary malformations come in a variety of forms.

SALMON PATCH (NAEVUS SIMPLEX; ERYTHEMA NUCHAE)

A salmon patch is a red macule present at birth, which most commonly involves the skin of the nape of the neck, the upper eyelids or glabella. It is usually central, does not follow a dermatomal distribution and will usually fade by 2 years of age, especially if it involves the skin of the face; the nuchal lesion is more likely to persist into adult life.

PORT-WINE STAINS (NAEVUS FLAMEUS)

Port-wine stains are well-demarcated vascular stains that are present at birth and increase in size commensurately with the child's growth. They are relatively uncommon and have an equal sex distribution. They tend to follow a dermatomal distribution and are usually unilateral, although they may occasionally cross the midline. Those involving the face are usually flat in early childhood but have a tendency to become thickened and nodular over time and may be associated with bony and soft-tissue hypertrophy. Most of these facial lesions occur as an isolated abnormality but some are part of a syndrome complex, for example, Sturge–Weber syndrome,[8] which describes the triad of a facial port-wine stain in a V1 distribution, an ipsilateral leptomeningeal vascular malformation and a choroidal vascular malformation of the eye that can cause glaucoma. MRI is helpful to document an intra-cranial abnormality, although only 10% of children with a port-wine stain in the V1 distribution will have the syndrome.

LOW-FLOW VASCULAR MALFORMATIONS

These have a varied clinical presentation depending on whether the lesions are focal or diffuse and which anatomical compartments are involved. They are present at birth, although they may not be apparent until adolescence or adulthood, and can fluctuate at certain times, for example, pregnancy. Venous malformations are the commonest low-flow entity, with a prevalence of 1% in the general population. These lesions are often described as having the 'iceberg phenomenon' as the portion clinically apparent is often the tip of the underlying abnormality.[9]

A detailed history and clinical examination commonly reveal the diagnosis and can help differentiate from other sinister pathology, for example, sarcoma. Clinical features are typically related to the focal mass and patients present with pain and swelling, often intermittent and associated with acute flare-ups lasting 3–5 days. Clinical features that are atypical for low-flow vascular malformations, including a short clinical history with rapid increase in size or pain, a poor response to treatment or atypical imaging, should lead to a percutaneous biopsy to ensure the correct diagnosis and to exclude the rare mimics of these malformations, for example, angiosarcoma, low-grade sarcoma, B-cell lymphoma, Ewing's tumour.

Vascular malformations tend not to respect anatomical boundaries and the prognosis, to some degree, depends on the tissues involved. The Birmingham classification[10] defined malformations dependent on the level of tissue involvement from skin to bone, eye and peritoneum and association with syndromes as identified on MRI imaging. The classification defined four types (1–4), which increased in complexity and difficulty in management (Table 20.2).

LOW-FLOW VENOUS MALFORMATIONS

Venous malformations consist of dilated venous spaces of varying size, within which blood flow is slow. They vary considerably in size and can be focal or diffuse. The morphology of venous malformations is dependent on the composition of degree and size of the vascular spaces to cellular matrix component. They can be subdivided into those with macrovascular spaces, matrix-rich (solid) or mixed lesions. This is an important distinction for treatment planning and prognosis. They occur anywhere in the body but are most common in the head and neck and limbs. Most commonly, the low-flow venous malformation (LFVM) causes a dull ache accentuated by activity, extremes of temperature, Valsalva manoeuvre or dependency. Frequently, there are more severe bouts of pain, secondary to localised thrombophlebitis. There is frequently a localised coagulopathy with low fibrinogen levels and raised D-dimers.[11] The extent of symptoms depends on the size, location and proximity to adjacent structures. Superficial lesions often exhibit a bluish discolouration and can be associated with dilated veins. On examination, the lesions are characteristically soft, compressible, non-pulsatile and demonstrate filling on dependency (Fig. 20.3). Phleboliths are pathognomonic and 75% progress during adolescence.[12] Most venous malformations are single, but they may rarely be multiple or combined with capillary, lymphatic and high-flow lesions or as part of

Table 20.2   **The Birmingham classification of low-flow vascular malformations**

	Limbs	Head and neck	Trunk
Type 1	Superficial (skin and subcutaneous tissue) (a) Localised (b) Diffuse		
Type 2	Fascia/muscle involvement	Fascia/muscle/mucosa involvement	Fascia/muscle involvement
Type 3	Bone/joint involvement	Bone/joint/airway involvement	Spinal/central nervous involvement
Type 4	Diffuse whole limb involvement ± hypertrophy (e.g., Klippel–Trenaunay)	Ocular/intra-cranial involvement	Intra-peritoneal involvement

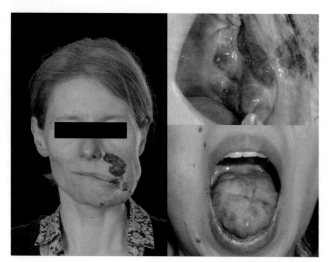

Figure 20.3 Typical clinical features of a low-flow venous malformation that affects skin and mucosal surfaces; blue discolouration with mass effect that exhibits dependency.

syndromes like the blue rubber bleb naevus or Bean syndrome. Most of these cases are sporadic, although some are inherited in an autosomal dominant fashion.

LOW-FLOW LYMPHATIC MALFORMATIONS

Lymphatic malformations are best subclassified into macrocystic and microcystic lesions; although there is no agreed definition, most authors consider macrocystic lesions as those that can be easily accessed with a small needle to administer therapy. Most are evident at birth, but some may not become apparent until early childhood. Macrocystic low-flow lymphatic malformations (LFLMs) most commonly affect the head and neck, trunk and extremities (90%); lesions do not exhibit dependency, are not compressible but transilluminate. Microcystic LFLMs can infiltrate tissues, most commonly skin and mucous membranes but they can also affect bone and organs. They have a typical clinical appearance, with multiple vesicles overlying the affected area, which often bleed, leak lymph and are frequently complicated by infections, which cause acute expansion and pain. LFLM lesions are most likely to progress during adolescence.

DIAGNOSIS AND IMAGING

The vast majority of low-flow vascular malformations are diagnosed with a detailed history and examination. Usually, one can differentiate them further into lymphatic and venous types based on anatomical position, features of dependency (LFVM) and transillumination (LFLM). Imaging is primarily required to identify the extent of tissue involvement, confirm the diagnosis and plan treatment options (conservative, percutaneous sclerotherapy or surgery).[13] The most useful imaging is ultrasound (US) and MRI. Angiography has no role and direct stick venography will be discussed later.

US is portable and can be performed in clinic at the time of outpatient attendance. A malformation typically appears as a low reflective or heterogeneous defined mass lesion, which can be unilocular, multilocular or solid (matrix-rich, or post-haemorrhage). Duplex US can help differentiate LFVMs from LFLMs by demonstrating low-velocity flow within the lesion, although in up to 20% of LFVMs no flow is

seen. It should be noted that US has limitations with depth penetration and assessment of associated structures such as nerves, bone and defining the extent of lesions not located in the extremities.

MRI is the imaging modality of choice as it has superior contrast resolution to identify soft-tissue involvement. The assessment with MRI can give prognostic information and should include a description of the extent – focal, multifocal or diffuse, tissues involved, including joint involvement, and evidence of prior haemorrhage. There are numerous MRI protocols described in the literature, but a simple approach is to optimise imaging to identify slow-moving fluid – lymph or blood. T1-weighted imaging defines anatomy and the presence of previous haemorrhage and fat suppression techniques (either fast spin-echo T2-weighted or short-inversion time inversion recovery) to increase lesion detection by suppressing the bright fat surrounding the bright LFVM (Fig. 20.4). The addition of contrast imaging is useful to aid differentiation of low-flow vascular malformations; LFLMs demonstrate peripheral enhancement whereas LFVMs enhance homogeneously throughout the lesion and help in identifying a differential diagnosis, for example, vascular tumour.

MANAGEMENT

A multidisciplinary team approach is essential for the best patient outcomes, with the aim of treatment to improve symptoms and the cosmetic appearance.[13,14] The management of LFVMs and LFLMs can be considered together as there is much overlap in the techniques, although the agents used for treatment may differ slightly. The majority of patients only require assessment and advice of the diagnosis and natural history, along with made-to-measure compression garments and treatment of complications, for example, infection, thrombophlebitis. When patients are particularly symptomatic, there are essentially two treatment options available: direct stick sclerotherapy (DSS) or surgery.

DSS is a minimally invasive technique that uses US and fluoroscopy to guide needle access into the vascular malformation to allow the safe and controlled instillation of a sclerosant agent. Once the needle has been image-guided into the lesion, contrast can be instilled under fluoroscopy to confirm intra-lesional position and outline the malformation. In LFVMs, this direct stick venography (DSV) classifies the malformation using the Puig system.[15] There are a variety of sclerosant agents used which aim to destroy the endothelial linings of venous and lymphatic malformations[16] (Fig. 20.5). Each agent has its own unique technique for use and safety profile, and it is essential that operators have a detailed knowledge of these agents to manage these patients.[13] Agents commonly used to treat these malformations are sodium tetradecyl sulphate,[17] ethanol, bleomycin,[18] doxycycline and picibanil (OK432). These agents are injected into the malformations in either their liquid form or more commonly in LFVMs as a foam using a 1:2 or 1:3 mix with air/CO_2 using the Tessari method.[19] Bleomycin can also be foamed with albumin to increase its volume and contact with the endothelium. In matrix-rich LFVMs and microcystic LFLMs, bleomycin treatment has become first-line;[4,17] furthermore, some authors are combining sclerosant therapies when lesions are mixed or contain both cystic and solid components. Bleomycin can also be administered

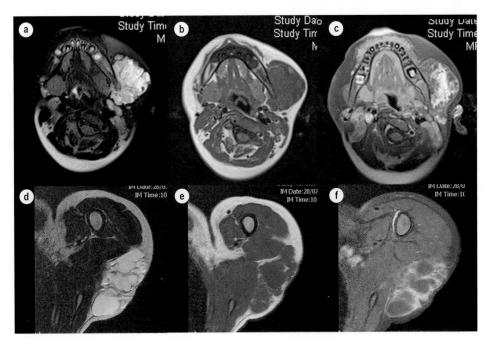

Figure 20.4 Magnetic resonance imaging (MRI) features of low-flow vascular malformations. Both show similar appearances on the T2-W (a, d) and T1-W (b, e) sequences. Venous malformations (a–c) demonstrate central homogeneous enhancement (c), whereas lymphatic malformations demonstrate peripheral edge enhancement post-intravenous gadolinium (f).

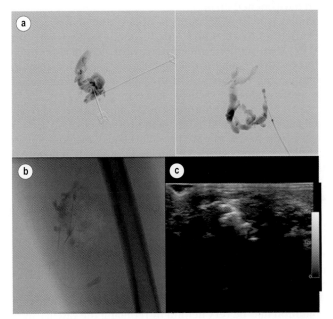

Figure 20.5 Direct stick sclerotherapy with needle placement into the venous malformation. Venography confirms intra-lesional position (a); post foam sclerotherapy air can be seen within the malformation on fluoroscopy (b) and ultrasound (c).

using cliniporation; a technique using adaptive electroporation technologies. A cliniporator machine is used to pulse voltages in the target area using a variety of multiple needle probes once the bleomycin has been administered. This increases cellular uptake of bleomycin by up to 5000% with subsequent improvement in clinical outcomes.

Surgery has traditionally been used to treat low-flow malformations and there are a number of surgical techniques used.[20] There is, however, a high recurrence rate for these lesions and surgery can potentially be quite morbid. The use of surgery after sclerotherapy for cosmetic reasons has been suggested and in very large malformations there is some logic to debulking surgery to prevent secondary compression effects and then treat remaining areas with DSS.

HIGH-FLOW VASCULAR MALFORMATIONS

AVMs are defects of the circulatory system that can arise during foetal development or be acquired after birth. Many, however, do not become apparent until puberty or even adult life. Progression of AVMs may also occur in response to pregnancy or trauma; trauma may be accidental or iatrogenic (e.g., surgery).

AVMs typically present clinically with a pulsatile soft-tissue swelling associated with pain and discomfort or because of symptoms caused by complications. Clinical examination with palpation demonstrates the high-flow nature of the lesion and the complications of AVMs, including thinning of the overlying skin, skin discolouration, frank ulceration, infection and bleeding, should be documented. AVMs are classified using a clinical classification developed by Schobinger (Table 20.3), which is a simple grading system (1–4) that aids decision-making in the timing of intervention. Biopsy should be performed only if there are any atypical history or clinical features to exclude differential diagnosis of a vascular soft-tissue tumour. An acquired post-traumatic arteriovenous fistula (AVF) may have an identical appearance on clinical examination to that of an AVM, except there is typically a history of previous blunt trauma or penetrating injury. A single fistulous communication is usually present, and this will sometimes be the first indication of this diagnosis; appropriate embolisation often results in a cure.

DIAGNOSIS AND IMAGING

The diagnosis of an AVM is typically clinical although deep-seated lesions may be less obviously pulsatile. US examination aids detection of an arteriovenous signal and reveals high flow with loss of normal venous damping on Doppler studies. MRI is the mainstay of diagnostic non-invasive imaging for AVMs for a number of reasons. AVM is a term that is commonly used (incorrectly) for all vascular malformations

Table 20.3 Schobinger clinical grading system for arteriovenous malformations

Grade 1	Quiescent – stable
Grade 2	Enlargement – growth
Grade 3	Symptomatic – pain, bleeding
Grade 4	Decompensation – high-output cardiac failure

and cross-sectional imaging with protocols similar to those used in low-flow vascular malformations will ensure the correct diagnosis, as well as identify combined complex malformations. AVMs typically demonstrate flow voids on both the T1- and T2-weighted sequences with lack of mass lesion; fatty hypertrophy and muscular atrophy are frequently associated. Gadolinium-enhanced magnetic resonance angiography (MRA) can be performed to identify the vascular anatomy, although the spatial resolution is poor when compared to formal angiography. New sequences are being developed and image quality is significantly improving, for example, Siemens TWIST (Time-resolved angiography With Interleaved Stochastic Trajectories). TWIST is a time-resolved three-dimensional MRA technique with very high temporal and spatial resolution that can capture multiple vascular phases.

Catheter angiography is an invasive procedure that is essential to understand the morphology of an AVM and plan treatment, which may be endovascular or combined with surgery following embolisation. The procedure can be performed just before treatment but more commonly is a separate investigation to allow all interested parties to understand and plan the treatment in these most complex patients.

AVMs are abnormal communications between an artery and a vein and are classified based on the level of communication using the Houdart system[21] described in 1993:

Type I: Arteriovenous. AVMs with a 'nidus' (first venous component) that is supplied by three or fewer arterial pedicles.

Type II: Arteriolovenous. AVMs with a 'nidus' (first venous component) that is supplied by more than three (often very many) arterial pedicles.

Type III: Arteriolovenulous. AVMs with communications that are minute and numerous such that they cannot be separately identified from multiple 'nidi' at a distance.

Cho et al. modified this classification system in 2006 by developing a type IIIa and type IIIb and linked classification type to clinical outcome following embolisation. The type III lesions were the commonest (60%) and the most difficult to treat.[22]

MANAGEMENT

AVMs that are quiescent, not associated with significant symptoms and cause little in the way of cosmetic deformity are usually best left alone. Patients should be informed that a change in the malformation might warrant re-evaluation. Patients with symptomatic AVMs who require treatment are often best managed by embolisation, although surgical excision or debulking, often combined with embolisation, may be necessary in some individuals.

The general principle of embolisation is that occlusion is performed at the site of the abnormal arteriovenous shunts; this is defined as the first dilated segment of vein and is referred to as the 'nidus' and acts as a venous sump that drives the AVM. This entity is paramount to the successful treatment of an AVM with embolisation. If one considers the 'nidus' as a traffic roundabout, with multiple roads entering and exiting the roundabout as feeding arteries and draining veins, then one can understand that only blocking the roundabout itself will prevent travel; blocking a feeding artery or draining vein will not. There are a number of access routes that can successfully be used to treat AVMs: transarterial, direct stick (DS) and transvenous (TV).[23,24] The best approach is to treat each AVM case by case, depending on site, Houdart classification and choice of embolic agent (Fig. 20.6). However, commonly DS or TV approaches best treat these lesions as they give the best access to the nidus (venous sump). When used with a liquid embolic agent such as sodium tetradecyl sulphate or absolute alcohol, then a long-term improvement in symptoms can be achieved with total obliteration. Type I and type II lesions are particularly suited to this form of treatment. New liquid embolic agents that are controllable and pushable are now on the market and have opened up opportunities to treat some of the most complex type III AVMs in the periphery and brain via a transarterial approach. Onyx (Medtronic), Squid (Balt) and PHIL (Microvention) are ethylene vinyl alcohol copolymers mixed with a radio-opaque agent for visualisation that are cohesive and can be pushed through very small arteries in the nidus segment to achieve success.

AVMs with a largely intra-osseous component are especially well suited to treatment by this method of embolisation because they usually have a type II (arteriolovenous) anatomy and are usually best approached by a direct, transosseous, puncture of the dilated venous component of the malformation.

With developments in embolic materials and catheter equipment, primary treatment of AVMs should be endovascular and surgery has a secondary role either as a planned staged procedure to improve the aesthetics following embolisation or to treat skin complications. These surgical techniques often require complex plastic surgery with the use of tissue expansion and muscular flap transfer techniques. Surgery is performed as a primary procedure only if the AVM can be totally excised and even then pre-operative embolisation may be very helpful by reducing the vascularity of the AVM. It is important not to embolise feeding vessels with coils or plugs even when distal embolisation has been performed with particles, as this will only hamper future angiographic assessment or treatment if the malformation recurs.

FOLLOW-UP AND OUTCOMES

The best results are achieved in dedicated specialist centres with multidisciplinary malformation teams able to provide all aspects of care in these complex patients. Treatment is mainly aimed at symptomatic improvement and prevention of progression/complications in this heterogeneous group of congenital anomalies. The outcomes of vascular tumours are highly dependent on early and accurate diagnosis and implementation of the appropriate treatment pathway. Within the vascular malformation group, the outcome is determined predominantly by patient education,

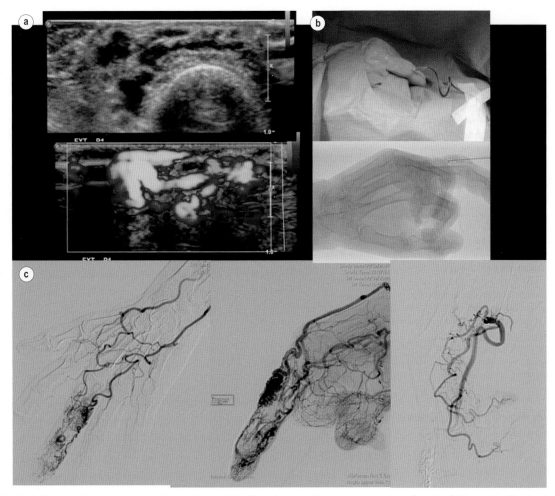

Figure 20.6   High-flow malformation of the finger demonstrated on duplex ultrasound and colour Doppler (a) treated with direct stick 'nidus' puncture (b) following placement of a super-selective catheter to outline the arteriovenous malformation (AVM) by angiography before and after Fibrovein (STS 3%) injection under orthopaedic tourniquet control (c).

managing patient expectations and treating the appropriate cohort of patients where the benefits of sclerotherapy or embolisation significantly outweigh potential serious complications, for example, skin loss, neuropraxia and muscle loss.

Sclerotherapy procedures for low-flow malformations frequently require a course of treatment rather than a single session to obtain satisfactory patient symptom improvement. Outcomes are better for localised malformations involving superficial structures or focal intra-muscular lesions. Those involving multiple compartments and that are multifocal fare worse, but treatment can still be focused on the symptomatic areas within. Microcystic LFLMs have always been a significant challenge, however, work by Muir et al. has demonstrated remarkable results using intra-lesional bleomycin injections.

AVMs represent a significant challenge, and it is clear that the outcomes are worse for the higher-type lesions.[21] Outcomes significantly improve with a full understanding of the AVM morphology and appropriate access to achieve nidal ablation. Whilst a significant number of type I and II lesions have good long-term success rates, in the type IIIa and IIIb AVMs, one can often only achieve a downgrading, in terms of Schobinger grade and angiographic complexity. This is very important for the patient but often means that repeat treatments are inevitable.

CONCLUSIONS

Vascular anomalies are simply classified into vascular tumours and vascular malformations. The common haemangioma of infancy makes up the vast majority of the former group and most of these will involute spontaneously without the need for active intervention.

Vascular malformations are difficult to treat successfully and a cure is unlikely. Patients with these anomalies are best treated in specialised units providing multidisciplinary expertise, including diagnostic and interventional radiology and surgery.

Key points

- Vascular anomalies are classified into vascular tumours and vascular malformations.
- The commonest vascular tumour is the infantile haemangioma.
- The majority of infantile haemangiomata require no treatment.
- Vascular malformations are inborn errors of vasculogenesis and persist throughout life.
- Vascular malformations are most conveniently classified into high- and low-flow lesions.
- A significant proportion of vascular malformations do not require treatment.
- Venous and lymphatic malformations may cause marked disfigurement.
- The main treatment of symptomatic venous and lymphatic malformations is direct stick sclerotherapy.
- Large venous malformations may have a localised coagulopathy with low fibrinogen and elevated D-dimers, which may result in severe bleeding during surgery.
- High-flow malformations are equally difficult to manage and may require multimodality treatment, including embolisation and surgery.
- An understanding of the angio-architecture of a high-flow malformation is essential as this influences the approach to treatment and predicts the likely response to embolisation.

References available at http://ebooks.health.elsevier.com/

KEY REFERENCES

[1] Mulliken JB, Glowacki J. Hemangiomas and vascular malformations in infants and children: a classification based on endothelial characteristics. Plast Reconstr Surg 1982;69:412–22. PMID: 7063565

[17] Perkins JA, Manning SC, Tempero RM, et al. Lymphatic malformations: review of current treatment. Otolaryngol Head Neck Surg 2010;142(6):795–1. PMID: 20493348

Index

Note: Page numbers followed by "*f*" and "*t*" refer to figures and tables, respectively.